HEALTHY WOMAN, HEALTHY LIFE

HEALTHY WOMAN HEALTHY LIFE

The Women's Book of Alternative Healing

GARY NULL, PHD

Project Editor, Amy McDonald

Seven Stories Press
New York • Oakland

Seven Stories Press
140 Watts Street
New York, NY 10013
www.sevenstories.com

Book design by Jon Gilbert

Library of Congress Cataloging-in-Publication Data

Names: Null, Gary, author. | McDonald, Amy, project editor.
Title: Healthy woman, healthy life : a woman's book of healing / Gary Null,
   PhD, project editor, Amy McDonald.
Other titles: Be a healthy woman!
Description: Seven Stories Press second edition. | New York : Seven Stories
   Press, [2016] | Revision of: Be a healthy woman! c2009. | Includes
   bibliographical references.
Identifiers: LCCN 2015046818 | ISBN 9781609806743 (paperback)
Subjects: LCSH: Women--Health and hygiene. | Women--Diseases--Alternative
   treatment. | BISAC: HEALTH & FITNESS / Women's Health. | HEALTH & FITNESS
   / Alternative Therapies.
Classification: LCC RA778 .N877 2016 | DDC 613/.04244--dc23
LC record available at http://lccn.loc.gov/2015046818
Printed in the USA.

9 8 7 6 5 4 3 2 1

Excerpts from the following books and websites are reprinted with permission from the publisher.

Null, Gary, *Be a Healthy Woman*. Seven Stories Press, New York: 2009.

Null, Gary, "Breast Cancer: These Natural Solutions Could Save Your Life." Gary Null Blog. 2014. http://blog.garynull.com/wp-content/uploads/2014/03/Breast-Cancer-Revised.docx

Null, Gary, "HPV Vaccines: Unnecessary and Lethal." Gary Null Blog. 2014. http://blog.garynull.com/wp-content/uploads/2014/03/HPV-Vaccines.doc

Null, Gary. "The Importance of Integrative Medicine in the Treatment of HIV/AIDS." PRN FM, Progressive Radio Network. Posted May 6, 2015. http://prn.fm/the-importance-of-integrative-medicine-in-the-treatment-of-hivaids-gary-null/

Null, Gary. *No More Allergies: A Complete Guide to Preventing, Treating, and Overcoming Allergies.* Gary Null Publishing, New York: 2014.

Null, Gary. *No More Cancer: A Complete Guide to Preventing, Treating, and Overcoming Cancer.* Gary Null Publishing, New York: 2014.

Null, Gary. *No More Diabetes: A Complete Guide to Preventing, Treating, and Overcoming Diabetes.* Gary Null Publishing, New York: 2013.

Null, Gary. *No More Menopause: A Complete Guide to Preventing, Treating, and Overcoming Menopausal Symptoms.* Gary Null Publishing, New York: 2014.

Null, Gary. *Reboot Your Brain: A Natural Approach to Fighting Memory Loss, Dementia, Alzheimer's, Brain Aging, and More.* Gary Null Publishing, New York: 2013.

Contents

III. Alternative Health Resources

Introduction

More than ever before, American women are living in a crisis. There is a perfect storm in their midst.

Job security is no longer guaranteed irrespective of a woman's education and skills. In fact, a woman may have worked for the past thirty years, earning a respectable annual income, and suddenly find her company bringing in people who are willing to take her job for a fraction of her salary. She may find she is at a place in her life where she is being challenged to reconsider the quality of her relationships, such as with her family and friends. And she may be facing the challenges of dealing with aging parents who may be threatened with dementia, Alzheimer's, or Parkinson's disease. Perhaps there is no one else to care for them and the burden falls upon her shoulders.

Many women reach a point in their lives when they are at a loss after becoming aware that they never intentionally planned to become ill. Rather it was an accumulation of multiple bad choices—junk food, alcohol, stress, lack of exercise—that have taken their toll. Now she discovers she is suffering from heart disease, arthritis, cancer, or diabetes. At one time, she was able to lose weight easily. Now it requires more effort to drop pounds and very often her attempts are unsuccessful.

At one time, a woman never thought about menopause. Finally a time dawns when she experiences hot flashes, night sweats, thinning hair, and a gradual loss of libido. Even if she desires to have sex with her partner, it is more difficult to do so. She never had trouble going to sleep but now wakes up several times a night. She looks at her skin and observes sagging, wrinkles, and a loss of elasticity. All of this concerns her.

Needless to say, there are no shortages of health and emotional concerns as we age or as the effects from living a poor lifestyle reveal themselves. As troubling as these scenarios are, there is good news: I have spent the last five years collecting research on state-of-the-art nontoxic and natural therapies for preventing these health conditions, for treating disease, and for improving women's quality of life. In the pages that follow, you will find a wealth of information, including interviews with dozens of the finest medical and alternative health minds in the country, who share their first-person wisdom, advice, and insights into how a woman can remain healthy and vibrant. An emphasis has been placed upon the more recent science of epigenetics, which essentially informs women that what they think and feel about diseases, illnesses, conditions, and healing processes in their bodies can either reduce or hurry their health conditions.

It is never too late. There is always something positive women can do.

EVERYDAY HEALTH

We are in a health crisis in the United States. When you consider the numbers, they are staggering. In 2015, the federal Agency for Healthcare Research and Quality estimated that 96 million Americans were living with chronic conditions. The country was projected to spend $3.2 trillion on health care of all types, or about $10,000 per person. Although the rate of spending has slowed in recent years, we still have to ask, what are we getting for all this money? With the Affordable Care Act, more people than ever now have insurance coverage, and this is great news. But we are by no means out of the woods. Medical care is costly, and there is no assurance that insurance companies will actually allow for people to get the treatment they need. Unfortunately, women bear the brunt of this predicament.

Compounding the crisis is the fact that despite the talk, we still do almost nothing in our society to prevent illness or truly acknowledge that lifestyle choices can affect health and well-being. There have been some changes, but the conventional medical establishment continues to minimize the role of diet, nutrition, exercise, emotions, and the environment in maintaining good health. Instead, it pushes more pills, more dangerous "quick fixes," and more profits for the ever-growing medical industry. In the women's health arena, menopause and the use of hormone replacement therapy provide a stark case in point. As described throughout this book, there are many other examples as well.

The natural healing community has a long tradition of providing safe, sensible, and cost-effective health solutions. More than two decades ago, I introduced health support groups to my radio audience. The health support group is meant to bring people together to show them that with just lifestyle modification, we can change the outcome of illnesses. I had people from every walk of life, from every state of health, from totally deteriorated health to very good health, and all ages and all races. We had a good melting pot. I started to apply principles that I had been using with individual patient for a long time. I put them on vegetarian diets. I excluded all meat, dairy, artificial sweeteners, refined carbohydrates, deep-fried and processed foods, and caffeine. I got them to go organic. They went through a really thorough detoxification, which generally took about a year. Then we used the supplements, herbs, and juices that were necessary to rebalance their body chemistries. What we found was that as long as people applied these principles and followed the protocols, there was tremendous benefit. If they only applied part of the principles and only did some of the things, they benefited somewhat, but not as completely by any means.

Later I started to do specific groups, such as arthritis, diabetes, high blood pressure, obesity, depression, skin, and hair. The results were astonishing. We presented our findings from the latter group at the World Congress on Anti-Aging Medicine before a group of thousands of scientists. We showed for the first time that lifestyle modification—in and of itself, with no drugs, no topical applications of any type of proprietary product—was able to reverse balding, thinning, and graying, and to sustain the reversal in a statistically significant number of individuals. These people also saw their pigmentations, wrinkles, and poor skin improve substantially. From their diaries, we noted that many also overcame or improved their arthritis, fibromyalgia, and high blood pressure.

A support group for menopausal and postmenopausal women also showed remarkable results. Nearly 260 women followed the protocol that included hormone rebalancing using plant therapy, the phytoestrogens from specific plants and herbs; elimination of dairy, meat, artificial sweeteners, and caffeine; and use of supplements. Within three weeks, people started talking about having more energy. Within two months, people who hadn't been able to lose weight were doing so, and keeping it off. Over time, the hot flashes subsided. The drying and chafing skin were reversed. Brittle and fungal nails were reversed. The night sweats were gone. The mood swings were gone. Hair started to grow where it was balding and thinning. About nine months to a year into the study women started noticing that their white or gray hair was growing in brown and black. There were major changes in their musculoskeletal system because human growth hormone was restimulated. Simple bone density studies showed that, across the board, women re-mineralized. There is nothing in orthodox medicine that can compare with the results these women achieved. The only side effects were positive.

These health support groups have continued throughout the years, with unbridled success. Testimonials from a number of recent participants are included at the end of this book, giving you access to first-person accounts of the power of natural healing. Throughout this book, you—like these women—will find practical and proven ways to apply lifestyle modifications on your road to optimal health and well-being.

Chapter 1

Diet and Nutrition

According to a 2015 report from a federal advisory panel on nutrition, about half of all American adults have at least one preventable, chronic disease related to diet and lack of physical activity. In addition, 37 percent of women are obese, and another 30 percent are overweight. The situation is not new. Many medical practitioners and the public at large are finally acknowledging what the natural healing community has known for ages: a good diet can not only promote health, but also prevent disease. Today it is customary to talk about how food choices affect overall well-being and help ward off heart problems, cancer, diabetes, stroke, osteoporosis, depression, and myriad other ailments. Most people are also aware that a healthy diet can decrease the risk of disease by reducing predisposing conditions such as obesity, high blood pressure, and high cholesterol.

Eating a balanced diet is the most effective way to ensure that our bodies receive the nutrients we need. Unfortunately, the typical American diet does not meet many of the requirements for good health. Part of the problem relates to the types and proportions of foods people eat. Just as important to our health is how the foods are grown and processed as they make their way to our grocery shelves and kitchen tables.

Eating properly means selecting unprocessed or minimally processed foods. You want to avoid pesticides, dyes, and wax coatings. Many of our diets need to be adjusted to include more complex carbohydrates, fewer proteins, and less fat. A wide assortment of whole grains, legumes, vegetables, fruits, nuts, and seeds supplies multiple nutrients. Sometimes supplements are necessary. Juices from watermelons, raspberries, pomegranates, and tomatoes are filled with phytochemicals that help repair DNA and prevent cancer. We should be thinking about our diets as part of our daily health routines.

Nutrition is the way the body makes use of foods to meet its needs for growth, repair, and maintenance. There are six major groups of nutrients: carbohydrates, fats, proteins, vitamins, minerals, and water. You need all of these nutrients every day. How much you require depends on your health as well as your energy needs. Along with an understanding of these basic nutrients, you also need to be aware of the air you breathe, the balance of enzymes in your body, and the function of antioxidants in helping your body to combat disease and degenerative processes.

Carbohydrates

Until recently, carbohydrates have gotten bad press. This is because the highly sugared and refined carbohydrates such as candy, soft drinks, and sweetened cereals have been lumped together with the complex carbohydrates such as fruit, nutritious starchy vegetables, whole grains, and tubers. We now know that we need carbohydrates. They are the most important source of energy for all of our activities. The foods in which they are found are also important sources of vitamins, minerals, and other nutrients.

Carbohydrates come in two forms: complex and refined. Complex carbohydrates are starches and fibers in foods such as cereals, legumes, nuts, seeds, vegetables, and tubers. They exist in these foods just as they are found in nature, having undergone minimal or no processing.

Refined carbohydrates, on the other hand, have been tampered with in a very substantial way. "Refined" may in fact be an overly refined way of putting it. Having been processed by machinery and industry, they are merely skeletons of the complex carbohydrates found in nature. Refinement is a recent innovation in our long history of evolution, food consumption, and food delivery. When carbohydrates are refined, they are stripped of their outer shell (the bran layer that contains most of the fiber), their oil, and a B vitamin–rich germ (found at their cores). Refined carbohydrates also may be bleached, milled, baked, puffed, or otherwise processed. Refined carbohydrates may not be good for us. What's worse, they may harm us. They contain little or no fiber, so overreliance on them as a source of energy can lead to poor intestinal health and myriad digestive disorders. Also, overconsumption of refined sugar, as discussed below, is linked to obesity, diabetes, and other blood sugar disorders.

Fats

Americans get nearly half their calories from fat. Over indulgence in fatty foods has taken its toll by contributing to weight gain as well as degeneration of the heart and blood vessels. The American Heart Association and others recommend that we reduce the amount of saturated fat and cholesterol in our diets to decrease blood cholesterol levels, prevent heart disease, and reduce the risk of certain cancers. However, we should not avoid fats completely; they are essential elements of a sound diet.

Fats contain an alcohol called glycerol and fatty acids. Certain fatty acids can be manufactured by the body. Others can only be obtained from foods. There are two types of fats: saturated and unsaturated. Saturated fats are found in animal food sources such as meat and dairy products. Although needed by the body in small amounts, they have been associated with increased blood levels of "bad" LDL cholesterol and an increased risk of developing cardiovascular diseases.

The unsaturated fats are primarily found in grains, legumes, seeds, nuts, and the oils derived from them. They provide us with the essential fatty acids that the body cannot make on its own, including the omega-6 family derived from plant oils, and the omega-3 family derived from fish oils, as well as some plants such as flaxseed. Both are important to good health. However, the standard American diet today contains too much omega-6 and too little omega-3, an imbalance that may be responsible for an increased risk of inflammation associated with heart disease, asthma, stroke, and cancer.

The unsaturated fats are further categorized as polyunsaturated and monounsaturated. Olive oil, which is high in monounsaturated fats, helps protect the heart by lowering "bad" LDL cholesterol levels and raising "good" HDL cholesterol.

Trans fats are created by partial hydrogenation, the process by which oils are made more solid. Many types of margarine, shortening, pastries, and prepared foods contain trans fats. They have been found to increase the risk of heart disease, stroke, and other ailments. Following the lead of state and local governments over the past decade, the Food and Drug Administration (FDA) in 2015 introduced restrictions on the use of trans fats at the national level, telling companies they will soon have to seek its permission to use the ingredient or find an alternative. Some manufacturers and restaurants have come up with healthier options to trans fats that work just as well.

Proteins

Meat has become the most prominent and expensive source of protein in the average American diet. Despite the belief by many people that we should be getting our protein from meat, there are a variety of other sources, including eggs, dairy products, grains, legumes, nuts, and seeds. In fact, there is no need whatsoever for any animal proteins in our diets. Plant-based proteins are completely compatible with our lives. Grains, legumes, nuts, and seeds are more than adequate.

Proteins are the building blocks of life. They are the basic materials from which all our cells, tissues, and organs are constructed. The optimal intake of high-quality proteins allows the body to grow and maintain healthy bones, skin, teeth, muscles, and nerves. Protein is also an important source of energy.

Amino acids are the chief components of protein. Some amino acids can be created by the body itself. Eight amino acids cannot be created by the body, and therefore must be obtained from the diet. Known as the essential amino acids, they are threonine, valine, tryptophan, lysine, methionine, histidine, phenylalanine, and isoleucine. Amino acids are vital for certain vitamins and minerals to be utilized. All the necessary amino acids must be present simultaneously in sufficient amounts so that cells can make the proteins they need to grow.

The current recommendation according to the US Institute of Medicine is that adults should consume 10 to 35 percent of their calories from protein. Pregnant and lactating women may need more.

Vitamins

Vitamins act as cofactors or catalysts in enzyme reactions throughout the body. They enable those enzyme reactions to proceed at a faster pace than they would if the vitamin was not present. Vitamins exist in one of two forms: water soluble and fat soluble. Water-soluble vitamins dissolve quickly and cannot be stored in the body. As soon as they are exposed to water or blood they dissolve and then are excreted. The fat-soluble vitamins are stored in the fatty tissues and don't dissolve. They can accumulate in the body. They do not need to be replenished every day but can accumulate into toxic doses in the fat tissues, and are harder to get out of the body. The fat-soluble vitamins are A, D, E, and K. All the rest are water soluble.

One-quarter to one-third of Americans currently take vitamin supplements. Thousands of different products are on the market today. Research has shown that supplements can not only help reverse nutritional deficiency, but also maintain physical as well as emotional health in many people.

Minerals

Minerals serve as the building materials for bones, teeth, tissue, muscle, blood, and nerve cells. They help spur many biological reactions in the body and maintain the fragile balance of fluids. We need minute amounts of minerals. They constitute only 4 or 5 percent of our total body weight. Among the important minerals are calcium, chromium, iodine, iron, magnesium, manganese, potassium, selenium, sodium, selenium, and zinc.

Water, Air, Enzymes, and Antioxidants

The environment from which we gain sustenance can also have an adverse effect on us. Consider the life-giving and life-supporting elements of the world around us. Although it comprises 50 to 70 percent of our body weight, water is too often overlooked or taken for granted when we consider amounts of water needed and proper balance of nutrients necessary for good health. Similarly, we must pay attention to the quality of the air we breathe and the very activity of breathing itself.

Antioxidants oppose the oxidation of substances within the body. They have been identified as important factors in helping us live longer, fight heart disease and lung problems, and combat cancer. They work, in part, by battling the degenerative processes associated with free radicals. Free radicals are the toxic agents produced by the processing of oxygen. They can damage a cell's DNA and have been linked to certain symptoms of aging. Antioxidants protect the body by trapping free radicals and preventing the degenerative processes associated with their reactions. Vitamin E is the most common antioxidant. Vitamins A, C, and D are less powerful antioxidants, as are selenium and sulfur-containing amino acids.

Federal Dietary Guidelines

According to the *Scientific Report of the 2015 Dietary Guidelines Advisory Committee*, which provides recommendations to the US government as it develops national nutritional policy, Americans are consuming too much sodium and saturated fats and not enough vitamin A, vitamin D, vitamin E, vitamin C, folate, calcium, magnesium, fiber, and potassium. Adolescent and premenopausal women are also deficient in iron. The report suggests that American adults maintain diets that are rich in seafood and plant-based foods such as vegetables, fruit, whole grains, legumes, and nuts; moderate in low- and non-fat dairy products and alcohol; lower in red and processed meat; and low in sugar-sweetened foods and refined grains. Recommended daily goals for the general population are less than 2,300 mg dietary sodium, less than 10 percent of total calories from saturated fat, and a maximum of 10 percent of total calories from added sugars. The report notes that research has shown that moderate consumption of coffee (three to five cups per day) can be included as part of a healthy diet as it is not associated with increased long-term health risks among healthy people, and has protective effects against the risk of type 2 diabetes, cardiovascular disease, and Parkinson's disease. The report also reverses previous guidance to restrict the intake of dietary cholesterol from foods like eggs and shrimp, stating that that the data does not support the link between dietary cholesterol and blood cholesterol in most people.

The Case Against Dairy

Dairy is the number one source for saturated fat in the average American diet. We're seeing an epidemic rise in its use. Susan Levin, director of nutrition education for the Physicians Committee for Responsible Medicine, is a registered dietician who has a master's degree in nutrition from Bastyr University. She is among the many who are concerned about the quantity and quality of dairy that we're consuming.

"Broadly speaking, I don't recommend the consumption of any dairy products," she says. "I take that back to watching over all of the species on this planet and how they act and what they do. No species drinks his or her mother's milk after weaning. It doesn't happen because they don't need it. Once they are strong enough to live with just consuming food products, they don't need mother's milk anymore.

"For some reason, our species has decided that, not only are we going to keep consuming milk, we're going to turn to a completely different species to get it. It's no wonder that we have so many problems. Milk is made, ideally, for a baby to grow very quickly. For a cow, specifically, to stand on his or her four legs and be as independent as possible, as quickly as possible. This is a product that makes everything grow very rapidly and it's no wonder it's so closely linked to some forms of cancer, hormonal changes, weight gain, and more." Among the cancers associated with dairy are breast and ovarian cancer.

The milk we drink has antibiotics and chemicals to make it safe for human consumption. It is pasteurized and homogenized, and often low in fat. But milk is not meant to be this way. It is meant to be fatty to help baby calves grow. "It's not even really milk that we're drinking," Levin says. "It's some sort of processed beverage that we've forced it to be to make it even slightly 'healthy.'"

The USDA recommends daily intake of dairy. This agency was originally created to support the agriculture industry, but now is relied upon for our nutritional guidance. You can imagine the conflicts of interest. Millions of dollars are spent in marketing the idea that dairy is needed to protect our bones, but at what cost to our overall health? In addition to milk, many people get their dairy from cheese. In fact, Levin says, the average American now consumes about 35 pounds of cheese every year. Cheese is high in fat, averaging about 70 percent, and also high in sodium and cholesterol.

"What I think people don't realize is that you can get the nutrients that promote bone health from healthier food sources," Levin says. "You can get it where the cow would have liked to have gotten it: from leafy green grass. You can get it from leafy green vegetables as well. Other sources include calcium from beans and greens, and vitamin D. Vitamin D, like vitamin A, doesn't naturally occur in dairy. It's added. You can get that from other sources and, ideally, from the sun, which would be the best source for vitamin D."

The Problem with Sugar

In 2015, researchers from Tufts University reported that sugary drinks are linked to 184,000 adult deaths worldwide each year. While most of these deaths were in developing countries, the US is affected at a rate of 125 per million. Today, the average American eats seventy-seven pounds per year, or twenty-two teaspoons daily. Volumes of scientific evidence implicate this sweet menace as a leading cause of America's epidemics of obesity, diabetes, Alzheimer's disease, cancer, and heart disease.

Despite its devastating effects on health, most of us continue to overdose on sugar every day. Unfortunately, it is not always easy to know when we are consuming added sugars. Most foods in the American grocery store have added sugar. The industry uses many other names for sugar on the food label, including mono- and disaccharides, lactose, evaporated cane syrup, dextrose, maltose, and intrinsic and extrinsic sugars. Products such as salad dressing, tomato sauce, bottled teas, frozen meals, and even sandwich breads are commonly manufactured with significant amounts of refined sugar. As such, it can be difficult even for the health-conscious consumers to find food that hasn't been laced with sugar.

Though many choose to write it off as simply "having a sweet tooth," sugar addiction is a well-documented condition that can be as difficult to overcome as some drug dependencies. One obesity researcher found that excessive sugar intake can lead to dependence, while the absence of it can create withdrawal symptoms, quantitatively similar to those associated with morphine and nicotine. An investigation carried out by the Oregon Research Institute examining the effect of sugar on the brain discovered that sugar produces a neurological response similar to that of highly addictive drugs, such as cocaine.

For the most part, calorie-free sweeteners are not a good alternative to sugar. Artificial sweeteners such as aspartame have been shown to contribute to weight gain, cardiovascular disease, and diabetes. In addition, artificial sweeteners have been shown to be addictive. One study found that when rats were given a choice between cocaine and the calorie-free sweetener saccharin, most favored saccharin. The best way to avoid excess sugar and artificial sweeteners is by eating an organic, whole foods diet.

Super Foods

What does it mean when we say a food is super? No, it's not that the foodstuff is so powerful that, as might happen in a Hollywood movie, a few bites will cure cancer or diabetes. Nature's products don't work that way, but move gradually to improve health where it is weak or to maintain it where it is strong. All natural foods have nutrients and work to boost different bodily processes. Super foods are those that perform these functions in a big way. Native traditions throughout the world have long known that certain vegetables, fruits, and grains are especially powerful purveyors of protective, preventative, and therapeutic health benefits. However, it was not until there were studies of these natural products by modern biochemistry, botanical science, molecular biology, and medical clinical research that many of these foods' extraordinary properties were more widely known.

APPLES

For thousands of years, apples (malus sylvestris) have been used for a wide variety of medical complications and diseases, including diabetes, fevers, inflammatory conditions, and heart ailments. In addition to having confirmed many of the healthful properties of apples, modern research has identified invaluable phytochemicals contained by the fruits. Phytochemicals are chemical compounds that are found in plants and have been used to treat illnesses. One of these found in apples is phloretin, a natural antibiotic. The fruits also contain pectin and pectic acids that provide essential bulk to a diet. The apple's tannins, quercetin, alpha-farnesene, shikimic acid, and chlorogenic acid promote health benefits, such as increasing production of the neurotransmitter acetylcholine, which helps offset cognitive decline due to oxidative damage. With high levels of phenols, polyphenols, and other antioxidant, chemoprotective properties, apples have been shown to help guard against a variety of cancers, including leukemia and those that target the colon, lung, breast, liver, and skin. Apples also provide essential nutrients to improve cardiovascular health, reduce the risk of coronary heart disease and stroke, and prevent atherosclerosis.

APRICOTS

This fruit had a long and rich history in the medical practices of China and India. In traditional Chinese medicine, apricots and their kernels are prescribed for treating asthma, cough, and constipation. The fruit is a stronghold of vitamins C and K, beta-carotene, thiamine, niacin, and iron. Japanese scientists have called attention to the apricot's ability to inhibit the pathogenic bacteria frequently associated with ulcers and acute gastritis.

BANANAS

Bananas are low in calories while providing essential nutrients, among them vitamin B_6, vitamin C, potassium, and manganese. They also stimulate probiotic activity, which sustains healthy gut flora. Bacteria in our gastrointestinal system are critical for proper digestion and absorption of nutrients. Bananas help keep this system on track. Recent findings have indicated that bananas may offer protection against kidney cancer, particularly in women, and aid renal function.

BERRIES

Many berries have health-boosting properties. Berries that are black, blue, and red are especially known for their possession of antioxidant nutrients. Blueberries specifically contain the antioxidant groups of flavonoids, phenolic and polyphenol compounds, all of which have shown some ability to reverse cellular aging of the cognitive and motor functions. In a study that compared the antioxidant levels of one hundred different foods, blueberries scored highest. Other examinations have shown blueberries acting to protect brain health, improve memory, and sustain coordination by, for one, enhancing communication between nerve cells. This activity provides protection from serious neurodegenerative diseases, such as dementia and Alzheimer's. On top of this, blueberries have anti-inflammatory properties that protect the skin, joints, and the cardiovascular and neurological systems. Eating this fruit has proven beneficial to those suffering from diabetes. Its consumption prevents bone loss and inhibits cancer cell proliferation, particularly in the cases of prostate and colon cancer.

BROCCOLI

What makes broccoli a super food is its high concentration of the phytochemicals diindolymethane and isothiocyanate, which are powerful immunomodulators, or substances that have strong effects on the immune system. Because it fosters immune system strength, broccoli helps to fight against cancer (breast and prostate cancer, in particular) and provides protection from bacterial and viral infections. Along with the phytochemicals, broccoli also contains other anticancer agents, such as glucoraphanin. Due to these observed properties, right now a substantial amount of research is being conducted on broccoli's mutagenic qualities.

This vegetable is rich in vitamins A, B_5, B_6, B_9 (folate), C, and K, and provides plenty of dietary fiber. It also provides moderate amounts of calcium, iron, phosphorus, and potassium. As with other leafy green vegetables, it contains lutein and zeaxanthin, which foster eye health. Since it has more calcium than even most dairy products, it can protect bones and increase bone mass.

CARROTS

Carrots can be looked to as chief provider of carotenoids, a family of antioxidants proven to block DNA and cellular membrane damage caused by free radical activity. They are rich in the phytochemicals alpha-carotene and lycopene, both shown to have anti-carcinogenic properties, fighting against cancer especially in the colon, lung, prostate, and stomach. The less-known black and purple carrots have high levels of anthocyanin, a powerful anti-cancer biochemical that has been found to slow cancer cell proliferation by as much as 80 percent. The vegetable has shown capacity in boosting brain function and decreasing cholesterol, as well as improving vision. Carrots are high in retinoids, which benefit ocular health. Since carrots are a good source of vitamin A, they should be kept in the diet of diabetics, given that vitamin A lowers blood sugar and aids in the development of insulin-producing cells in the pancreas. One cup of raw carrots can provide almost 700 percent of the daily recommended consumption of vitamin A and 220 percent of vitamin K, a substance critical for bone health. Thus, we have to dub carrots another superhero among edible plants.

GARLIC

While garlic contains phytonutrients similar to those found in onions, it also possesses selenium, a substance that, according to some studies, offers protection against various cancers and damage from free radicals. It has been shown to guard against heart disease and arterial calcification (hardening of the arteries), and to reduce cholesterol and blood pressure. Since it is a source of the flavonoid quercetin, it contains antibiotic properties that empower it to fight colds, stomach viruses, and yeast infections.

GINGER

Ginger is already widely employed throughout the world by anyone who wants to cure stomach upsets, reduce gastrointestinal gasses, and relieve nausea that arises from pregnancy, seasickness, and chemotherapy drugs. Ginger is largely composed of fragrant essential oils, which gives it a distinctive aromatic flavor. One of these oils, gingerol, makes it a natural sedative for calming the gastrointestinal tract. This oil also provides some protection from pathogenic bacteria that upset the stomach. New evidence suggests that ginger helps lower cholesterol, and works as a mild immune booster, warding off colds and flus, sinus congestions, and coughs. There have also been some preliminary findings in animal studies suggesting that ginger may help to treat diabetes.

GOJI BERRY

Also known as wolfberry in its native Europe, the plant is found through much of Asia. The berry is a common ingredient in traditional Chinese medicine, dating back thousands of years. The oblong red goji berry has a high concentration of phytochemicals, amino acids, vitamins B and C, and beta-carotene. Additionally, it contains eleven essential and twenty-two trace dietary minerals, is moderately high in alpha-linolenic acid, and is an outstanding source of the antioxidant lycopene. One can look to the goji berry for extra protein, dietary fibers, calcium, zinc, and selenium. Among its many health-lifting effects are protection against cardiovascular and inflammatory diseases, age-related vision disorders such as glaucoma and macular degeneration, cancer, liver problems, and sexual dysfunction.

GREEN TEA

The ingredient in tea—in green tea particularly—that has stirred the most scientific interest is catechin. Approximately 25 percent of a dry tea leaf is catechin. Although traces of catechin are also found in chocolate, wine, and other fruits and vegetables, it is tea that offers the greatest amount of this super nutrient. The multi-tasking catechin not only reduces the plaque buildup that is part of atherosclerosis, but also protects against infectious bacteria and reduces oxidative stress. In our polluted world, tea catechins are also useful in improving DNA replication and guarding against genetic damage from environmental toxins. Studies have noted its inflammatory properties and suggested it can play a role battling cancer. Green tea can improve bone density and cognitive function, reduce the risk of developing kidney stones, and strengthen heart function. There is also some evidence showing that green tea's polyphenols protect against the brain cell death that is associated with Parkinson's and Alzheimer's diseases.

LEGUMES

When I mention legumes, most people think of beans, peas, and lentils. However, alfalfa, clover, peanuts, and cashews are also legumes. These vegetables and grains are excellent sources of cholesterol-lowering fiber important for gastrointestinal and colon health. When you consume a legume, its fiber content helps you manage blood sugar levels. One cup of lentils can provide as much as 65 percent of the minimum daily necessary dietary fiber.

Legumes in general contain energy-boosting protein and iron. Black beans are rich in the potent antioxidant anthocyanidin, which promotes heart and vascular health. Green beans are excellent sources of vitamins C and K. Garbanzo beans, commonly known as chickpeas, are a superb source of molybdenum, which strengthens teeth and preserves tooth enamel. Another important legume is the adzuki bean. Originally from the Himalayas and standard in East Asian cooking, it is a rich source of magnesium, potassium, iron, zinc, and B vitamins. Very high in soluble fiber, the adzuki helps eliminate bad cholesterol from the body. In Japan, it is treasured for its kidney and bladder health-promoting function, and used in weight-loss programs.

To maximize the benefits of legumes in the diet, combine them with whole grains. The reason for this is that legumes are very low in methionine, an essential amino acid that supports cellular life, while whole grains are replete with this amino acid, but low in lysine, which is abundant in legumes. A wholesome, integrated vegetarian diet will contain a balance of legumes and grains.

LEAFY VEGETABLES

Dark green, leafy vegetables include spinach, kale, cabbage, arugula, Swiss chard, collard greens, and watercress. They are high in carotenoids and other antioxidants that guard against heart disease, cancer, and problems in blood sugar regulation. They also have individualized, singular health benefits. Spinach is one of the best sources of iron. Per gram, it generally contains over 30 percent more iron than a hamburger. (Any diet heavy in spinach should include sufficient vitamin C to help assimilate the iron.) Spinach is also an excellent source of folic acid, calcium, copper, zinc, selenium, and omega-3 fatty acids. One cup of cooked kale provides over 1,300 percent of the daily requirement of vitamin K needed for maximum bone health. It is also rich in calcium and manganese, other nurturers of bone density. As does broccoli, kale contains the anti-cancer phytochemical sulforaphane. Cabbage contains glutamine, an amino acid that contributes to anti-inflammatory activities in the body and protects against infectious complications due to human papilloma virus (HPV). The juice from cabbage will quicken the healing of peptic ulcers. Watercress, a superb source of phytochemicals, has been shown to be a diuretic and digestive aid, protect against lung cancer, and strengthen the thyroid. Collard greens supply ample quantities of immune response modulator diindolylmethane.

MUSHROOMS

My friends who have traveled to the Yunnan province in China mention that some of the most prized eatables there are the wide varieties of mushrooms. Where an average, un-health conscious American would find his or her greatest culinary delight in choosing between cuts of steak, the Yunnan citizen is delicately discriminating between different mushrooms. A wealth of growing peer-reviewed science shows that many edible mushrooms are among the more important immune builders in the plant kingdom. In particular, medicinal mushrooms inhibit tumor growth, have antipathogenic and blood-sugar-lowering activities, and strengthen immunity. Different mushrooms have shown some effectiveness against pathogen from polio, hepatitis B, influenza, candida, Epstein-Barr virus, streptococcus, and tuberculosis. The scientific literature also notes how mushrooms can be enlisted in the fight against leukemia, sarcoma, and the bladder, breast, colon, liver, lung, prostate, and stomach cancers, even in advanced stages. Among approximately two hundred different varieties whose health-enhancing skills have been noted are the chaga, cordyceps, maitake, oyster, portobello, reishi, shiitake, and turkey tail mushrooms. Although it is possible to find all of these in fresh or dried form, in the US the shiitake mushrooms are the easiest to obtain.

ONIONS

A rule of thumb is that the more pungent the onion, the greater its health benefits. It's as if you could smell its disease-thwarting power. Onions are particularly important to include in diets for diabetics, for one, because they are rich in chromium, a trace mineral that helps cells respond to insulin. Moreover, refined sugar depletes the body's chromium levels, so for anyone who has this sugar in her diet, onions are an excellent source of replacement. Onions are also rich in vitamin B_6, vitamin C, manganese, molybdenum (essential in preserving tooth enamel), potassium, phosphorous, and copper. They are also just about the best source of quercetin, which works hand in hand with vitamin C in helping the body eliminate bacteria and strengthen immunity.

Onions help lower blood pressure and cholesterol, and strengthen bone health. They also can reduce symptoms related to inflammatory conditions, such as asthma, arthritis, and respiratory congestion. Some studies have noted that they lessen the adverse effects from colds and flus.

ORANGES

The orange is a vitamin and mineral-packed treasure chest of a fruit, rich in vitamins A, B, and C, potassium, and calcium, as well as an excellent source of fiber. One phytonutrient in oranges that boosts it into the super-food category is the flavonoid hesperidin. This biochemical works to support healthy blood vessels and reduce cholesterol. The orange is stocked with vitamin C, an important antioxidant that limits free radicals while also building the immune system. Vitamin C's healing properties are well known and have been repeatedly validated scientifically. These include the lessening of arterial plaque as well as protecting from Alzheimer's, Parkinson's, and Crohn's diseases, arthritis, and diabetes.

PEPPERS (CAPSICUM)

Native American folk medicine, which has so many features we can still learn from, gave a prominent place in its pharmacology to peppers of the capsicum family, which includes bell and chili peppers. Recent work suggests that the nutrient capsaicin, found in these peppers, is a natural analgesic and a neuro-inflammatory blocker that relieves aches and pains to joints and muscles. This is one reason why Native American medicine prescribed a topical application of pepper to painful areas of the body.

Promising research has explored the uses of capsaicin in the treatment of type 1 diabetes, leukemia, and prostate cancer. Some scientists have noted that it helps with weight loss, stimulation of insulin-producing cells, and prevention of LDL cholesterol oxidation. Another benefit recently uncovered is that the nutrient protects from stomach ulcerations and induces apoptosis (cancer cell death) in lung cancer.

Setting aside the value of capsaicin, peppers can also be prized because they are rich in the antioxidant vitamins A as well as in vitamins B_1, B_6, E, and K. They are also high in potassium, magnesium, and iron. Yellow peppers are rich in lutein and zeaxanthin, which protect from eye disease and blindness.

SOY

Studies that have considered dietary reasons for the lower cancer rates in the East as compared to the West always point to soy as one of the major foods that distinguishes these global eating patterns. A number of studies show that the phytochemicals in soy protect against the genesis of cancer. Isoflavones, including genistein and daidzein, which are major constituents in soy, seem to be some of the active ingredients that provide natural protection against various cancers: breast, colon, endometrial, and prostate. One important Japanese study involving more than twenty-four thousand women found those who had the highest soy content in their diet were best protected against breast cancer. A later Japanese study noted the soy isoflavones could reduce breast cancer risk by up to 54 percent.

Along with this exciting attribute, soy has given evidence of an ability to lower blood LDL cholesterol and promote good HDL cholesterol, improve cardiac function, strengthen bone mass, and stabilize blood sugar.

In vegetarian diets, soy-based foods are an excellent replacement for animal protein. Soybeans are also high in iron, omega-3 fatty acids, phosphorus, riboflavin, magnesium, and potassium.

TOMATOES

Tomatoes are the best source for lycopene, a carotenoid biochemical that gives them their red color and is packed with positive properties. It has been estimated that approximately 80 percent of the lycopene consumed in the US derives from tomatoes and tomato-based foods. There is a vast body of scientific literature confirming lycopene's antioxidant and antimutagenic properties. This chemical is noteworthy for its protection against and treatment of various cancers, including that of the bladder, breast, cervix, lungs, mouth, ovaries, prostate, and stomach. Because diabetics often have low levels of lycopene in their blood, tomatoes should become a regular part of their diets.

Tomatoes have been shown to prevent cholesterol oxidation, lower blood pressure, and decrease the risk of atherosclerosis. Other benefits include improved renal function. Tomatoes also have antiviral and antibacterial qualities. In particular, lycopene can protect against human papillomavirus, one pathogen that has been associated with cancer.

Tomatoes are rich in most of the B complex vitamins as well as in potassium, manganese, chromium, folate, and iron. You can look to the tomato as an excellent source of the amino acid tryptophan, which is important for neurological health and can improve sleep.

WHOLE GRAINS

By now most Americans are aware that whole grain breads and pastas are healthier than those made from white flour, and brown rice is higher in nutrients and health benefits than white rice. However, once a person has changed over to brown rice and whole grain breads, she still has a rich world of whole grains to explore, each of which offers unique health benefits and phytonutrients.

As with legumes, whole grains are rich in fiber. Take spelt, which is being used in breads and pastas and will provide 75 percent of the recommended daily requirement for vitamin B_2. Spelt is highly water soluble, which means its nutrients are easily absorbed. There is evidence that spelt is a good choice for diabetics. Another grain, barley, is distinguished by being an excellent source of selenium, a substance that reduces the risk of colon disorders and colorectal cancer. Because barley is high in tryptophan, it will aid in sleep regulation. A third important grain, millet, is high in manganese, magnesium, and phosphorous, all of which support cardiovascular health.

Two less-familiar grains also deserve mention. The Glycemic Research Institute in Washington, D.C., has trumpeted the value of kamut for its low-glycemic properties, which makes it an ideal super food for diabetics, athletes, and people suffering from obesity. It is also an excellent substitute for those with wheat allergies. Quinoa has been identified as a super food among grains for its ability to balance blood sugar and provide high quality fiber and protein to the diet. It is higher in calcium, phosphorus, iron, and zinc than are wheat, barley, and corn. In addition to balancing insulin resistance, quinoa protects against atherosclerosis and breast cancer, and acts as a probiotic to foster the good micro-flora in the gut.

Chapter 2

Weight Control

No doubt about it, if we continue on the current path of increasing obesity among children and youth, the future looks grim. Extrapolating from childhood obesity rates in 2000, researchers estimate that by 2020 as many as 44 percent of American women and 37 percent of men will be obese. The increased incidence of obesity has paralleled the skyrocketing cases of diabetes as well as other illnesses. According to the Centers for Disease Control and Prevention, when compared with people of healthy weight, obese adults have seven times the risk for diabetes, four times the risk for arthritis, three times the risk for asthma, and two times the risk for high cholesterol.

One may well ask what catastrophic change in our society has brought about this epidemic of obesity. A variety of factors seem to be involved. Increased consumption of "empty calories" from junk foods and sedentary lifestyles are two major culprits. Others include possible genetic predisposition, a commercial structure of advertising, and an instant gratification philosophy that encourages unhealthy eating.

When looking at weight control, diet is generally the first place to start. Knowing about options is a theme you will see throughout this book. It applies to being a healthy woman in so many ways, and diet is no exception. Take the simple caloric restriction diet. It seldom works because people think their only option is a blanket curtailing of calories. They don't realize they can selectively reduce their calories by differentiating, for example, between calories from the sugar of as apple, as it naturally occurs, and calories from white, granulated sugar, in its unnatural form. Without knowing about the option of choosing a selective calorie reduction diet, a person wanting to lose weight is often drawn to a diet that is doomed to failure.

The typical diet also considers only one desire of an adherent: to lose weight.

But that means that other desires and feelings, such as the loneliness that may be compelling a person to binge on junk foods, doesn't enter the picture. Maybe the reason that so many diets, including ones with tens of millions of followers, which often look good on paper, have only had marginal success is because they have not tried to work with the whole gamut of issues related to losing weight, which involve emotional and physical needs as well.

Hormones and Food Intake

In understanding the etiology of weight gain, it is important to look at how hormones regulate food intake. When a person's stomach is relatively empty, the hormone ghrelin is released, telling the brain it is hungry and needs to eat. Once food has been consumed, leptin, a hormone made by fat, goes to the brain and tells the body to stop eating. From the brain's end, this is controlled by a number of integrated entities, including the hypothalamus. It has been theorized that some people with a genetic disposition toward obesity do not have enough leptin or they do not have the receptors to bind to the leptin so their brains are not getting a proper message telling them that they are full.

Surprisingly, as demonstrated in a study with mice, higher leptin levels were found to be associated with obesity. On the surface, it might appear that leptin should be scarce, not abundant in cases of extreme weight gain. However, the research showed that excessive leptin can result in leptin resistance, which essentially means that the body stops reading weight-suppressing messages from the hormone, even though it is present at high levels. Another study exploring the role of leptin in rats found that while the hormone had some effect on weight control in lean animals, no weight-loss benefits existed when the subjects were overweight, unless an exercise regimen also was involved. This led the researchers to conclude that exercise can reverse leptin resistance.

Eating Patterns

When to eat and how much have been the subject of ongoing medical debate over the past thirty years. Some physicians have argued that overweight people, as well as those with diabetes, insulin resistance, or the metabolic syndrome conditions, should have many small meals per day. Others have contended that three meals should be the norm.

Recent research on this topic makes a decisive contribution to the discussion. Dr. Markus Stofell and colleagues in late 2009 published the results of their study, based on an analysis of physiological processes, which determined that eating three "high-quality" meals with no snacks was the preferred pattern because fasting between meals was necessary. The research centered on transcription factor FOXA2. As explained in a summary, "Transcription factors are proteins that make sure that other genes are activated and converted into other proteins. The control element for FOXA2 is insulin in both the liver and hypothalamus. If a person or animal ingests food, the beta cells in the pancreas release insulin, which block FOXA2. When fasting, there is a lack of insulin and FOXA2 is active." So what is FOXA2 doing when it is active in the bloodstream? For one thing, it moves into the brain where it assists in the formation of proteins that sharpen awareness. As the scientists pointed out, "If mammals are hungry [which means FOXA2 is being produced], they are more alert and physically active." However, if one is constantly snacking, there is little downtime in which FOXA2 can course through the body. Insulin is released with every snack, thus suppressing FOXA2, which in turn means that we do not feel the need for activity, such as exercise." Considering the danger of a deficiency in FOXA2 brought on by too much insulin in the body, the researchers concluded it is healthy to get hungry between meals.

Food Selection

Now that we know how often during the day we should eat, we can take a look at what foods are best. In the previous chapter, we discussed diet and nutrition, and provided a list of super foods, which are packed with immune system boosters and natural energizers. Too many women today are asking their bodies to run on the wrong fuel: refined carbohydrates. Surrounding themselves with wholesome choices that consist mostly of fruits, vegetables, grains, and legumes is the key to staying healthy and fit. A woman taking this dietary route will arrange her day something like this: In the morning, she chooses a cereal that contains whole grain ingredients and no artificial sweeteners. Later in the day, she may supplement lunch with a green smoothie, made from blending and juicing leafy green nonstarchy vegetables. Fresh vegetables usually contain fewer carbs than fruit, many contain fiber, and they are naturally low in fat and sodium. For dinner, our health-conscious woman enjoys vegetables by lightly steaming or sautéing them.

She adds shredded cabbage or coleslaw to salad; and includes beans and legumes in a soup or salad to meet daily protein requirements.

When looking at weight management and considering what carbohydrates to put into your diet, it is worthwhile to pay attention to the Glycemic Index (GI). This ranks foods based on how quickly carbohydrates raise blood glucose. A high GI number indicates that carbs break down quickly into blood sugar. In general, the higher the fat and fiber content, the lower the GI of the food. By contrast, the more cooked or processed the food, the higher the GI will tend to be. Watching your carbs in terms of their GI value will not only help you lose weight, but will curtail the blood sugar surges that commonly occur after meals packed with high GI foods. Chronic insulin overload caused by such a diet leads to further weight gain and is associated with all types of age-related diseases.

It is important to keep in mind that GI value does not say anything about portion control. Portion size is crucial for managing blood glucose and for losing weight. Moreover, a simple GI value doesn't tell the whole story since many foods break down more quickly or slowly when they have been eaten in combination with certain other foods as opposed to how they release glucose when they are consumed by themselves alone.

In discussing the danger of inrushing blood sugar, let me tag the way food producers have played on Americans' proclivities to sell them a bill of goods, in liquid form. Americans always have an eye out for a bargain. So when they hear or see one of the billboard or TV ads saying, for instance, "Drink Super Fizz Apple Juice, made of 100 percent juice," they rush to buy it. Why? For one, they think they are getting a bargain, since instead of buying, say, five apples, they are getting five apples in one glass. Moreover—and this is the insidious part—they want to be healthy and have been told, by the commercials, that these fruit juices and concentrates are good for you because they contain the nutrients found in fruits.

In fact, the very idea that the fruit is coming to you concentrated should warn you of what's wrong with this message. When you eat a whole apple or other fruit, the sugar in the food enters the bloodstream gradually as the stomach breaks down the item. If, however, a number of pieces of fruit are concentrated, the natural sugar in them is also concentrated, and put in liquid form so that there is a quick release of the fructose that can spike serum insulin.

While these advertised juices are unhealthy, fruit itself is filled with attractive qualities. There are adequate amounts of folic acid, vitamin C, fiber, carotene, and nutrients in whole fruits as well as in frozen fruit, both of which are crucial to a healthy diet.

I might add that while these juice concentrates are of little value, there are other extracted forms of fruits and vegetables that can do great good for the body. To give a single instance, I recently learned of the value of mulberry leaf powder, which decreases fasting glucose levels and raises the levels of good cholesterol in the body. In studies conducted in both India and Japan, researchers found that in patients who took mulberry leaf powder daily with their meals there was a reduction in harmful lipids (which boost cholesterol) as well as a diminution of free radicals.

Having mentioned the misleading advertising used to sell fruit juice—I find food commercials are more often misleading than downright false—let me turn attention to the blandishments that are put forth in relation to another product line. Food companies plaster certain products with the labels "fat free" and "low fat," representing such commodities as always beneficial. Not so. Look at the labels. Many of them are loaded with sugar calories in the form of high fructose corn syrup, sucrose, and cheap, fortified processed ingredients. Whatever value might have been in the food in its untouched form is undermined or cancelled out completely by this raft of additives and sweeteners. A good example is green tea, which is a strong health promoter in its natural form, but is often sweetened with sucrose. Salad dressings also see their natural ingredients sabotaged when they are combined with high fructose corn syrup.

On the topic of fats, let me mention that here again a distinction has to be made. Recognizing and monitoring the quality and type of fat consumed is essential to maintaining a healthy weight. Most people have heard about the dangers of eating transfatty acids. While some of these can be found in beef, the majority are created by food processing, so that they are highly present in junk foods, baked goods, and fried food, such as French fries and fried chicken.

How dangerous are such transfats? In a recent study, scientists found the risk of diabetes in women to increase by nearly 40 percent from a "miniscule" 2 percent increase in calories from transfats. This compared with a 37 percent reduction in diabetes risk from a 5 percent increase in calories from polyunsaturated (good) fats. You can have a rich and healthy diet by replacing transfats with flax oil, extra virgin olive oil, sesame oil, hemp oil, avocados, almond oil, coconut oil, and pumpkin oil.

Eating Your Way to Reduced Weight

If we want to think of diet in terms of calories, then cutting calories by three hundred to five hundred per day should lead to a loss of between one and two pounds per week. Some may say such a cut in calories is difficult to achieve for an overeater. In my experience, though, this is a realistic target. Others may say the one- to two-pound-per-week reduction is too slow. It may seem that way, but it would add up to a weight loss of more than fifty pounds in a year, of which one can be proud.

To achieve this calorie reduction, switch off the fats, which contain more calories per serving than what is found in carbohydrates and proteins. For nutrition, lean heavy on the whole grains, beans, fruits, and vegetables. Here are some rules of thumb that will help you achieve the weight loss goal:

- Eliminate alcohol from the diet
- Replace sugary treats in between meals with whole grain snacks, fruit, or green juices
- Learn to eat smaller portions mindfully
- Do nothing else during the meal. Stop multitasking and eating on the go
- Eliminate coffee and all caffeinated drinks
- Replace milk products with soy or rice-based dairy foods
- Enjoy ice water with lemon, lime, or orange rather than drinking your calories by consuming fruit cordials

Finally, don't be tempted to skip breakfast or any meal to lose weight. While skipping a meal will reduce your calorie intake for that moment in time, it will leave you much hungrier later on. When it comes time to eat, you will be tempted to overeat to compensate. Irregular eating habits also disrupt your body's metabolism, which makes it harder to lose weight in the long run.

On this diet, it will take a week or two before you notice any changes, but they will steadily appear. After about thirty days, you will notice your clothes are looser, your energy is greater, and your self-esteem is increasing. Keeping your motivation up is one of the most difficult aspects of dieting. There will be days when you backslide. Perhaps, you go to a party and see a table overflowing with junk food. Everyone else is eating it. The host offers you a platter and without thinking you chow down. It happens. Healthy eating has gone out the window for that one night, only to be continued the next day. There may be weeks when due to such lapses you may not lose much or any weight. But remember at such times that weight loss is a process that with this change in eating habits will be slow but sure. Even if you only lose one pound in a single month, it's preferable to putting that one pound on.

Celebrate the new you as it achieves weight-gain goals one by one. What pleasure can top that of stepping on the scale and seeing the weight drop? Your only regret will be you have to restock your wardrobe as you drop in pants or dress size.

Lifestyle Changes

I use the word *diet* to describe the change in eating patterns I'm advocating, but that's really not the right word, at least with the connotations that word has now. Think about it: going on a diet usually suggests taking a temporary detour away from normal eating patterns. For the time being, while on a diet, the person eats foods that are healthy but generally not liked. As soon as the weight is off, provided the diet is a success (which, in fact, is not that likely), the person can rush back to eating junk food again.

You can see that is not what I envision for weight losers. My "diet" is not a temporary aberration from one's normal eating. Instead, it is a lifestyle change. What I am prescribing are the eating habits you should keep for your whole life, provided you want that to be a long and healthy one.

Lifestyle changes will make the difference when diets don't make the grade. But the lifestyle changes laid out in this book do not stop at eating. Eating is part of an integrated, multi-layered program. The typical diet is food only. It has no other components, such as advice on how to cope with emotional crises. As explained before, people often eat as a way to face emotional difficulties, rather than because they're hungry. For example, after a bad day at work or after a row with a loved one or as an end to a long week, a woman will "allow" herself a junk food meltdown, as it were, in which she overeats chips or ice cream or another guilty pleasure.

Dieting does nothing to cope with the possible emotional roots of eating. If anything, it makes people more depressed because it becomes one of the issues that causes overeating. When a person "falls off the wagon," and breaks her diet plan, this may engineer later meltdowns, in which, unable to deal with the self blame for the violation of the plan, she binges once again. The only people who lose weight and keep it off are those who make permanent changes to their (and to their family's) eating and exercise habits. They, to borrow a phrase from Leonard Cohen, are the "beautiful losers."

Among the other lifestyle changes important to weight management, as well as overall health and well-being, are exercise, bodywork, meditation, detoxification, and living mindfully.

Chapter 3

Exercise and Physical Fitness

Exercise and physical fitness are critical to maintaining good health. As you will see throughout this book, regular physical activity can not only help control weight, but also can prevent or delay the onset of disease, increase energy, enhance mood, and boost longevity. Unfortunately, as reported in a 2013 survey from the Centers for Disease Control and Prevention (CDC), only about 18 percent of American women and 23 percent of men get the recommended amounts of both aerobic and muscle-strengthening exercise per week.

Types of Exercise

Women need different forms of exercise for total body fitness. Aerobic exercise is especially good for the heart. It keeps your cardiovascular system in good shape. Studies show that as little as thirty minutes of exercise twice a week actually creates collateral circulation in the coronary arteries. For maximum benefit, aerobic exercise should be done three or four times a week for at least twenty to thirty minutes. Start slowly, increasing the amount of time and intensity by about 10 percent every two weeks. Among the specific aerobic activities are fast walking, jogging, swimming, bicycling, and jumping rope.

Weight-bearing exercises help to build up your bones, and prevent osteoporosis. They work your bones and muscles against gravity. Weight-bearing activities include walking, jogging, tennis and other racquet sports, and weight training with free weights or machines.

Yoga and qi gong are among the age-old methods that have been gaining popularity in recent years. Yoga has been found to help build and fortify bones, keep muscles strong and flexible, improve posture, and help with balance and coordination. Qi gong is an ancient Chinese practice that uses aerobic exercise, meditation, relaxation techniques, and isometrics to control the vital energy of the body. Like many Asian therapies, it emphasizes the unity of mind, spirit, and world. Qi gong is useful in relieving hot flashes and night sweats associated with menopause, menstrual irregularities, breast pain, kidney dysfunction, and sexual energy problems.

Health Benefits

Dr. Joseph Pizzorno, past president of John Bastyr College of Naturopathic Medicine in Washington, says that strengthening exercises are the best defense against the increased frailty women face as they age. "It turns out that the majority of the debility of old age is simply due to people not using their muscles. The full strength of what one had at twenty and thirty is almost completely returned with weight-strengthening exercises. Weights are used in a very, very controlled, very, very intense way to get maximum effects from the exercise. I am quite impressed with what I have seen."

Chiropractor Mitch Proffman says that traditional cultures have long appreciated the connection between physical fitness and longevity, making athletic activities a part of women's ritual ceremonies. "In Navajo society," he explains, "women would run three times daily as a formal part of the four-day rites of passage after the onset of menstruation. The first run was at dawn, and each subsequent run would be for a longer distance. It was believed that the total distance a woman could run would determine her longevity."

Research supports the connection between exercise and a longer life. "The *Journal of the American Medical Association* has reported that exercise increases people's life spans," Proffman says. "Women walking forty to fifty minutes, three to four times per week, live longer. The same article claims that exercise decreases the chance of dying from all known diseases. This can be attributed to the fact that most major diseases, such as cancer, diabetes, and heart disease, are stress-related, and exercise reduces stress."

Another important function of exercising is improving mental state. There's research in this area as well. "In a study at the University of Illinois," Proffman explains, "Dr. William Greenboro studied four different groups of rats. One group led a sedentary life. Another group played aimlessly on wood and plastic in their cages. A third group was on a special motorized wheel, and a fourth group walked through intricate mazes and ropes. The finding was that all rats that exercised in any manner had more capillaries in their brains and better brain function. This suggests that exercise fuels the brain with more oxygen and increases natural growth factors, in humans as well as in rats."

For people with mental health concerns, exercise is especially critical. "It is important for depressed people to get up and get dressed," said the late holistic medicine pioneer Dr. William Goldwag. "They should not walk around in pajamas or nightgowns because this maintains that connection to the bed and the bed means inactivity. That's the thing you're trying to overcome. Exercise may take the form of walking, walking the dog perhaps, or going outside to do some simple gardening. These are all very important for overcoming that feeling of lassitude that is so characteristic of depression.

"Another benefit of exercise is a feeling of accomplishment. Even doing a little bit of exercise will make you feel more energized later on. Finishing an exercise routine, even one that's fatiguing, after a brief period of rest, will give you a feeling of revitalization, of energy, and a psychological feeling of accomplishment. It gives a feeling of, 'I've done it. It's completed.' For the depressed individual, the boost to self-esteem that this can give is important."

An exercise program must be tailored to the individual. "There is no one exercise that is good for everybody," said Dr. Goldwag. "Some people can just do a little bit; some can push themselves much further. Ask anybody who has gone from a relatively sedentary life to an exercise program and they will all report the same thing: more energy, more interest in what is going on, a clearer mind and less stress. Being active, therefore, is an integral part of any kind of medical program, particularly for people who are having mental disturbances."

Dr. Judith Sachs agrees that exercise "triggers all of these brain stimulants that make us feel good, these natural opiates. This is another system we have in the brain that takes away pain and gives us pleasure. A lot of people who run say, 'Well it feels so good when I stop,' but even people who are not crazy about that kind of exercise are finding that they feel better. They feel efficient, like the body is not just this house that they happen to live in, but has actually become an integral part of their mind, their spirit, the whole way that they approach themselves and other people. That can really turn around a lack of self-confidence, a lack of self-esteem. When you've said 'all I could do was to walk down to the mailbox to get my mail' and suddenly you are able to run up five flights of stairs or run a mini-marathon—that can make you feel very effective as a person."

Chapter 4

Pain Management

Pain is associated with a host of diseases and injuries. Millions of people suffer from acute or chronic pain at some point in their lives. When something hurts, a typical reaction is to reach for a pill. Over-the-counter medications for everyday aches and pains are standard fixtures in home medicine cabinets. For more severe pain, doctors have many additional drugs to offer.

In 2014, Americans received 259 million prescriptions for narcotic painkillers. This represents 80 percent of the global supply. More than one-third of women aged fifteen to forty-four enrolled in Medicaid and more than a quarter with private insurance filled a prescription for a pain medication each year between 2008 and 2012. Every day millions of people wake up knowing they are going to contend with pain, and many believe they have to pop pills, undergo surgery, or else live with their condition. Unfortunately they do not realize that there are varied ways of treating pain naturally.

In this country we need a different approach to acute and chronic pain. We need to go from treating just the symptoms to treating the sufferer holistically. This includes getting proper nutrition through sensible eating and taking natural supplements, including minerals and herbs. Other methods of pain management include chiropractic, shiatsu, acupuncture, and the Trager and Alexander techniques.

One Physician's Personal Experience

Dr. Art Brownstein, author of *Healing Back Pain Naturally* and *Extraordinary Healing: The Amazing Power of Your Body's Secret Healing System*, is a former assistant clinical professor of medicine at the University of Hawaii who also teaches yoga. He was a back pain patient himself for twenty years. Like many of the 50 million Americans who have chronic back pain, he ended up on an operating table in a futile attempt to relieve his suffering. He describes his experience and how it bolstered his views on alternative healing.

"I've got two vertebrae that are only halfway there, and I was getting worse after the surgery to the point where I couldn't work for three years as a physician. I got hooked on the narcotic pain pills, and I was depressed and suicidal. At the end of the three-year period I was offered another operation, at which point I remembered my professors in medical school saying, 'Physician, heal thyself.' To make a long story short, I ended up traveling around the world several times during the next three- to seven-year period and discovered some very simple, ancient mind-body healing techniques, including yoga, which allowed me not only to heal my own back pain naturally but also to help thousands of others."

Dr. Brownstein's back pain protocol emphasizes the importance of the muscles in supporting the health of the back. "When people have back pain, they automatically assume, because it is so painful, that there must be a problem with the discs or the bones. And that is what conventional medicine focuses on with its diagnostic tests such as MRIs and X-rays. Muscles don't show up on MRIs or X-rays, so in performing these tests, physicians are simply bypassing the most important system."

Often, Dr. Brownstein says, the back problem relates to the condition of the muscles. "If you look at other cultures that have very little furniture and very low-tech kind of societies, they have virtually no back pain. We spend so much time sitting down, sitting at our jobs, sitting while we are driving, that these muscles in our back just don't get used . . . We have to really tone our muscles in our backs and stretch them . . . Yoga is an effective strategy for this."

Stress management is part of his program. When people are under mental stress, the nerves are overstimulated. This can cause the muscles, including those of the back, to tighten and contract. If you have pain in your back, it will get worse. "If you don't have pain," Dr. Brownstein says, "you are an accident waiting to happen. Just bending forward and picking a paperclip off the floor can send your back into tremendous spasms." Among the stress management techniques Dr. Brownstein uses are breathing, relaxation, meditation, and visualization.

Diet is also part of Dr. Brownstein's program. He explains: "I've discovered a very strong connection between what you put in your body and not only every cell and tissue of your body but particularly your back."

Take coffee, for example. "I had a patient who had been to the top specialists all over the country—the Mayo Clinic, Johns Hopkins, Harvard," Dr. Brownstein says. "[T]hey were all recommending surgery for him. I asked him about his diet and it turned out he was drinking eight to ten cups of coffee a day. I asked him if he would be willing to quit, and reluctantly he agreed. Of course he had the caffeine-withdrawal headaches, but after two to three days he got over that. Within three weeks his back pain was totally cleared up. So it can be something that simple."

Diet

As Dr. Brownstein's example shows, one of the most important ways of combating back and other types of pain is by guiding your diet to avoid abrasive foods and concentrate on those that build up the body's biochemistry. You should eat the same way you should drive—defensively.

It seems that people are really taking a new look at diet, especially people who used to think that relief from aches and pains could come only from a jar or bottle or from even more drastic remedies such as surgery. Not in every case, but in many cases, we're finding that diet can be the most powerful medicine.

One physician who has been looking is Dr. Neal Barnard, author of *Food That Fights Pain* and president of the Physicians' Committee for Responsible Medicine, a nationwide group that promotes preventive medicine and addresses controversies in modern medicine. As he sees it, there are four ways pain is manifested in the usual course of an illness. He uses arthritis as an example. First, there is some type of injury. Second, there is inflammation with redness, swelling, and stiffness. Third, there is irritation of the nerves that transmit the pain signals to the brain. Fourth, the brain receives the signals.

Dr. Barnard explains that there are three steps that must be taken in using diet to help with health problems. First, it is necessary to look for possible trigger foods. These are foods that commonly set off pain: dairy products, wheat or citrus for some people, tomatoes, meat, and eggs. "We want to do a little detective work and see which one is a trigger for an individual, because the triggers may be different for each person," Dr. Barnard counsels.

The second step is to find out which foods are safe to eat. "We focus on the pain-safe foods, which is fairly simple to do."

The third step, which Dr. Barnard believes is especially necessary for women, is to use foods to balance hormones. Because low-fat, vegetarian diets reduce hormone swings, they can dramatically reduce pain.

FOODS THAT WEAKEN RESISTANCE TO PAIN

In contrast to normally innocuous foods such as strawberries, which may trigger a pain reaction in certain people, some foods may reduce pain but also weaken the body's ability to resist pain. Coffee is one of those foods.

Dr. Barnard mentions sugar as another substance that lowers a person's pain tolerance. "Sugar never gets good press, and I'm sorry I have to add to the list of its problems. In a research study, people have taken volunteers and put a little metal clip on the web of skin between the fingers. Then this clip is hooked up to an electrical generator. The participants are given a little bit of electrical energy, which is gradually increased, and asked when they can feel it and when it becomes intolerable. Those numbers are written down. Then they are given sugar and the progression is repeated. These studies find that after ingesting the sugar, they feel the pain sooner and it becomes intolerable sooner.

"I've been so struck by the fact that people would start their breakfast with a cup of coffee, which, as a vaso- and cerebrodilator, temporarily reduces pain, then add a little sugar, which will increase pain sensitivity. It goes on for the rest of the day, where we are mixing up foods that cause and reduce pain."

PAIN-SAFE FOODS

Pain-safe foods include rice—any kind of rice, but especially brown rice—and cooked green vegetables such as broccoli, Swiss chard, and spinach. If you get an upset stomach from broccoli, cook it a little longer; this knocks out some of the vitamins, but the proteins in the broccoli are what cause stomach irritation in some people. Also, cooked orange vegetables such as sweet potatoes and carrots are pain-safe. Cooked yellow vegetables such as squash are also good. For fruits, pick the noncitrus ones, especially dried or cooked.

PAIN-REDUCING FOODS

Dr. Barnard has also found that some overlooked foods are especially good for dealing with pain. "One of the things we like to use is hot peppers, jalapeño peppers. The zing in the jalapeño is from a chemical called capsaicin. This doesn't just make your mouth hot, it actually changes what happens in the nerves. It stops the nerves from being able to conduct pain. Pharmaceutical manufacturers have taken this capsaicin straight out of the pepper and mixed it into a cream, which is applied externally. Two brands of capsaicin cream in the United States are Capsin and Zostrix.

"At first when you put on the capsaicin, it tingles and may even burn a little just as a hot pepper would. Do it day after day, and gradually the pain will diminish. You will still feel touch and pressure, but you won't feel pain. Give it a couple of weeks to work."

VITAMINS, MINERALS, AND OTHER SUPPLEMENTS

Most people know that minerals are essential for building up the body, maintaining the body's fluid balance, and helping with many chemical reactions. Let us look specifically at how minerals and vitamins have proved effective in treating pain.

Magnesium salts are useful for those with pain from the torso or joint aches. Many people are already deficient in magnesium. This calmative mineral is obtained from nuts and seeds that are raw and not roasted. Nuts are also beneficial in that they contain essential oils, including the omega-3 fatty acids, which also have mild anti-inflammatory properties that help reduce pain. For torso and joint problems, intake of magnesium citrate salts should be 400 milligrams per day, divided into doses of 100 to 200 milligrams.

Sound sleep is an essential part of good health. For people who have trouble sleeping due to headaches or other pains, there are a number of useful supplements. Valerian, hops (the same element found in beer), skullcap, or passionflower can be used. These supplements, which can be mixed, should be taken a half hour before going to sleep, in either capsule (one or two) or tincture form. You might also try taking 1 milligram of melatonin before sleep.

General musculoskeletal pain can be relieved by a number of substances. L-carnitine allows the body to burn fats and soak up excess lactate, which may be causing pain. Also helpful with muscle aches are the methyl donors, such as DMG (dimethyl glycine) and TMG (trimethyl glycerin), taken in doses of 100 milligrams per day.

To reduce the soreness after exercise, one should take vitamin E (400 to 800 IU/day), which prevents the leakage of enzymes from the muscles.

A final way to approach pain is to modify the way the brain perceives it. DL-phenylalanine (DLPA), which is a synthetic amino acid, slows down endorphins, making the ones you have work better. Taken in a dosage of 500 milligrams three times a day, it reduces chronic pain while getting the sufferer off analgesics.

Chiropractic

Chiropractic treatment involves the manual manipulation of vertebrae that become misaligned, causing nerve pressure and energy blocks to various organs. This manipulation is called an adjustment. It involves the chiropractor's gentle application of direct pressure to the spine and joints. The chiropractor may squeeze or twist the torso, pull or twist the limbs, or wrench the head or back. What the chiropractor is doing is readjusting the spinal column to restore the normal vertebral relationship. This eliminates the body's energy blocks and keeps life-sustaining energy flowing freely to the vital organs.

Chiropractic is effective in dealing with pain and as a preventive treatment because it relieves nerve pressure. The buildup of this pressure is cumulative in its erosion of the health and integrity of specific body organs or regions. If one vertebra is out of relationship to the one next to it, a state of disrelationship is said to exist. This disrelationship throws off that vertebra's environment, that is, the blood supply and detoxifying lymphatic drainage surrounding it. When this occurs, a congestion of blood, toxins, and energy creates pressure that upsets both local and systemic homeostasis, or balance.

Tissues all need normal nerve functioning in order to transport required nutrients to the cells. Insofar as the vertebrae are misaligned, the blood becomes congested and slow in its delivery, creating the absence of this nutrient supply. The cell's normal activity is thereby hindered, and it becomes irritated. Moreover, once the cell's metabolic processing is interfered with, its waste-removing lymphatic servicing to that area is diminished. This leads to toxic buildup that causes further irritation and inflammation. The chiropractor is concerned with alleviating all these problems.

Acupuncture

Acupuncture sees pain as being derived from blocked energy or qi (chi). In treating this blockage, the practitioner has to determine whether it stems from an overabundance or a deficiency in energy, so that treatment can be adjusted depending on whether it is necessary to strengthen or decrease qi.

The acupuncturist first records the patient's medical history in the manner of a conventional doctor. Then, with the patient lying down or seated, depending on the area to be treated, fine-gauge, stainless steel needles are inserted into significant points and meridians to exert different physiological effects on the body and induce both relaxation and energization. The patient will remain in this position for twenty to thirty minutes, though an appointment with an acupuncturist may last up to an hour, since part of the time will be spent consulting about the employment of other traditional and herbal treatments that might be recommended. Bodywork and massage may also be included in the session.

Dr. Christopher Trahan notes that the treatment will have analgesic and anesthetic effects, block pain, and accelerate recovery from motor nerve injury. Moreover, it enhances the immune system, which has a sedative effect; helps with muscular spasms or neurological problems; has a homeostatic effect in that it helps balance blood pressure; and has positive psychological effects, acting directly on brain chemistry.

Many patients with chronic low back pain find that acupuncture will not only help break the pain cycle, it will also allow them to reduce pain medications and participate more vigorously in physical therapy. Dr. Emily Kane, a naturopath who practices in Juneau, Alaska, says in an article on the website of the American Association of Naturopathic Physicians (www.naturopathic.org) that experiments have shown that acupuncture stimulates the nervous system to release endorphins as well as other chemical pain relievers in the body. Some people get immediate relief from low back pain after the first acupuncture session, but she recommends having six or eight sessions within a short period of time before assessing whether or not it is working for you.

Bodywork

SHIATSU

Shiatsu is also based on the principle that qi (chi) flows through the body. The primary cause of pain is an imbalance of this energy. The goal of the healer is to balance the client's energy so that pain and discomfort do not manifest or, if they do appear, will be relieved.

As bodywork practitioner Thomas Claire explains it, thumbs, fingers, palms, forearms, elbows, and even knees are used to apply pressure to specified points in the body to modulate the flow of energy. During a shiatsu treatment, the client lies on the floor on a comfortable padded surface, such as a futon, fully clothed or undressed to her level of comfort. What the client feels is pressure, which can be gentle or deeper at the places where the practitioner is working.

As the pressure continues, the patient generally feels relaxed and energized at the same time.

Shiatsu is good for treating a variety of different pains. It is especially beneficial in combating chronic pain in the back, neck, or shoulders, but it has also proved effective in treating whiplash, herniated discs, and problems affecting the nervous system, such as Bell's palsy.

A shiatsu healer concentrates on certain pressure points that have metaphoric names that tell us something about what they do or how they are to be worked with. The first point of interest is on the ankle and called Spleen 6. It is at the meeting of three yin meridians and is the most powerful point for tonifying the feminine energy in the body. It can be located by placing the little finger on the border of the inside ankle and counting up four fingers. At the very top of these fingers, and at the center, is Spleen 6. To modulate the energy, you can put pressure on this point with your thumb, pushing three times in succession for seven to ten seconds each time. This pressure will also help a woman control PMS and irregular cycles.

The corresponding point for male tonification is called Stomach 36. To locate this point, find the indentation just outside the kneecap. Put one finger at this indentation and go down four fingers. There you'll find Stomach 36, which is also known as Leg 3 Mile. This second name is given since, it is said, if you have a strong Stomach 36, you will have enough stamina to walk three miles with no trouble. For women, this point can be used to ease childbirth and labor pains.

A third important point, located at the middle of the web of the hand, is Large Intestine 4, also called Meeting Mountains. The latter name is derived from the "mountain of flesh" found jutting up between the thumb and index finger when you close your hand. To locate this point, find the highest point on that protruding flesh and then open your hand. This point should be pressed three times running for seven to ten seconds to tonify the upper body. Pressing this point can also help with nausea, vomiting, colds, and constipation.

TRAGER TECHNIQUE

The Trager technique is a way of working with the mind and body simultaneously. According to the philosophy behind this technique, pain comes from the accumulated action of the patient frequently tightening her movements and posture. To correct it, the practitioner uses gentle motions to increase the patient's pleasure in the quality of the tissues and decrease the restriction and the sense of holding. The practice works by reaching into the functional subconscious with particular qualities of movement, posture, and sensation. Gentleness is emphasized so that no message will be sent to the body alerting it that pain is on the way or causing the patient to tighten up. The movement reaches into the central nervous system with a motion at once pleasurable, lengthening, softening, and opening, conveying this sensation to the tissues and joints. The movements can be very small and internal or can be done at the periphery of the body in the limbs. In the latter case, the limbs are used as handles to reach the core.

Roger Tolle, a Trager practitioner, says that some clients will feel results immediately, as the touching allows them to release pain. In other cases, it takes a repetition of the information into the body and mind, which will gradually allow the client to relearn how to go about daily activity with a different quality of motion.

The Trager method works particularly well against pain in the temporomandibular joint (TMJ), neck, back, pelvis, and carpal tunnel.

ALEXANDER TECHNIQUE

Jane Kosminsky, an Alexander technique teacher, describes this modality: "The Alexander technique is an educational tool that teaches us first how to balance our heads well at the top of the spine. It teaches the correct use and relationship of the head to the spine and the spine to the limbs. We deal with the problems of the lower back, the arm, or the leg by focusing first on the balance of the head and its relationship to the spine."

Actual exercise is not part of the Alexander program. "In Alexander we don't do exercise, we don't try to fix ourselves," Kosminsky says. "We notice what we are doing and then we make the decision to say no to a habit that is not good for us. For example, we note excessive tension, crunching in the spine, pulling in the shoulders, and then we use the technique of visualization to effect change."

ROLFING

According to the practitioners of Rolfing, pain is due to chronic shortenings in the tissue. Correction of this pain can be accomplished through soft-tissue manipulation. This manipulation acts to create order in the body so that the client stands tall and free of restriction.

David Frome, a physical therapist, states that Rolfing is done in a ten-session series designed to address all the shortenings in the structure systematically. Each session works in a different area. In the first hour, for instance, concentration is on the trunk, shoulders, and hips. In the second hour, work is done on the back and lower leg. Going through the complete series allows the therapist to work through all the body's shortenings. During a session, a patient may experience a tingling sensation and a sense of release. The patient should strive to draw the deepest possible breath to aid in treatment.

The major goal of the treatment is not pain relief per se, but it has been found to help with TMJ pain, frozen shoulder, tennis elbow, carpal tunnel syndrome, chronic hip problems, sciatica, cervical neuropathies, and knee, foot, and ankle problems.

CRANIOSACRAL THERAPY

The sacral region is at the bottom of the spine. Between it and the cranium (skull), there should be a balanced rhythmic motion maintained for the health of the organism. When pain arises, it may be due to a restriction that disturbs the harmony between these two regions or between them and the rest of the body.

In craniosacral therapy, the practitioner places his or her hands on the client's body in such a way as to try to bring the cranium and sacrum back into alignment, reestablishing a natural rhythm. Charles A. Kaplan, the founder and director of the Center for Pain Management, points out that this hands-on technique usually centers on touching the head or lower back but can be done anywhere, such as on the fingers or toes. Some patients will go through a first treatment and not feel anything, but most will leave the treatment table feeling very relaxed and stress-free.

Craniosacral therapy is recommended for dealing with muscular and skeletal pain, headaches, pains in the back and neck, sports injuries, sciatica, and nerve pain. It can also be beneficial to those recovering from pneumonia or bronchitis, helping by loosening the rib cage. Craniosacral therapy is a tremendous stress reducer.

MAGNET THERAPY

With an ancestry as old as that of acupuncture and shiatsu, magnet therapy also acts to influence the body's energy. Dr. Jim Joseph mentions that the healing power of magnets was known in China over four thousand years ago. Such ancient fathers of medicine as Galen and Aristotle discussed magnets, as did Paracelsus, one of the founders of chemistry. Mesmer and others in the nineteenth century also elaborated on the value of magnet therapy, and it is still being developed and practiced today.

Down through history, magnets have been used to deal with the causes of various ailments. As Dr. Joseph remarks, "Pain is a messenger. We don't want to kill the messenger but find the cause."

Pain in the body can be caused by positive energy being drawn to the site of injury. To bring about this transfer, the brain sends out a negative signal. Using the negative side of a magnet can augment and assist that reaction. Furthermore, around an injury there will be an acidic buildup. The negative side of the magnet is an alkalizing force that can help alleviate the pain accompanying this acidity.

A second source of pain arises when a person is overworked or suffering from undue stress, causing that person's cells to be overly positively charged. Putting a negative magnet on a weakened area will repolarize the cells, restoring the balance between positive and negative charge.

The distortion of the cells' polarity and resultant pain may also be caused by our technological environment. We are swamped with positive electromagnetic pulses coming from televisions, radios, electric clocks, and all the other electrical devices around us. The pulses of their fields are not congruent with the one found in our body and can throw us into disharmony and disease.

Magnets can be obtained in a plastiform case that can be molded and shaped for a particular area. They last indefinitely and are low priced. A medium-sized magnet may cost twenty dollars. Healing magnets are color-coded with the negative pole green and the positive red. The positive side of the magnet is active and sun-oriented; the negative side is relaxing and earth-oriented. All the treatments discussed here utilize the negative pole. One must be careful with the positive pole, since positive magnetism causes growth in any biological system, even cancer. Treatment should last from twenty minutes to overnight. The magnet's power should be from 1,000 to 6,000 gauss.

A magnet can be wrapped with Velcro on the area to be covered. Special wraps in which the magnets are inlaid in Velcro are available. These wraps can be placed on most parts of the body, though they should not be used on the eyes. Negative magnetism attracts fluids and gases, and a negative magnet placed near the eye would draw out its fluids. If work is to be done on the eyes, the magnet can be placed off to the side. From this position, magnetism can be exerted on cataracts to reduce oxidation and free-radical development. The magnet's value in reducing oxidation is due to the fact that oxygen is paramagnetic. When you breathe, you are pulling negative energy from the earth into your body.

At night, it is useful to lie on a magnetic bed pad and put magnets behind the head, where they will bathe the pineal gland in energy. This will induce a restful night's sleep. By using a magnet, one can feel rested even after sleeping fewer hours than one normally does. Magnets have also been known to increase sexual abilities.

Magnets can help with shoulder pain, pain in the rotator cuff, and aches in the lumbar region of the back. They can be attached to the head or neck to deal with hypothyroidism, depression, migraine headaches, and problems with the vestibular system. For depression, the magnet should be placed near the occipital lobe.

The Mind-Body Connection

Some therapists such as Dr. Art Brownstein, mentioned earlier, recommend a more eclectic approach, one that looks for and relies on the often-overlooked synergies that flow between the mind and the body. Dr. Ron Dushkin brings up a number of points to consider in dealing with pain. He notes, first, the importance of relaxation, which will quiet and calm the nervous system. Remember that when we feel pain, we are also feeling a layer of stress on top of that pain. If the layer of stress is relieved, the pain will diminish significantly.

Human touch can also play a part in relieving pain. As babies we like to be touched and as adults we still find this important.

A third overlooked factor in healing is humor. The late writer Norman Cousins tells the story of how he was hospitalized with a critical health problem. As he saw it, a lot of his physical deterioration was due to stress and negative thoughts from that stress. He reasoned that if we can create disease with stress, then by alleviating stress through means such as humor, we can cure disease. He had a movie projector brought into his hospital room and began showing Marx Brothers' films and other comedies. Soon his room became a place of congregation for other patients who wanted to enjoy the shows. It got rather chaotic because so many people were coming into his room and laughing. You're not supposed to laugh in a hospital. Some people were scandalized. Cousins said that the doctors would give him blood tests before and after he had been laughing at a humorous film and would find an improvement after the film. He also had less pain after laughing.

Guided imagery is also an element of the mind-body connection. With this technique, a sufferer places a hand over the injured area and invites the other cells in the body to go to the aid of the damaged area. After all, the body's cells always work together, and this is one way to encourage their interplay.

All the methods mentioned as part of the mind-body connection get the patient to take charge of personal recovery. Many people are strong in many areas of life—pursuing a career, forming good relationships, playing sports—but when it comes to their own health, they turn over all control to a doctor. To really escape pain, the patient must play a big role in the recovery process.

Chapter 5

A Home Detoxification Program

Toxic substances abound in our air, water, soil, and food. A healthy person can often eliminate harmful substances through the liver and other organs. But a person whose health is compromised, or on a diet that is too high in fats, processed proteins, sodium, refined sugars, and other refined foods has a reduced capacity to rid the body of toxins. When this happens, the toxins accumulate.

Frances Taylor, coauthor of *Natural Detoxification*, tells us more: "As we journey through life the way most people do, we become overloaded with the toxins that absorb in the body. Unless we do something to get rid of these things, our bodies become overloaded and our health suffers. We develop symptoms such as headaches, digestive problems, sluggishness, after-meals fatigue. Many health benefits can be obtained by simply detoxifying the body."

Taylor says there are many ways to detoxify at home. Her guidelines are presented below.

Water

One of the first things people need to do is make sure they consume enough water. Taylor says, "Some people do reasonably well with city water, tap water, which of course contains a number of additives. Most people will do considerably better if they use some type of filtered or ionized water or reverse osmosis water."

Detox Bath

Taylor uses a lot of detox baths with her patients. "We jokingly refer to detox baths as a poor man's sauna," she says. "Hot water increases the blood flow in the capillary action near the surface of the skin and causes a faster release of toxins."

Anybody who has a bathtub can do a detox bath. Taylor explains the procedure: "First of all you need to start off with an absolutely clean bathtub. You wash your body thoroughly before you take your bath. Then you fill the bathtub with water as hot as you can tolerate it without burning your skin. You need to cover the overflow valve so the water will be high enough for you to immerse your body up to your neck.

"This next step is very important. You begin with a five-minute soak in the hot water. Some people say, 'Oh, gee, it felt so good I stayed in for fifteen minutes.' These people frequently cannot get out of bed the next day because their body releases toxins more rapidly than the liver can detoxify them, so they don't feel well. It's very important that you stay in the plain hot water bath for five minutes only the first time.

"After your bath you must take a shower and scrub every square inch of your skin to get off any toxins that may have been released. If you don't do this, these [toxins] will be reabsorbed into your body."

If you don't have any symptoms after the five-minute bath, increase bath time by five minutes more the next day. Gradually increase your time until you can sit in the plain hot water for thirty minutes. Most people need to do a detox bath only about three times a week. It's a good idea to drink an eight-ounce glass of water during your bath because you are going to be sweating. You can even take some vitamin C both before and after your bath because this will help your body remove the toxins that are released into your bloodstream.

Taylor recommends the use of Epsom salts in the bath. "The sulfur component in Epsom salts helps detoxify," she says. "It works as a counter irritant on the skin to increase the blood supply and it changes the pH of the skin surface. Begin with only a fourth of a cup of Epsom salts and gradually increase it over time until you are using about four cups per tub of clean hot water."

Again you want to do things very gradually so that your body won't detoxify too rapidly. You don't want to exceed the capacity of your liver and your detox system to get rid of the toxins.

Apple cider vinegar, baking soda, clay, and herbal teas may also be added to a detox bath, following the same principles as Epsom salts. With apple cider vinegar, Taylor says to start with the plain hot water bath first, then add 1/4 cup of apple cider vinegar, and over a period of time increase this to 1 cup. Baking soda baths are particularly beneficial for people with weeping open sores. Combining baking soda and salt is effective if you have had an X-ray or been exposed to radiation. "We routinely have our patients take a salt and soda bath if they have to have any X-rays done," Taylor says. "You will use equal amounts of the soda and noniodized sea salt and you build up until you use a pound of each."

For clay baths, Taylor recommends a cup of clay to a tub of water. Clays can be purchased at many health food stores.

Among the herbal teas that can be used in a detox bath are catnip, peppermint, blessed thistle, and horsetail. Use 1 cup of brewed tea per tub of hot clean water. Taylor says use only one of these teas per bath. In addition, "some sensitive people may not tolerate the tea."

Diet

Diet is important when detoxifying. Taylor says, "You want to eat clean food. Food that has not been pesticided, has not been dyed, doesn't have a wax coating on it. If you have food allergies, of course, you don't want to eat your food allergens. Rotation diets will help people with allergies. Some people even find that fasting is helpful. One word of caution about fasting: if you do have numerous food allergies and you start fasting, you could have withdrawal symptoms because people are allergic to the foods or they are addicted to the foods to which they are allergic. If a person has a very heavy load of food allergens, they may not feel very well if they try a fast."

Following are some foods that can help build good health:

SPROUTS—Sprouts are one of the most nutrient-rich, powerful, health-building foods in nature. They will help cleanse and rebuild your entire system.

What kind of sprouts should you try? Don't stop with just common sprouts like alfalfa or mung beans. Expand your cuisine. Try high-protein buckwheat sprouts; the sweet sunflower sprout; the aromatic fenugreek sprout; clover sprout; and for a little bite and pinch, try a radish sprout. A mustard sprout tastes as good as mustard, and yet is subdued enough in flavor to fit in better with a salad.

More than twenty different seeds for sprouting are available commercially. They're inexpensive and versatile. You can make salads out of them, put them into pita bread, use them in casseroles, and put them in soups.

MISO—Miso should also be on the list of detoxifying and rebuilding foods. For more than 3,000 years, this nutritionally superior food has been helping people build better health. Miso is a fermented product. Like yogurt, its bacteria work well in the intestines. Miso should be used sparingly, however, because it does have a high sodium content.

VEGETABLE JUICES—Vegetable juices are important detoxifiers. Generally speaking, Taylor says, drink no more than one glass of carrot juice per day. Beta-carotene is a precursor of vitamin A in the body. If you drink too much carrot juice, you'll be overloading the liver with vitamin A and your skin may turn yellow or orange. One glass will give you all the benefits of the vitamin. Celery, cucumber, cabbage, parsley, and sprouts can be added. For people who've never really enjoyed vegetables, juices are another way to get good-tasting, high-quality nutrition into the diet.

GRAINS—Grains are another group of foods that help the body cleanse itself and rebuild its strength. It is unfortunate that most Americans never taste whole grain. They eat refined carbohydrates in white bread or white rice, but not brown rice or whole grain bread. Whole grains are loaded with far more nutrition than their refined counterparts. The grain family includes rice, corn, buckwheat, rye, oats, and millet, as well as less well-known, newly available grains like triticale, amaranth, and quinoa, a light, fast-cooking grain from South America.

SEA VEGETABLES—The next group of foods to include as part of your health-rebuilding program is the sea family of vegetables. These include hijiki, a form of seaweed that tastes salty like fish. You can buy seaweed dry and store it for months. There are many types, including kombu, wakami, and nori. You can cut it into pieces, flake it, or put it into casseroles or soups. Include seaweed in your miso soup to increase its nutritional value. You can wrap seaweed around rice like grape leaves. Seaweed is so versatile that entire books are devoted to its use in cookery.

Seaweed is loaded with minerals. By dry weight, hijiki has ten times more available calcium than cow's milk.

BEANS—Beans, or legumes, are a group of healthy, detoxifying foods that many Americans deliberately avoid. The main reason we have kept ourselves away from one of nature's most important sources of vitamins, minerals, and fiber is that we have never really understood how to cook it. Most people, and most restaurants, do not soak beans overnight. This diminishes their digestibility. During digestion, gas forms in the colon, causing indigestion and flatulence. That uncomfortable feeling needn't be. All you have to do is soak beans overnight and then boil them for one or two hours. That usually takes care of most gas-producing properties. Then be sure to combine them with the right foods: don't eat fruit or sugary foods with a bean meal.

Legumes have more protein than grains or seeds. They are also high in fiber. There are more than sixty different legumes.

Nutritional Supplements

Taylor also recommends supplements. "We encourage our patients to take bowel tolerance vitamin C," she says. "I'm talking about a clean, pure vitamin C that is free of the common allergens such as wheat, yeast, corn, and sugar."

Taylor explains the procedure: "To do bowel-tolerance vitamin C, you start off with a gram, which is 1,000 milligrams, with each meal, and at bedtime. The next day you would add another one at breakfast. Then the next day you would add another one at lunch. The next day you would add another one at bedtime and so on. You know when you have reached bowel tolerance when you develop diarrhea. Most people can take much larger amounts of vitamin C than they would ever imagine. If a person is very, very toxic or has a lot of allergies they may be able to take 10 to 20 grams, that is 10,000 to 20,000 milligrams, of vitamin C a day. Between meals we encourage people to take buffered C, which is an ascorbic acid to which calcium, magnesium carbonate, and potassium bicarbonate have been added. This helps with detox but also helps with digestion. You would continue adding vitamin C, a gram a day, until you develop diarrhea and then you would back up 1 gram and that is the amount you would take in divided doses throughout the day."

Other nutrients are important for detoxification. These include the B vitamins. "You need to take a multimineral also because detoxification in the body is an enzymatic process and all of the enzymes require a metal to make them work," Taylor says. "Organic germanium is also good because it helps the body oxygenate at the cellular level. It is a little expensive but is very, very well worthwhile."

Chapter 6

Natural Medicine Cabinet

Many times we want to be able to go to our home medicine cabinet and find what we need for our day-to-day ills and problems. In this section you will find some of the components of a well-stocked natural medicine cabinet.

Herbal Antibiotics

The widespread use of antibiotics in this country has created a serious problem. The danger now is that bacteria have become immune to some of our most common antibiotics. The way this happened is that bacteria communicate with each other and actually teach each other how to become immune to medications. Now that they have become resistant to so many antibiotics, what does this tell us about further attempts to create stronger antibiotics? Steven Harrod Buhner, author of *Herbal Antibiotics*, explains that millions of people a year are coming down with antibiotic resistant infections. The Centers for Disease Control and Prevention (CDC) and many epidemiologists are warning that in the next twenty years most of our antibiotic arsenal will fail. "People will have to turn to more natural alternatives that are more ecologically sound, as herbs are. Things that naturally stimulate the immune system, that help keep us from getting ill in the first place.

"As our antibiotic arsenal fails, it becomes more and more important for everybody to stimulate their immune system and to keep it healthy and balanced. Whether it is bubonic plague or Ebola river virus, some people never become ill because their immune system is potentiated and healthy.

"We only get sick when our bodies are out of balance. Our natural immune system should deal with almost all diseases we encounter. Plant medicines are not something bacteria can become resistant to. Herbal medicines are so much more effective than antibiotics and are a lot gentler on the body."

To identify the most useful herbal antibiotics, Buhner studied each individually. "When I assessed the most powerful herbs, I had three criteria. One was the length of time it had been used in different cultures. Second was the degree to which it was used by indigenous and folk practitioners around the world. Third was the effectiveness in clinical trials and laboratory studies." Below are his recommendations, and more.

ALOE—Aloe, which comes from a southwestern American plant, is directly effective against staphylococcus bacteria, even resistant staph bacteria. When aloe is used on burns, it also acts as a softener and moisturizer.

ASTRAGALUS—Astragalus reduces tumor cell growth and reverses cancerous conditions. It is found in America as well as in China, where it has been used since ancient times to strengthen the body. Like echinacea, it increases the number and activity of immune cells in circulation, and has been shown to reduce the frequency and duration of colds.

BURDOCK ROOT—One of the best-known cleansing herbs, Burdock root works as a liver and bile stimulant, and also increases digestion.

CRYPTOCOCCUS—This West African plant has been used traditionally for malaria for thousands of years. It may also be effective against antibiotic-resistant bacteria.

DANDELION—Dandelion root helps to stimulate the liver, gallbladder, and bile secretion. Dandelion leaves are useful in a detoxification program because of their diuretic properties. The leaves also have high levels of potassium.

ECHINACEA—Also known as purple coneflower, echinacea has long been known for its powerful immune-stimulating properties. It has been shown to increase the number of developing immune cells in the bone marrow and lymphatic system. Echinacea is popular as a liquid extract, but also comes in capsules and tablets.

ESTONIA—Estonia, a lichen that grows on trees throughout the world, has been found to be more powerful than penicillin. The inner white thread is an immune enhancer and an immune stimulant, and the outside green part is strongly antibacterial.

GARLIC—Garlic not only stimulates the immune system but also serves as an antibacterial, antiviral, and antifungal element. It is a mild natural antibiotic, which increases the activity of natural killer cells so they are better able to fight off viruses and tumor cells. It is beneficial to take garlic every day as a preventive measure and to enhance your well-being. You can take tablets or use it when cooking.

GOLDENSEAL—Goldenseal benefits the mucous membrane system, and has been found to be useful for *E. coli* infections, which can cause severe, sometimes bloody diarrhea that can be fatal in children.

GURMAR—Gurmar, known scientifically as gymnema, was used in Ayurvedic medicine in India more than six hundred years ago for the treatment of what they called "honey urine." This was their name for the modern-day diabetes. Scientific studies of extracts of this plant have confirmed that its properties are beneficial to people with diabetes. It has been found to be effective in reducing blood sugar and repairing damage to the kidneys, liver, and pancreas.

LICORICE—Some preliminary evidence shows that licorice root fosters anti-HIV activity. You can buy it in liquid abstract form, in capsules, and in tablets, or as a whole herb.

MILK THISTLE—Milk thistle has long been known to protect and regenerate the liver. One milk thistle compound, called silverin, is an injectable drug used as a life-saving treatment to stop the progress of fatal or potentially fatal mushroom poisoning.

PANAX AND SIBERIAN GINSENG—Both ginsengs are known to build stamina, energy, and endurance by stabilizing the body. They are popular with athletes and with people who suffer from conditions that zap them of their strength and energy, such as chronic fatigue syndrome.

PAU D'ARCO—This herb has wonderful immune-enhancing and antifungal properties and works as a blood cleanser.

PHILANTHUS—Also called life plant, philanthus has been shown to act against hepatitis B and is now being researched for its antiretroviral and anti-HIV activity. It is a new herb in this country and may be hard to find.

RED CLOVER—Many cleansing programs include red clover, partly because of its high nutritional content and its anti-free radical effect. It protects liver cells and cells in other organs from oxidation damage, and thereby promotes rejuvenation and longevity.

ST. JOHN'S WORT—A common weed found in California, St. John's wort is now being studied by AIDS researchers because it seems to help prevent infections of T cells by making it harder for the AIDS virus to get into cells. In addition, the National Cancer Institute is looking at hypericum, a chemical found in the weed, because researchers believe it to be the active component of the plant. Unfortunately, a clinical trial of hypericum was altered when the project's natural source of hypericum was replaced by a semisynthetic form. Thus the effects of hypericum taken in its natural context could not be observed.

USNEA AND LOMATIUM—Both new to the marketplace, usnea and lomatium are known for their specific antiviral activity. They seem to help fight off influenza and chronic fatigue syndrome, and may promote antifungal activity against candida.

Other natural antibiotics include colloidal silver, wild oregano oil, manuka honey, olive leaf extract, black cumin seed oil, coconut oil, and bee propolis. Use as directed.

Natural Antihistamines

Histamine is a protein produced by the body in response to an allergen. It is responsible for the sneezing, congestion, and itchy eyes caused by exposure to pollen, dust, and other substances. Commonly known side effects associated with the over-the-counter antihistamines found in most people's medicine cabinets include drowsiness, confusion, dry mouth, and constipation. A 2015 study published online in *JAMA Internal Medicine* revealed even more alarming news: several popular antihistamines may also increase the risk of dementia in older adults.

Among the many evidence-based natural therapies for blocking the release of histamine are vitamin C, quercitin, bromelain, N-acetylcysteine (NAS), and *Petasites hybridus* (butterbur extract). According to a 2014 article in the *Townsend Letter*, nettle leaf (*Urtica dioica*) is also useful. "In vitro, a nettle extract inhibited several key inflammatory events responsible for seasonal allergy symptoms," the authors stated. "In one double-blind randomized study of 98 subjects with seasonal allergies, 58% of the subjects reported relief of most of their symptoms and 48% rated nettle leaf as being more effective than other over-the-counter medications."

Homeopathic Remedies

A number of homeopathic remedies also belong in the natural medicine cabinet. Homeopathy is based on the idea that the cure for an illness is similar to its cause. Homeopathic remedies, all made from natural substances, are given in microdoses.

According to Food and Drug Administration regulations, a natural remedy cannot be labeled safe and effective for treating a specific ailment even if study after study has proven that it is more effective than over-the-counter or doctor-prescribed medications. Therefore the average American will only see television commercials for products such as Anacin or Tylenol to treat a headache, even though a simple homeopathic remedy may be safer and just as effective.

Millions of Americans suffer from a myriad of everyday health conditions and do not know about natural remedies. Dr. Lynne Walker is a doctor of pharmacy and homeopathy, and has a master's degree in Chinese herbology and acupuncture. She has specific recommendations for what ought to be in everyone's medicine chest, especially if your access to a doctor or medical care is limited.

TEA TREE OIL—Dr. Walker's first recommendation—although this is not, strictly speaking, a homeopathic remedy—is tea tree oil. "Tea tree oil is an oil from Australia, also called melaluka oil. It is a strong antiviral, antifungal, and antibacterial. You could use it on any cut, for any kind of fungus in the mouth, and for fungus under the nail. It works as a gargle for sore throat and for gum problems. There is a tea tree oil toothpaste for those with ongoing gum problems. It works on canker sores, cuts and abrasions, insect bites, and even as an astringent for the face. Tea tree oil is a good basic remedy to have around the house."

RESCUE REMEDY—Rescue remedy is a Bach flower essence, which is actually a combination of five flower essences. It is useful in stress relief, and can be calming in times of emergency. This remedy is safe for children and animals. "When there is a crisis," Dr. Walker says, "I recommend that every member of the family, not just the sick one, take rescue to see things a little bit more clearly."

BITING INSECT—This remedy actually prevents insect bites. It is useful against fleas, mosquitoes, and other bugs. It is not as effective in the case of spider bites. If you know you will be exposed to bugs, Dr. Walker suggests 10 drops, three times a day.

PEPPERMINT OIL—Peppermint oil can be mixed in warm water and consumed for a stomachache or rubbed directly on the forehead for a headache. Again, although not strictly speaking a homeopathic remedy, peppermint oil is an enteric-coated herbal remedy.

BLACK OINTMENT—Made by Nature's Way and some other companies, black ointment can be used to draw out a splinter or any little sliver that won't come out. "It is also a very healing salve for any kind of cut, " Dr. Walker says.

ARNICA—Arnica homeopathic in low potency, either a 6x or 30x, can be used for any kind of trauma to the body. Dr. Walker explains, "It stops the body from overreacting to the trauma. It's good for muscle aches and pains, such as on days when you have worked really hard physically. Some people take it before surgery, but just take one dose to help your body not overreact."

TRAUMA OINTMENT OR TRAUMED OINTMENT—These combinations of homeopathic remedies are designed particularly for trauma, and can be used on sore muscles.

CALENDULA TINCTURE—Calendula tincture is an oil made from marigold flower, which is recommended for cleansing wounds and promoting healing.

NUX VOMICA—Dr. Walker recommends this preparation in a low potency, 6x or 30x, for hangovers as well as stomach discomfort from overeating or over-drinking. It also works well for hemorrhoids.

CALENDULA HYPERICUM—This ointment, especially the brand made by Boron, promotes healing and relieves pain. It can be used to quickly heal cold sores, other sores on the face or mouth, cuts, or abrasions.

GUNPOWDER 6X—"One of my favorites is not well known," Dr. Walker says. "This is for any minor infection like tooth abscesses or any infection on the skin. I find it useful for those who are getting their ears or bellybuttons pierced and they get infected. You can't get any sustainable antibiotic levels at those sites if you get an infection there. Take three gunpowder pills three times a day and the infection will resolve in two or three days."

VACTICIME DROPS—Made by Complemed, these drops help in fighting bacterial infection by boosting the immune system. Dr. Walker suggests 10 drops, three to five times a day.

ABC DROPS—Popular in Europe, ABC drops are a combination of aconite, belladonna, and chamomile homeopathic medications. They are beneficial against colds and earaches.

Aphrodisiacs

Aphrodisiacs enhance sexual desire, arousal, and performance. Certain foods, herbs, vitamins and minerals, amino acids, hormones, and aromatic oils can directly affect our biochemistry and hence our sexuality. There are over a dozen herbs that act as aphrodisiacs; they work in various ways and produce different results. For example, there are fast-acting herbs, which affect one or more of the stages of sexual response. Then there are herbs that, if taken over a long period of time, boost a person's overall physical and emotional readiness. Although herbal preparations do not carry the same risk as pharmaceuticals taken to enhance sexual performance, it is important to understand how to take them for maximum effectiveness. Overall, herbs can vary tremendously in their strength and effectiveness depending on where they are grown, when they are harvested, how they are processed, and so on. It can be challenging to sort it all out.

Nancy Nickel, the author of *Nature's Aphrodisiacs*, has studied food, nutrition, and alternative therapies for more than thirty years. Using her expertise as an educational writer, lecturer, and researcher in nutrition and molecular therapy, she offers a review. "Natural aphrodisiacs have been a source of legend for centuries," she says. "Oysters and shrimp actually contain nutrients that benefit the reproductive system. There have been some scientific studies of natural aphrodisiacs but not too many. Most research is done by pharmaceutical manufacturers and it doesn't pay them to research a product they cannot patent. But we have some scientific evidence on why several natural products and natural aphrodisiacs work."

As we all know, sex is hardly ever just about sex. Emotions and psychological health have a direct impact on sexual health. Feelings such as anger, worry, tension, and depression all affect sexual encounters for both women and men. There are quite a few herbs that are useful for addressing this aspect of sex and pleasure.

Nickel helps us to identify what they are and how they work: "To reduce anxiety and elevate mood, there is kava kava, valerian, gotu kola, lemon balm, angelica, skullcap, and vervain. These work quickly. (St. John's wort is also very good but takes several weeks to have an effect.) Kava kava tea has a physical effect on sexual performance; however, it is also an unbeatable tension reducer. It makes you feel happy, relaxed, and sociable. You can buy tea bags or make it from an extract. Put 10 to 30 drops in juice or water. It is fairly safe although slightly narcotic. Because it affects the nervous system, it should not be used by people who have Parkinson's disease or those taking an antidepressant."

Gotu kola is a nerve tonic that stimulates the central nervous system, decreases depression and fatigue, and enhances the sex drive. "If you take it regularly, which you can do, gotu kola tea has a cumulative effect as a sex drive booster," Nickel says. "Unlike herbs that contain caffeine, it doesn't cause insomnia or nervousness. You can take one to three capsules a day. As an extract, you can mix 5 to 10 drops in a liquid and drink it. Take it about three times a day. Excessive doses can make you feel faint and sometimes it can cause a headache."

Lemon balm is an excellent aphrodisiac that can be grown in your own garden. It works by relaxing the nervous system and elevating mood. Further, Nickel says, "It is one of the gentlest herbs and one of the most pleasant tasting. In Europe it is customary to drink lemon balm tea to calm stress and frayed nerves. It is available as a tea, a dried herb, and an extract. If you buy it as an extract, mix 1/2 to 1 teaspoon in liquid. Use the dried herb to make tea. Avoid lemon balm if you have a thyroid condition because it could interfere with a hormone that stimulates the thyroid. They are not sure about this, but I say be on the safe side.

"Angelica is a versatile herb that increases blood circulation. It acts as an aphrodisiac and is especially good for tension headaches. The dose is between 10 to 30 drops in a liquid. It should not be used by pregnant women because in strong doses it can bring on a period. And because it contains sugars, diabetics should not use it."

Skullcap is an herb with tranquilizing properties. "It is called skullcap," Nickel says, "because the flower looks like a little cap. It is excellent for relieving stress or nervousness associated with sex, or any kind of performance anxiety. It is very safe and mild, relaxes the muscles, and produces inner calm."

Other useful herbs are damiana, yohimbe, and muira puama (also called potency wood).

Nickel offers words of caution. "Because these herbs are potent and have chemical compounds that work, there are side effects, so you have to be careful."

The Problem with Medications

Over the past several years, the pharmaceutical industry has increased sharply its attempts to downplay, and even discredit, supplementation and healthier diets. Drug companies seem to view the growing inclination of Americans to take control of their health as an attack on their turf. Some people have fallen for the rhetoric. Unfortunately, what people don't often realize is that many medications actually deplete nutrients, which in turn can wreak havoc on the body.

"I have been really shocked at how much depletion occurs relative to the drug someone's taking that actually makes the condition worse," says Dr. Hyla Cass, a board-certified expert in the fields of integrative medicine, women's health, and psychiatry, and the author of many books including *Supplement Your Prescription: What Your Doctor Doesn't Know about Nutrition*. "For example, statins and coexzyme Q10. Statins are given to people with heart problems. However, depleting CoQ10 makes heart problems worse and can lead to cardiac failure. This doesn't make sense."

Other medications that have similar negative effects include the blood sugar-lowering drugs, which deplete some of the B vitamins that are needed for processing sugar and glucose; bone density medications, used to protect against osteoporosis; the bipolar drug lithium, which has been found to deplete inositol, a secondary messenger that makes serotonin and some of the other neurotransmitters believed to influence mood regulation; and heartburn drugs.

"When you take something for heartburn the assumption is that you have too much stomach acid," Dr. Cass says. "Often, it has to do with low stomach acid. So you end up taking an acid blocker, a prescription or an over-the-counter acid blocker, and then you don't have the hydrochloric acid that you need to break down and absorb essential nutrients like vitamin D, B_{12}, folic acid, calcium, chromium, iron, zinc, and phosphorous.

"When you have heartburn, it's about what you're eating. You have a sensitivity, a food sensitivity. It could be how you're eating or how much you're eating. It has to do with your diet rather than let's take a pill for every ill."

Antibiotics used for stomach infections such as *H. pylori*, a common cause of peptic ulcers, can also drain the body of nutrients. "Antibiotics cause depletion in guess what: the natural probiotics, our gut flora, the four or five pounds of wonderful friendly bacteria that live in the gut that help our immune system," Dr. Cass says. "These are very important for really everything. We know that when people have the right probiotics or the right friendly bacteria in the gut it can affect their mental state. People who have been depressed or even psychotic or autistic, when their gut biome—that is the population in the gut of these friendly bacteria —when it's balanced and robust and really working, a lot of these symptoms will clear up."

Dr. Cass has found healthy alternatives in the natural medicine cabinet. For bone loss, she recommends magnesium, calcium, boron, strontium, and vitamin D. For stomach infections, she suggests bismuth, zinc carnosine, and probiotics. Instead of antidepressants, she recommends B vitamins, probiotics, and amino acids.

How to Purchase Vitamins, Supplements, and Herbal Remedies

When I am talking with people in my travels, one of the questions they most frequently ask me is, "How can I be sure I am choosing a high-quality supplement?" With the rise in popularity of nutritional supplements, it can be confusing.

Natural health stores or groceries stock most of the vitamins, supplements, and herbs I recommend in this book. Even some mainstream grocery stores carry many of the vitamins and supplements mentioned. If you are able to use the Internet, it is easy to research and purchase supplements and herbal remedies online.

When shopping for vitamins and supplements, there are a few important questions you should ask:

- How does the manufacturer select its ingredients?
- What is the specific formula of the vitamin or supplement?
- What is the potency level of the vitamin or supplement?
- Does the manufacturer test for quality control, and if so, how?
- Are the vitamins natural (i.e., from food sources) or do they include added ingredients?

You may wonder whether it is better to choose tablets, capsules, powders, or liquids when purchasing vitamins and supplements. Generally speaking, tablets have a long shelf life, but can contain fillers and stabilizers that may cause allergic reactions. Capsules are generally used for fat-soluble and powdered supplements. The powdered type is most rapidly absorbed and generally contains no additives. The liquid forms may contain coloring agents or sweeteners.

Multivitamins may be useful in combining vitamins and minerals that are more effective when taken together (e.g., a B-complex vitamin). Most multivitamins combine vitamins and minerals in complementary doses. In some of the protocols given earlier in this book, I recommend doses higher than those found in multivitamins. For that reason, with the exception of a B-complex vitamin, I recommend buying vitamins and supplements individually.

Finally, when purchasing supplements, remember these important points:

- Buy from organic sources whenever possible. Avoid artificial ingredients.
- If you have food sensitivities, buy hypoallergenic products. Avoid wheat, yeast, and corn.
- Always examine the expiration date before purchasing.
- If you have any questions or doubts about a product, never

hesitate to contact the manufacturer and ask questions. A reputable company will not hesitate to address concerns.

If you are taking herbs, it is essential to take them in proper dosages, because they contain powerful ingredients. For centuries, people have been taking herbs to treat various conditions. When taken in the correct manner, herbs do not have the side effects that traditional medicines may cause. If herbs are used randomly or indiscriminately, however, they may produce unwanted side effects. If you are taking prescription or over-the-counter medications, you should talk with your health care provider before taking any herbal remedies, because some may have adverse interactions with medications. Herbs may be taken in their natural forms of leaves, barks, or roots by brewing them in teas. More commonly, herbs are taken in capsules or tinctures. Herbs can be used in compresses, applied externally with essential oils, or infused in teas, ointments, or salves.

For more information on vitamins, supplements, and herbal remedies, including hundreds of scientific studies on the efficacy of herbs for impacting various conditions, along with recommended dosages, go to my website: www.garynull.com.

Chapter 7

Colds

So far there has been no cure for the common cold even though billions of dollars have been spent on medical research. Keeping healthy in the first place is the best defense. A healthy immune system can tackle a virus better than any antibiotic or medication. Among the things you can do to boost your immunity are wash your hands often, exercise, eat a balanced diet, reduce stress, and get enough sleep.

Dr. Ray Sahelian is a board-certified family practice physician and graduate of Thomas Jefferson School of Medicine. In his book, *Finally the Common Cold Cure*, he recommends an approach for getting rid of the cold.

Immune System "Busters"

As Dr. Sahelian points out, the primary cause of the cold is a virus. There are at least several hundred types of viruses that cause colds. But, as we know, not everybody comes down with the common cold when they are exposed to the virus. The most likely reason people don't get sick is that they are maintaining healthy living habits. Dr. Sahelian has identified four immune system "busters" that cause people to get sick: lack of sleep, stress, smoking, and unnecessary use of antibiotics.

We should be getting at least six to eight hours of restful sleep, Dr. Sahelian says. "It is during the time of our deepest sleep that the immune cells are regenerated. One particular type of immune cell, called the natural killer cell, is very important. It is during deep sleep that the natural killer cell is activated. If it is not activated, then we are more vulnerable to getting a cold. Everyone is going to be exposed to the virus sooner or later, by shaking the hand of someone who has a cold or being exposed to children who are sneezing or coughing. If we have a good, activated immune system it is going to knock out that virus."

Stress can come from a variety of sources, including personal relationships, financial problems, work, athletic competition, and illness. It can temporarily decrease immune functioning, thereby allowing the virus to get a foothold.

The third immune system buster is smoking. "Smoking damages the lining of the respiratory tract," Dr. Sahelian says. "There are hairlike structures called cilia that are constantly sweeping out the germs that we inhale. If the cilia are damaged from smoking they are not going to be able to sweep out the bacteria or viruses, which then settle in to start a cold or another type of infection."

The final immune system buster is taking antibiotics when you don't need them. Dr. Sahelian explains, "Whenever someone comes down with a cold, as a rule they wait it out a day or two, take some over-the-counter pills if they are not into natural medicine, and then go to their doctor. The doctor examines them, and says, 'You have a cold, take some more over-the-counter medicines, and you are going to be okay in a week.' Well, the patient is not satisfied if they made the effort to go all the way to the doctor, wait in the office waiting room, pay $60 to $200, and then be told to use an over-the-counter medicine. So they are going to request an antibiotic prescription.

"Even though 90 percent of all upper respiratory infections are caused by a virus, over 50 percent of the time the patient will come out with a prescription for an antibiotic. *Antibiotics do not kill viruses.* And antibiotics are harmful because they can cause side effects, such as yeast infections, killing all the good bacteria in the gut. They can also cause fatigue, allergic reactions, diarrhea, and sometimes even more harmful things. So that is not the answer."

Immune System Boosters

What is the answer, then? According to Dr. Sahelian it involves maintaining a healthy diet, and taking supplements such as vitamin C and vitamin E, juices, and fish oils.

The late Gail Ulrich, founder of Blazing Star Herbal School in Shelbourn Falls, Massachusetts, and the author of *Herbs to Boost Immunity*, told us more: "Our culture's diet is high in fats, refined sugars, and sodium. We now know that these foods produce free radicals in the body that create toxicity and weaken immunity. It is important first of all to eliminate refined sugar and flours, as well as caffeine, cigarettes, alcohol, and processed or deep-fried foods. It goes without saying to avoid tobacco and commercially raised red meats, especially because of the high pesticide and hormone content in these products, and to minimize alcohol consumption.

"An immune-enhancing diet would include a wide variety of organically grown fruits and vegetables or wild fruits and vegetables as well. You also need whole grains and legumes along with adequate amounts of protein from soy, grains, or fish. The more you get back to a simple diet based on whole foods as they occur in nature, the better off you will be. It is important to include super-foods or nutrient-dense foods such as miso soup, garlic, and sea vegetables such as kelp. Wild foods are important, as are greens such as dandelion greens, mustard greens, watercress, astragalus, and steamed nettle greens. There are some delicious medicinal immune-enhancing mushrooms such as shiitake and reishi. Yogurt that contains acidophilus is important for balancing the garden of the intestinal flora, if you don't have lactose intolerance. Other immune-enhancing foods include dates, almonds, buckwheat, chicken soup, chickpeas, burdock root, and parsley."

Other lifestyle changes may be in order. "They always say, eat like a king at breakfast, a prince at lunch, and a pauper at dinner. Drink at least eight glasses of pure water daily and exercise adequately," Ulrich said.

A variety of herbs can be used to enhance immunity. "Echinacea is well known," Ulrich said. "I also recommend garlic, osha root, and milk thistle. These protect the mucous membranes and stimulate production of white blood cells. There are also deep immune tonic herbs that would be helpful to build the bone marrow and increase deep immunity. These are astragalus, Siberian ginseng, and shiitake and reishi mushrooms. These are especially helpful when we have immune deficiency and long-term stress on the immune system."

Adaptogens are herbs that help the body cope with physical as well as environmental and emotional stress. They include Siberian ginseng, panax ginseng, Korean ginseng, licorice, borage, and milk thistle.

Natural Remedies

What should you do at the first signs of a cold? "Sometimes a cold can come on mildly—a scratchy throat, a runny nose, or even just a tingling sensation in the nose or throat," Ulrich explained. "But as soon as you notice the very first symptom, do not wait to act. Immediately take between 3 and 5 grams of vitamin C. You may wish to keep the 500 milligram capsules on your kitchen counter and take about six to ten of these, which would equal about 3 to 5 grams of vitamin C. Right after that immediately put a zinc lozenge in your mouth. The zinc lozenge should contain between 10 and 25 milligrams of zinc. Many people chew it and within a brief period swallow it, but this is a mistake. The zinc is fighting the cold by acting locally in the throat and palate and the nasopharyngeal area. It has to stay in the mouth for as long as you can tolerate it, generally five to ten minutes. You can bite it, but keep the pieces in your mouth before you swallow it. Keep these at home because you never know, a cold can start at two o'clock in the morning and by the time you have gone to the health food store in the morning to buy these supplements, the cold might have gotten a foothold."

It is also important to take the supplements for an appropriate amount of time. "A common mistake is stopping the medications too soon," Ulrich said. "The symptoms may have eased and then you forget to take the supplements. They have to be taken continuously. With the vitamin C you can lower the dose from 3 to 5 grams to 1 to 2 grams every few hours. I recommend the zinc at least every hour or two for the first half day and then every six hours after that. The maximum time for this protocol is a few days. The problem with the zinc lozenge is that it can irritate the palate and cause soreness. But I would rather have that than allow the virus to settle in. These suggestions are crucial, and timing is very important here.

"You may travel somewhere where zinc and vitamin C are not available, so I recommend taking them with you. I also recommend using the zinc lozenge right before you go to bed. If you wake up, take it again. Don't let six or eight hours pass without doing it."

How can you tell the difference between a virus, bacteria, or allergy? "Even doctors have trouble differentiating them because the symptoms overlap," Ulrich said. "Viruses and bacteria will give fever but allergies do not. Runny nose is common with the common cold virus and allergies, but bacteria will rarely if ever give you a runny nose. Nasal congestion is common with the virus and allergies, but bacteria rarely. Another way to differentiate viruses from allergies is muscle aches and pains. If you have bad muscle aches and pains, it is more commonly a virus and hardly ever an allergy. Allergies will rarely give you yellow-green mucus, but bacteria commonly will as will all the viruses.

"It is not inevitable that we all come down with colds. By eating the right foods, getting a good night's rest, reducing stress, not smoking, taking some of the supplements on a regular basis, like vitamin C and fish oils, garlic, onions, and then taking the immediate steps right away when coming down with a cold, you can, as a rule, either eliminate or greatly decrease the frequency of viruses."

Chapter 8

Headaches

A pounding headache afflicts most people at some time in their lives. It interferes with daily activities and keeps us from functioning at our best. Doctors offer powerful medications that may or may not help and have side effects of their own. What are the main types of headaches? What causes them? And how can we get rid of them without making ourselves sicker?

In her book *No More Headaches, No More Migraines*, Dr. Zuzana Bic has some of the answers. Dr. Bic is a lecturer for the Public Health Program in the College of Health Sciences at University of California at Irvine, and is in private practice. In her research and work using integrative lifestyle medicine in the prevention of chronic diseases, she has been able to identify headache "triggers." There are many things that trigger headaches. If we know what they are, we can avoid them and cut down on headaches without pain medications. She describes changes we can make in our day-to-day lives to make headaches a thing of the past.

"Where my research is unique," says Dr. Bic, "is in trying to identify the common denominator for all the lifestyle factors. I have a group I call diet-related triggers. In this group belongs all food that is high in fat, high in refined sugar, most processed or refined food, and food that is low in complex carbohydrates. A related group is obesity, which is connected to not eating properly, and also hypoinsulinemia or insulin resistance, one of the first signs of diabetes. Hypoglycemia, which means low levels of sugar, is another trigger for headaches. Prolonged hunger and dehydration can cause headache, as can alcohol and caffeine intake."

What is the common factor? "This is the question I have addressed in my studies," Dr. Bic says. "What I have found I try to explain to the patients. As you know, the cells in the blood—platelets, red blood cells, and white blood cells—

all coexist in the blood vessels. A high level of fat in the blood will crowd up the vessels, similar to a crowded freeway with one car bumping into another car. A process like platelet congregation occurs and there is a little bit of damage to the platelet, causing it to release serotonin. The body acts to excrete this excess serotonin and thus you have lower levels of serotonin. Serotonin is a very important neurotransmitter, and its lack is an important factor in triggering headache."

Other lifestyle triggers include smoking, a sedentary lifestyle, and exhausting physical exertion. "Some patients who suffer from anorexia nervosa or bulimia exercise excessively, and this is the type that can result in headache," Dr. Bic says, adding that "stress, oral contraceptives, or hormone replacement also trigger headaches."

Dr. Bic identifies imbalanced diet as one of the main headache triggers. She found it effective to put her patients on a low-fat diet with a lot of fruit, vegetables, grains, beans, and a higher amount of fiber. She also recommends increasing the daily intake of water. "They think they drink enough water, but if they monitor it in their food diaries, they find that there is not enough water. They are always surprised.

"I also recommend starting an exercise program or increasing the level of physical activity. Start walking ten minutes in the morning and ten minutes in the evening. Or park the car as far away as possible and walk to the office. To cut down on stress, I recommend meditation or one-minute relaxation techniques such as breathing exercises or changing how they perceive situations to a more objective point of view."

In her research, Dr. Bic also elucidates the timing of the trigger and the headache. "Some of my patients are more sensitive and can have a headache immediately, one hour after the trigger. For others it can be seventy-two hours after the trigger. I think it is the accumulation of unbalanced lifestyle factors. It is possible for a person to be sedentary, eat a high-fat diet, have a very stressful situation, and not be drinking enough water. All these things accumulate and they can have that headache from three hours to seventy-two hours."

Dr. Bic points out that some types of headaches are not caused by triggers and therefore are unaffected by lifestyle changes. These include headaches resulting from trauma, infection or tumors in the brain, or problems with eyes or ears.

Types of Headaches

There are several types of common headaches. For information on migraines, see chapter 45.

Tension Headaches: Tension headaches are characterized by a dull, aching pain that radiates throughout the entire head. Some sufferers describe the feeling as having a tight band wrapped around their head. Tension headaches can start in the shoulders and neck and move upward to the back of the head. Stress, arguments, repressed anger, poor posture, depression, social problems, or major life changes can induce tension headaches. Tension headaches may also be a symptom of depression, especially in the elderly who have experienced a potentially traumatic or stressful event, such as retirement, forced relocation, reduced mobility or independence, or a serious illness.

Cluster Headaches: Cluster headaches come in groups. They can last for extended periods of time for days, weeks, or even months. Sufferers usually experience one or more headaches per day. Each headache may be relatively brief, lasting for thirty to ninety minutes, and may escalate in intensity during that time. In general, cluster headaches affect one side of the head, and the pain is centralized in the eye area on the affected side.

Exertion Headaches: Exertion headaches are connected to physical activities such as exercise, sex, laughing, and coughing. They generally occur during or just after the activity. In and of themselves they are not dangerous, but frequent exertion headaches may indicate an underlying physical state conducive to stroke or another serious condition.

Organic Headaches: Headaches that are the symptoms of a serious underlying physical condition, such as high blood pressure or brain tumors, are considered organic headaches. In addition to the headache pain, the sufferer may have fever, confusion, and/or trouble speaking or moving. The pain tends to grow worse, increasing with each headache or striking more frequently.

Hypnic Headaches: This newly described type of headache, which occurs in elderly patients, is easy to recognize. Hypnic headaches—so called because they arise out of sleep—present as bilateral pain that lasts for thirty to sixty minutes, awakening patients from sleep one or two times each night. Hypnic headaches occur primarily in individuals over age sixty-five and respond well to treatment with medication (most often lithium, taken at bedtime).

Diagnosis

Keeping a daily journal of headache occurrences may help you and your doctor to understand what is causing your headaches. A number of medications, many of which are commonly prescribed as we grow older, may cause headaches. If you are worried about your headaches, or if they are disruptive to your daily functioning, you should consult with your health care provider. If your headaches follow a recent head injury; are associated with seizures; are so severe they prevent you from doing activities you want to do, wake you from sleep, cause blurred vision, eyespots, or other visual changes; or are associated with fever, vomiting, stiff neck, or tooth, jaw, or sinus pain, you should consult with your doctor immediately. Chronic headaches, or headaches that change in character or suddenly develop in an older person, should be carefully evaluated. They may be the result of a drug interaction or carbon monoxide poisoning. Headaches may also be the symptom of a more serious condition, such as giant cell arteritis (a condition of the arteries of the optic nerves that can result in blindness), brain tumors, spinal degeneration, lung disease, or even a warning sign of stroke.

Natural Therapies

Lifestyle and nutrition play important roles in headache prevention and treatment. Other alternative therapies include homeopathy, acupuncture, bodywork, and aromatherapy.

LIFESTYLE
Attention to specific areas of your lifestyle can be crucial in preventing headache. Any behavior that promotes a healthful lifestyle, such as regular sleeping schedules, managing stress, practicing relaxation techniques, and staying physically fit, can reduce the frequency and intensity of headaches. When the pain is in your brain, the importance of the mind–body connection becomes paramount.

Studies have shown that moderate exercise can release endorphins and natural cortisol, which act to elevate mood and reduce stress. Aerobic exercise, such as dancing, walking, biking, or swimming, can help reduce the frequency of tension headaches. Gentle exercises, such as stretching, yoga, or even walking, can reduce discomfort while releasing stress. Exercise is also beneficial in normalizing sleep patterns and enhancing self-confidence. To ensure that you stay on a regular exercise regimen, I suggest that you choose a pleasurable activity and stick with it.

Meditation acts to calm the mind and relieve stress. Twenty minutes, twice a day, of mindful meditation is recommended to prevent and reduce tension and stress. Engaging in breathing exercises and being generally aware of your breathing patterns throughout the day can be beneficial in eliminating headaches. Focusing on the positive aspects of life and nurturing an optimistic outlook will reduce the effects of stress on the body and aid in coping with headaches.

It may sound simple, and it is. Standing and sitting correctly can keep your muscles from tensing and triggering a tension headache. Good posture supports and protects all of your body, allowing you to move efficiently and with less fatigue. When standing, make sure your weight is evenly distributed on both feet, hold your shoulders back, and tuck in your chin. Pull in your abdomen and buttocks. When sitting, make sure your thighs are parallel to the ground and your head is not slumped forward. Try to avoid standing or sitting in one position for long periods of time. Take frequent breaks to move around and stretch. Make sure your shoes fit correctly, and do not make a habit of wearing high heels regularly.

NUTRITION

Studies indicate that a poor diet may be a significant factor in triggering headaches. One of the most important steps is the elimination of caffeine from your diet. Caffeine and caffeinelike substances found in coffee, tea, and many soft drinks can cause symptoms of anxiety, such as nervousness, fear, heart palpitations, nausea, restlessness, and tremors. Caffeine overstimulates the adrenal system and can deplete your body of important B-complex and C vitamins. It can cause stress and anxiety reactions in users. One study shows that patients with anxiety experienced a degree of anxiety that directly correlated with their consumption of caffeine. Even more astonishing, this report suggested that the persons most at risk for suffering from anxiety effects have a heightened sensitivity to the effects of just one cup of coffee.

Ironically, the process of eliminating caffeine from your diet may cause withdrawal headaches, as your body compensates for the lack of caffeine by producing more adenosine, a neurotransmitter that helps to regulate the diameter of the arteries in your head. As adenosine levels increase, your arteries dilate, and the excessive blood flow can then cause a throbbing headache. Once your body begins to regulate adenosine levels, however, the withdrawal headache will cease and you should remain headache-free.

Hypoglycemia (lowered blood glucose levels) is also directly correlated to headache and its related symptoms. To compensate for lowered glucose levels, your body releases insulin, a hormone that encourages glucose to move from the bloodstream into the cells. A sudden drop in blood sugar may cause the arteries in your brain to constrict, contributing to high blood pressure and headache. Maintaining proper blood sugar levels by avoiding refined carbohydrates is essential to controlling headaches.

Another common trigger for headaches is sensitivity to certain chemicals in foods. These chemicals include monosodium glutamate (MSG), a common flavor enhancer found in many processed foods; artificial sweeteners found in diet foods and diet soft drinks; nitrites, preservatives found in processed meats and some cheeses; and amines, a common compound found in a wide range of foods, including spinach, tomato, potato, tuna, liver, dark chocolate, and alcohol.

Headache sufferers should be conscious of the foods they eat. Choose organic, chemical-free foods and eat regular meals to avoid hypoglycemic reactions. Keep a food journal that lets you see if there are food-related patterns to your headaches. When a headache occurs, review the foods you ate in the seventy-two hours prior to its onset to see whether you can identify any trends. If you suspect a particular food may cause headaches, try eating that specific food for a week and see whether it triggers a headache. If it does, avoid it in the future.

HOMEOPATHY

The following remedies may be used for both temporary and acute cases of headache. When dealing with a chronic condition, homeopathic remedies must be used in conjunction with other therapies, as prescribed by a qualified health professional. Consult with your health care provider before taking any homeopathic remedy, and follow your provider's recommendation for the appropriate dosage. Always inform your medical practitioner of any homeopathic remedies you may be taking.

- Bryonia is indicated when the headache is left-sided, over the left eye or forehead, and worse when coughing.
- Ferrum is suggested for a continuous headache lasting two to three days. Headache can be in one spot on the left temple or a general frontal headache.
- Gelsemium is used for a headache that begins at the neck and gradually moves to the forehead.

ACUPUNCTURE

Acupuncture may provide relief from chronic headache pain. By listening to your symptoms and examining your appearance and pulse, acupuncturists can diagnose and impact headaches. Acupuncture releases tension in the muscles. It causes a relaxation response in the body, resulting in lowered blood pressure and heart rate. Acupuncture increases the flow of blood, lymph, and nerve impulses to affected areas and decreases stress while promoting feelings of well-being and energy.

BODYWORK

A variety of treatments involve the transfer of energy from the practitioner to the patient, which can help relieve pain and anxiety. In one study, massage reduced anxiety and lowered saliva cortisol levels (a key measurement of stress). Massage can be very effective at removing tension from the muscles and may provide relief from headache pain.

Reiki employs a powerful, hands-on healing technique in which the universal life force energy is channeled through the practitioner and transferred to the patient. Chronic stress and anxiety can deplete the energy in our bodies. Reiki is used to support the body's natural ability to heal itself. It releases spiritual and emotional blocks and brings a feeling of harmony and vitality.

Massage can enhance general relaxation and provide an outlet for stress and tension. Massage therapy can reduce feelings of anxiety, promote better sleep patterns, and increase feelings of well-being.

Shiatsu combines traditional Chinese medical theory and various Japanese massage techniques. The therapist uses direct pressure with hands and fingers to redirect the flow of energy throughout the body. Shiatsu treatment is deeply relaxing and can be beneficial in both chronic and acute conditions.

Many people who experience tension headaches also grind their teeth during sleep—a practice called bruxism. A device called an NTItension suppression system (NTItss) is created and fit by a dentist and is worn while sleeping as a guard against tooth grinding and jaw clenching.

Craniosacral therapy is a hands-on healing technique that manipulates the soft tissues and bones of the head (cranium), the spine down to its tail (sacrum), and the pelvis, as well as the membranes and cerebrospinal fluid that surround these areas. The practitioner uses an extremely light touch to palpate, or feel, areas to detect a fluctuation in the cerebrospinal fluid, and then manipulates the area to clear blockages and correct the flow. This therapy is beneficial in reducing stress, improving the quality of sleep, and enhancing the general functioning of the body's organs.

AROMATHERAPY

Essential oils can be used in baths or inhaled to provide rebalancing effects. Do not apply essential oils directly to the skin; they must be mixed with carrier oils. Some of the scents that may be effective in easing headache pain include euca-lyptus, ginger, lavender, peppermint, rosemary, sandalwood, and wintergreen.

Hangovers

The alcohol hangover is an old problem. It's even referred to in the Bible: "Woe unto them that rise up early in the morning, that they may follow strong drink" (Isaiah 5:11). The doctors call it by a fancy name: veisalgia, meaning "uneasiness following debauchery" and "pain." The symptoms are headache, nausea, diar-rhea, and fatigue, combined with decreased cognitive and visual-spatial skills and work loss.

Alcohol in high doses can be toxic. It can dehydrate the body and have effects on the heart. It also negatively impacts the brain, liver, and kidneys. Anyone who drives a car or has to operate machinery is going to have a problem when they have a hangover. Anyone who has to run a meeting or get the chores done is going to have a problem the next day. These people are going to feel lousy even after the alcohol is gone from their bodies. The alcohol leaves behind its toxic effects when you drink too much.

We know it has something to do with what's in the alcohol. Dark-colored liquors, like brandy, wine, and whiskey, produce a bad hangover. Vodka, gin, or other clear liquors do not cause the worst symptoms. Sulfites found especially in dark wines can make you sicker. Alcohol causes a diuresis, or excessive fluid excretion.

Are there any ways to prevent hangover? In one study, an herbal preparation called Liv.52 from the Himalaya Drug Co. in Bombay decreased hangover symptoms. How did it work? The investigators thought it might be because the herb blocked the conversion of ethanol to acetaldehyde. Acetaldehyde is created from the by-products of ethanol (which is alcohol) in our stomachs. It can act like a poison in some people. Women are more susceptible to this because they have lower levels of the enzyme needed to convert alcohol to something less toxic.

In another study, vitamin B_6 was given before, during, and after parties where the participants drank enough to get intoxicated. Those who took the vitamin reduced the number of hangover symptoms by 50 percent.

One thing everybody agrees on is to drink lots of fluids before, during, and after drinking alcohol. It helps to dilute the alcohol in the first place and replaces the fluids that are excreted by the kidneys.

GARY NULL'S PROTOCOL FOR HEADACHE

The following chart summarizes the supplements I recommend adding to the protocol for overall brain health found in chapter 16. This protocol is designed for individuals who suffer from, or are specifically concerned about, headache. If you are concerned about conditions discussed in other chapters, consult with a health professional about how you can safely impact multiple conditions.

If you are taking medications—whether prescription or over-the-counter—or have any food restrictions, consult with your doctor before beginning any supplement program. Your health care provider should always be up-to-date on all vitamins, supplements, and herbal or homeopathic remedies you are taking. Supplement overdoses are rare, but possible, and certain combinations may affect individuals adversely.

SUPPLEMENT	DOSAGE	CAUTIONS
5-HTP (5-hydroxytryptophan)	50–100 mg three times daily	Several months of treatment may be needed for maximum benefit. Nausea is the main side effect, but if it occurs, it usually dissipates within several days.

		Do not combine with prescription antidepressants. If you are taking prescription medication for depression, you should consult your doctor before taking 5-HTP. Excess levels of serotonin in the blood can be dangerous in case of coronary artery disease.
magnesium	Up to 1,000 mg	May take six weeks or more for effects to be felt.
melatonin	300 mcg–1 mg two to three nights per week	Tolerance may develop with regular use. Long-term effects of nightly use are unknown.
vitamin B2 (riboflavin)	Increase daily dosage from 50 mg to 150 mg. Do not exceed a daily supplement of 150 mg.	Must build up to a therapeutic level. May not show results for several months.
vitamin B3 (niacin)	At the onset of migraine aura, take 100–150 mg .	High doses of niacin may cause a "hot flash" sensation. Some varieties are advertised as "flash free" and prevent this effect.
fever few	As directed	
black cumin seed oil	1 tsp	
cayenne pepper capsules	As directed	

Chapter 9

Insomnia

According to a 2012 congressional briefing, 50 to 70 million Americans suffer from insomnia, with women 1.4 times more likely than men to be affected. Thirty-five to 40 percent of menopausal women report sleep problems, but they can occur at any age. Clearly, insomnia is a common concern, which can accompany many of the disorders discussed elsewhere in this book. People with sleep-onset insomnia have difficulty falling asleep, while those with maintenance insomnia wake frequently throughout the night or very early in the morning.

As women get older and their hormones change, it becomes more difficult to have a good night's sleep. One of the hormones that is particularly important for sleep is progesterone, says Dr. Hyla Cass, a board-certified expert in the fields of integrative medicine, women's health, and psychiatry, and the author of many books including *Eight Weeks to Vibrant Health*. Because older women make less progesterone, this can affect their ability to sleep.

Pregnancy is another time in which insomnia may be common. "Pregnant women can't fall into their usual sleep positions or have their usual contact with their bed mates," says Dr. Samuel Dunkell, a psychiatrist and sleep clinician working in an insomnia outpatient clinic, and former director of the American Sleep Disorders Association. "There is also an increase in insomnia caused by the pregnancy toward the end of the pregnancy period. Postpartum, women often have difficulty falling asleep for a number of days or weeks."

Insomnia can be associated with a variety of physical, mental, and behavioral conditions. Among the common causes are pain, anxiety, tension, illness, indigestion, caffeine, and drugs. A major cause of insomnia, especially if it's chronic, is reactive hypoglycemia. This is frequently exacerbated by eating late at night, especially foods with a high glucose level, such as pastries, candy, or even fruit juice.

Such foods cause blood-sugar levels to go up and then plummet, a fluctuation that can contribute to insomnia. Also, overindulging late at night in highly fatty foods can cause sleeplessness. That's because foods with a lot of fat take four to five times longer to empty from the stomach and be digested than simple or complex carbohydrates do.

Another important cause of insomnia is intake of stimulants. Most of us are aware of the caffeine in coffee, tea, chocolate, and colas. Alcohol, although generally considered a depressant, can have stimulant effects in some cases. In addition to food and drink, certain medications can be culprits in insomnia. Drugs that can interfere with the natural sleep cycle include Prozac, the newer drugs related to it, and Xanax.

Exercising in the late evening is another possible bane for the insomnia-prone in that it can overstimulate adrenal levels and excite the musculoskeletal system, resulting in difficulty getting to sleep. Likewise, stress and overstimulating the mind by thinking about unresolved conflicts can be a problem when the goal is sleep.

Clinical Experience

CONVENTIONAL TREATMENT

Many people with insomnia often use over-the-counter or prescription drugs to help them sleep. Benzodiazepines and tricyclic antidepressants are among the medications that may be prescribed by a doctor. Potential side effects include daytime sleepiness, loss of muscle coordination, and addiction.

HERBAL REMEDIES

A variety of herbs can be a real help to those challenged by insomnia. Unlike sleeping pills, herbs won't leave you in a fog in the morning, or feeling like you haven't really slept. Most of these herbs address the underlying cause of the insomnia, a depleted nervous system that cannot settle itself down.

Herbalist Terry Willard, in an article posted on the HealthWorld Online website (www.healthy.net), offers some recommendations:

REISHI MUSHROOM (*Ganoderma lucidim*)—This herb provides daytime calm, decreases anxiety, and adjusts sugar metabolism. It helps to resolve what the Chinese call disturbed shen qi (a disturbed mental spirit). It has also been found to boost the immune system and reduce cholesterol and hypertension. Take three 1-gram tablets three times daily.

HOPS (*Humulus lupulus*)—This age-old sedative can be taken as a tea or combined with other dried herbs in a sleep pillow. To make the tea, mix 1 teaspoon whole hops into a cup of boiling water. Some people may have an allergic reaction to hops.

VALERIAN (*Valeriana officinalis*)—Valerian has been used as a sedative for more than 2,000 years. In Europe it is the most commonly used over-the-counter drug for sleep disorders. Willard recommends that valerian be taken only for short periods or intermittently, when insomnia is at its worst. This is because the herb can become habit-forming, and increased doses may be required if used for a long period. Too much valerian can also make you nauseated. About an hour before going to bed, take a dose of 300 to 400 mg of valerian product standardized to 0.5 percent oil.

SKULLCAP (*Scutellaria lateriflora*)—This is a powerful nerve tonic and sedative herb. It can be taken as a tincture of 15 to 40 drops two to three times a day; in combination with reishi, hops, and valerian; or as a tea, using 1 to 3 teaspoons of the root for every cup of water.

PASSIONFLOWER (*Passiflora incarnata*)—This is an important relaxant herb. You can find tinctures and extracts in health-food stores. You can make a cup of tea by pouring 1 cup boiling water over 1/2 teaspoon dried passionflower. If you're being treated for depression, Willard issues a warning: this herb can reduce the effects of monoamine oxidase inhibitors.

LEMON BALM (*Melissa officinalis*)—Lemon balm is used to relax the body and help with sleep. It can be taken as a tea, by steeping 1 to 2 tablespoons in a cup of hot water.

KAVA KAVA (*Piper methysticum*)—This powerful anxiolytic (antianxiety agent) and sedative "will probably become one of the most important healing herbs in the next few years," Willard says. Its active compounds, called kavalactones, apparently work directly on the limbic system, which regulates emotional feelings and behavior. A clinical study in Germany found that patients receiving 100 mg of kava extract three times daily experienced a significant reduction in anxiety symptoms after only one week of treatment. Willard cautions that you should not take this herb if you are depressed, pregnant, nursing, or operating machinery.

CHAMOMILE (*Matricaria chamomilla*)—Chamomile not only relaxes and calms the body, but also strengthens the nervous system. Chamomile tea is a commonly used before-bedtime sedative. You can also take it as a tincture, 10 to 40 drops three times a day; or in capsule form, six 300 to 400 mg capsules daily.

HERBAL SLEEP PILLOW—Rosemary Gladstar, former director of the California School of Herbal Studies and author of *Herbs for Reducing Stress and Anxiety*, tells how to make an herbal pillow that can be placed next to your head while you sleep: Fill a 4-by-4-inch piece of fabric with dried hops, rose petals, lavender blooms, and chamomile flowers. You might want to put a few drops of lavender oil on top of the pillow as well.

NUTRITION AND SUPPLEMENTS

Tryptophan has been found to benefit people with insomnia. Foods with high amounts of naturally occurring tryptophan, such as turkey, fish, eggs, and dairy products, may help you sleep. Tryptophan breaks down into serotonin, the brain chemical that regulates sleep, and also enhances the brain's ability to produce melatonin, the hormone that regulates your body clock. I recommend taking 1,000 milligrams half an hour before bed.

Melatonin, produced in the pineal gland, aids in sleep and setting circadian rhythyms. Low levels can cause interrupted or restless sleep. To prevent insomnia, I recommend taking 300 micrograms to 1 milligram half an hour before bed, two or three nights a week.

Other options include calcium citrate and magnesium citrate, 1,000 milligrams of each taken any time after dinner; up to 30 milligrams of zinc; and 10 to 15 milligrams of iron; 50 milligrams of the B complex; and 200 milligrams of inositol. Also, 200 micrograms of chromium in the evening will help stabilize your blood-sugar level. Niacinamide, 70 to 280 milligrams daily, has been found to help some people.

Dr. Cass adds the following recommendations: In menopausal women, it may help to enhance progesterone using herb vitex and over-the-counter natural progesterone. To address stress-induced high levels of cortisol in the body, which can cause nighttime wakefulness, use supplements of phosphatidylserine or phosphoralated serine. To address waking due to low blood sugar, you can also keep a small protein snack by your bed.

HOMEOPATHY

Homeopathy is based on the principle that "like cures like." Homeopathic remedies are prescribed in minute doses. The homeopathic remedy chosen should correspond to the symptoms described; only one should be used for best results. Sometimes it's a matter of trial and error; if one does not work, try another. Judyth Reichenberg-Ullman and Robert Ullman, naturopathic and homeopathic physicians, describe some of the most commonly used remedies for insomnia in an article posted on HealthWorld Online (www.healthy.net):

ARSENICUM ALBUM—Recommended for insomnia caused by anxiety, with waking after midnight and restlessness.

NUX VOMICA—Used for insomnia from overuse of stimulants, stress, worries about work. The person usually wakes up in the middle of the night and stays awake.

COFFEA CRUDA—Recommended when you find yourself wide awake at three o'clock in the morning, feeling jubilant, excited, with a racing mind.

Other homeopathic remedies include arnica, aconite, cocculus, ignatia, kali phosphoricum, pulsatilla, and sulfur.

OTHER NATURAL THERAPIES

A gentle neck and head massage for fifteen minutes may do the trick in conquering insomnia, and fifteen minutes in a warm bath may be helpful as well. Along the lines of positive affirmation, writing in a diary shortly before bedtime can be extraordinarily beneficial. It can be a way of really seeing what you've done that's affirmed your mental, spiritual, and physical health, as well as any deeds you've done that have had positive effects on others. If a woman spends some time at the end of each day reflecting on what she's done in the past twenty-four hours that's been positive, and on plans for the next day, she gains a sense of completeness about the day. In a sense, then, diary-writing legitimizes going to bed; it's as if you can now see that you really deserve the good night's sleep you're about to get.

It's important to prepare for sleep. Choose a time for bed and stick with it. Get ready for bed by unwinding slowly. Your bedroom should be "soothing and comfortable, dim and quiet," say Judyth Reichenberg-Ullman and Robert Ullman. Make it a "peaceful sanctuary" used simply as a place for sleeping.

Dr. James Pearl, who is a member of the Sleep Panel at the Presbyterian St. Luke Medical Center in Denver and in private practice as a psychologist, has additional recommendations. "If you are feeling like you are under a lot of stress and a lot of anxiety, it's important to take a look at that either with a self-help book or with a therapist to see what you can do to minimize the problems. One powerful way to improve your sleep is to maintain a regular sleep-wake schedule. Getting up at the same time every day is helpful, even on weekends. Some sleep experts say you should go to bed at the same time every night and some say go to bed only when you're sleepy. Do whatever feels right for you. But it is really good to try to get up at the same time every day.

"Sunday night insomnia is a common problem, especially for people under forty. Let's say you normally go to bed at 11:00 and get up at 7:00. On Saturday, if you sleep in an extra hour, your body rhythms are one hour behind. If you sleep an extra hour on Sunday, until 9:00, then your internal sleep-wake rhythm is two hours behind. Sunday night, if you try to go to bed at 11:00, you are not sleepy because your body clock is two hours behind. If it is really important for you to sleep in on weekends, don't go to bed that Sunday night until you feel sleepy. You might sleep one or two hours less than usual but that won't hurt you."

Light therapy can be useful. Dr. Pearl explains, "Studies show that people who spend a lot of time indoors away from windows, away from sunlight, have a disproportionate amount of insomnia. They have difficulty sleeping for the same reason that blind people do. Nine out of ten blind people have severe sleep problems because they are not getting sunlight into the retina of their eyes, into the brain to tell the brain that it is time to be awake during the day. The more light stimuli you can give your body during the day, the stronger your sleep-wake rhythm will be. I am talking about sunlight in particular. Indoor light is not going to make any difference. You need to expose yourself to bright sunlight—just your eyes. There are artificial sun boxes that are commercially available. But if you have insomnia, get outside as much as you can, during your lunch hour, during your breaks. Don't wear sunglasses, unless you've got an eye condition that requires it."

Exercising in the late afternoon or early evening may help some people with insomnia. "When you do aerobic exercise for half an hour, you raise your body temperature," Dr. Pearl says. "Five or six hours later, your body temperature drops. So working out after work or before dinner is an ideal way to get your body ready for bed. A lazy way to get that same benefit is soaking in a hot bath. It has to be really hot, at least 102 degrees. When you use passive body heating, the drop in body temperature occurs just about three hours later.

"A lot of people intuitively know that stressful experiences during the evening can disturb nighttime sleep and research has confirmed that. So it is important to think of the evening as a transition period between the day's troubles and the night's rest. Get ready to wind down. Try to leave your work at the office. If you have to bring it home, get it done early in the evening. Do stressful things like planning your schedule early in the evening or else wait until the morning."

Physical stress can interfere with sleep. "If your muscles are tense and tight or your breathing fast and shallow, try abdominal breathing," says Dr. Pearl. "Take breaths that are increasingly deep and slow, so deep that it makes your abdomen push out. Hold it for a few seconds and let it out slowly, breathing away the tension.

"Finally, if you can't sleep despite everything you have tried, do something else. Switch on the light and read; watch a tape or clean out a drawer. A lot of people think that missing sleep is going to hurt their health, but losing sleep has very few effects. Many studies show that when people sleep less than normal, their performance the next day in most cases is just as good as when they had a good night's sleep. Highly creative tasks do sometimes become more difficult when you have lost sleep, but, for most of us, even if we go a whole night without sleep, we can get along fine the next day. Don't be afraid of insomnia. Don't lie in bed trying to sleep. Some people like to imagine sleep as a wave in the ocean and themselves as a surfer. Position yourself in this warm ocean and wait. The wave will overtake you and sweep you away."

GARY NULL'S PROTOCOL FOR INSOMNIA

The following chart summarizes the supplements I recommend adding to the protocol for overall brain health found in chapter 16. This protocol is designed for individuals who suffer from, or are specifically concerned about, insomnia. If you are concerned about conditions discussed in other chapters, consult with a health professional about how you can safely impact multiple conditions.

If you are taking medications—whether prescription or over-the-counter—or have any food restrictions, consult with your doctor before beginning any supplement program. Your health care provider should always be up-to-date on all vitamins, supplements, and herbal or homeopathic remedies you are taking. Supplement overdoses are rare, but possible, and certain combinations may affect individuals adversely.

SUPPLEMENT	DOSAGE	CAUTIONS
calcium (from citrate)	1,200 mg from citrate taken in four equal doses.	
iron	15 mg daily for menstruating women; 10 mg daily for men and nonmenstruating women.	
L-tryptophan	100 mg taken a half hour before bed. May take an additional 200 mg if awakened during the night.	
magnesium	900 mg taken in four equal doses along with calcium.	May take up to six weeks or more for effects to be felt.
melatonin	300 mcg–1 mg taken a half hour before bed.	Tolerance may develop with regular use. Long-term effects of nightly use are unknown.

Chapter 10

Skin Care

The state of your body on the inside has a direct effect on the appearance and texture of your skin. Certain nutrients, foods, and herbs are important for healthy skin. Stephanie Tourles, a certified herbalist, aromatherapist, and reflexologist, and the author of *Naturally Healthy Skin*, tells us more:

"Nutrition is very important for skin care. I don't care what you put on the skin topically, if you are feeding yourself garbage, your skin is going to reflect that. What you eat is reflected on your face and body. In my daily quest for natural beauty, health, and vitality, I am in awe of what Mother Nature has to offer us. She provides everything you need to encourage and support the healthy functioning of your skin, but it is up to you to partake of these offerings.

"My personal recommendation is that you try to eat a very balanced diet, preferably vegetarian with minimally processed whole foods in their natural state. Include approximately 40 to 60 percent complex carbohydrates, 20 to 30 percent lean proteins, and 10 to 20 percent fat. This all depends on your activity level and your state of wellness."

Tourles also recommends a number of vitamins, minerals, and fats.

Vitamins

Five essential vitamins provide antioxidant benefits and healing agents that enhance your skin: A, B complex, C, D, and E. "Vitamin A is essential for growth and maintenance of epithelial tissue, which is your skin tissue, and for the proper functioning of the mucous membranes," Tourles says. "This vitamin helps prevent dry, rough skin, and premature aging. It speeds healing, especially of acne and impetigo, which is caused by staph or strep infection that results in pustules around the nose and mouth. Vitamin A also boosts your general immunity. Deficiency symptoms of this vitamin include premature wrinkles; acne; pimples; blackheads; cirrhosis; and dry, rough, itchy, scaly, or cracked skin, especially on the feet and the hands. An early symptom of deficiency is what I call chicken skin: small raised bumps on the back of the neck, upper arms, back, and shoulder."

The B complex vitamins can be obtained from brewer's yeast, whole grains, alfalfa, almonds, sunflower seeds, all the soy products, green leafy vegetables, blue-green algae, fresh wheat germ, molasses, peas, and beans. "This is your anti-stress vitamin," Tourles explains. "It helps prevent premature aging and acne, and promotes healthy circulation and metabolism. It is very essential to wound healing such as sunburn, bruises, and infection. It aids in new cell growth and increases your vitality. Deficiency symptoms of this vitamin include a sore mouth and lips. Where your top and lower lip meet will get cracks and become red and very sore. Other deficiency symptoms are eczema, skin lesions, dandruff, a pale complexion, pigmentation problems, and premature wrinkling."

Vitamin C sources include rose hips, citrus fruits, tomatoes, berries, pineapples, apples and persimmons, bell and hot peppers, and papayas. Tourles says, "Vitamin C helps to produce collagen in your connective tissue. Collagen is what keeps your skin plump and firm, and keeps you from getting wrinkles. Vitamin C also strengthens the capillary walls, speeds healing, and helps battle environmental stress and toxins. If you have a deficiency in vitamin C, you will probably bruise more easily, your gums can become spongy, wrinkles form more quickly, you will notice sagging skin, premature aging, pyorrhea (which is a gum disease), and slowed healing."

Vitamin D can come from milk or fish liver oils, as well as fortified soy milk, alfalfa, watercress, and sunshine. In combination with vitamin A, vitamin D helps to treat acne. "It also treats herpes simplex, the little sores that show up around and just inside your lips," Tourles says. "It helps slow premature aging and enhances bone mineralization and calcium absorption. This is great for your fingernails. Deficiency symptoms of vitamin D are a lack of vitality, very slow growth, and bone problems."

Vitamin E is the last essential vitamin that benefits the skin. According to Tourles, "Outstanding sources are the cold-pressed vegetable oils, not the vegetable oils you normally find in your grocery store. Those have been heated too high and heavily processed, so you need to get the cold-pressed oils. Whole grains, alfalfa, parsley, sprouted seeds, nuts, fresh wheat germ, and green leafy vegetables are good vegetarian sources. Skin care benefits for vitamin E are that it oxygenates the tissues and increases body stores of vitamin A, slows premature aging, helps to block the formation of tumors, and speeds healing of severe burns and chronic skin lesions. It may also decrease scarring."

Vitamin E also enhances red blood cell formation. "If you are deficient in vitamin E, there will be a degeneration of epithelial cells, which are your skin cells in the organs, and skin germinating cells," says Tourles. "This results in tissue-membrane instability and collagen shrinkage, which leads to premature aging and the sagging of your skin. Your skin can look very lackluster. You can be very tired because you are not getting oxygen in your body. Remember I said vitamin E helps to oxygenate the tissues. You will also have an increased tendency to bruise as a result of the fragility of the red blood cells."

Minerals

Tourles also recommends four minerals for healthy skin. "The first one is iodine," she says. "Outstanding vegetarian sources for iodine are blue-green algae, sunflower seeds, kelp, iodized salt, and sea salt. If I use salt at all, it is sea salt. Fish and shellfish are also great sources. Skin care benefits of iodine are that it aids in healing skin infections, increases oxygen consumption and the metabolic rate in the skin, and helps prevent roughness and premature wrinkling. Deficiency symptoms of iodine include slow growth and healing, slow metabolism, very poor skin tone, and dry skin. There is a contraindication for iodine: It may aggravate acne. If you have acne you may want to drastically decrease fish, cut down on your blue-green algae, and maybe switch over to barley grass instead. You may see good results by doing that.

"The next mineral is silicon. A good source for that is horsetail herb, which is very good to combine with nettle and blue-green algae in capsule form. Echinacea root is very good; dandelion root, alfalfa, kelp, flax seed, barley grass, wheat grass, all varieties of apples and berries, onions, almonds, sunflower seeds, and grapes are all good sources. Silicon aids in collagen formation, helping to keep the skin taut, tight, and uplifted. It helps to strengthen your bone and skin tissues and aids in wrinkle prevention. Deficiency symptoms include premature wrinkling, lack of skin tone, and sagging skin."

The third mineral is sulfur. "Sulfur can be found in turnip greens, dandelion greens, radishes, horseradish, string beans, onions, and garlic," Tourles says. "All of these foods have a strong flavor. Cabbage, celery, kale, soybeans, and asparagus are milder. Asparagus is particularly high in sulfur. Sometimes sulfur is called the beauty mineral. It really helps to keep the skin clear and smooth. Deficiency symptoms of sulfur include dry scalp, rashes, eczema, and acne."

The last mineral is zinc. Tourles says, "Good sources are blue-green algae and barley grass, alfalfa, yellow dock root, echinacea root, any of the seaweeds such as kelp, fresh wheat germ, all variety of seeds, brewer's yeast, and all kinds of nuts and green leafy vegetables. Zinc aids in wound healing, promotes cell growth, and boosts immunity. It helps treat acne when combined with vitamin A and B. Deficiency of zinc includes slow healing, dandruff, and lowered resistance to infections."

Essential Fats and Fatty Acids

The essential fats and fatty acids are important for healthy skin. "Fat in the diet is very vital to your skin's health and beauty," Tourles says. "Without fat your skin has no contour, no roundness. It cannot be beautiful without at least a thin layer of padding to support it and give it shape. Fat is a necessary requirement if you desire radiant and moisturized skin."

Omega-3 and omega-6 are essential fatty acids that have many benefits for the skin. Coldwater fish such as bluefish, salmon, mackerel, or tuna are good sources of omega-3. "If you want a vegetarian source," Tourles says, "use ground flax seeds or flaxseed oil. Flaxseed oil is sometimes called the vegetable alternative to fish oil. Walnuts and walnut oil and Brazil nuts are other sources. Omega-3 helps with proper wound healing, is reported to relieve arthritis symptoms, aids in healing eczema and cirrhosis, and helps to balance the sebum or the oil production in the skin. A deficiency symptom of omega-3 is dry, scaly skin, eczema, inflammatory skin conditions, and slow healing."

Omega-6 can be obtained from evening primrose oil, borage oil, black currant seed oil, and blue-green algae. "Skin care benefits are smooth, healthy, moisturized skin and proper joint function and flexibility," Tourles says. "Deficiency symptoms include dry, flaky skin; eczema; and painful stiff joints."

Herbal Formulas

Stephanie Tourles has formulated an herbal tea that is "a delicious way to boost your energy levels as well as your natural immunity." This tea contains 2 tablespoons lemon balm, 1 tablespoon lavender flowers, 1 tablespoon peppermint leaves, 1 tablespoon chamomile flowers, 1 tablespoon rose petals, 1 tablespoon nettle, 1 tablespoon alfalfa, 1 tablespoon rose hips, 2 teaspoons dandelion leaves, 2 teaspoons raspberry leaves, 1/2 teaspoon gingerroot (or you can substitute cinnamon bark).

"Combine all of these herbs in a medium-size bowl," Tourles says. "Blend the ingredients and store this mixture in a tightly sealed tin, jar, or plastic tub and store it away from light in a very cool, dry location. It is best if used within six months.

"For each cup of tea you need 1 teaspoon of the dried herb. Bring a cup of water to a boil in a small saucepan. Remove this from the heat and add 1 teaspoon herbs. Cover this and allow it to steam for ten or fifteen minutes and strain before you drink it. You can add honey, lemon, cream, or maple syrup to enhance the flavor. This recipe yields approximately 30 cups of tea if you use 1 teaspoon of formula per cup."

Tourles also describes an herbal ointment you can make yourself for soothing skin irritations, cuts and abrasions, and even diaper rash. It has four simple ingredients: 1/2 cup vegetable shortening, preferably 100 percent hydrogenated soybean oil; 10 drops calendula essential oil; 10 drops everlasting or spike lavender essential oil; and 5 drops orange or lemon essential oil.

"Start with the vegetable oil at room temperature and add all the essential oils at once," Tourles says. "Whip all the ingredients together until thoroughly combined. It can be stored in a glass or plastic container with a tight lid and will keep, if refrigerated, for up to one year. To use, clean the infected area and apply the ointment; use as necessary to help heal and prevent infections. It is great for a nightly treatment for dry hands and feet and also as a cuticle treatment. It will have a beautiful orange color and it smells really nice, too."

Regular use of sunscreen is the most effective way of protecting your skin from sunburn, aging effects, wrinkles, and cancer. Start with a sunscreen with an SPF of 15 or higher. SPF stands for sun protection factor. It means that you can stay out in the sun fifteen times longer before burning than you would be able to without sunscreen. Put it on your face and hands after you wash your hands. If you are older and beginning to see age spots, use an even higher SPF. Use it every day all year round.

Psoralens are chemicals found in certain foods that make your skin more sensitive to the sun so that it burns more easily. Psoralens are found in foods such as parsley, limes, and parsnips. Be sure to use a sunscreen with a high SPF if your diet includes a lot of psoralens.

Some perfumes cause age spots, especially those with musk or bergamot oil. Small age spots can be bleached away with hydrogen peroxide. With a cotton swab use 30 percent hydrogen peroxide daily for several weeks. Another choice is hydroquinone, which interferes with your skin's production of melanin. It works very slowly but can fade age spots.

Tourles has another herbal formula for cleansing the skin. "I call it my Pure Cream Cleanser," she says. "This is great for all skin types except oily. It is a wonderful emollient, leaving skin soft and hydrated, and removes eye and lip makeup if you happen to wear those. It has only two ingredients: 1 tablespoon heavy cream and 1 drop carrot seed essential oil or rose essential oil. Rose oil can be very expensive. Mix the ingredients in a tiny bowl and apply the cream with a flannel cloth or a very soft washcloth in gentle circular motions over the entire face, neck, and chest. Rinse well, pat dry, and follow with your favorite herbal toner and moisturizer if you desire. There is so much fat in heavy cream that frequently you won't need an additional moisturizer unless it is the dead of winter and the air is very dry. This amount yields one or two treatments."

Cosmetic Laser Surgery

Cosmetic surgery continues to increase in popularity, for women as well as for men. What are the pros and cons of the various procedures? Dr. Debra Sarnoff, a graduate of Cornell University and George Washington University's School of Medicine, is one of the premier laser surgery experts in North America, specializing in cosmetic dermatology and dermatological surgery. She sees lasers as a great tool. "New methods and uses for laser surgery are emerging almost every month. Lasers can't do everything, but they have truly made a difference in cosmetic surgery, particularly in relation to what may seem minor problems, such as broken blood vessels on the face and around the nose, brown spots, age spots, liver spots, whatever you'd like to call them, on the tops of the hands or in the chest area." Lasers have proven helpful with problems such as removing tattoos. They are also useful for spider veins on the leg, acne scars, and wrinkles.

Lasers are essentially beams of light applied to the skin. Unlike a scalpel, which actually cuts the skin and causes some bleeding, a laser beam will pass through the skin without causing any bleeding. It has a particular target that it is trying to eradicate. There are certain problems that only lasers are capable of solving, just as there are certain problems only scalpel surgery can solve. For example, Dr. Sarnoff says, "There's no way that pulling and stretching and tightening the skin, through surgery, can change the quality of the skin. If your problem is that something is wrong with the quality of the skin, very often a laser can help that."

One cosmetic surgery procedure that can be done well with lasers is skin resurfacing. We all develop wrinkles as we get older. After smiling, laughing, and expressing ourselves with our faces for all these years, most of us develop lines around the eyes—crow's feet—as well as lines on the upper lip.

Dr. Sarnoff says that even the best face-lift in the world will not eradicate those lines. Something has to be done to resurface the skin. "In the old days, we used a machine called a dermabrader, which was like a little sanding machine that people used to try to peel off the top layers of the skin. In other cases, doctors used acid as a chemical peel. The theory was that when the skin healed, it would be much smoother and the wrinkles would not be as apparent."

Then, says Dr. Sarnoff, "Along came this generation of lasers. The laser can be used to peel off the top layers of skin as opposed to using a chemical or a dermabrading machine."

This procedure involves going to a reputable physician, preferably a dermatologist or plastic surgeon who is experienced in this technique, and having the top layers of skin removed in a controlled way with a laser. Healing will take at least ten days, during which the recovering patient has to lie low. She will look like she's had the worst sunburn ever. The skin will be red, moist, and chapped. She won't be able to put on makeup for at least ten days.

AGE SPOTS

Many people have sun spots or age spots, also known as photodamage, from all those years of baking in the sun before we knew that ultraviolet rays were potentially harmful. Dr. Sarnoff explains: "A lot of that sun damage will be entirely reversible if the beam of light can be used to strip off those top layers of skin.

That type of laser resurfacing is a fairly involved procedure that really takes a commitment and a healing time. It's not the kind of thing you just pop in to have done as if you were going to the deli and do a little laser over your lunch break. That laser resurfacing is a bigger deal."

BROKEN BLOOD VESSELS, HAIR REMOVAL, TATTOO REMOVAL

There are many other uses for lasers in skin care, including lightening stretch marks, removing birthmarks, and removing tattoos. "For something like a tattoo," she says, "usually several visits are needed. They would be spaced about six to eight weeks apart, and it would not be unusual to need up to eight treatments to clear a tattoo completely."

Procedures such as zapping broken blood vessels and removing little brown spots are simpler; the side effects are usually no more than a little bruising, crusting, or scabbing, something you might want to wear a small bandage over or apply a little antibiotic ointment to, but nothing that would keep you out of work or prevent you from functioning. Many times people have these procedures and go right back to work.

Lasers can also be an alternative to electrolysis for hair removal. The procedure can be done very rapidly, and the patient can immediately return to her activities.

RISKS AND BENEFITS

Dr. Sarnoff insists that a savvy consumer must ask the right questions. You must learn whether a procedure is a one-shot deal or will have to be repeated. And you should ask how long the improvement will last. Certainly you want something that is going to be cost-effective. Some laser treatments are really long-lasting. With hair removal, by contrast, very often the hair will grow back in a few months. Dr. Sarnoff stresses that you have to know that before you commit. "I think it is very important to ascertain ahead of time approximately how many treatments are needed and what you should expect."

There are risks, Dr. Sarnoff cautions. One is that you may pay good money and be disappointed because your underlying problem will still be there. "Something else that consumers have to be aware of is scarring. It's usually not the case that scars occur, and with a doctor who is well trained and experienced, I think the technique is very safe. Nonetheless, it is a topic that definitely needs to be addressed before the procedure is done."

Sometimes there are some temporary changes in pigment. As the skin is healing, it can become a little darker or lighter than the surrounding skin. You must be aware how often this happens and know whether it is in fact only temporary or could be permanent.

There are very different types of lasers. Each beam of light accomplishes a different purpose, and the potential hazard from each is different. Still, there are some universal precautions that all competent laser providers follow. You need the correct eyewear, for example. Each laser is set at a very specific wavelength, and the protective eyewear needs to be specific to that wavelength.

Postoperative instructions make a difference, too. If you're removing tattoos or broken blood vessels, there is usually nothing else to do. However, with skin resurfacing, Dr. Sarnoff cautions that it is extremely important that patients follow the protocol afterward so that they heal properly and do not get any kind of infection.

The number-one fear people have about lasers is that they involve harmful radiation. But, as Dr. Sarnoff explains, the word *radiation* in the spelled-out version of laser actually refers to the verb *radiate*, meaning "to give off light." Most of the beams of light used in lasers are in the visible light range. That is, they are part of normal light. The only unique thing about lasers is that they are monochromatic. You might have a red beam or a yellow or green one, as opposed to natural light, which is a blend of all the colors of the rainbow. Laser light is non-ionizing; it's basically safe, as opposed to X-rays or ultraviolet light from the sun, which are ionizing. Ionizing radiation may change our cells and damage our chromosomes. We can get in real trouble with that type of radiation, but most lasers are not in that part of the electromagnetic spectrum.

Research Update

An increasing body of evidence is showing the benefits of natural modalities to overall health and well-being. Following is a sample of recent peer-reviewed scientific studies in the area of skin care.

In 2012, the Institute for Natural Healing cited findings that aloe vera reduces the signs of aging: a report in *Annals of Dermatology* found improvement in both facial elasticity and collagen production in all thirty women who were given supplements of either 1,200 mg or 3,600 mg per day for ninety days; and in the *Indian Journal of Dermatology*, researchers found that amino acids in aloe vera hardened skin cells, and zinc from the plant had astringentlike properties that tightened pores. A 2011 article in *Life Extension Magazine* stated that resveratrol, an antimicrobial substance produced by plants in response to stress, infection, or strong ultraviolet radiation, has been found in many studies to reduce inflammation and oxidative stress associated with skin aging. Research has also shown that polyphenols in green, white, and black tea, and the herb *Aspalathus linearis,* have similar antioxidant and anti-aging properties. Reports in *Toxicology and Applied Pharmacology* (2011) and *PLoS One* (2010) described the actions of other plant polyphenols in combating free radical damage that undermines the health of the skin.

Chapter 11

Dental Care

Famed dental researcher Weston Price wrote a book, which he worked on in the 1920s and 1930s, based on studies of the teeth of people in native cultures. People who followed traditional ways, eating simply prepared food indigenous to the region where they lived, had healthy teeth. As soon as they adopted a Western diet of canned, processed food with white sugar and white flour, their dental health deteriorated. Children born to parents on a Western diet had occlusion and malformed teeth. Price even saw that children born before the introduction of Western foods had healthy teeth, while children in the same family born after the new diet was instituted had poor teeth.

The first thing to think about when it comes to healthy teeth is diet. A good diet will be reflected in the condition of the gums and teeth. Think of the general practitioner of yesteryear. One imagines this doctor making a house call on an ailing patient. His first request on seeing this patient was "Stick out your tongue." He wanted to see the tongue's color.

Dr. Victor Zeines, the author of *The Natural Dentist*, reminds us that this practice, far from being quaint and outdated, can still be used to make a good first diagnosis of medical problems. In fact, Chinese doctors, who also ask to see the patient's tongue, have a book that discusses 280 diseases that can be detected from the state of the tongue. For example, a white tongue indicates that toxins are coming out of the body (this will be observed in people with a cold or the flu), cracks in the tongue indicate vitamin deficiency, a yellowish gray or yellowish green tongue indicates gallbladder or liver trouble, and a brownish or grayish green tongue indicates intestinal or stomach problems.

The mouth is indicative of the body's general state of health. If you have a cavity, it is the end result of general physical problems of the whole body, not just the isolated tooth. When a person is not eating properly, the body becomes acidic. Minerals are pulled out of the mouth to travel into other parts of the body. The teeth weaken in an acid environment, while acid-based bacteria increase. A cavity may arise from a mineral deficiency followed by an invasion of bacteria.

Sugar is a primary culprit in this process, though not in the way popularly understood. Many people believe sugar gets in the mouth and sits on the tooth, wearing it down. The real problem with sugar is that it reverses the fluid flow. This flow normally goes from the tooth's pulp chamber into the mouth. Sugar alters this process, sending materials in the mouth into the tooth's internal environment, irritating the inside of the tooth.

Many Americans contend daily with high levels of stress, pollution, and a deficient diet. Food often comes to us shipped over long distances, losing many of its nutrients along the way. We need to make up for those lost qualities with vitamins and minerals.

Calcium and magnesium are especially important for healthy teeth. Folic acid can help the body utilize nutrients. Coenzyme Q10 and vitamin C are also recommended.

Green leafy vegetables and carrot juice are high in calcium. Traditional culture held that chewing on kale was the fastest way to get white teeth. This idea is probably based on recognition of kale's high calcium content. Kale can be juiced and mixed with carrot or apple juice, perhaps with a drop of lemon.

The Truth about Mercury Fillings

Mercury has been widely used in common dental fillings. The "silver" amalgam filling is actually a mixture of silver, tin, copper, and mercury. Mercury makes up about 50 percent of the filling. Eighty-five percent of the American population has these fillings.

For well over 150 years we have been told these fillings are safe, the most durable available. This is not true. Until 1985, the American Dental Association (ADA) repeatedly declared that mercury never escapes from fillings. Then they had to acknowledge that it did leak. Still, even with the leakage, the ADA still declares the fillings safe.

In a guidance document in 2009, the US Food and Drug Administration (FDA) issued a final rule stating that "clinical studies have not established a causal link between dental amalgam and adverse health effects in adults and children age six and older." However it reclassified mercury from a "least risk" class I device to a "more risk" class II device, and categorized dental amalgams as a class II device. Among the potential risks of dental amalgam were exposure to mercury, and toxicity and adverse tissue reaction. In addition, the rule stated that dental amalgam releases low levels of mercury vapor. In high levels, mercury vapor is associated with adverse effects in the brain and kidneys.

SYSTEMIC EFFECTS OF MERCURY

Dentist Flora Para Stay, in an article posted in the HealthWorld Online website (www.healthy.net), summarizes some of the research on mercury in dental fillings going back more than forty years. One of the first reports, published in 1970 in the *Journal of the American Dental Association*, concluded that mercury is not stable but rather "vaporizes at ordinary temperatures." In 1985, a report in the *Journal of Dental Research* stated that mercury vapor from fillings travels through the body and accumulates mostly in the brain, kidneys, and gastrointestinal tract.

According to Dr. Stay, researchers have also described a "battery effect" that occurs when mercury gets into the saliva. She explains that "currents are generated, causing mercury molecules from the surface of the fillings to be released into the tissues."

Mercury can also damage the immune system. Dr. Stay cites another report from the 1980s that concluded that amalgam- and nickel-based fillings are associated with a reduction in the number of T lymphocytes, a type of white blood cell.

The effects of mercury toxicity range from a metallic taste in the mouth, brittle nails, and dry skin, to fatigue, anxiety, depression, headaches, memory loss, gastrointestinal problems, kidney disease, heart problems, and more. Mercury can stop nutrients from entering the cells and prevent wastes from being eliminated. High mercury levels have been found in people with multiple sclerosis and other autoimmune diseases. Mercury can also produce spontaneous abortions. Because of these wide-ranging symptoms, mercury toxicity often goes undetected.

REMOVAL OF FILLINGS

Many people aware of the dangers of amalgam fillings have had them removed and replaced with safer alternatives. Gold, porcelain, or composite restorations may be used. Upon removal of the silver filling, they often see improvement, although it may be constrained by the mercury already in the body. Complementary physician Dr. Michael Schachter has seen patients whose blood tests have gone from abnormal to normal once silver fillings were removed. He has also seen people with multiple sclerosis and chronic fatigue syndrome markedly improved once fillings were taken out. Dr. Zeines has seen improved memory, better sleep, and less nervousness in patients following removal of mercury fillings.

Removing these fillings is not an easy task and the process is potentially dangerous since taking out the amalgam could accidentally release mercury.

Dr. Howard Hinton, a holistic dentist, stresses that the removal must be done under the care of both a physician and a dentist. The patient must be on a good diet and should undergo laboratory tests to determine how he or she is eliminating the mercury. Ideally, the removal should be carried out in a sterile bubble chamber—a round room with a Laminar Air Flow or hepafilter circulating through the space; negative ion generators, to charge particulates in the air; and processed water and air. A rubber dam is used in the mouth to reduce exposure, and the filling is removed with extreme care. (The highest absorption in the body is in the mouth.) During the procedure, high suction and a lot of water are used to reduce the presence of mercury vapor.

Once the fillings are removed, the body should be detoxified. A lack of health improvement may be due to the fact that mercury is still in the body.

Dr. Elmira Gadol, another practitioner of holistic dentistry, says that garlic supplements will help the body eliminate the existing mercury toxins, and selenium can be taken to neutralize the metal. Once the fillings are removed, hair analysis should be done to see what other heavy metals are in the body. These metals interfere with cell processes, such as the oxygen going in and the carbon dioxide going out. These metals also have to be drawn out or problems will remain.

Some patients can be helped by taking intravenous vitamin C. Also, various chelating agents can be prescribed. These agents will attach to the mercury and take it out of the body in urine or feces.

Hot baths with Epsom salts and baking soda are also recommended as a way of bringing out the mercury. In working on detoxification, various methods should be tried alone and in combination.

The Fluoride Debate

We don't have to look too far to find fluoride these days—it's there in our toothpastes, our mouthwashes, and much of our drinking water. In fact, about 75 percent of people in the US who are served by public water systems drink fluoridated water. Proponents of fluoride say we need it to prevent tooth decay. But many health experts say otherwise. Finally, the US government is waking up too: in 2015, for the first time in fifty years, federal health officials cut by almost half the maximum amount of fluoride that should be added to drinking water. Although a step in the right direction, this move doesn't go nearly far enough. Moreover, the reason cited for it—an increase in fluorosis, or white spots on the tooth enamel—is nowhere near the crux of the problem.

We have been led to believe that fluoride is a safe and effective method of protecting teeth from decay, but this is, in fact, a fraud. In recent years it's been shown that fluoridation is neither essential for good health nor protective of teeth. Dr. David Kennedy, from the International Academy of Oral Medicine and Toxicology, puts it quite well when he states that fluoride is a poison. It kills rats and insects so, certainly, it will kill bacteria if it is scrubbed on the teeth. What fluoride does is poison the body. We should all at this point be asking how and why public health policy and the American media continue to live with and perpetuate this scientific sham.

Dr. Mark Breiner, the author of *Whole Body Dentistry*, who has been practicing holistic dentistry for more than thirty years, says that putting fluoride into toothpaste or mouthwash will probably cut down on decay somewhat because it is such a potent toxin. However, he asks, while it may cause a decrease in tooth decay, what else is it causing? "I think there are better ways to prevent tooth decay, the main way being proper nutrition and if need be, some supplementation. But to go and use a potent toxin like that just doesn't make any sense."

TOXIC EFFECTS OF FLUORIDE

The health hazards of fluoride are known, and have been for some time. In 1977, an executive of the National Cancer Society documented that there was a 5 percent increase in cancer in communities that began fluoridating their water. An even more notorious study, and an attempt to suppress it, involved Dr. William Marcus, a senior science adviser at the Environmental Protection Agency's Office of Drinking Water. He read a study that was done to test the dangers of fluoridation. It concluded that there was an increase of bone cancers in animals that were given fluorides. In April 1990, Dr. Marcus went to a meeting where the National

Toxicology Program was to review the study and found that the program's staff had downgraded every cancer reported. An investigation found that scientists at the program had been coerced into making these downgrades.

Some of the ailments that may be caused or exacerbated by the accumulation of fluoride in the body include a depressed immune system, musculoskeletal problems, genetic damage, cancer, and kidney and thyroid problems. Other effects of fluoride include abdominal distress, tremors, convulsions, skin eruptions, headaches, increased thirst, and disturbances of calcium metabolism. Mottling of teeth, marked by white and brown patchy areas, may also occur.

HOW TO AVOID FLUORIDE

To limit your exposure to fluoride, drink bottled or filtered water and use non-fluoridated toothpaste. Dr. Breiner offers some additional recommendations. "I like something called Tooth and Gum Tonic, which is made without alcohol or any chemicals. It is an herbal product and has a number of really good ingredients such as echinacea, peppermint, thyme, and eucalyptus. This will also kill bacteria."

For a mouthwash, you can also use plain salt water. Dr. Breiner says, "Use nonfluoridated water and take some salt and swish that around in your mouth. It is good for the gums. You can take some baking soda and mix that with a little peroxide and make your own toothpaste. You don't have to go to the store and buy something."

Chapter 12

Hair Care

A beautician who has treated hundreds of people's hair was asked whether she sees any connection between a woman's diet and lifestyle on the one hand, and hair health on the other. She replied, "Definitely, I see that when people eat well, the hair is healthy looking. It's a reflection of what they eat and the habits they have. Everything is shown in the hair."

Another hairstylist added, "Your hair is fed by the bloodstream, so if there are any difficulties in that area, it will be carried through into the hair and skin. You could be losing your hair; it could be brittle or dull. Nutrition has an effect on everything in your body, and your hair is an appendage of what is going on. It is a reflection of who you are."

Nutritional Approaches to Better Hair Health

Dr. Danise Lehrer, a licensed acupuncturist and a doctor of homeopathy, confirms the statements quoted from the hairstylists above. She notes that in traditional Chinese medicine, hair health is viewed as a sign of the health of the kidneys, liver, and blood.

One clinical nutritionist tells us that for hair and overall body health, we should consume six freshly prepared green juices a day with organically grown vegetables. Increased circulation to the scalp is important, so exercise should be part of any program.

In a 2012 article posted on www.naturalnews.com, Danna Norek tells about the nutrients known for promoting hair health. Biotin, a water-soluble B vitamin, prevents hair loss, boosts growth, and may be useful against loss of hair pigmentation. Natural sources include Swiss chard, liver, halibut, and goat milk. Panthenol, a form of vitamin B_5, is often used externally as a moisturizer and lubricating compound in shampoos and other hair products. A deficiency of vitamin B_{12} can lead to anemia, which stunts hair growth. Sources of this vitamin include grass fed beef, egg yolks, and free range poultry. Antioxidant vitamins C, E, and A are also important, as they "increase the health and efficiency of the entire body, thereby 'freeing up' the resources to feed your hair the nutrients it needs on a daily basis."

Among the herbs that have been shown to be effective are horsetail, rosemary, lavender, and hops. The active substance in horsetail is silica, which strengthens hair, reduces breakage, and decreases thinning. Silica also increases shine, body, and volume. Rosemary is used topically to stimulate hair growth and increase circulation to the scalp. Lavender makes hair shiny and cleanses it of dulling deposits. Hops, the main ingredient in beer, is used as a natural hair conditioner and softener.

Gary Null's Protocol for Healthy Hair

I recommend the following four-stage program to provide increased vitality to your hair and scalp:

Stage 1
Daily Protocol for the First Three Months
    B complex (50 mg)
    B12 (1 mg)
    Garlic (500 mg twice)
    Aloe (1 oz three times)
    Protein (0.9 g per kg of body weight)
    6 glasses dark green vegetable juice or 6 scoops chlorophyll-rich powder

Stage 2
Daily Protocol for the Second Three Months
    Sea vegetables (1 serving)
    Flaxseed oil (1 tbsp)
    Evening primrose oil (500 mg)

Choline and inositol (500 mg twice)
PABA (100 mg)
Folic acid (400 mcg)
Biotin (500 mcg)

Stage 3
Daily Protocol for the Third Three Months

Sea vegetables (1 serving)
Zinc (50 mg)
L-cysteine (500 mg twice)
Evening primrose oil (500 mg twice)
Pantothenic acid (100 mg twice)
Vitamin E (400 IU twice)
Coenzyme Q10 (200 mg twice)
Biotin (500 mcg)
Choline and inositol (500 mg)
B complex (50 mg of each)
B12 (1 mg)
Silica (150 mg)
PABA (250 mg)
Folic acid (800 mcg)
6 glasses dark green vegetable juice, or 3 glasses dark green vegetable juice
    plus 3 glasses green plant extract, or 6 scoops chlorophyll-rich powder

Stage 4
Daily Protocol for the Fourth Three Months

PABA (500 mg)
Pantothenic acid (500 mg)
Garlic (1,000 mg)
Onion (1,000 mg)
Sea vegetables (6 oz)
Biotin (500 mcg)
Choline (1,000 mg)
Inositol (1,000 mg)
Niacin (250 mg)
Borage oil (500 mg)

Omega-3 oil (1,000 mg)

Cayenne (5 mg)

Protein (0.9 g per kg of body weight)

6 glasses dark green vegetable juice, or 3 glasses dark green vegetable juice plus 3 glasses green plant extract, or 6 scoops chlorophyll-rich powder

Chapter 13

Adolescence

The time of life between childhood and adulthood poses many challenges and rewards. Michael Gurian, therapist, social philosopher, and author of *The Wonder of Girls*, says that biology, hormones, and brain development all must be taken into account when exploring this critical period of a girl's life.

Brain development in adolescence extends over a period of five to seven years, maybe more. A lot of changes are taking place, hormones are being produced, and different parts of the brain are growing at different rates. This creates missteps, self-esteem issues, and relational problems. Most of the time, these concerns are within a normal range. When someone has an actual disorder, such as anorexia or bipolar disorder, that can become clear. But, Gurian says, "a lot of girls are being pathologized, underserved, and under-nurtured because we're thinking there is something wrong with them and we're not looking at what's going on with the brain."

An area that is not addressed sufficiently is hormones. "There is a fear of dealing with hormones, and the fear comes from hormones having been misused in the past," Gurian says. "With people saying, 'Well, you know women are just hormonal,' or 'That's just PMS,' we've avoided the issue. But we can't because—and I say this as a father of two very successful daughters—we have to look at the fact that hormones fluctuate, and there are periods of time of different strength for each girl in which she can experience feeling sort of nuts. We need to help her to look at why that is, and if she needs biological help we have to give her that.

"I tell the story in *The Wonder of Girls* about a woman whose daughter was sent from school to school and from psychologist to psychologist, and they weren't looking at hormones. They were looking at self-esteem drops and was there a systemic problem in the family because she was incredibly angry and manifesting—she was also not eating. They finally found someone who looked at it hormonally and they noticed that her progesterone levels were not in sync with her estrogen. They got her on a progesterone patch, and within two weeks the behavior was altered. They had been going two years through these other systems. So sometimes going right to the biological is crucial, and especially if one notices a daughter who is going up down, up down, up down starting at puberty."

Among the "conflicts" that take place in the brain during adolescence is the one between the chemical oxytocin and the cingulate gyrus. While oxytocin stimulates bonding, the cingulate gyrus causes reactions to stimuli that make girls feel that they can't bond. "This creates a powerful, powerful disconnect," Gurian says. "And if we don't tell them about this, they think there's something wrong with them. They're trying to bond. They can't bond. People hate them. People love them. They feel unattractive. All of these things are going on, and a lot of it's biochemical.

"Now with the Internet, people have to be very careful. If we don't understand this chemistry and we say to a twelve- or thirteen-year-old girl, 'Go ahead and go on the Internet unsupervised,' we need to expect that she's going to have problems. She's not going to know how to handle this bonding tool—which the Internet is—and she may well get involved in cyberbullying. She may be bullied or she may become a bully and not even realize it because what she's trying to do is bond, and she's paying attention to these internal signals of bonding and of personal attractiveness and self-esteem."

Clinical Experience

Among the strategies that work best for girls during adolescence are close relationships with parents, close relationships with other caregivers in the extended family, and the setting of limits. "Girls are definitely taking in toxins, and they're eating foods that are bad for them, and we're not controlling that," Gurian says. "There are a lot of toxins now, pollutants and very bad foods that mess with female biology. Estrogen receptors in food: there is a lot of that. The girls are gaining weight in ways that are not appropriate, and then we're not telling them that they're twenty or thirty pounds overweight. We think we'll hurt their self-esteem. We need a strong family and extended family that says, 'Here's what's dangerous to you. Don't eat these foods. Eat these foods. In our house, these are the foods we eat.' Excessive freedom or excessive liberty for any child to do whatever they want is dangerous in adolescence.

"Girl drama is a lot about biology and helping girls through it means helping them understand their hormones and their brain. You know it's not just nature, but how it all works together."

Addressing these issues from the appropriate standpoint is critical. Unfortunately, there are too many people looking toward pharmaceuticals for the answer. "It's no exaggeration to say that there are more children in school on psychiatric drugs today than there used to be in psychiatric hospitals for children years ago," says Dr. Peter Breggin, a leading psychiatrist, expert on clinical psychopharmacology, and author of many books including *Talking Back to Prozac* and the new *Medication Madness*. "Years ago you'd go into a psychiatric hospital for disturbed kids and they'd be loath to give out psychiatric drugs. Back in the fifties we even had many of the same drugs like Ritalin and the other stimulants. But we rarely gave them out to kids, even in the hospitals. Instead we tried to work with the families. Tried to work with the schools. Tried to help empower the child. Now you've got higher rates of kids in our schools getting psychiatric drugs than in the mental hospitals before the psychopharmaceutical industry took over. The schools then become triage centers, and of course this has expanded and is going to continue to just mushroom over our culture because there is practically no opposition at all."

Columbia University's TeenScreen Program, which may sound to many people like a good idea, is another quick-fix idea that should be avoided, says Dr. Breggin. TeenScreen is a nationwide mental health and suicide risk screening program that claims it is not affiliated with or funded by any pharmaceutical companies. In actuality, says Dr. Breggin, "it's totally a pharmacologically based concept. It's a concept of the drug companies to get consumers. One of the inspirational points for the whole screening process comes out of Columbia, headed by a woman who has been a lifelong associate of the drug companies working to promote their interests.

"As a parent, if you hear anything going on in your school that you're supposed to sign up for, to have your child screened in any way that looks like it has mental health or psychological consequences, you should absolutely refuse; if, by chance, it slips through the cracks and your kid ends up getting screened without you even knowing it, do not follow up on any recommendations. It is nothing more than a conduit toward clinics that will give psychiatric drugs to your child."

Chapter 14

Aging

The aging of America is a statistical reality: by 2050, the population aged sixty-five and over is expected to reach 84 million, nearly double that of 2010. The number of women will increase from 24 million to 46 million. Despite apparent strength in numbers, older women face challenges. Society glamorizes so much of what it means to be youthful, and young women are always projected as the ideal. If you see an older woman in the media, it is not usually in a positive light; it's about incontinence, or dementia, or how to get your life insurance together. Instead of honoring a woman as she becomes wiser and more mature, it almost positions her to seem irrelevant, and that is especially true for senior citizens, who are given virtually no credibility for having anything left to put on the table that others should be interested in.

In the fourth book of *Gulliver's Travels*, the hero comes to an island near Japan, where a race has realized mankind's dream of living forever. The irony is that these immortals all wish they were dead because, though they have lived hundreds of years, these have been miserable years, since they have all the infirmities of the aged, such as blindness, deafness, arthritis, and senility. Jonathan Swift's satirical thrust can be applied today, when we consider the following facts: people are living longer than ever before, but many are unable to enjoy longevity because its potential pleasures are canceled out by the prematurely early encroachments of aging.

The idea that aging inevitably means gaining weight and having high blood pressure, high cholesterol, and arthritis is widely accepted. Since so many people have these problems, we think of them as normal. Even doctors are likely to say that when we get to be a certain age, these conditions are to be expected and, since they are irreversible, accepted.

Fortunately, recent research has given us a better understanding of the causes of aging; in particular, several theories have led to new therapies offering women opportunities not only to improve their health but to actually slow down the aging process. We now know that it's possible to live to a hundred and beyond and to stay healthy throughout our life spans, thus "rectangularizing" the aging curve.

Dr. Martin Feldman, a traditionally trained physician who practices complementary medicine, supports this stand. "We need to have optimum energy as we grow old, not accept the diminishment many find encroaching as they grow older," he says.

Dr. Saralyn Mark, a geriatrician and endocrinologist, tells about the process of healthy aging. "So many people live to die," she says, "and it's such a horrible way to think about your existence." Instead, Dr. Mark says, we should be highlighting the positives. "Every day is a gift," she says, and we need to think about how to make each day special and how to take charge of our lives.

Dr. Feldman cites joint disease as an example of a condition that medicine has accepted as inevitable, a condition that is reversible. There is now an epidemic of joint disease in the United States. Osteoarthritis, the most common form, afflicts 21 million people in the United States, more than 15 million of whom are women. Conventional doctors call osteoarthritis a "wear-and-tear disease," as if the joints wear out like the parts of a car. That sounds plausible, but it is nonsense. The disease is a product of deficiencies and occurs when the joint is not being nourished. A nourished joint will remain healthy. Dr. Feldman has seen marathon runners in their seventies and eighties who use their joints ten-fold or even fifty-fold more than a normal person does, yet their joints remain robust.

Causes

FREE RADICAL DAMAGE

It is widely accepted that aging and degenerative diseases are the result of cellular damage brought on by free radicals, molecules that have become unstable after losing one of their orbiting electrons. The unpaired electrons make the molecules highly reactive, and in an attempt to restore balance, a free radical will steal electrons from other molecules, causing cellular damage and destruction.

Free radicals are produced through normal metabolism in the body, but increase with exposure to animal fat, alcohol, cigarettes, and other toxic chemicals. Dr. Christopher Calapai, a proponent of complementary medicine who has a medical practice in New York, gives an example of how this damage can occur: "Free radicals generated by cigarette smoke are huge in number. They steal healthy electrons from the lining of the lungs, thereby oxidizing lung tissue.

When lung tissue is oxidized, cells break down and die. As hundreds of thousands of cells become oxidized and damaged, tissues and organs throughout the body are affected. Aging and disease are magnified."

Stress is perhaps one of the greatest causes of accelerated aging in our society. "It affects every cell in our body," Dr. Mark explains. "It affects our immune system. It affects the cells in our body that can help us fight cancer. Every day we're exposed to environmental toxins and our body has cells to go out there. They're sort of our soldiers on the front line to protect ourselves. To protect ourselves from the free radicals in the environment, from the toxins that we potentially might eat or drink."

Dr. Mark shares what she has learned about aging through her work with astronauts at NASA. "When you go into space you begin to see changes in the body almost immediately that you see [over a longer term] with the aging process on earth. For example, bone mass declines. In normal aging, it's 1 percent per year. In space it can be up to 1 percent per month. We see changes in the amount of red blood cells and white blood cells, and bone marrow suppression. We see changes in muscle and fat. What is really exciting for me is that we see these changes when you go into space, but when you come back the body adapts to the environment here and you basically get back to your state that you were in before you went. So in a sense it's reversing aging. It's very, very exciting. And we're learning now how to do that even better."

LOW THYROID FUNCTION

The thyroid gland located in the middle of the neck produces thyroid hormone, described by Dr. Mark as "a master hormone that helps keep our bodies in sync." About 10 percent of women have antibodies to the gland that make it sluggish; this condition is known as hypothyroidism. Hypothyroidism may cause people to feel tired and cold; develop dry, brittle hair and skin; gain weight; and have difficulty concentrating.

Low thyroid function can prompt diseases associated with aging. Dr. Ray Peat, a distinguished research scientist from Eugene, Oregon, says that doctors in the first part of the twentieth century were better informed than today's doctors about the importance of correcting this condition. "Most of the basic research on the thyroid was done before World War II. Pharmaceutical companies came in after the war with what they thought was the latest word in understanding the thyroid. It turns out they were wrong. Until 1940 it was accepted that 40 percent of Americans benefited from taking thyroid supplements. After faulty tests were established, it was believed that only 5 percent of Americans needed or benefited from thyroid supplements. In the 1930s indications of hypothyroidism included such things as too much cholesterol in the blood, insomnia, emphysema, arthritis, and failure of the immune system. Many conditions now considered mysterious diseases were recognized as traits of low thyroid. Very often these conditions would simply disappear when thyroid supplements were given.

"When the thyroid is low we have to rely on emergency systems—such as the production of adrenaline and cortisone—to adapt to stress. Cortisone and adrenaline are now recognized as factors that cause damage, setting degenerative diseases in motion and causing damage to the lining of blood vessels and brain cells, but very often people don't realize that it is the thyroid that keeps us from relying excessively on these stress hormones."

BIOLOGICAL CLOCK

Another theory on aging holds that women have a built-in cellular "biological clock" that is set so that cells self-destruct after a certain amount of time. Dr. Lance Morris, a naturopathic physician from Tucson, Arizona, notes that since the theory was first described, the proposed upper limits for the clock's running time have increased. "At this time," he says, "there is a feeling that the top limit is pushing 140 years. Individuals have actually lived to that age, and even longer."

SHRINKING THYMUS GLAND

Atrophy of the thymus gland, which plays a role in maintaining a healthy immune system and fighting infection, may also be involved in the aging process. As Dr. Morris explains, "When we are born, this gland covers a part of our chest. As we grow older, it diminishes in size, a process known as thymic involution. One of the theories of aging is that if we could stop thymic shrinking we could stop the aging process altogether."

MERCURY

The late Dr. Hal A. Huggins of Colorado Springs, Colorado, highlighted another cause of premature aging, the mercury in silver amalgam fillings. According to Dr. Huggins, the mercury in your fillings does not just sit there—you inhale it and it goes into your lungs. Every time you eat and chew, minute amounts of mercury get into your stomach and digestive system and from there to cells in all parts of your body, where it can undergo oxidation, forming methyl mercury, a highly toxic substance.

OTHER THEORIES

Dr. Elson Haas, an integrated medicine physician, is director of the Preventive Medical Center in San Rafael, California, and author of *The Staying Healthy Shopper's Guide*, among other best-selling books. In an article on the HealthWorld Online website (www.healthy.net), he summarizes a few other theories of aging: errors in DNA, possibly caused by free radicals; alterations in brain function; imbalance in the hormonal and nervous systems; a breakdown in immune system function; and stress. His own theory, he explains, is that all these processes combine in various ways in each person to result in aging, with the key factor being "stagnation of bioenergy circulation and stagnation of the digestive tract and bowels."

Symptoms

A variety of gradual bodily changes are associated with aging, such as an increased susceptibility to weight gain and fatigue. But there is no physiological reason why women should become obese or get tired more easily as they grow older: these are society's, not nature's, norms. It can be just as natural, for example, for a woman to eat and sleep a little less as she grows older, compensating for any slowing down of metabolic processes and thus maintaining stable weight and energy levels.

The risk of contracting degenerative diseases such as cancer and heart disease, and suffering from thyroid dysfunction, musculoskeletal problems, and gastrointestinal disorders, also typically increases with age. As women get older, they may suffer from elevated blood sugar, an increase in cholesterol and triglycerides, and other chemical imbalances. Decreases in memory, concentration, and sharpness may occur. Typical signs of aging also include changes in skin, hair, nails, and connective tissue. Again, it is not inevitable that these changes take place.

Clinical Experience

DIAGNOSING PROBLEMS

Aging well means being healthy and balanced from within. To check that all systems are running optimally, Dr. Calapai recommends a full spectrum of diagnostic tests, with special attention to adrenal function, vitamin and mineral levels, blood chemistry, pancreatic enzymes, and stool. "The adrenal glands produce our antiaging hormones. With age, some people start producing less. This can be from free radical damage, excessive stress, injuries, and all sorts of reasons. As a result we see changes in memory, concentration, skin, hair, hormonal fluctuations, and energy levels. We start to see problems with immune response and increases in blood sugar, cholesterol, and abdominal deposition of body fat. So we need to look at adrenal function.

"Certainly, tests should look at vitamin and mineral levels to check our digestive and absorptive abilities. Looking at the basic blood chemistry tells us how well we are absorbing protein. We need to look at the fat-soluble vitamins and cholesterol, triglycerides, and the ratio of good HDL cholesterol to bad LDL cholesterol, which can provide information about our fat absorption. I also recommend looking at enzymes of the pancreas to assess function and having a comprehensive stool analysis done to see whether or not there are too many undigested particles in the stool. If parasites are present, this can decrease our absorptive ability. These are some of the main tests we need to perform to get a thorough picture of the individual."

ANTIAGING DIET

A basic healthy diet will vastly improve the quality of life and reduce the aging process in women of all ages. This diet should consist of high-quality organic foods, reduced caloric intake, emphasizing complex carbohydrates such as beans and whole grains, fruits, and vegetables. Adolescents, who are still growing, may need more of certain nutrients, and people in specific age groups may have specific nutrient requirements that can be addressed through supplements.

Anti-aging diets contain no animal proteins. Let me repeat that. Not a little bit, not a moderate amount, but zero animal products. Eliminate all pro-inflammatory food & beverage, i.e. pizza, deep fried food. What you do want are high-fiber foods, more organic raw food and juices. This means about 50 to 60 grams of fiber a day, soluble and nonsoluble. High-fiber diets help prevent common afflictions associated with aging, such as constipation, hemorrhoids, pressure in the intestines, ulcers, high blood pressure, colorectal cancer, and overall body toxemia. Reduce advanced glycation end products and eliminate all processed sugar.

One of the principles of longevity is eating to the point of being not quite full. As we get older, it is advisable to eat small servings more frequently. I'd rather see you eat three small servings a day than one big meal because your body requires energy throughout the day and if you only eat one meal, your body is not going to be able to sustain its energy. You'll think it's normal to be fatigued about four hours after you've eaten your meal when what's happening is your blood sugar level is simply low. It takes you twice as long to digest food when you're older because your whole metabolism is slowed down.

Many senior citizens suffer from dehydration because their intake of fluid is inadequate. Dehydration adversely affects the body's electrolytes, which carry electricity and are important for normal functioning of the nervous system. You should drink at least ten 8-ounce glasses of liquid daily. I don't want you drinking tap water. It's too polluted, no matter what your public health official says. I've done so much work showing what's in a glass that you can't even see. In addition to water, either filtered or distilled, you should be drinking juices. There is a proper way to take the juices so you don't overwhelm the system. Start with one glass of juice per day for the first month. Then add a glass a day per month until you reach six glasses a day at the end of six months. The juice floods the body with phytochemicals and chlorophyll, which are really important for healing.

SUPPLEMENTS

The first thing to look at as a means of reversing the symptoms of aging is supplements. Many people do not understand the effective use of vitamins and minerals as dietary supplements. Basically, you must follow the law of compensation. If you are a woman who smoked, and used sugar, caffeine, or alcohol; if you were an angry person who held in your anger; if you have not honored the life force; if you have not exercised; or if you have felt unfulfilled, you must work to compensate for these deficiencies.

One-a-day supplements are the easy way out. I have met people who say, "I eat meat. I eat sugar. But it's all right because I take my one-a-day vitamin." My friend, that does not work. The body cannot be lied to. After thirty or forty years of the body being debilitated by an unhealthy lifestyle and environment, a little pill will not do the trick. You need to detoxify and cleanse the body.

You have to know what your bodily state is and plan accordingly. I would suggest one level of usage for healthy women who know they are healthy, and a very different level for those processing diseases. A person becoming conscious of her health will need to consult a nutritionist who can design a personalized supplement program to meet her individual needs.

The reason that supplements are even more crucial as we get older is that as we age, certain fatty acids, amino acids, and members of the main groups of nutrients are lost. Scientists looking into this issue already know that choline, tyrosine, glutathione, cysteine, vitamin E, zinc, and chromium are poorly absorbed and deficient in older people. Meanwhile, as these substances grow scarce, there is a buildup of heavy metals, such as aluminum and lead. These metals can be removed from the body through a process known as chelation. Vitamin C and zinc are also useful in flushing them out. Most importantly, all the nutrients that are lost, for whatever reason, must be restored for optimum physical and mental functioning.

At the same time, the free radicals in our bodies, which grow in number as we age, have to be fought. Remember, when you eat meat, drink alcohol, and are exposed to pollutants, the body creates free radicals. They cause the skin to wrinkle in the sun, and they foster cancer, arthritis, and heart disease. However, antioxidants, such as beta-carotene and vitamin A, are able to neutralize the effect of the free radicals, slowing down the aging process.

ANTIOXIDANTS

Dr. Morris calls aging a catch-22: "Oxygen is the great substance that sustains and gives life, but unfortunately it is also the substance that destroys us through oxidation." For this reason, antioxidants are essential. Here are the most important ones:

VITAMIN E—400 to 1,600 IU, taken at the largest meal. Women with herpes, chronic fatigue syndrome, hepatitis, and even AIDS have dramatically improved after taking large doses of this vitamin on a regular basis. Vitamin E is best in its natural form (as a mixed tocopherol or d-alphatocopherol). Synthetic vitamin E (dl-alpha) should be avoided.

BETA-CAROTENE—25,000 IU per meal. Beta-carotene can be obtained in all the green, red, and orange fruits and vegetables. They help slow down aging and lessen cancer risk. They are nontoxic, since the body converts beta carotenes into vitamin A and will not convert more than it can use.

VITAMIN A—5,000 to 10,000 IU per day. Vitamin A is a fat-soluble vitamin essential for healthy bones, skin, eyes, digestion, and immune function. Blood tests will determine whether or not a woman is getting too much vitamin A, which can be toxic.

VITAMIN D3—5,000 IU per day.

SELENIUM—100 mcg once or twice a day. One cause of premature aging and even death, particularly in professional athletes, is cardiomyopathy, an enlargement of the heart. This is usually associated with selenium deficiency. Adequate amounts of this critical nutrient are needed to help the body produce the antioxidant enzyme glutathione peroxidase, which is on the front line of aging defense.

ZINC—15 to 25 mg daily. Zinc feeds more than one hundred enzyme systems in the brain, as well as various systems throughout the body. It is essential in the formation of stomach acid; without sufficient zinc, malabsorption syndrome occurs. Malabsorption is the failure of the body to absorb at the cellular level the nutrients that have been ingested. Most older people are zinc-deficient.

VITAMIN C—The single most important dietary supplement is vitamin C. I generally suggest people start at 1,000 mg a day. Then, in divided doses of 500 mg several times a day, you start to gradually take yourself up to 10,000 mg a day. This process takes several months. To really fight disease, you may have to take 200,000 mg daily via intravenous drips, under medical supervision of course. The benefits of this vitamin are multiple. Vitamin C is important for the skin, giving it youthful elasticity. This is because it produces collagen, a type of connective tissue that holds the muscles and skin together. It helps the body produce interferon and increases white blood cell disease-fighting activity. It aids the thymus gland, the liver, and the brain, and acts to prevent arthritis, cataracts, and heart disease.

At the Healing Center of New York City, drips of vitamin C and other nutrients are used to counteract the aging process. Dr. Howard Robins points out that toxins and free radicals are stressful to both the body and the mind. A body in pain, fatigued, and under attack from heavy metal and other pollutants is weakened, and the mind is adversely affected. Dr. Robins asserts that intravenously administered vitamin C cleanses the body. The Healing Center also uses drips with other nutrients, such as EDTA (ethylenediaminetetra-acetic acid) to cleanse the heavy metals from the body, and destroy viruses and keep them from replicating. These drips will also help boost energy levels.

GRAPESEED EXTRACT—100 mg per day and up to 200 mg per day for people in a disease state. This is a bioflavonoid, a water-soluble substance that ensures the strength and proper function of the capillaries, helps manufacture collagen, and protects the cells against attack and invasion by viruses and bacteria. It has the highest known antioxidant properties of any nutrient.

SUPEROXIDE DISMUTASE (SOD)—This important antienzyme nutrient is produced by the body. It is not effective when taken orally unless it is enteric-coated. According to Dr. Haas, manganese and copper, together with zinc, support the action of superoxide dismutase.

HORMONES

Dr. Richard Ash has talked to his large New York City radio audience about the revivifying power of DHEA (dehydroepiandrosterone), which is a key ingredient underlying the normal functioning of the adrenal gland. He tells us that when the body is under stress, the adrenal gland requires higher amounts of cortisone and adrenaline. If these hormones are overused, they will become depleted, as will DHEA, their precursor.

An eighty-year-old woman may have only one-twentieth of the DHEA she had at age twenty. According to Dr. Ash, this can result in all sorts of negative consequences for the immune system, leading to a weakened capacity to fight diseases. One of the earliest signs of DHEA depletion is an inability to get REM sleep, which can lead to insomnia and chronic fatigue. An uninformed doctor may prescribe sleeping pills for a patient with insomnia, which will not get at the root of the problem. Other symptoms of low DHEA levels are hyperglycemia (an excess of glucose in the blood), palpitations, sweating, confusion, poor concentration, and the inability to cope with everyday stress.

Another effect of low DHEA is a reduction in salivary IgA, an antibody that fights infection in the gastrointestinal (GI) tract. When IgA is depleted or absent, there will be more antigen penetration in this area as well as increased sensitivity reactions to foods and chemicals. There may be inflammation of the GI tract, a condition called "leaky gut," in which certain foods and chemicals are not absorbed but pass out into the bloodstream. When the body tries to defend itself against these unexpected intruders, autoimmune disease may arise. Dr. Ash notes that by administering DHEA and building back up salivary IgA, we can diminish food sensitivity, lower toxic load, and repair the GI tract, restoring normal immune system functioning by treating the cause, not the symptoms.

Dr. Eric Braverman, director of the Place for Achieving Total Health (PATH) in New York and Philadelphia, and the former chief clinical researcher at the Princeton Brain Bio Center, has found that counteracting the aging process has to be undertaken on an individual basis. His treatments are personalized on the basis of each patient's specific hormone balance, brain function, attention span, memory capacity, and cardiac and exercise capacities. Once these have been evaluated, the patient's nutritional needs are assessed. He recommends natural yam extract, which contains progesterone, estrogen, and testosterone (PET), the three hormones he considers essential. Progesterone has anticancer properties and helps calm the brain. Estrogen strengthens the bones, has anticancer effects, especially in the colon, aids memory, and gives cardiovascular protection.

Testosterone reduces the side effects of other hormones, and helps keep the sex drive vigorous through a person's fifties, sixties, and beyond. For a woman, the ovary produces all three of these substances, but, as Dr. Braverman puts it, "If the ovary dies, you must resurrect it. If you permit an organ to die, you allow yourself to die. We must stop this if we want abundant life. We replace depleted hormones with PET, and missing adrenal with DHEA."

BIOFLAVONOID COMPLEX

Another invaluable supplement group is the citrus bioflavonoid complex, which can be obtained from lemons, plums, and oranges, among other fruits. With an orange, one can cut open the skin and right below is the nutrient, the bioflavonoid. Another good bioflavonoid is rutin, which comes from buckwheat. To take the bioflavonoid in pill form, I recommend 300 mg per day for a healthy woman, while someone in poor health should take 500 to 1,000 mg. As for the rutin, the proper dosage for a healthy person is 25 mg per day, while the ill person may take up to 50 mg.

OTHER SUPPLEMENTS

BLUEBERRY AND RED CABBAGE EXTRACTS—Blueberry extract is good for the eyes. During World War II, the Royal Air Force gave this to its pilots to improve night vision and strengthen the immune system. Red cabbage extract is also important. There are cultures that lack a variety of foodstuffs, but those people eat cabbage and obtain its antibacterial, antiulcer properties. Cabbage, eaten juiced or steamed, is very healthful.

CALCIUM—Calcium protects against osteoporosis and colon cancer, is important for strong teeth, and helps energy production as well as heart and nerve function.

CHROMIUM—Chromium supports glucose tolerance, decreasing the craving for sugar, and plays a role in preventing atherosclerosis by helping to lower blood cholesterol.

COENZYME Q10—200 mg daily. Every cell in the body needs this coenzyme to create energy and build stamina.

CYTOKINE SUPPRESS WITH EGCG—300mg.

RESVERATROL—200mg.

GRAPE SEED EXTRACT—200mg.

PYCNOGENOL—200mg.

GREEN TEA—If you lived in China, you would probably be drinking green tea and taking green tea extract. We know it has anticancer properties. It is an immune system stimulator. Decaffeinated green tea is very beneficial.

GLUTATHIONE—Glutathione is good for the immune system, but it is not easily assimilated by the body, so it should be taken with something that produces it in the body, such as N-acetyl-cysteine (NAC). Generally you need 500 mg of NAC and 500 mg of reduced glutathione.

L-CARNITINE—L-carnitine, a nonessential amino acid involved in fat metabolism, may help reduce fat and weight.

L-CYSTEINE—This amino acid, which scavenges free radicals, protects the tissues from chemicals and aids detoxification, partly by helping the liver produce and store glutathione. Most often it is taken with vitamin C to prevent the formation of kidney stones of cysteine, which is produced when cysteine is metabolized. Take 250 mg with a gram of vitamin C twice a day. When you take L-cysteine on a regular basis, you should also take a formula that contains the other amino acids the body needs.

DIGESTIVE AIDS—Lactobacillus acidophilus, along with other intestinal bacteria, may be needed occasionally to support the balance of bacteria in the colon. Similarly, supplements of hydrochloric acid and digestive enzymes aid digestion and metabolism of food, and thus prevent both nutritional deficiencies and free-radical formation due to food reactions.

ESSENTIAL FATTY ACIDS—Essential fatty acids, such as EPA (eicosapentaenoic acid) and DHA (docosahexaenoic acid), diminish the risk of cardiovascular disease. Omega-3 fatty acids, derived primarily from plant oils, help regulate blood cholesterol and promote the health of the immune, cardiovascular, and nervous systems. Flaxseed oil is a superb source of omega-3. Omega-6 fatty acids, which come from fish oils, are important for blood clotting and constriction of blood vessels.

FOLIC ACID—Folic acid also helps in RNA, DNA, and red blood cell synthesis.

MAGNESIUM—Magnesium supports the cardiovascular system and decreases nervous tension.

L-CARNOSINE—1,000–2,000 mg daily.

MOLYBDENUM—Molybdenum is a trace mineral that may help prevent cancer.

NIACIN—Niacin, a form of vitamin B_3, decreases cholesterol and helps improve circulation.

NADH (NICOTINAMIDE ADENINE DINUCLEOTIDE)—Also known as coenzyme 1, NADH is a naturally occurring substance in the body that supplies energy to the cells, allowing them to live longer.

RNA—RNA, taken in blue-green algae, spirulina, chlorella, and wheatgrass (all of which are also rich in chlorophyll), can decelerate the aging process.

SEA ALGAE—This is high in trace elements, antioxidant cofactors, flavonoids, and carotenoids.

THYMUS EXTRACT—Pure oral thymus extract enhances immune function and helps reverse the aging process.

TYROSINE—Strengthens the thyroid and adrenal glands, protecting against stress.

VITAMIN B12—Vitamin B_{12} boosts energy and protects the fatty sheaths that cover the nerves. It is involved in synthesis of red blood cells and DNA and RNA, which are needed for important rebuilding processes.

HERBS

Herbs are an important part of any anti-aging nutritional protocol, and can be taken as capsules, powders, teas, or tinctures.

CAPSICUM—This stimulates elimination, and circulation, and its mild diuretic properties help cleanse the kidneys.

FO-TI—Fo-ti rejuvenates the endocrine system and is an excellent digestive tonic.

GARLIC—This is antiviral, antibacterial, and antifungal. It boosts energy but—unlike coffee—helps lower cholesterol and blood pressure. Garlic also stimulates liver and colon detoxification and may have anticancer properties.

GINKGO BILOBA—The ginkgo tree has survived for hundreds of thousands of years due to its powerful immune system. An extract of the leaf of the tree improves circulation to the microcapillaries of the brain and heart so that needed nutrients and oxygen can get to all the tissues.

GINSENG—Ginseng is the best-known longevity herb. For centuries, the Chinese have revered ginseng for its rejuvenating effects. Research has shown that ginseng can stop the free radical damage associated with aging. It helps people focus better when under stress and increases overall energy levels.

GOTU KOLA—Gotu kola is useful for increasing vitality and endurance, and may lower blood pressure.

HAWTHORN BERRIES—Hawthorn berries support circulation and cardiac function.

MILK THISTLE—Milk thistle protects liver function. The liver releases toxins from the body, promoting health and youthfulness.

YAM—Wild yam supports adrenal gland production of DHEA, a building block for the development of estrogen, progesterone, testosterone, and cortisols, which decrease with age. As an adaptogen, wild yam balances the body's hormonal functions. It has been shown to ameliorate numerous chronic conditions, including heart disease, cancer, arthritis, and autoimmune diseases. DHEA is extremely safe, with no known side effects.

DETOXIFICATION THERAPIES

The more toxic we are, the faster we age. Cosmetic changes such as face-lifts and hair dye may temporarily make women appear younger, but they do not make a real difference. To keep youthful and healthy, we must address what is happening inside.

"Everyone needs detoxification," says Susana Lombardi, founder and president of the We Care Health Center in Palm Springs, California, and author of *Ten Easy Steps for Complete Wellness*. "I am vegetarian, and I take care of myself. Do I still need detoxification? Yes, because the air that we breathe is polluted, the water that we drink is full of chlorine, the clothing we wear is made of artificial fabrics and chemicals, the lotions and shampoos that we use all contain chemicals. Once these chemicals are inside us, we never fully eliminate them unless we go through a detoxification procedure."

Lombardi recommends rejuvenating the system from the inside out by, once a week, limiting food intake to fresh raw vegetable juices. She and many other practitioners also recommend the following simple, yet effective, detoxification therapies.

JUICE FASTING

Juice fasting gives the digestive system a rest and speeds up the growth of new cells, which promotes healing. (If you have any medical problems, do not fast without medical approval and supervision.)

On a juice fast, a person abstains from solid foods and drinks juice, water, and herbal teas throughout the day. "We should be drinking every half hour to an hour," advises Lombardi. "If we go for long periods of time without drinking anything, then a little glass of juice will not be able to sustain us. But if we are constantly drinking, the day will go by very smoothly."

Lombardi recommends a combination of the following:

CARROT JUICE—High in the antioxidant beta-carotene and full of wonderful enzymes.

CELERY JUICE—High in sodium, not the artificial type poured from the saltshaker, which is bad for you, but the good, natural kind that promotes tissue flexibility.

BEET JUICE—Beets nourish the liver, one of the most important organs in the body, with hundreds of different functions. If your liver is functioning well, most likely everything else in your body will too.

CABBAGE JUICE—Cabbage juice is high in vitamin C.

Mix the juice from each vegetable in equal proportion and drink this combination throughout the day. A little cayenne, which increases circulation, sending blood to every corner of the body to promote healing, can be added for flavor. Lemon juice in water and different herbal teas—some good ones are parsley and dandelion tea for the liver and kidneys and pau d'arco for blood purification—can be added for variety. "Any herbal tea free of caffeine will be good," Lombardi says. "Since you need to drink on an hourly basis, you don't want to drink the same thing over and over."

Other juices that I recommend, not necessarily as part of a fasting program but important to your daily health regimen, include tomato, watermelon, cherry, blueberry, and raspberry. These contain phytochemicals, such as lycopene and anthocyanin, the blockbuster antioxidants that protect against cancer, heart disease, and other ailments.

CHELATION THERAPY

Dr. Martin Dayton, who is board-certified in family medicine, chelation therapy, and clinical nutrition, says that chelation therapy has multiple benefits, and long life is one of them: "Dramatic increases in life span are found with chelation. While there are no longevity studies per se, this conclusion is implied indirectly by studies that show a lessening of killer degenerative diseases. In fact, chelation favorably impacts all four major causes of death in the United States [heart disease, cancer, cerebrovascular disease, and lung disease]."

During the chelation process, many beneficial changes occur at the cellular level. A synthetic amino acid called EDTA is administered to the patient via intravenous drip. Once in the bloodstream, EDTA attaches itself to heavy metals such as lead, cadmium, and mercury and holds onto those toxic substances until they exit the body through the urine. Dr. Dayton explains why removal of these substances is vital to good health: "The toxic material prevents normal function and repair. For example, lead prevents normal enzymatic processes so that the body cannot function properly and repair itself. This leads to premature aging and the premature development of disease. Removal of toxic material through chelation keeps the body functioning optimally."

Dr. Dayton notes that even an excess of iron, which is necessary for life, accelerates free radical production and causes harm: "Periodic purging of iron from the body via menstrual bleeding is thought to protect women from hardening of the arteries. However, this protection is lost at menopause with the cessation of menstruation. At this time, arterial clogging accelerates. Chelation removes this excess iron."

Since modern people are overwhelmed by pollutants, Dr. Dayton recommends chelation therapy for anyone over the age of thirty. "Lead is found everywhere, in the air we breathe, the water we drink, the food supply. It is even found at the North Pole. Lead and other toxic pollutants are hard to avoid in today's world. As a matter of fact, the concentration of lead found in the human skeleton now is several hundred times greater than that found in our preindustrial revolution ancestors. In one study, where lead was thought to be involved, in eighteen years following chelation therapy a ten-fold decrease in cancer death rate was found for those who had the treatment versus those who had nothing."

Aside from its overall benefits, chelation therapy specifically helps aging individuals by improving brain function. Dr. Dayton cites the following evidence: "Research shows that circulation improves greatly in the brain and to the brain. One study of fifteen patients who had twenty infusions of chelation therapy found that fourteen out of fifteen demonstrated significant cerebral blood flow. Some showed dramatic improvement in cognitive abilities. In another study thirty patients with carotid blockages were given thirty chelation treatments over a ten-month period. The carotid artery extends from the chest through the neck to the brain. It is the brain's main source of blood flow. Blockage decreased between 20 and 40 percent.

"Unclogging carotid blockage is vitally important because the American College of Physicians states that patients with an obstruction of 70 percent or greater are at a high risk for stroke. People who have carotid artery disease improve as their arteries open up. I see this happen over and over again."

COLON CLEANSING

Colon cleansing is an ancient and time-honored health practice for rejuvenating the body; it was used in Egypt more than 4,000 years ago. Later, Hippocrates taught these procedures in his health care system. The large intestine is restored to its natural size, normal shape, and correct function.

Colon therapist Anita Lotson explains the procedure and some of its physical and psychological benefits: "There are several stages of therapy. The first segment involves cleansing, a thorough washing of the large colon. The colon is irrigated by a technique whereby water is gently infused into the large bowel, flowing in and out at steady intervals. Through this method, water is allowed to travel the entire length of the colon. The walls of the colon are washed and old encrustations and fecal material are loosened, dislodged, and swept away. This toxic waste material has often been attached to the bowel walls for many, many years. It is laden with bacteria, which set up the perfect environment for disease to take root and entrench itself in the system, wreaking havoc. As this body pollution is eliminated, many conditions—from severe skin disorders to breathing difficulties, depression, chronic fatigue, nervousness, severe constipation, and arthritis—are reduced in severity, providing great relief, especially when augmented with dietary changes and other treatment modalities.

"The next phases are healing, and finally restoration of a healthy colon, functioning at maximum efficiency for the final absorption of nutrients, and the total and timely elimination of all remaining waste materials. During the healing phase, we begin to infuse materials into the bowel that will cool inflamed areas and strengthen weak sections of the colon wall. Flaxseed tea, white oak bark tea, and slippery elm bark tea all soothe, lubricate, and introduce powerful healing agents directly into the large intestine. These herbal teas may be taken orally as well. Simple dietary changes have been made by now, such as the addition of water. This simple measure spells the difference between success and failure in alleviating many bowel conditions. I ask all my clients to double their intake of water.

"I love to see people's change in attitude from the time they come in to the time that they leave. Sometimes people are very irritable when their bowels are backed up. They're often depressed, and sometimes nasty. By the time they leave, you can see a smile and a bounce in their step. It's a different person altogether."

ENZYME THERAPY

Nina Anderson, author of *Over Fifty, Looking Thirty: The Secrets of Staying Young*, attributes slow aging to sufficient enzyme levels: "Many scientists say that people get old before their time due to enzyme exhaustion. Some people are old at forty because of the lack of enzymes, while others are young at eighty because of an abundance. Above all else, I would advise anybody who is trying to avoid looking and feeling older as they get older to take supplemental enzymes."

She goes on to explain that enzymes allow nutrients to be used. For example, you have enzymes in the heart that allow magnesium to be used. Without those enzymes, magnesium cannot get to the heart: "Enzymes are molecule catalysts found everywhere in your body. In fact, there are over thirteen hundred different ones. They make everything happen. In my book I use this analogy: minerals are the building blocks of your body. They are the nose, eyes, ears, bones, all the things that hold you together. Something has to build this. Enzymes are the construction workers that facilitate everything in the body going together."

Anderson recommends that women eat more raw foods, mineral supplements, and digestive plant enzymes to increase enzyme levels. Raw foods are loaded with enzymes. Fruit and vegetable juices are filled with enzymes. When food is processed, the first things taken out are enzymes. Why? Because the enzymes are what allow the food to ripen. However, if the food becomes too ripe, it rots. To stop it from ripening and rotting so that it can be sold longer, these enzymes must be destroyed. But if you destroy the enzymes, you lessen the food's life force. It will have proteins, carbohydrates, vitamins, fats, and minerals, but less life force.

"The mineral supplements to take," Anderson adds, "should be in crystalloid form, with electrolytes. The crystalloid form goes right into the cell walls. This fortifies your body.

"Plant enzymes assist in the digestion of food right on through the intestinal tract. You want to help the digestive process for the whole length of the digestive tract. With supplemental enzymes, you won't have an upset stomach anymore or feel bloated and exhausted after a big meal. The skin will start to improve too. The skin manifests everything that happens inside. If your inner organs start to degenerate, if they are not functioning properly, this kind of stress shows up on your face. The first thing people do when they start getting older is look in the mirror and go, 'Oh my God, I've got wrinkles.' They spend millions trying to get rid of them. But what they have to realize is that wrinkles start from inside. You have to work on the inside to get the outside to reflect that good health.

"Without the proper enzymes, none of the other good things you do matter. For example, the fat-soluble vitamins A, D, E, and K require fat for absorption. That fat has to be broken down by an enzyme, lipase. If lipase is not present in sufficient quantities, that fat will not be broken down. If the fat isn't broken down, the vitamins will not be released. Therefore, you can spend a fortune on vitamin pills, and if you don't have the proper enzymes to release those vitamins into your system, they are just going to be flushed out."

Enzymes can be used externally as well as internally for youthful effects. Anderson explains, "There are amazing enzyme treatments for the skin. Papaya enzymes are wonderful. Or you can mix a plant enzyme powder and put it on as a mask. Not only does it take the lines out of your face, but it fills them in and builds up collagen. It can also get rid of age spots and shrink moles. When you use enzymes as a mud pack when you come in from the sun, it fights free radicals that otherwise might foster melanoma."

EXERCISE AND BREATHING

When we exercise, we detoxify as we sweat through our skin and exhale from our lungs. Some good exercises include jogging or daily brisk walks, yoga stretches, and jumping on a minitrampoline, which exercises every cell in the body. Exercise slows down the aging process because it stimulates detoxification.

Recent research supports the connection between exercise and a longer life, more stable moods, and decreased risk of disease and injury.

Breathing exercises combined with physical activity increase the action of lymphatic cleansing. Detoxification expert Susana Lombardi explains: "For lymphatic cleansing, you want to synchronize your breathing with the movement of your legs and arms. When you are walking or jumping on the trampoline, inhale four times and exhale four times. Move your arms and legs each time you take a little breath. Inhale through your nose and exhale through your nose or mouth.

"This breathing technique was learned from the Taromaro Indians, who live in the northern part of Mexico. They are famous for their fantastic health. They have less need of hospitals or homes for the elderly. They have less disease."

STRESS RELEASE

"In my personal opinion, the single most important factor influencing aging and disease is stress," says Dr. Morris. "We need to control emotional anxieties and tensions, and learn how to not let life get to us. It is important to learn to let go and enjoy life." Methods Dr. Morris and others suggest to overcome stress include deep breathing exercises, Reiki, skin brushing, saunas, and magnetic healing. Tai chi, yoga, meditation, qi gong, massage, biofeedback, and the Feldenkrais method are also recommended.

Since exercise increases oxygenation, it also has the potential to foster free radical damage. To prevent undesirable effects, women may want to combine exercise with sufficient amounts of antioxidants in the diet and/or as dietary supplements.

REIKI

Reiki is a type of massage therapy or bodywork in which pressure point techniques are used to move energy through the body, achieving balance and harmony. Reiki therapist Nilsa Vergara reports below on her clients' experiences with Reiki therapy.

"My first example is a fifty-nine-year-old woman who came to our healing circle feeling old and tired. She suffered from aches and severe pain in her neck and knee from car accidents. She was also going through job changes, and was estranged from her adult son. Each week she received a fifteen-minute session, and she quickly began feeling better. She released a lot of emotional toxins via crying and verbal expression of what she was feeling. She decided to take a Reiki class so that she could give herself daily treatments. Within a month, her changes were quite dramatic. She had a tremendous increase in energy and vigor. She told me she now feels like she is twenty-eight. With the Reiki, she now has very little pain. She feels emotional and vital. Her attitude has changed. She feels self-fulfilled and in control of her life. Her relationship with her son has greatly improved. To quote her, 'I feel like my whole life is as it should be.'

"My next client is a sixty-five-year-old woman. When she first came to see us, she was depressed. She had been in therapy for years, but nothing seemed to lift the depression. She felt tired all the time and would catch colds easily. Emotionally, she felt like a victim, and others treated her like one.

"After her first fifteen-minute session she felt immediately better. She knew that something powerful was happening. She returned and eventually studied Reiki. Today, she reports feeling much healthier. She has more energy and an optimistic outlook. She no longer feels like a victim, and if anyone tries to put her in that role, she is no longer afraid to set limits. In addition, she is much more able to tolerate cold weather, which indicates that her body has improved its oxygen intake.

"One of my students has an eighty-three-year-old mother who fell and broke her hip bone as well as bones in her wrist and arm. She decided to give her mother

Reiki regularly, and her mother responded quite well. She began feeling stronger and stronger. Within four weeks she was out of her cast, walking with just the aid of a cane, not a walker."

SKIN BRUSHING

Using a natural brush on dry skin removes dead cells and leaves pores open, so that more toxins can be expelled. Lombardi explains why this is so important: "We are supposed to eliminate toxins through the pores of the skin. Due to pollution, smog, the creams we use, the clothes we wear, and so forth, our pores are more closed than open. Always brush toward the heart."

SAUNAS

The sauna is a good follow-up to dry skin brushing because it pushes toxins out through the skin. The main thing to remember with saunas is to be prudent. You want to perspire but not remain there for too long. Nor do you want too much heat. "Follow the directions," says Lombardi. "And wear a cooling drape on your head. You don't want to heat up the brain area."

There are multiple benefits from sauna detoxification, explains Lombardi: "You will look and feel better. Your skin will be clear and you will not have constipation. Your nails will improve as well as your heart and digestive system. It will clear your mind and improve concentration. Nothing will de-stress your body like a sauna."

MAGNETIC HEALING

Susan Bucci is a holistically trained nurse who has spearheaded the development of magnetic healing products. "Magnets oxygenate tissues and allow cell walls to absorb more oxygen," she explains. "They promote mental acuity and normalize pH balance by increasing alkalinity. Restorative sleep is enhanced. Therapeutically, they stop pain, fight infection, and reduce inflammation and fluid retention. Over time, fatty and calcium deposits dissolve and the circulatory system opens up. Put that all together and you've got enhanced health. Take that a step further: if you achieve optimal well-being, you can actually live a long, productive life."

In addition, magnets can eliminate many specific signs and symptoms of old age. Bucci reports these antiaging benefits from her own use of magnetic healing techniques: "My energy level has increased. I used to have chronic fatigue in the worst way, but now that's gone. My immune system is functioning much better, so my susceptibility to viruses and colds has decreased dramatically. Allergies are basically gone, and there are no more killer sinus headaches. My circulation has improved so that I withstand weather a whole lot easier. Wounds heal quickly, and my spider veins have disappeared. Also, I was headed for an early menopause, but now my menstrual cycle is very much on track, very regular.

"Hair, skin, and nails have definitely improved. My hair grows faster and has a much better quality to it. Within two weeks of using magnets on a daily basis, I was able to see new, thick, dark hair growing. My grays started falling out and disappearing. I was going to color my hair about four years ago, and I still haven't touched it with an ounce of anything. My skin definitely looks and feels younger. And my nails grow so well that if I break one, it doesn't upset me. I know that it will grow right back."

How can magnets do so much? Simply stated, magnets confer a wide range of benefits because we are magnetic beings who derive energy from the earth's magnetic field. Magnets create overall benefit by restoring internal harmony.

It is important to realize that not just any magnet will do. The negative pole restores health and good energy to the system, while exposure to the positive pole is detrimental. This has been proved repeatedly in studies where a variety of creatures, from earthworms, mice, and chickens to larger animals, live longer as untested control groups when exposed to negative field magnets. Bucci recommends unipolar magnets, marked by the Davis and Rawls system with an *N* or the word *negative* and a green label. "That's the healthy side, and that's the one we face toward the body." Negative field ions support biological systems, which help the body to heal itself. "The body is an amazing machine with a remarkable capacity to cure itself," Bucci says. "Give it a boost in the right direction and it does the rest on its own. The negative field is completely safe and risk-free."

Bucci finds that magnets work best when worn on a daily basis. During the day she wears a magnet over her heart to improve circulation and oxygenation. "It keeps the heart open and flowing and sends all that wonderful oxygen throughout my body," she says. At night, she takes the magnet off and sleeps with her head on a magnetic mattress pad. She does this because the most important benefit while sleeping is increased melatonin production from the brain's pineal gland: "People are running out to buy melatonin, but guess what? We can encourage our own melatonin production.

"People ask me how long magnets should be worn. Generally speaking, the longer you wear them, the more healing takes place. You can wear them all night and during the day. Generally, the body will tell you when it has had enough. It also will tell you when a condition has healed, although you should check with a physician just to make sure."

Research Update

An increasing body of scientific evidence is showing the benefits of natural modalities to overall health and well-being. Following is a sample of recent peer-reviewed literature in the area of aging.

A 2012 *Life Extension Magazine* article cited numerous studies indicating that supplements of the coenzyme PQQ (pyrroloquinoline quinone) protect against mitochondrial dysfunction, heart degeneration, brain injury, and cognitive decline, among other degenerative conditions. Reports in 2010 and 2012 in the *Journal of Bioscience, Journal of Neurotrauma*, and *Journal of Biological Chemistry*, for example, cited evidence of PQQ's neuroprotective effect, its versatile role in biological processes, and its ability to activate cell signaling pathways that have the potential to reverse cellular aging. In a 2014 study published in *Antioxidants and Redox Signaling*, researchers from the University of Warwick reported that sulforaphane in broccoli and quercetin in onions are capable of increasing movement of Nrf2, a protein that regulates antioxidant response and is important for cellular health. Caloric restriction has now been established as the one provable anti-aging therapy.

Chapter 15

Epigenetics

There has been a lot of excitement recently about epigenetics, the study of the molecular processes that regulate our genes. Although DNA sequences do not change, alterations on genes can change the way DNA is read and expressed. These alterations occur as a result of interactions with the environment. Chemical markers on the genome show which parts of DNA turn on and off not only as the result of disease progression, but also in response to changes in stress, diet, exposure to toxins, and other external factors. To date, scientists have found epigenetic changes associated with cancers, depression, addiction, and more. There is even research indicating that epigenetic marks can be passed from one generation to the next.

While people may have certain genetic dispositions toward a variety of health risks, it is actually our environment that pulls the trigger. It should come as no surprise that lifestyle, state of mind, and diet can essentially instruct our genome to regulate disease-related genes. Despite the lack of acknowledgement by the cancer establishment, for example, there is a significant body of scientific research indicating that cancer is caused largely by environmental variables. The notion that cancer is actually an epigenetic disease is in stark contrast to mainstream medicine's view that it is a genetic disease brought on by DNA mutations within the cell. The epigenetic theory is backed by numerous studies carried out around the world that strongly suggest that genetic mutations associated with cancer development occur after a cell has been transformed by physiological stressors such as chemicals and ionizing radiation.

Dr. Dawson Church, founder of the National Institute for Integrative Healthcare in California, and author of *The Genie in Your Genes: Epigenetic Medicine*, provides some background. "The dominant way of understanding genetic activity in modern medicine has been genetic determinism," he says. "It's in my genes. I have this gene and therefore I'm highly likely to get this disease. This association between genes and disease has been one of the foundations of science for the last seventy years. This has been regarded as the cornerstone of the way our cells work and our bodies work, and yet it's completely not true.

"There are certain genes that are fixed and those are genes for things like eye color and hair color. My eyes are gray. They'll never be blue. They'll never be brown. So those genes are fixed, but they only represent about 15 percent of the genome. The other 85 percent of the genome is being expressed in collaboration with factors not just from outside the cell, but often from outside the body. Often something happens totally outside of our bodies and our bodies translate those external events into internal molecular messengers, which literally switch genes on and off. So, yes, you might have a gene but in the vast majority of cases, it is in fact being affected from outside the genome."

With epigenetics, we are able to see scientifically how lifestyle changes, yoga, meditation, and exercise affect the expression of thousands of genes. "A fascinating study was actually published just last week on this," Dr. Church says. "It showed the effect of listening to a piece of soothing music for 20 minutes. They found that up to 97 genes changed their configuration when you just listened to a piece of music. Some of those genes have to do with inflammation and some with immunity. So there was this beneficial shift in gene expression just as a result of listening to music."

Science is proving the holistic effects of natural therapies. "Our bodies are a whole and they are not a collection of parts," Dr. Church says. "A drug company aims to find the magic bullet that will affect one molecule that will shut a gene down or turn it on. Holism is exactly the opposite. When you, meditate, do EFT [Emotional Freedom Technique, a self-help method that combines cognitive therapy, exposure therapy, and acupressure], HeartMath [which emphasizes the heart-brain connection], or mindful thinking, what's happening isn't just that you're affecting one molecule, or synthesizing one protein. You aren't just affecting the expression of one gene. You're affecting the expression of many genes throughout your body. Our minds, our bodies, our spiritual lives, all of these things are having a dramatic impact on which genes are expressed."

The Role of Stress

The scientific community performing epigenetic research tends to focus on the role of the environment on gene alterations contributing to disease, but most of this research is looking at environmental toxins that surround us constantly and are found in our food and in our products at home. For example, in 2015 the World Health Organization condemned Monsanto's weed-killer Roundup (glyphosate) for its serious health risks. While toxins are important, they are by no means acting alone.

"I don't want to discount the effect of mechanical changes to the genes brought about by things like environmental toxins," Dr. Church says. "There is a very real concern about those, but we human beings are remarkably resilient creatures. If you look at the whole sweep of evolutionary biology you will see that, as a species, we have been able to survive enormous climate changes, social changes, and technological changes, and this is going back hundreds of thousands of years. I believe that we underrate how strong we are and how capable we are of surviving challenges. I think people worry a whole lot about things like nutritional influences, environmental toxins, and so on, and they don't realize that their stress level is often affecting them dramatically more than those potential threats to their health. Your stress level has a huge effect."

Dr. Church describes recent scientific investigations relating to stress. "In an astonishing piece of research I describe in *The Genie in Your Genes*, receptors for adrenaline were found on the surface of cancer cells. So you have high adrenaline, high cortisol, and high levels of your stress hormones, and you're literally feeding the cancer. If you're a woman at risk of any of these kinds of inherited diseases, your stress level is literally going to contribute to the sustenance and the triggering of those cancer cells. If you do all you can to reduce your stress, then you can be having this holistic overall effect on your health. Again, I'm not saying to discount environmental toxins, and by all means pay attention to nutrition, but your stress level is your huge lever. This lever can be affecting the expression of thousands of genes at a time, and it's the big leverage you have over your health."

How Consciousness Affects the Genome

Convincing scientific evidence supports the idea that consciousness can be an important factor of regenerating and repairing DNA. Dr. Church tells how times have changed in the past thirty years. "If we had gone to a medical conference in the early '80s and proposed that consciousness—your thinking and world view, your beliefs, your view of the universe—that all of these things affected the genome, we would have been tarred and feathered and thrown out, and they would have thought we were totally ridiculous. But now we have these tools like these gene chips, like these DNA microarrays that actually measure gene expression, and we're discovering that consciousness has profound effects on the genome. Again, not just on one or two genes but on cancer genes, inflammation genes, immunity."

Dr. Church tells about one of his exciting projects in this area, a triple-blind, randomized, controlled study published in the oldest psychiatric journal in America. "We analyzed the cortisol levels of people who got EFT, who got talk therapy, and who got rest. Three groups and one session each—just one session each—and we found that cortisol dropped dramatically in the EFT group. We found that anxiety and depression dropped twice as much in the EFT group as the other two groups, and that there was a correlation between the reduction in anxiety and depression, and the reduction in cortisol."

These findings are significant because they show that as people change their thoughts, beliefs, and world view, and reduce stress, anxiety, and depression, they are actually changing the expression of the genes that code for cortisol. "The result is that much less cortisol is being made," Dr. Church says. "The positive side effect of that, too, is that the two precursors for cortisol are the main precursors for DHEA. DHEA is your main cell repair and youthening hormone. As you down-regulate those cortisol genes, you up-regulate your DHEA genes. Automatically, you're having a rise in DHEA as you're having a drop in cortisol, and that was from just one session."

Caution: Invasive Surgery

Although certain genes carry high risks for cancer and other diseases, caution is urged in how we respond. The actress Angelina Jolie had a double mastectomy and removal of her ovaries after learning that a mutation in the BRCA1 gene gave her an 87 percent risk of developing breast cancer and a 50 percent risk of ovarian cancer. She determined that this was the right course of action in her particular case and correctly implores other women to get advice and consider all of their options before making any of their own decisions. In a *New York Times* commentary in March 2015, she stated, "A positive BRCA test does not mean a leap to surgery. . . . There is more than one way to deal with any health issue. The most important thing is to learn about the options and choose what is right for you personally."

This case raises an urgent question regarding invasive surgery as a preventative medical procedure due to certain genes associated with disease. This risk model used is a mathematical model that does not take into account if we changed the circumstances of our lives. Change our diets. Change our attitude. Change our exercise. Change our stress levels. There are so many options. For more discussion on this topic, see chapter 24.

Chapter 16

Baseline Wellness Protocols

First, a word of caution. When it comes to protocols, or specific programs, it is important to remember that they are designed to be done in an incremental fashion, under medical supervision. The following baseline protocols, and the other protocols indicated for specific ailments that will be presented throughout this book, are not in any way to be construed as prescriptions to cure the conditions, but as suggested nutritional components only. Each protocol was requested by physicians for specific patients, and they should only be employed under a physician's directions.

There are three important things to note about following these protocols: First, a patient's diagnosis, treatment, and medications must be considered in determining if any of the suggested vitamins, minerals, foods, and herbs are inadvisable. Special considerations should be given to pregnant and nursing mothers.

Second, each protocol must be implemented in gradual steps. Begin with low doses of one or two items of the protocol's suggested items to determine a patient's acceptance and tolerance. Once it is determined that the patient has adapted, the dosage should be increased in gradual steps.

And finally, a word about dosages. This will be repeated later, but it is extremely important. It will be given in the form of an example: If you have high cholesterol, heart disease, and hypertension, and each has a protocol calling for garlic at 1,000 milligrams, this does not mean that you are to take 3,000 milligrams. You take only the amount called for in one protocol. In other words, these protocols are not additive. Generally, you would follow the protocol for the primary condition. Let us say you have five illnesses. Take the illness that seems to be the most threatening, and follow that protocol. Once you have followed this protocol for a year, and you see the condition improving, chances are great that the other conditions are improving as well.

Your whole body, at this point, should be stronger and healthier, and your immune system should be working better. The energy-enhancing vitality of one protocol will, no doubt, help you with your other conditions. However, if you still find you need help, go to the second protocol (the one for the next troublesome condition). Try that one for a year as well. Never take three protocols for three conditions at once. That would overwhelm the system.

I also want to stress again that in suggesting alternative treatments, I am not claiming that these treatments are absolute cures, only that they can have some beneficial effect on the conditions. I am not asking you to give up whatever your doctor is suggesting, if you decide to go with any of these protocols. These are complementary, augmentative treatments. That is why they should be followed under medical supervision.

Baseline Wellness Program

The following baseline wellness protocol is a one-size-fits-all program of supplementation based on the work I did in health support groups and represents one of the pillars of my Wellness Model. You should work with your doctor to make sure that the supplements listed below are right for you. This is particularly important if you are taking any medications. Moreover, you should not be taking all these supplements at once.

Vitamin A	15,000 IU
Vitamin C	2–10,000 mg
Vitamin D	1–5,000 IU
Vitamin E	4–800 IU
Vitamin B1	75 mg
Vitamin B2	50 mg
Vitamin B3	150 mg
Vitamin B6	50 mg
Folic Acid	800 mcg
Vitamin B12	1 mg
Vitamin K	2 mg
Biotin	400 mcg
Pantothenic Acid	500 mg

Calcium	600 mg
Iodine	10 mcg
Magnesium	600 mg
Zinc	20 mg
Manganese	25 mg
Chromium	200 mcg
Selenium	100 mcg
Molybdenum	125 mcg
Potassium	100 mg
Copper	2 mg
Astaxanthin	25 mg
L-Carnosine	1,000 mg
Rosemary Leaf Powder	25 mg
Tocotrienols	25 mg
Raspberry Leaf Powder	5 mg
Citrus Bioflavonoid	300 mg
Rutin	25 mg
Red Wine Concentrate	100 mg
Grape Skin Extract	150 mg
Decaffeinated China Green Tea Leaf Powder	400 mg
Cabbage Leaf	25 mg
Carrot Root	25 mg
Para Amino Benzoic Acid	200 mcg
Mushroom Complex	300 mg
Milk Thistle Leaf Extract	25 mg
Bilberry Fruit Powder	25 mg
Lycopene	20 mg
Grape Seed Extract	150 mg
Coenzyme Q10	300 mg
Quercetin	1000 mg
Ginkgo Biloba Leaf Powder	150 mg
Broccoli	300 mg
Acerola berry	200 mg
Hesperedin	100 mg

Glutathione	500 mg
Linolenic Acid	100 mg
Ginger Rhizome Extract	100 mg
Superoxide Dismutase	25 mg
Alpha-Lipoic Acid	600 mg
Trimethylglycine	200 mg
Phosphatidylserine	200 mg
Isoflavone Genistein	200 mg
Inositol	250 mg
Lutein	25 mg
Citrus Bioflavonoids	300 mg
Methylsulfenyl Methane	400 mg
L-Taurine	500 mg
N-Acetyl Cysteine	500 mg
Orthinine Alpha Ketoglutarate	500 mg
Choline Bitartrate	500 mg
Phosphatidyl Choline	500 mg
Acetyl L-Carnitine	500 mg
Bromelain	15 mg

Supplements for Best Brain Health

Supplemental vitamins and minerals, as well as smart nutrients and drugs, can be extremely beneficial to brain health when used in combination with a healthful diet. Keeping track of the proper dosages can be difficult. To help you in that goal, I have provided the following chart that summarizes the supplement program I recommend.

The plan that follows is intended to promote brain health and protect your brain. When recommending protocols for specific conditions, as I do later in this book, I am assuming that you are already following the supplement program in the chart that follows.

Again, do not combine this protocol with any other protocol from this book. If you are taking medications, or have any food restrictions, you should consult with your doctor before beginning this or any supplement program. Supplement overdoses are rare, but possible, and certain combinations may affect individuals adversely.

VITAMINS AND NUTRIENTS	DAILY DOSE	COMMENTS
Acetyl L-carnitine (ACL)	2,000 mg in two divided doses	
Alpha-lipoic acid	300 mg in two divided doses	
B-complex vitamins	• 100 mg thiamin (B1) • 50 mg riboflavin (B2) • 100 mg niacin (B3) • 300 mg pantothenic acid (B5) • 75 mg pyridoxine (B6) • 250 mg inositol (B8) • 800 mcg folic acid (B9) • 1 mg vitamin B12 • 60 mcg biotin • 200–300 mg trimethylglycine (TMG) • 500 mg choline • 100 mg para-aminobenzoic acid	A B-complex vitamin should contain the dosages I recommend.
Carnosine	1,000 mg	
Coenzyme Q10 (coQ10)	100–300 mg with meals	
Dehydroepiandrosterone (DHEA)	25–50 mg	Must be prescribed by health practitioner. Individuals with hormone-related cancers should not take DHEA.
Dimethylaminoethanol (DMAE)	150 mg	May be overstimulating for some people. Headaches, muscle tension, and irritability may occur. Do not take if you have epilepsy, a history of

		convulsions, or bipolar disorder. If you have kidney or liver disease, consult your doctor before taking this supplement.
Essential fatty acids (EFAs)	• 4,000 mg borage oil (equals 920 mg GLA) • 2,000 mg fish oil extract (equals 1,000 mg DHA) • 400 mg EFP	
Glycerylphosphorylcholine (GPC)	600 mg	
Hydergine	5–10 mg	
Lecithin	1 gram	About 1 heaping tablespoon of granules.
Phosphatidylcholine	500–1,000 mg	
Phosphatidylserine (PS)	300 mg	Do not use if you have a bipolar disorder. Do not use if you suffer from depression.
Pregnenolone	50 mg	Individuals with hormone-related cancers should not take pregnenolone.
Proanthocyanidins	200 mg	Naturally occurring in grape seed extract and pine bark extract.
Selenium	200 mcg	
Vinpocetine	10 mg two times daily with meals	

Vitamin C	1–8,000 mg	
Vitamin E	• 4-800 IU • 200 mg (gamma tocopherol) • 65 mg (palm oil–derived tocotrienols)	Mixed tocopherols with an emphasis on gamma.

II.

Specific Health Concerns

Chapter 17

Addiction

The recent public battles with addiction of high-profile celebrities, including Whitney Houston, Lindsay Lohan, and Amy Winehouse, have opened many people's eyes to the growing problem of drug and alcohol problems among women. According to a 2012 article published in *Psychology Today*, an estimated 2.7 million American women are substance abusers. Other addiction problems may involve caffeine, sugar, and food. Although women tend to fare better than men in treatment, they are often less likely to get themselves the help they need.

General Considerations

There are a number of alternative approaches to beating addiction, including detoxification, hypnotherapy, and diet/nutrition.

DETOXIFICATION

Detoxification is a process whereby the body is cleansed of the toxins created by the addictive substance. Dr. Elson Haas is a practicing integrated medical physician and the director of the Preventive Medical Center in San Rafael, California. He is the author of several best-selling books on health and nutrition, including *The Detox Diet*. Dr. Haas describes the best times to detox: "Right now, I'm on day six of my twenty-fifth annual spring cleanse, so I've been doing juices and broth. I usually cleanse in spring. That's one of the best times. Seasonal change times are usually fraught with problems, and a cleanse can help a person. Going into autumn is another good time.

In embarking on a detox program, there are other considerations besides the seasonal. It may be a good idea to begin when you experience congestive problems or are having regular headaches or sluggish intestines. Dr. Haas adds, "Other good times to start are when allergies are kicking up, when blood pressure is getting too high and the cholesterol is rising. Those are times when I, as a physician, would use detoxification as one of my medical treatments. When I see people who have problems of toxicity and congestion, and other things stemming from or related to addictions, I see that detoxification works better therapeutically than almost anything I can do for them. So we have both the time of the year and also the individual time for people when it's appropriate."

Various levels of detoxification can be used. Juice cleanses, dietary changes, drinking more water, getting more exercise, and doing steams or saunas may all help in the detoxification process.

Dr. Haas's prescription for the type of detox regimen to follow depends on a person's level of toxicity. "If you treat somebody too extremely," he explains, "and she has too much toxicity, then she'll have more symptoms come up and more problems. In any kind of diet change—and the detox diet particularly—there's usually a couple of days of transition during which, as you're starting the diet, you may feel headachy, a cold, irritable. Usually by the third day, you start to click in. It's much like aerobic exercise. The first few minutes are difficult, but as soon as you get into that aerobic state, you think, 'Wow, this feels good. I'm moving forward.'"

Note, however, that people who are pregnant, convalescing from illness, or taking medications, as well as those who have diabetes, hypoglycemia, mental problems, or metabolic imbalances should not undertake any type of cleansing program unsupervised. First they must determine that any proposed supplements or juices are not contraindicated by their medical program. During the program, if the person becomes weak, faint, or dizzy, she should have a protein drink made of high-quality soy- or rice-based protein containing anywhere from 20 to 35 grams of protein. Grains such as brown rice, millet, or barley, beans, or a serving of fish may help while cleansing to maintain blood sugar. Eating these foods does not detract from the cleansing program.

Dr. Haas says detox is broadly helpful. "Anybody," he says, "can benefit from a detox program if it is done in the right way at the right time. That's why I wrote *The Detox Diet*, to show people how they can take very simple steps that most anybody can handle. The detox diet provides nutrition for people with fruits and grains and vegetables, which provide many vitamins and minerals. With this diet, you are being nourished while you are detoxing."

HYPNOTHERAPY

Another health practitioner with experience dealing with addictions is Michael Ellner, a medical hypnotherapist and co-author, with Dr. Richard Jamison, of *Quantum Force*. His treatment begins when the addict decides she wants a change of behavior. The next step is to develop the self-confidence and self-esteem necessary to move forward.

"I use hypnotic conditioning to help the person create a shift. The shift would make the desire [for example] to be smoke-free much more important to the person than any impulse to smoke. Ordinarily, the impulse to smoke is much stronger. The hypnosis enables the person to make choices rather than respond to preconditioned reflexes."

To some people, the very word hypnosis has a stigma attached to it. Ellner comments: "If you ask fifty of the leading experts in the world about what hypnosis is, then you'd probably get fifty different answers. When I use the word hypnosis, I'm talking about a way to help a person change neurological patterns. This is done through imagery, metaphor, and the power of suggestion."

Hypnosis is actually a communication tool. "There are a number of practices that are quite popular and are in fact hypnosis, but the practitioners avoid using the word. An example would be guided meditation. Guided imagery and visualization are also forms of hypnosis. Many meditation practices are forms of self-hypnosis. I myself am working very hard to educate the public to understand the word and to appreciate that hypnosis is one of the most powerful self-help tools available."

Ellner's clients who are dealing with smoking addiction often find relief in just one session, especially if they also have some adjunct sessions with an acupuncturist. "These two systems work very well together to help a person stop smoking very quickly and with little or no withdrawal.

"With food issues, it could take between four and eight sessions. There are a lot of additional areas that have to be worked with that involve building self-esteem, building a better self-image, helping a person gain confidence."

For people with alcohol and drug addictions, Ellner tries to get the person involved in another rehab program and to act as an adjunct. "I will recommend different programs for helping a person stop using drugs and stop drinking. Then the hypnosis would take the edge off. It would give the client a higher quality of motivation."

A substance abuser may find that it's not so difficult to stay off drugs in the rehab environment, but going back home is a different story. When the person goes home, all of the things that contributed to the problem in the first place may still be there. Ellner says he could help the person address this hypnotically in such a way as to "create space and disassociate from those triggers that ordinarily lead back to the addiction."

Situational triggers produce anxiety and the anxiety says, 'Hey, I need a drink. Maybe I need a drink and a cigarette,'" says Ellner. "With the hypnosis, the same stimuli can now create a relaxation response. Instead of anxiety overwhelming the person in that situation, suddenly the person feels calm and peaceful. Suddenly, speaking to the people in front of her is as natural as taking a deep breath. The person is in the same situation, but the triggers don't provoke the same response, don't produce the old unwanted behavior. In that respect, in conjunction with a program and a support system, most people can turn these behaviors around rather quickly and dramatically."

Ellner speaks passionately about how thought processes can have a negative impact. "To me, the biggest and most dangerous addiction is toxic thinking. People are very often addicted to negative beliefs, negative opinions about themselves and the world they live in. This addiction really diminishes one's quality of life. Instead of having fun, life is always a drag. Very often, that primary addiction gives rise to all the secondary addictions that people put all their time and energy into. One of the first things I do is make people aware of the nature of toxic thinking. Then I help them do a mental detox and change the way they think.

"As part of that I use meditation, creative visualization, and other forms of hypnosis. One of the most engaging forms of hypnosis comes about when a person has some kind of creative pursuit, whether it's strumming a guitar and going into an enhanced state of consciousness, or reading a very exciting book, or taking a walk and having contact with nature. All those things are hypnotic experiences. All those things involve moving from one state of consciousness to another. I encourage a person to get very active in everyday life."

DIET/NUTRITION

Diet and nutrition are also used in addiction treatment. "When I am working as an adjunct to the acupuncturist," Ellner says, "I have the acupuncturist also do nutritional counseling. If I am not working with her, I would refer the client to a nutritionist. One of the more popular programs I recommend is to join one of Gary Null's study groups, which provides peer support and a firm education about nutritional issues and gives people something to do that is a good use of their time. This is very important in making this kind of change."

A 2011 article in *Life Extension Magazine* describes the success of Dr. Marvin (Rick) Sponaugle in treating addiction the natural way. Board certified in both anesthesiology and addiction medicine, Dr. Sponaugle uses an approach called nutritional and rapid detox in which intravenous amino acids, vitamins, and minerals are administered to address biochemical imbalances, and intravenous sedation and other medications are used to address symptoms of physical withdrawal.

Alcohol Addiction

One out of every thirteen Americans ages twenty-one and older has an addiction to alcohol. Four million American women have alcohol problems, and the number is expected to grow. Surveys conducted in 2013 found that 12.5 percent of adult women, or one out of every eight, engaged in binge drinking an average of three times per month; in teenage girls, the rate is one in five, which is nearly as high as that of boys. Alcoholism can affect all aspects of a woman's life, including health, career, and relationships. Symptoms of alcoholism include a craving for alcohol, loss of control, increased tolerance, and physical dependency.

Excessive drinking has serious negative nutritional consequences. "Alcohol doesn't have a lot of nutrients in it," Dr. Haas explains. "People will say wine has a little bit of vitamin C and some nutrients from grapes. Beer has some B vitamins. Yet the levels aren't really that significant. Alcohol is also a diuretic. It causes loss of nutrients through the urine."

Dr. Haas does not espouse teetotaling, however. "When people have a drink here or there and they are eating a healthy diet, it will not cause a problem. In fact, studies show that people who drink wine tend to have a better, more Mediterranean-like diet" and the associated better health, "whereas people who drink beer and other kinds of alcohol tend not to eat as conscientiously."

He adds, "One thing I've seen over the years is that bad habits tend to multiply. People who tend to abuse any substance, whether sugar, alcohol, nicotine, or caffeine, tend to also be less conscientious about how they take care of their bodies. They have other habits that are undermining their health."

Alcohol also irritates the liver, and people who drink more tend to consume more calories. Dr. Haas explains, "Alcohol is a sugar that gets absorbed relatively directly into the body and causes an overstimulation of insulin. Then you are dealing with problems in the whole sugar metabolism. These heavy drinkers then tend to consume less nutrient-rich foods. They get depleted that way. Those are some of the ways that alcohol endangers the body."

What is the best detox program for getting off alcohol? Dr. Haas advises, "You want a nutrient-rich program. If you have been taking a lot of alcohol, you will definitely need professional guidance and intervention to help get through the period of withdrawal." Dr. Haas finds that the best daily combination of supplements for getting off alcohol is vitamin B, vitamin C, and a combination of calcium and magnesium, which helps alleviate the agitation that accompanies withdrawal. Chromium is another substance that can help in sugar metabolism. He advises a person to take either chromium picolinate or another form of chromium. "You'll need at least 200 micrograms, which is the way they usually come in capsules. Take these a couple times a day to help with processing the sugar."

Another amino acid that can really help is L-glutamine, which affects brain chemistry. "Remember, a lot of the addictions we have are related to the opiate receptors, which oversee addiction in the brain," Dr. Haas says. "L-glutamine seems to help feed the brain the nourishment it needs. It appears to reduce both sugar cravings and alcohol cravings. It's been used successfully in several alcohol clinics for people with more serious problems. The amount of glutamine that people might use is 500 to 1,000 milligrams, two to three times a day. If you have cravings, you can take more. It's safe. I never see problems with it."

Dr. Haas does suggest that "with any amino acid or any B vitamin, you don't want to use one substance for a long time by itself because you can throw the body off balance a little bit. So if you are using the amino acid or B vitamin for more than a few weeks, you may want to use a whole complex."

The late orthomolecular psychiatrist Dr. Abram Hoffer had this advice: "For alcoholism the basic treatment starts with Alcoholics Anonymous. Bill W., the cofounder of Alcoholics Anonymous, first showed that when you added niacin to the treatment of alcoholism, you got a major response that you did not see before." Today, there are a large number of very good alcoholism treatment programs in the United States that combine AA's twelve-step approach, various social aids, good nutrition, and the right supplements.

Caffeine Addiction

Too much caffeine is bad for you, particularly over time. In the short term, it raises your blood pressure. It can also make you hyperagitated, increase anxiety, and affect sleep. In the longer term, because caffeine is a diuretic, it causes the loss of many minerals, such as calcium, magnesium, and potassium. The result of these losses is a more permanent increase in blood pressure, as well as weakened bones, and a variety of other problems. In women, Dr. Haas notes, caffeine seems to increase the incidence of all kinds of cystic problems, such as fibrocystic breast tumors and uterine fibroids. Studies on the relationship between caffeine use and cancer have produced conflicting results. However, a number of studies suggest that caffeine does increase the risk of certain types of cancer.

Dr. Haas observes that "most people, when they go off caffeine, will have some secondary effects, usually a headache, at least for twenty-four hours. Sometimes they will feel agitated or fatigued. They are going through a short-term withdrawal. If they have a very large habit, it may last forty-eight hours, but usually it's only twenty-four hours." Dr. Haas says that some people can mitigate the withdrawal headache by taking an over-the-counter aspirin, but he thinks it's better to avoid that chemical medication if possible.

Dr. Haas recommends that you begin a detox diet the day before you start getting off caffeine. You can either go cold turkey or try to reduce your intake so that over a week you get down to maybe half a cup a day or less. If you do it gradually in this way, you will have fewer symptoms. According to Dr. Haas, "Many of the withdrawal symptoms happen because of elimination of acid from the foods and chemicals that we're cutting out.

"Doing the detox diet will reduce the withdrawal. I advise that you take additional nutrients, as follows: 2,000 to 10,000 milligrams of vitamin C from calcium ascorbate, 1,200 milligrams calcium and magnesium from citrate, 400 milligrams potassium, 400 milligrams alpha lypoic acid, 200 milligrams ginkgo, 1,500 milligrams essential fatty acids, a 20-milligram capsule of cayenne pepper, 200 milligrams ginseng, 400 international units (IU) vitamin E, 500 micrograms vitamin B_{12}, and 200 milligrams nonflush niacin.

"Drinking lots of water helps. Also make sure the bowels move. Some people like caffeine because it gets their bowels to move in the morning. It stimulates the intestine's peristaltic activities. For these people caffeine withdrawal may cause constipation. Now, not moving your bowels enough can cause more toxins to back up, and you will feel worse. So it's really important to do what you can about this. Even a day or two after you go off caffeine, you might get something from the natural food store such as laxative tea or laxative tablets or find other means of cleansing the bowels."

Sugar Addiction

Many people may debate whether sugar is addictive in the same way as nicotine and alcohol, but it is definitely a hard habit to break. Dr. Haas notes: "When I talk to people about cleaning up sugar because there are so many books out now recommending lowering sugar intake and mentioning the problems with refined sugar, I find that it is an emotional problem above all. People were trained so early on that sugar is a reward. Sugar is sweet. All the love-talk words involve sugar. You're 'sweet on someone,' the person is your 'honey' or 'sweetie.' Sugar is associated with love and reward. So it's hard to break that emotional pattern."

Yet getting rid of sugar improves health. "When women who have problems with their menstrual cycle, who are irregular, who have pain, who have PMS clean that sugar out of their diets, often within a couple of months they are feeling a lot better, as long as they are taking some other nutrients," says Dr. Haas.

Not only does sugar affect behavior and moods, it is responsible for quite a few health problems. As Dr. Haas tells it, "Although some studies have refuted these findings—studies sponsored by the industry, I might add—researchers have found that sugar causes problems in kids in their focus and behavior. I think it causes increases in candida and parasites. It causes weakness in the digestive tract. Clearly, it's a cause of tooth decay. It has some causal relation to obesity, diabetes, and chronic digestion problems, as well as menstrual irregularities. It also hooks into alcohol abuse."

He has seen psychological problems that he believes had strong roots in the patient's sugar intake. "I've had a number of young women patients who came in. They were on medicine for depression and other low moods. When I interviewed them about their diet, which their psychiatrist never did, it turns out they were drinking a quart of cola or one of those heavily sweetened beverages a day. So they were getting in the neighborhood of 40 to 50 teaspoons of sugar a day. Those intakes were really influencing their moods. The women whom I've gotten to pay attention to their diets and get off sugar have been able to reduce their medicines and be more stable without these psychoactive drugs."

He echoes a theme that recurs throughout this book: "I think there's a lot to be said about how lifestyle and these habits affect our health and sanity. One of the key overall views is that when people don't feel well, they need to look at their lifestyle first and see if there are factors in the way they are living that may be contributing to their decline. Then they should look at natural remedies. Lastly, I would tell them to turn to medicines, which I still use in my practice because I think that's part of being an integrated doctor. I use any system that I think is going to be of benefit to my patients. Sometimes people do need prescription medicines to help them get out of trouble. If they lived better, however, they wouldn't be getting into that trouble in the first place."

To really eliminate sugar, he encourages people to read labels and work on cleaning up their diet as a whole. He commonly sees people who have some form of yeast infection, or candidiasis. They also have problems with moods, energy, and brain function, secondary to the yeast fermentation process in their intestinal tract, which causes toxins to get into their bodies. A key to recovery for such a person is to eliminate alcohols and sugars to stop feeding the yeast.

"Usually, within three or four days of cutting out the sugar, the person will feel a change. She doesn't have any symptoms in the way she would from alcohol withdrawal, but for the first couple of days she may feel headachy and moody. This will only last a day or two.

"Again, if you drink more water and you take your extra Bs and other supplements, you'll have a smoother transition. Typically, by the third day and definitely within the week, you'll notice smoother and more balanced energy and better brain function."

Dr. Haas is not against sweets per se. Breaking sugar addiction, he says, "doesn't mean we can never eat anything sweet. Fruits are sweet, and they are some of the purest foods we have. Most sweet foods are based on extracts from either grains, such as corn syrups, or from other plants that are naturally sweet. Overall, we just want to balance out the diet."

Food Cravings and Addictions

Jerry Dorsman makes the unusual point that food addictions are harder to kick than drug or alcohol addictions. He's a certified addiction counselor from

Oakton, Maryland, and the author of *How to Quit Drinking Without AA* and *How to Quit Drugs for Good.*

"Let me begin by saying that in my clinical experience, it is harder to get people to change their diet than to break an addiction to drugs and alcohol," Dorsman says. "I've seen statistics on this recently that show we have a 30 to 40 percent success rate for people breaking addictions to substances; but there is only about a 5 percent success rate for people who are trying to change diet and get away from bad food habits.

"The reason for this, I think, is that we have deeply ingrained addictions to food. Our body has come to expect certain foods in our diets. We have a metabolic expectation. If we don't get those foods, we begin to crave them. If you take a look at it, we've been eating foods since we've been one year old, whereas, typically, drugs or alcohol aren't started until we are in our teens or early twenties. So they have had a shorter period in which to change the body. I think it's a longer-term, more deeply ingrained pattern that creates the difficulty in changing diet."

To break food addictions, one has to get a handle on cravings. According to Dorsman, "The more balanced we can make our diet, the healthier it becomes. The addiction causes a certain imbalance in the body. The body has to be constantly prepared to metabolize this substance that it's experiencing over and over again. This creates a severe imbalance. Our natural response is to balance it. The place to start is dealing with this physical part of cravings. By changing the diet based on the contractive/expansive as well as the acid/alkaline balances, we can really begin to settle our metabolism and find greater peace based on diet alone. In fact, in my opinion, changing diet is the number-one stress-reduction technique available.

"A second way to handle cravings is to just wait it out. Most cravings, according to scientific studies, last for only about five to ten minutes. Once we know that up front, that particular piece of knowledge can help us beat the cravings. You can think to yourself, 'Hey, I just have a few minutes here to wait this out and manage it.'"

The basic difficulties in resisting cravings—and this applies to any type of addiction, from food to drugs to alcohol—can, in Dorsman's opinion, "be broken into two categories: problems that substance use caused and problems it concealed. The most common problems that substance use causes are the physical problems, because of the biological effects of the drug or alcohol or food on the body, which are very devastating at the cellular level and to the nerve cells. The problems that are concealed are emotional ones. Those are problems that, when a person drank or used drugs or binged on food, tended to go away, because the person could ignore such things as depression, anxiety, and anger. Those emotional difficulties a person ignored when drinking or drugging or bingeing will come back up when the person puts down the addictive substances."

Using Addictions to Battle Depression

If you are taking a substance because you are depressed, your depression may be physiologically induced, perhaps due to some form of brain imbalance. You might have an underactive thyroid, for example, or a blood-sugar imbalance—whether high or low blood sugar. Either of these conditions can be manifested as depression. In order to get away from the chronic feeling of emptiness that frequently accompanies depression, people will start to drink.

One of the reasons people drink is that it takes away the feelings: both the highs and the lows. It gives the drinker a sense of being in a never-never land. The same is true of many drugs. People take drugs because it gives them a euphoria they wouldn't have achieved on their own or that they may have had but could not sustain. So they keep going back to it. Once you get used to that, it's quick and easy to just stick a needle in your arm or put some form of narcotic up your nose. You drink it or ingest it. None of this helps us resolve the underlying conflict, which may be biological, psychological, or a combination of the two.

I have found that the best way to approach this is to get the person into a systematic cleansing program—and there are many—where the person actually breaks all physical addictions, and not just to one thing like sugar, but also every other thing they could be allergic to. That seems to be a major first step. The person's energy comes back. A very big thing about any addiction withdrawal is the lack of energy. So when you substitute for the energy they had been getting from the drug by giving it to the person naturally, through the body's own process of metabolism, the person feels better.

Then you start to rebuild the center of the brain with phosphatidyl serine, 500 milligrams; acetyl L-carnitine, 500 milligrams; phosphatidyl choline, 500 milligrams; and with certain herbs that are known to have an impact, such as feverfew and green tea. Also flood the body with flavonoids. The person should also juice, juice, juice, taking anywhere from four to six glasses of fresh-made organic vegetable juice a day. Within six months to a year, I have seen people who have been totally addicted clear up about 80 percent, stay off, and not come back.

Research Update

An increasing body of scientific evidence is showing the benefits of natural modalities to overall health and well-being. Following is a sample of recent peer-reviewed literature in the area of addiction.

A 2012 study published in the *Journal of Ethnopharmacology* found that ginger prevented the development of morphine analgesic tolerance and physical dependence in rats. In addition, treatment with ginger reduced almost all of the naloxone-induced withdrawal signs, including weight loss, abdominal contraction, and diarrhea. Yoga was found to have positive effects on alcohol and drug abuse in women with posttraumatic stress disorder (PTSD) in a 2014 report in the *Journal of Alternative and Complementary Medicine*. It was associated with reduced symptoms of PTSD, decreased risk of alcohol and drug use, and increased interest in psychotherapy. A 2014 study in *Evidence-Based Complementary and Alternative Medicine* concluded that acupuncture diminished withdrawal-induced behaviors in rats during protracted abstinence following chronic morphine exposure.

Chapter 18

Adrenal Fatigue

The adrenal glands are two small glands located near the top of the kidneys. They release hormones, including cortisol and adrenaline, which help regulate vital bodily functions, including metabolism, response to stress, sexual maturation, and maintaining pregnancy. Problems can occur when the glands make too many or not enough hormones. Among the adrenal disorders that are diagnosed and treated by conventional medical practitioners are Cushing's syndrome, Addison's disease, congenital adrenal hyperplasia, and tumors. But there's another disorder that is even more prevalent that has long been ignored and untreated by mainstream doctors: adrenal fatigue.

Simply put, says Dr. Martin Feldman, "adrenal fatigue is an area where traditional medicine has no clue as to what to do."

Causes

Adrenal fatigue is a collection of symptoms caused by the inability of the adrenal glands to meet the demands of emotional and/or physical stress. It can also be caused by infection.

Symptoms

Among the symptoms of adrenal fatigue are low energy, tiredness, body aches, nervousness, sleep problems, and digestive difficulties. Given that these symptoms are common to a variety of conditions, Dr. Feldman tells how to determine whether adrenal dysfunction is the culprit. "There are some symptoms, which are very, very telling, which have very high correlation with the adrenal weakness," he says.

Fatigue despite adequate sleep is a primary symptom. "You get a full night's sleep—let's say, eight hours sleep—and you wake up and you're tired," Dr. Feldman says. "Tired in the morning is a key issue regarding adrenal."

Feelings of dizziness also occur. Usually this happens when the person moves from a sitting to a standing position, or from lying down to sitting. "When we are moving from one level to another in terms of gravity, or even just bending down and standing up, we need to have that pressure modulated to fix for the change of position. The adrenals modulate much of that, so that's another very good sign if you get this type of dizziness," Dr. Feldman says.

The Ragland blood pressure test can be useful. Dr. Feldman explains the procedure: "You take your horizontal lying blood pressure. So let's say it's 115 over 70, which is a normal, fairly good pressure. This is a resting five-minute pressure. Then rapidly sit up or stand up, and retake the pressure immediately. Now when you're moving from horizontal to vertical, the blood really has to increase blood pressure to get up to the brain. You need a higher potential push against gravity. Lying down, the gravity is not important because the heart and the brain are on the same level. In a healthy person, the systolic, or upper level, is supposed to go up by at least ten points. But in many people with beginning or advanced adrenal fatigue, the pressure may actually fall or certainly won't go up. They may say, 'Oh gee, I'm getting dizzy. I've got to lie down again.' That's a very simple test. Doctors do it in America hardly at all. It gives a very important simple beginning idea of whether you have low adrenals."

Other tests include pupil response to light; saliva testing for DHEA, a major hormone produced by adrenal glands; and adrenal energy fields.

Clinical Experience

In treating adrenal fatigue, it is necessary to decrease stress, reduce the glycemic load by avoiding sugars and carbohydrates, and eliminate caffeine. Dr. Feldman recommends several vitamins and herbs, including zinc, vitamin C, vitamin B complex, vitamin E, pantothenic acid, and DHEA. Among the herbs he uses are de-glycyrrhizinated (DGL) licorice, Siberian ginseng, rhodiola, ashwagandha, sarcode, black cohosh, and chaste berry.

Dr. Raphael Kellman, a physician in New York City who has been practicing alternative and complementary medicine for two decades, tells about the importance of emotional balance in increasing energy and relieving stress. "There is a concept called over-caring. Well-caring, if it's done from the right place, will always give you more energy. It will always increase your vitality and your energy. However, when you're in a state of over-caring then it will actually be depleting. In certain situations or with certain people, it's impossible to enter into an interaction or dialogue that will be sustained with a state of caring. It ultimately will have an adverse effect on the caregiver because if you look closely, really their motivation is not pure. It's not coming from a real loving perspective. It's coming more from an ego perspective even though it looks like it's coming from a giving perspective.

"You always have to balance giving and receiving, and you can only give to somebody who is capable of receiving. If they're not capable of receiving what you want to give them, then why bother giving it to them? You've got to think about why you're trying to give when they're not capable of receiving. So it's not just about giving. It's really about balancing giving and learning to withdraw and not to give in certain situations because if you give too much and you're not in a balanced state, it will have an adverse effect on you and on your ability to withstand stress. It will ultimately adversely affect your adrenal gland and it will absolutely adversely affect your immune system and your immune system's ability to counteract disease."

Research Update

An increasing body of scientific evidence is showing the benefits of natural modalities to overall health and well-being. Following is a sample of recent peer-reviewed literature related to adrenal fatigue.

Swedish researchers reported in a 2009 study published in *Planta Medica* that repeated administration of a standard rhodiola extract reduced fatigue, increased mental concentration, and decreased cortisol response to awakening stress in patients with fatigue syndrome. Participants received 576 mg per day of the extract, and no adverse effects were noted.

Chapter 19

Alzheimer's Disease

Alzheimer's disease is the leading cause of senile dementia in this country. It is slow but progressive and wipes out many functions of the brain, especially memory. The heartbreaking tragedy of Alzheimer's disease is that it steals the person by taking away who they are.

According to *2015 Alzheimer's Disease Facts and Figures*, published by the Alzheimer's Association, 5.3 million Americans are living with the disease, nearly two-thirds of whom are women. By 2050, it is projected that as many as 14 million people in the US will have Alzheimer's. From 2000 to 2013, the number of Alzheimer's deaths increased 71 percent.

More than a century after it was first identified, the cause of Alzheimer's disease remains the subject of intense scientific scrutiny. Many experts believe that cell death as evidenced by shrinkage in the brain is related to a sticky, waxy protein called amyloid plaque, but whether the plaque causes cell death or is a by-product of it is unclear. A second feature of Alzheimer's disease is neurofibrillary tangles consisting of tau protein, an essential protein in the infrastructure of neurons. Plaques and tangles obstruct the electrical messages that allow us to think, remember, talk, and move. As neurons begin to die, the amount of acetylcholine, a crucial chemical in the brain, decreases. Acetylcholine is necessary to carry the complex messages governing reactions and movement. Thus, as Alzheimer's progresses, physical impairment begins to occur along with cognitive losses.

Causes

Alzheimer's is believed to be the result of a combination of factors. As you look at the various risk criteria outlined here, it is worth noting that many of them can be addressed proactively.

CHEMICAL RISK FACTORS

Imbalances in neurotransmitters, nutrient deficiencies, and metabolic deficits have all been implicated:

- Hyperhomocysteinemia, or high homocysteine levels, which is significantly correlated with low levels of the nutrients folic acid and vitamins B_6 and B_{12}
- Altered taurine metabolism—the body's ability to metabolize taurine, a nonessential amino acid necessary for the proper development and maintenance of the central nervous system—which may contribute to the memory loss that is characteristic of Alzheimer's when altered
- Low levels of DHEA, an adrenal hormone that declines with age
- Low levels of acetylcholine, serotonin, GABA, dopamine, and norepinephrine, which are all key neurotransmitters
- Estrogen imbalance

ENVIRONMENTAL RISK FACTORS

External factors include exposures to neurotoxins, such as mercury, lead, pesticides, and excess iron; alcohol abuse; free radical damage; and aluminum exposure.

SOCIAL RISK FACTORS

Factors such as lower levels of education, lack of social contact, poor word fluency, emotional stress and/or poor stress-coping mechanisms, and the lack of willingness to learn new information and face mental challenges have all been implicated in the development and progression of the symptoms of Alzheimer's disease.

PHYSICAL RISK FACTORS

Possible physical risk factors include advanced age, a history of Parkinson's disease or Down's syndrome, head trauma, depression, reduced blood flow, stroke, olfactory deficits, gum disease or other markers for inflammation, or coronary disease.

Diagnosis

The presence of amyloid plaques and neurofibrillary tangles are the only definitive way to make a positive diagnosis of Alzheimer's disease. Progress is being made in using advanced imaging technologies and novel biomarkers to detect disease and dementia before they reach the moderate stages. Unfortunately, even the powerful imaging tools used by doctors today cannot reliably scan for these markers. Only a brain biopsy or an autopsy can provide positive confirmation that Alzheimer's disease is the cause of an individual's dementia.

Early detection of Alzheimer's disease is extremely difficult. Most clinical diagnoses are made in patients who have already developed a considerable amount of mental difficulties. The Alzheimer's Association has developed a list of warning signs. If you or someone close to you exhibits several of the symptoms listed below, you should see a doctor for a complete examination.

- memory loss, especially forgetting names, objects, places, times and dates; and inability to recall recently learned information
- difficulty performing everyday tasks and forgetting to maintain personal hygiene
- problems with language and noticeable intellectual decline
- disorientation to time and place, and tendency to wander from home or office
- poor or decreased judgment
- problems with abstract thinking, and an inability to follow simple instructions or stay focused on a task
- misplacing objects or putting things in unusual places
- changes in mood or behavior, especially rapid, unwarranted changes in emotion
- changes in personality, exhibiting extreme confusion, suspicion, fear, or dependence
- loss of initiative, depression, excessive sleeping during daylight hours

Medical tests might include imaging scans, such as an MRI or CT; laboratory tests, such as blood and urine; neuropsychological tests, such as tests of memory, vision-motor coordination, and language function; and even a psychiatric evaluation to assess emotional factors. Some medications prescribed for other conditions can cause side effects that mimic some symptoms of Alzheimer's disease. It is important to remember that hormones are closely related to brain health. Hormone levels fluctuate with age, and the importance of consulting with an endocrinologist to assess hormone levels and balance in treating memory deterioration should not be underestimated. Hormones related to memory function include human growth hormone, vasopressin, DHEA, and pregnenolone.

Conventional Treatment

There is no cure for Alzheimer's disease. Treatment is aimed at alleviating symptoms, and halting or preventing progression of the disease. Mainstream medicine emphasizes the use of medications to improve memory and thought processes, as well as other conditions that may co-occur, such as depression, anxiety, hallucinations, or delusions. The FDA has approved use of two types of drugs to lessen or stabilize the cognitive symptoms: cholinesterase inhibitors and memantine. Although it has not approved the use of antipsychotic medications for treating associated psychosis or agitation, due to safety concerns, these drugs are often used on an off-label basis. Research funded by the National Institute of Mental Health (NIMH) to determine the risks and benefits of using antipsychotics has yielded mixed results.

Natural Therapies

Remembering and forgetting things is a perfectly normal part of daily life, but we need not fear that the extreme and progressive cognitive decline that is a symptom of Alzheimer's disease will be an inevitable part of our aging process. There are a number of things we can do to positively impact our brain health and overall mental abilities as we age. In late-stage Alzheimer's there is little that can be done to influence the mood swings, long-term memory loss, verbal outbursts, or delusions that are the hallmarks of the latest stages of the disease. There are several simple ways to prevent the onset of Alzheimer's, however, or to reduce the severity of symptoms if your doctor has diagnosed your memory loss as probable Alzheimer's disease.

Dr. Marwan Sabbagh, a board-certified neurologist and author of *The Alzheimer's Answers: Reduce Your Risks and Keep Your Brain Healthy*, is among the physicians who view Alzheimer's as a preventable disease. "The fact is that people start to develop Alzheimer's changes in their brains twenty to thirty years before their first day of forgetfulness. So by the time you are getting a little bit of 'where did I put my car keys?' you've been already accumulating changes in your brain for many, many years."

ENVIRONMENT

It is important for your environment to be free of hazardous toxins, particularly heavy metals that can accumulate in the body. High levels of aluminum and mercury are found in the brain cells of Alzheimer's patients. Limit your exposure to cookware, deodorants, antacids, and food additives that contain aluminum. Mercury is found in thermometers, thermostats, and dental amalgams. It is recommended to remove all silver fillings from your mouth. Chelation therapy—which uses certain amino acids to form strong ionic bonds with the toxic metals in your body, allowing them to be excreted from the system—may be useful in removing toxic metals and other chemicals from your body. Bentonite, a claylike substance that is used in a drink, may be taken at night to draw out toxins from the colon and assist in the detoxification process. Installing charcoal filters on all water sources used for drinking or cooking can reduce or eliminate harmful toxins that are found in the water from our reservoirs.

SOCIAL ACTIVITY

Continued community involvement and frequent contact with friends and family may reduce your risk for Alzheimer's disease. In a paper presented at the Alzheimer's Association International Conference on the Prevention of Dementia, Jane Saczynski, PhD, of the National Institute on Aging, and colleagues presented data from a longitudinal study, conducted since 1965, that showed that subjects with decreased social activity from mid- to late life had a statistically significant risk of dementia.

EXERCISE

Physical activity seems to play a role in slowing or preventing the progression of Alzheimer's. A National Institutes of Health news release cites research demonstrating that long-term physical activity increased the learning ability of mice and decreased the level of plaque forming beta-amyloid protein fragments in their brains. Remaining physically active throughout our lifetimes offers immeasurable benefits to both body and brain. Physical activity does not have to be rigorous. Walking, dancing, or practicing yoga helps safeguard our brains against the type of cognitive decline that is a symptom of Alzheimer's disease.

MEMORY SKILLS AND BRAIN BOOSTERS

In addition to an active body, it is important to have an active mind. A study published in the *New England Journal of Medicine* supports the theory that mentally demanding activities can help stave off dementia. The study involved 469 people ages seventy-five and older. Those participants who read, played games of strategy (e.g., checkers, backgammon, or chess), played musical instruments, or danced at least twice a week were significantly less likely to develop dementia. Those who did crossword puzzles four times a week were also found to have a significantly lowered risk. It seems clear that participating in mentally stimulating hobbies and being willing to learn new information and challenge our brains on an ongoing basis provide important benefits in preventing the symptoms of Alzheimer's disease.

COPING STRATEGIES

If you or someone close to you has been diagnosed as being in the early stages of Alzheimer's, there are some strategies for coping with the symptoms of memory loss that may be the first hallmarks of this disease. These coping strategies will help relieve the stress and tension that arise from memory problems and can help lessen the impact of such problems on day-to-day life. Remember, in addition to practicing the strategies outlined below, you should make the lifestyle and nutritional changes I recommend in this chapter to slow or reverse the progression of these early symptoms.

- Establish a regular routine in familiar surroundings.
- Make mental associations, such as using landmarks, to help you find things.
- Repeat names when you meet people.
- Put important items, such as your keys, in the same place every time. Label or color-code doors and exits to keep from getting disoriented. Draw a map for simple routes. Write down directions.

- Make lists, use a calendar, and keep notes of important dates and financial matters.
- Set realistic daily goals.
- Keep track of when medicines are taken; use a chart or special pill box to stay current.
- Tell your doctor about all medications or supplements you are taking. Keep a list of important names and numbers near the telephone.
- Stay in frequent contact with family and friends.

DIET

What researchers are beginning to say now is something that I have said over and over again: Deficiencies of essential nutrients can lead to a variety of health problems and leave us vulnerable to serious conditions such as Alzheimer's. The good news is that it is never too early to start good nutritional habits that will help to protect the brain over a lifetime. And it is never too late to benefit from good nutritional habits.

The best success that we have had helping people with Alzheimer's is to shift their diet to 75 percent raw and 25 percent lightly cooked. We begin with one 16-ounce glass of fresh, organic juice. The juice should have its primary volume filled with celery, cucumber, or apple. Then you can add into each different glass of juice any combination of grapes and berries. Begin with one 16-ounce glass per day for the first week. Add one additional juice per day for each additional week until you are at ten juices per day or as close to that many as possible. Juicing lettuce, radish, ginger, sprouts, and garlic also enhances its power. Supplement each juice with up to 1,500 milligrams of vitamin C (start with 500 milligrams until you achieve bowel tolerance).

Various studies support the efficacy of antioxidants as a method of preventing or reversing cognitive decline. Vitamins E and C are proven free radical fighters and are readily available in foods such as citrus fruits and juices; dark green, leafy vegetables; nuts; and sunflower seeds. The B vitamins, which play an important role in fighting the symptoms of Alzheimer's disease, are found in beans and animal proteins. Trace minerals, such as zinc, magnesium, and potassium, are easy to add to our diets by using whole grains, nuts, dried beans, bananas, and milk. Essential fatty acids (EFAs) such as omega-3 and omega-6 fats, which are found in flax oil and walnuts, have significant anti- inflammatory properties and may be important in preventing Alzheimer's. It has been suggested that a dietary deficiency in fatty acids may be a risk factor for Alzheimer's. Other studies have looked at the use of EFAs in impacting Alzheimer's and found them to be beneficial.

SUPPLEMENTS

Certain vitamins and minerals are important in fighting the symptoms of Alzheimer's disease. A number of other naturally occurring nutrients also have a beneficial impact.

MAGNESIUM. Magnesium is well known for its calming properties in people with anxiety symptoms, but proper amounts of magnesium are generally lacking in the average American diet. For impacting the symptoms of Alzheimer's, I recommend a daily supplement of 500 to 1,000 milligrams of magnesium, taken in two equal doses on an empty stomach.

POTASSIUM. Potassium is depleted from our bodies in times of stress, thus upsetting the delicate balance of neurotransmitter communication in our brains. It can interact with some drugs, so if you are taking prescription medications, consult with your doctor before taking potassium supplements. If potassium is safe for you, I recommend a daily supplement of 500 milligrams.

VITAMIN B-COMPLEX. It is important that your daily vitamin B-complex contain sufficient amounts of both vitamin B_9 and B_{12}, as deficiencies in these vitamins can develop as we age, and these deficiencies can contribute to the symptoms of Alzheimer's disease. If your doctor has determined you are deficient in B vitamins, you may want to ask about receiving intravenous or injected supplements of vitamin B-complex to combat symptoms of Alzheimer's.

VITAMIN C. Vitamin C may help delay the onset of Alzheimer's and slow the progression of symptoms. For best impact on the symptoms of Alzheimer's disease, I recommend increasing your daily supplement from 500 to 1,000 milligrams to 10,000 milligrams, taken in three divided doses. Do not exceed a daily supplement of 10,000 milligrams.

VITAMIN E. Vitamin E has beneficial antioxidant properties, and treatment with high doses has shown initial promise in slowing the progression of symptoms in individuals with moderately severe Alzheimer's. High doses may be associated with the risk of bleeding and interaction with anticoagulants and other medications often taken by elderly people. If you are not at risk, I recommend increasing your daily supplement of vitamin E from 268 milligrams to 536 milligrams, taken in two divided doses. Do not exceed a daily supplement of 536 milligrams.

ZINC. Many people who suffer from dementia have deficiencies in zinc. I recommend a daily supplement of 30 milligrams.

ACETYL-L-CARNITINE. This versatile nutrient is able to permeate the blood–brain barrier to stimulate and fortify the brain's nerve cells. Acetyl-L-carnitine is a type of carnitine produced naturally in the brain. For best impact on Alzheimer's symptoms, I recommend increasing your daily supplement from 2,000 milligrams to 3,000 milligrams, taken in three equal doses. Do not exceed a daily supplement of 3,000 milligrams.

DIMETHYLAMINOETHANOL (DMAE). This nutrient, found in sardines, is a powerful brain stimulant that increases acetylcholine, a neurotransmitter essential for short-term memory function and concentration. Some side effects associated with DMAE in Alzheimer's patients include drowsiness, high blood pressure, and increased confusion. If you experience these symptoms, stop taking the supplement for a few days, then return to your lower daily dose. I recommend increasing your daily supplement from 150 milligrams to 300 milligrams, taken in two equal doses with meals. Do not exceed a daily supplement of 300 milligrams.

L-GLUTAMINE. Glutamine is converted into glutamic acid and increases GABA, a neurotransmitter essential for proper mental function. There are two types of glutamine supplements: D-glutamine and L-glutamine. L-glutamine is the form that more closely mimics the glutamine in the body. I recommend supplementing with 500 milligrams, taken three times daily.

MELATONIN. Melatonin is a hormone manufactured by the pineal gland in the brain. It is involved in synchronizing the body's hormone secretions and setting daily biorhythms. To stabilize the sleeping cycle for Alzheimer's patients, I recommend supplementing with 300 micrograms to 1 milligram, taken nightly a half hour before bed.

N-ACETYLCYSTEINE (NAC). This amino acid protects the brain from damaging free radicals by boosting quantities of glutathione, one of the body's most powerful antioxidants. I recommend a supplement of 500 milligrams, taken three times daily.

NICOTINAMIDE ADENINE DINUCLEOTIDE (NADH). An enzyme that helps improve neurotransmitter function, NADH is present in all living cells and plays a critical role in energy production. It helps prevent cellular degeneration and may increase concentration and memory capacity. I recommend a supplement of 2.5 milligrams, taken twice a day for two or three days of the week.

PHOSPHATIDYLSERINE (PS). PS helps the brain use fuel more efficiently. Studies have revealed that supplementing with phosphatidylserine slows down and even reverses declining memory and concentration, or age-related cognitive impairment, in middle-aged and elderly subjects. For impact on memory loss, I recommend increasing your daily supplement from 300 milligrams to 400 milligrams. Do not exceed a daily supplement of 400 milligrams.

S-ADENOSYLMETHIONINE (SAME). SAMe promotes cell growth and repair and maintains levels of glutathione, a major antioxidant that protects against free radicals and reduces homocysteine levels. Alzheimer patients have extremely low levels of SAMe in their brains. SAMe should not be taken if you are taking MAO inhibitor antidepressants. I recommend a daily supplement of 400 to 1,600 milligrams daily, taken in four equal doses.

Also recommended are omega-3 fatty acids (2000 mg), EPA/DHA with sesame lignans, olive extract, krill, astaxanthin, PQQ (20mg), Magnesium L-Threonate (150mg), L-Carnitine tartrate (500mg), curcumin rhizome extract (700mg, 3x day), cytokine suppress (300mg), EGCG (green tea, 300 mg), black cumin seed oil (1 tsp, 3x day), coconut oil (1tsp, 2x day), probiotics (5 billlion, 2x day).

HERBAL REMEDIES

Some herbal extracts and homeopathic treatments have properties similar to conventional medications, but are gentler and may lack the drugs' side effects. Always inform your medical practitioner of any herbal remedies you may be taking.

- Butcher's broom is an herb that promotes clearer focus and enhanced memory. I recommend a daily supplement of 850 milligrams, taken in two equal doses.

- Bacopa monnieri is a potent antioxidant that has been used in Ayurvedic medicine for centuries as a brain tonic to enhance memory, learning, development, and concentration. I recommend a daily supplement of 200 to 400 milligrams, taken in two equal doses.

- Ginkgo biloba is a potent antioxidant that may be beneficial in impacting dementia-related symptoms by stabilizing abnormal neurotransmitter communication in the brain. If ginkgo is safe for you to take, for prevention of Alzheimer's disease I recommend a daily supplement of 120 milligrams, taken in two equal doses.

- Kami Untan To (KUT) has been used for centuries in Japan to combat neuropsychiatric problems. KUT is a blend of thirteen different herbs and should be taken as directed by the manufacturer.

- Huperzine A is a compound isolated from a Chinese herb called *Hyperzia serrata*. It increases acetylcholine activity in the cortex and hippocampus sections of the brain, and aids in improving memory as well as cognitive and behavioral functions. I recommend taking a daily supplement of 100 to 200 micrograms in two equal doses.

- St. John's wort (hypericum) is very popular in Europe, so much so that it is actually covered by German health insurance as a prescription drug. I recommend taking a daily supplement of 300 milligrams twice per day.

- Vinpocetine is a derivative of an extract taken from the periwinkle shrub. It enhances circulation to the brain and may prevent or improve mild cognitive impairment. I recommend taking 10 milligrams twice daily with meals.

HOMEOPATHIC REMEDIES

The following remedies may be used to impact the symptoms of Alzheimer's. When dealing with a chronic condition, homeopathic remedies must be used in conjunction with other therapies, as prescribed by a qualified health professional. Consult with your health care provider before taking any homeopathic remedy, and follow their recommendation for the appropriate dosage. Always inform your medical practitioner of any homeopathic remedies you may be taking.

- Alumina is indicated for dealing with great weakness or loss of memory in cases where consciousness of personal identity is confused.
- Anacardium is used for absentmindedness; memory for names is most affected
- Calcarea may help when the person is elderly, is wandering, and finds words difficult to remember.
- Sulphur can be used when there is difficulty remembering words or names.
- Curcumin, an extract from the spice turmeric, contains powerful anti-inflammatory properties that have been studied extensively in recent years. Research suggests that this compound inhibits the buildup of amyloid plaque in Alzheimer's patients. I recommend taking a daily supplement of 400 to 800 milligrams. Do not take if you have gallbladder problems or gallstones. Consult with your doctor if taking anti- coagulant or anti-platelet medications or have a bleeding disorder.
- Fish Oil's essential fatty acids are vital to healthy brain function. Studies demonstrate that these fats exert neuroprotective effects on the brain and may help slow the progression of Alzheimer's Disease. I recommend taking a purified fish oil supplement containing 1400 milligrams of EPA and 1000 milligrams of DHA daily. Consult with your doctor if taking anti-coagulant or anti-platelet medications or have a bleeding disorder.

■ Resveratol, an antioxidant found in grapes and red wine, may help curb Alzheimer's Disease and dementia. It has been shown to selectively target toxic amyloid plaque in brain tissue. I recommend a daily dose of 250 milligrams. Consult with your doctor if taking anticoagulant or anti-platelet medications or have a bleeding disorder.

AROMATHERAPY

Essential oils can be used in baths or inhaled to provide an energizing or soothing effect. Do not apply essential oils directly to the skin; they must be mixed with carrier oils. Experiment with various scents to see which help to alleviate the symptoms of Alzheimer's and increase mental clarity: bergamot, clove, frankincense, lavender, and lemon balm.

Research Update

An increasing body of evidence is showing the benefits of natural modalities to overall health and well-being. Following is a sample of recent peer-reviewed scientific studies in the area of Alzheimer's disease.

According to 2015 research published in *Clinical Pharmacology and Therapeutics*, cannabinoids decreased neuroinflammation, oxidative stress, and formation of amyloid plaque and neurofibrillary tangles in people with late onset Alzheimer's disease. In a 2015 report in the *European Journal of Medical Chemistry*, scientists demonstrated that derivatives of scutellarein-O-alkylamine, a natural flavone, had multifunctional properties in the treatment of Alzheimer's disease, including metal chelating ability, acetylcholinesterase inhibition, and antioxidation.

A comprehensive study released in 2011 by researchers at the Oregon Health and Science University in Portland and the Linus Pauling Institute showed that seniors who consumed a diet high in the B vitamins, as well as vitamins, C, D and E, performed significantly better on mental ability tests and exhibited less brain shrinkage than did those who ate a poorer diet. The results also suggested that higher consumption of omega-3 fatty acids improves the health of the brain, while eating trans-fats has the opposite effect. A 2012 study at Brown University that found that excess levels of insulin resulting from a diet rich in fatty and sugary foods decrease the brain's response to the hormone and, in turn, disrupt normal cognitive function. Studies published in the *Journal of Alzheimer's Disease* in 2012 revealed that vitamin D3 and curcumin worked synergistically to help eliminate the buildup of amyloid, and that low blood serum levels of vitamin C and beta-carotene were associated with a higher incidence of mild dementia among seniors.

In research presented at the 2012 Alzheimer's Association International Conference, a group from Japan's National Center for Geriatrics and Gerontology shared new data showing that routine aerobic, strength, and balance exercise over the course of a year significantly improved language skills in adults with mild cognitive impairment over age forty-seven. Another study presented by researchers at the University of British Columbia found that just six months of resistance training exercise boosted objective measurements of attention and memory in women ages seventy to eighty.

A 2012 analysis undertaken by a team at the University of California, Berkeley, found that those individuals who were mentally active over the course of their lives had significantly less buildup of the beta-amyloid protein.

Chapter 20

Anemia

More than three million people in the United States have anemia, with women and those with chronic illness at greatest risk. Anemia is a health condition characterized by red blood cells deficient in hemoglobin, the portion of the blood containing iron. Hemoglobin enables the blood to transport oxygen from the lungs and circulate it throughout the body, and to carry away carbon dioxide. The listlessness, pallor, and shortness of breath experienced by a person with anemia reflect a lack of oxygen and buildup of carbon dioxide in the tissues.

Causes

Dr. Dahlia Abraham, a complementary physician from New York City, describes three major classifications of anemia, each of which is associated with a specific cause:

EXCESSIVE BLOOD LOSS—This can result from conditions such as hemorrhoids and a slowly bleeding peptic ulcer, or in association with menstruation.

EXCESSIVE RED BLOOD CELL DESTRUCTION—Dr. Abraham explains: "Normally, old and abnormal red blood cells are removed from the circulation. If the rate of destruction exceeds that of manufacture of new cells, anemia can result. A number of factors can cause excessive red blood cell destruction, such as defective hemoglobin synthesis, injury, and trauma within the arteries."

NUTRITIONAL DEFICIENCIES OF IRON, VITAMIN B12, AND FOLIC ACID—This is the most common type of anemia, with iron deficiency the most frequent.

Dr. Abraham further explains: "People require extra iron during growth spurts in infancy and adolescence. Pregnancy and lactation are other times when women need iron supplementation. During the childbearing years, many women experience anemia caused by an iron deficiency."

Do supplements help? "Supplementation may not solve the problem because many people have difficulty absorbing iron," Dr. Abraham says. "They lack enough hydrochloric acid, the stomach acid that helps the body assimilate iron. This is common among the elderly, who generally produce less hydrochloric acid." Chronic diarrhea also may cause decreased iron absorption.

A defect in absorption is the most common cause of a vitamin B_{12} deficiency. Dr. Abraham remarks, "Vitamin B_{12} must be liberated from food by hydrochloric acid and bound to a substance called intrinsic factor, which is also secreted in the stomach. For B_{12} to be absorbed, then, an individual must secrete enough hydrochloric acid and enough intrinsic factor." For this type of anemia, supplements of vitamin B_{12}, hydrochloric acid, and intrinsic factor may help.

A deficiency in folic acid may also cause anemia. Alcoholics and pregnant women are particularly at risk. "Folic acid is vital for cell production in the growing fetus and prevents birth defects, such as neural tube imperfections," Dr. Abraham says. "This is why prenatal vitamins must contain this nutrient. In addition, a number of pharmaceutical drugs, such as anticancer drugs and oral contraceptives, can drain the body of folic acid."

Dr. Pat Gorman, an acupuncturist and educator in New York City, explains anemia and other blood disorders in women from an Asian perspective. "In women, blood has an actual cycle that rises and falls every month. There is a building phase that occurs for about a week after the menstrual period. Then there is a peak phase where the blood reaches its richest moment; that's the moment you ovulate. This is followed by a storage phase. (If you are pregnant, the blood is stored.) A week before the period, you go through a cleansing phase where your organs release toxins into the blood. That's the week before your period, when you can go through a PMS hell if the toxins are not being properly released. Next is the purging of the actual period."

Using this philosophy as her framework, Dr. Gorman holds that women become anemic when they are out of touch with their monthly cycles. In a fast-paced society, one of the major reasons for this condition is that women do not rest at the appropriate times. "Women work all the time. They show no vulnerability and just keep on going no matter what. There is no respect for the actual rhythm of the cycle. I believe that we need to bring back the menstrual hut. When you are bleeding, you need to stop working for a day or two. I know I am saying things that sound impossible, but if you have anemia—and 60 to 70 percent of the women I see do—you need to face the fact and work with it."

Another major reason women become anemic is that they approach pregnancy incorrectly: "There is a law called the one-month, one-year law," Dr. Gorman says. After a pregnancy is terminated, whether by abortion, miscarriage, or birth, one month of absolute rest is needed. Women say, 'That's not possible. I just gave birth, but I have other children. I have to take care of things.' The Chinese say this is a straight road to a severe problem with anemia.

"The one-year aspect is the avoidance of pregnancy for at least another year. Women who try to conceive and who then miscarry often frantically begin again. They need to build up the blood for an entire year's cycle before trying to conceive again. It is very difficult for me to help anxious patients relax and understand that this is the way to overcome anemia and to have a really healthy baby."

Additionally, Dr. Gorman warns that birth control pills disturb the integrity of the blood's cycle. They trick the body into believing that it is continuously pregnant by locking blood into its storage phase. By eliminating the cycle of building, peaking, storing, cleansing, and purging, oral contraceptives may create many problems.

Symptoms

The general symptoms of anemia are weakness and a tendency to tire easily. When there is a vitamin B_{12} deficiency, the symptoms may also include paleness; shortness of breath; a sore, red, swollen tongue; diarrhea; heart palpitations; and nervous disturbances.

Clinical Experience

DIAGNOSIS

According to Dr. Abraham, the treatment of anemia is dependent on proper clinical evaluation by a physician. Too often, physicians assume that anemia is caused by an iron deficiency, but this is just one possible reason. "It is absolutely imperative that a comprehensive laboratory analysis of the blood be performed. Do not be satisfied when your physician offers a simple diagnosis of anemia," she warns. "Insist that your doctor investigate the underlying causes."

While Dr. Gorman agrees that clinical studies help confirm the diagnosis, she adds that Asian physicians are trained to detect anemia and other blood disorders through observation: "In Chinese medicine, you examine the body. Look at your tongue. Is it pale? Look at your lips. Are they pale? See if the mucous membranes under the eyes are pale. These signs indicate whether you are anemic."

DIETARY REMEDIES

Green, leafy vegetables are high in iron and folic acid. It is best to purchase organic vegetables, since pesticides interfere with absorption. Eating vegetables raw or lightly cooked preserves their folic acid content. Soy or shoyu sauce, miso (a fermented soybean paste), and tempeh (another soybean preparation) are rich sources of vitamin B_{12}.

Proteins should be eaten every day, preferably vegetarian proteins such as those from grains and legumes such as rice and beans or oatmeal with soy milk. When animal protein is eaten, it should be from fish. Caffeine and alcohol are detrimental to healthy blood and should be eliminated.

Also recommended are wheat grass, barley grass, chlorellla, and spirulina (2 ounces, 2x day).

SUPPLEMENTS

According to Dr. Abraham, iron, vitamin B_{12}, and folic acid should be prescribed as needed. Additionally, hydrochloric acid and intrinsic factor are often required to aid the absorption of these nutrients.

Naturopath Dr. Tori Hudson, in a column in *Prevention* magazine, advises that iron citrate and iron aspartate are forms of iron supplementation that are less likely to cause constipation. She suggests taking 1,000 to 3,000 milligrams of vitamin C with the iron to enhance absorption.

HERBS

Dr. Janet Zand, a naturopathic physician, acupuncturist, and doctor of traditional Chinese medicine, in an article posted on the HealthWorld Online website (www.healthy.net), suggests an herbal program that anemic women can use to build the blood. It is meant to accompany iron and iron-synergistic nutrient supplementation as directed by a health care practitioner. Dr. Zand bases her herbal regimes for women on the shifting hormonal balance over the four weeks of the menstrual cycle.

During all four weeks of the cycle, red raspberry leaf and dong quai are used to build blood and balance hormones. These herbs can be taken as a tea, tincture, capsule, or tablet three times a day. Then, during the specified weeks, one also takes the herbs listed below:

FIRST WEEK—Take yellow dock leaf (*Rumex crispus*) and chlorophyll as a tea or tincture three times a day.

SECOND WEEK—Take American ginseng (*Panax quinquefolius* root), a blood builder, as a tea or tincture three times a day.

THIRD WEEK—Take nettle (*Urtica dioica* leaf) and chlorophyll as a tea or tincture three times a day.

FOURTH WEEK—Take alfalfa (*Medicago sativa* leaf), with chlorophyll as a tea or tincture three times a day.

AYURVEDA

Swami Sadashiva Tirtha, who founded one of the first certification programs on Arurveda, says that practitioners of Ayurvedic medicine consider anemia an imbalance of the blood that can have a number of causes. Too many sour, salty, or hot foods; drinking alcohol; poor nutrition; injury; excessive menstruation or bleeding; liver disorders; pregnancy; excessive sexual activity; and fevers are all factors that can cause a disorder in the kidneys, blood, and ojas (life force) and lead to anemia.

Swami Sadshiva recommends certain foods that help build blood. These foods include organic milk, pomegranate or black grape juice, boiled black sesame seeds, and molasses. Otherwise, people should follow the diet that is appropriate for their body type, according to Ayurvedic guidelines. Ayurveda uses meat as a medication only when anemia is extremely severe.

Women should use blood-building herbs after the menstrual period. To properly assimilate iron supplements, take them with ginger or cinnamon. You can take two or three teaspoonfuls of chyavan prash twice daily with warm milk as well as turmeric and ghee.

Aloe vera gel and triphala are very gentle laxatives that regulate the bowels and thus can help remove excess bile from the liver, a common reason for thinning of the blood. Other Ayurvedic herbs used to treat anemia are saffron, shatavari, manjishtha, and punarnava.

PATIENT STORY

I was born in Nicaragua, and I used to be a very healthy person. [One day] I went to the emergency room. My hemoglobin was down to 2.8; the normal count for a woman is between 12 and 14. There I was with aplastic anemia, meaning that my bone marrow was not making any blood cells: no red cells, no white cells, no platelets. I almost had no blood.

The doctor said that my sickness was idiopathic, meaning that they didn't know what caused it. They said that one possible cause was the use of an antibiotic. But the only time I had ever taken one was fifteen years earlier. Another possible cause was exposure to chemicals or pesticides. A lot of towns in Nicaragua are surrounded by cotton plantations where cotton growers use a lot of pesticides to spray their crops.

I was referred to a bone marrow transplant unit and was put on a medication, a kind of chemotherapy. After one month of treatment, the medication failed to work. Then the doctors wanted to do a bone marrow transplant. I have seven siblings, so I had donors, and one of them was a perfect match. But I had reservations. A bone marrow transplant is very costly. Also, you get bone marrow that is working, but because of the chemotherapy or radiation, your liver, kidneys, pancreas, and so forth, pay a terrible toll.

Before my sickness I was following a macrobiotic diet. I was starting to use alternative medicine, and I knew about the power of the body to heal itself. I decided to stay on my macrobiotic diet and was able to more or less clean myself of the chemotherapy. During this time I did not even get a cold. I didn't sneeze through all my sickness.

I was clean, but my blood counts were still very low. I needed a transfusion every ten days. The transfusions were very helpful, and I was grateful to be able to get them. But through transfusions I was also receiving a lot of genetic and other information completely foreign to my body. I could not control what the person who donated that blood was eating. So I was trying to clean my body of toxins, and I decided to look for help.

I went to a naturopath, who helped me a lot. Then I read an article on Ayurveda. It said that Ayurveda is very specific, even with the use of grains and vegetables. There are grains and vegetables that are not appropriate for your body type. I went to an Ayurvedic doctor. He gave me a very gentle treatment consisting of diet, aromatherapy, massage, and meditation. After three weeks of following that treatment, my blood count went up for the first time.

I keep up with this treatment still. My last checkup at the hospital showed normal white cells. Red cells were a little bit low. They were 3.83, and the normal count is 4. But they are increasing day by day. My energy level is excellent. I went back to work three months ago and am now leading a completely normal life. I am very grateful to Ayurveda.

—Yolanda

Research Update

An increasing body of evidence is showing the benefits of natural modalities to overall health and well-being. Following is a sample of recent peer-reviewed scientific studies in the area of anemia.

A 2010 cross-sectional study in *Annals of Hematology* confirmed the suspected link between vitamin D deficiency and anemia. In 2013, researchers from the Johns Hopkins Children's Center reported in the *Journal of Pediatrics* that examination of blood samples from more than 10,000 children revealed that vitamin D levels of 30 nanograms per milliliter or less nearly doubled the risk of developing the condition. According to a 2010 report in the *Journal of Nutrition*, a micronutrient supplement taken two times per week for twenty-six weeks significantly increased hemoglobin levels in girls with nutritional anemia. In 2011, *BMC Public Health* showed that pregnancy outcomes were similarly affected. A case report and literature review in the *Journal of Pediatric Hematology and Oncology*, also in 2011, found that high dose vitamin D supplements completely eliminated pain symptoms in a patient with sickle cell anemia. Several other studies have documented the oxidative stress-reducing activity of N-acetylcysteine (NAS) in patients with anemia.

Chapter 21

Anxiety

According to 2015 data from the National Institute of Mental Health, more than 40 million American adults experience an anxiety disorder over their lifetime, with women 60 percent more likely than men to be affected. Anxiety disorders include generalized anxiety disorder, panic disorder, and social phobia. They often co-occur with other mental and/or physical conditions. Although each disorder has a different set of symptoms, common to them all are excessive, irrational fear, and dread.

"A good definition of anxiety is that it is abnormal and overwhelming sense of apprehension or fear of misfortune that can be accompanied by physiologic signs like increased sweating, heart pounding, and muscle tension," says Dr. Marcey Shapiro, a board-certified family physician specializing in integrative medicine, and the author of *Freedom from Anxiety: A Holistic Approach to Emotional Well-Being*. "But I prefer the Buddhist teacher, Thich Nhat Hanh's, explanation of anxiety, which is: anxiety, the illness of our times, comes primarily from our inability to dwell in the present moment. I prefer that because that kind of shows us a way out the door of anxiety."

Mainstream medicine seeks to alleviate anxiety by using drugs to calm the nervous system. Unfortunately, as Dr. John Douillard, Ayurvedic physician and author of *Body, Mind and Sport*, explains, "Giving a sedative in this situation will only suppress symptoms and may deplete the nervous system further, making the situation chronic." Instead of being depleted, "the nervous system must be built up and rejuvenated so that it can put itself to sleep, stabilize its energy and moods, and stay that way." Recent scientific studies have shown the value of the natural approach: omega-3 fatty acids, magnesium, and adaptogenic herbs such as rhodiola can help the body deal with anxiety by harnessing its stress response mechanisms, and the B vitamins and amino acids can help with neurotransmitter synthesis and signaling.

Causes

Anxiety can have many different causes. Psychiatrist Helen Derosis, author of *Women and Anxiety*, talks about external pressures on people who lead busy lives and have never learned to plan properly and set priorities: "Practically everyone I encounter in this country is anxious to some extent. One can be slightly anxious or very anxious, anxious occasionally or continuously. The most devastating type involves being anxious all the time over the little things we have to do every day. People worry that somehow things will not turn out right for them."

Dr. Derosis continues, "A woman about twenty-five years old came to me who was very bright and educated and was working for a large TV company. She wanted to be a producer, but was only a gofer, though at a very good salary. She was very upset, disappointed, and angry. She would cry to her husband every night when he got home. Yet as soon as she realized it wasn't possible to achieve that goal so quickly and saw that life was not as easy as she thought, she calmed down.

"Earlier, a doctor or psychiatrist would have treated her with Valium and said her problems were not real, all in her head. Remembering those older treatments, a patient will come in today asking for medication, which is not a solution. Getting over anxiety involves growing. If you can keep growing, you will have problems, but the constant activity of being alive, thinking about what you want to do next, and planning how to achieve it will keep you from being bogged down in anxiety."

ENVIRONMENT

Dr. Shapiro tells about her recent research on the impact of the environment on our genes. "There's a constant barrage of environmental toxins that we are exposed to that can turn on different genes, and make it more difficult to overcome depression and anxiety," she says. She has been focusing on catechol-O-methyltransferase (COMT), a protein-coding gene that is involved in breaking down hormones such as epinephrine and norepinephrene. "Those things are associated with fight or flight, so when people have a gene mutation for COMT, and that is turned on by environmental factors or emotional milieu, then it's very difficult to break down fight or flight hormones."

GLUCOSE METABOLISM

From the perspective of orthomolecular psychiatry, practically any nutritional deficiency that affects the mind—and almost all do in one way or another—can cause anxiety as a symptom.

A glucose tolerance test is important in determining whether sugar is being properly metabolized. Anxiety attacks can occur when sugar levels get too low, as in hypoglycemia. Hypoglycemia can also cause a rebound effect when adrenaline is secreted to raise blood sugar levels. This adrenaline rush also causes anxiety. Orthomolecular psychiatrist Dr. Michael Lesser checks out sugar tolerance "rather than getting involved immediately in looking for Oedipal or pre-Oedipal fantasies," because in a recent review of his cases he found that 92 percent of people with neuroses had abnormalities in the glucose tolerance test.

Dietary recommendations based on the results of a glucose tolerance test may help a patient far more effectively, quickly, and safely than either psychotherapy or drug treatment will. The main objective is to create stability so that sugar levels neither drop nor rise too sharply or rapidly. For a person with hypoglycemia, a high-protein diet is recommended by Dr. Lesser because it digests very slowly, sending just a small trickle of sugar into the bloodstream so that the blood sugar is kept stable for a long period of time. Then, when the patient eats frequently, the blood sugar remains stable. "I have these patients eat six or seven times a day, small snacks so as not to put on weight," he reports. "Actually, they can handle more calories than they could if they were eating one, two, or three large meals a day because the body is set up to metabolize the small meals frequently. When you have a large meal, you cannot metabolize all that nutrition, and the body turns a portion of that into fat."

DIGESTION

Dr. Walt Stoll, a board-certified family practitioner who combines his traditional Western training with holistic healing practices, has found that anxiety disorders are often linked to an inability to completely break down proteins during the digestive process into their amino acids.

"Just three or four amino acids still hooked together (peptides), if they get through the intestinal lining, can stimulate the immune system to make antibodies against them. Since the body is also made up of peptides hooked together to make proteins, these antibodies can attack us. To an antibody, a peptide is a peptide. It frequently doesn't matter whether the peptide came from outside the body or is a part of the body. It is now being found that many of the chronic diseases that are so baffling to the allopathic disease philosophy of conventional Western medicine are related to autoimmune processes.

"In addition, some of these peptides have been found to be identical to certain brain hormones (endorphins) that are associated with panic attacks, depression, manic depression, schizophrenia, and other conditions. In these cases—with more certain to be discovered—there is no need for the immune system to be involved; the effect is direct. The two first examples to be discovered were peptides from imperfectly digested casein (milk protein) and gluten (wheat protein). Of course, these are the two most commonly eaten foods in our culture."

Dr. Stoll usually sees patients after they have tried a number of different therapies. "These patients come with stacks and stacks of records documenting that nothing seems to have worked in spite of every imaginable test having been done and every imaginable treatment having been tried. Psychoactive drugs either have worked poorly or have even caused the problem to worsen because the side effects exceeded the benefits.

"Since every other conceivable cause has been ruled out by the time I get to see them, I am free to look for the things that have not been evaluated. One of the first things I look for is how well the lining of their intestinal tract protects them from their environment. I frequently find that either they don't have the normal bacterial balance in the colon or they have gone beyond that stage to having candidiasis. Candida can escape from our control only if the normal bacteria are not under control. If candida has converted from the yeast form, which is a normal part of the intestinal flora, into the disease-causing fungal form, it further damages the lining so that the leakage of peptides is much greater.

"The greater the amount of peptide leakage, the more likely it is that the brain will interpret these protein particles as being identical to the endorphins it produces during panic attacks, depression, and the like. This leakage is responsible for the increasing sensitivities we see in patients who are sensitive to environmental substances other than foods. In most cases, it is much simpler to correct the leakage than it is to eliminate the substance. But why not do both?"

According to Dr. Stoll, dramatic improvement is often seen once the reason for the leakage is corrected. "The antibodies involved last only for seventy-two hours. Once the leakage is stopped completely, symptoms lessen substantially in just a few days; even a reduction of the leakage helps. There are many patients today who have had that kind of experience. Not everyone's mental symptoms are caused by poorly digested food playing tricks on the brain. However, in my experience it is the most commonly missed diagnosis and one that is relatively easy to resolve."

LIFE EVENTS

In Dr. Derosis's plan for reducing anxiety, the first step is to identify one thing that causes anxiety or creates tension, guilt, anger, and so on. One of the main problems in anxiety is that the person cannot discriminate between "distracting and anxiety-producing components" of life.

"For example, one of my patients had a teenage son who was troubling her a great deal. She said her son was coming to the dinner table that summer without any shoes, in his underwear, and with dirty, unkempt hair. She would yell at him, then they would argue, and he would get up and stomp out. Then she'd feel bad because she was kicking him out. In other words, those little details of life. So I asked, 'What is it that bothers you the most?'

"She responded, 'It's his wearing underwear to the dinner table.' Then she added, 'But he does so many things to get me mad.'

"I stopped her and said I wanted only one thing. Then I asked, 'What could you do about that one thing?' This was the second step. Once you have isolated a problem, you have to plan what you are going to do about it.

"I also suggested that she behave in a low-key way, for she had been carrying on just as her son did, and it never got her anywhere. In fact, it made things worse.

"She was able to keep quiet for quite a while and then she thought, 'What if I got him some summer shorts. Maybe he might wear them.'

"So she asked him if he might like them and he said, 'Yes.' She did that, and he wore them all summer. Every once in a while, she would grab them and put them in the washing machine. As a result, their whole relationship changed. But this change involved one of the little details that can make life easy or anxiety-filled."

IMMUNE SYSTEM

Medical science shows repeatedly that anxiety is deeply associated with the onset of a variety of stress-related illnesses and immune-compromised conditions. The immune system is actually linked to positive mood, and proper functioning is associated with overall good health. "The endorphin system, our natural opiates, really boost the function of the immune system, while stress and anxiety suppress it, leading potentially to a host of diseases, particularly, the inflammatory diseases that are so prevalent and at the basis of many different health problems today," Dr. Shapiro says. "If there are ways to change your set point, if there are ways to relieve anxiety and find more serenity and more ease, then you can profoundly affect not only your health but also the well-being of those around you."

Diet and Nutritional Remedies

Dr. Lesser stresses that good nutrition is also important, since junk foods can spur anxiety. Simple, processed carbohydrates such as white sugar and white flour products may give a quick lift to the a person with hypoglycemia, but this is followed by excessive insulin secretion that drives the blood sugar down again, only to be pumped up once again by an adrenaline rush. This episode leaves a person with cold hands, jitters, anxiety, and panic.

Special nutrients can help alleviate this problem, especially chromium—also called the glucose tolerance factor–which helps normalize blood sugar. Zinc and the B vitamins, especially thiamine and vitamin B1, are also beneficial. Niacin, has also been identified as an antistress factor. It lowers cholesterol and triglyceride levels, which are increased by anxiety, and affects the brain in ways that are similar to the effects of tranquilizers. Dr. Lesser is convinced of the efficacy of this nutritional approach, but emphasizes the need to be patient when looking for results.

It may take months for the condition to begin to clear because "the body has often been run-down for a number of months or years, and you have to gradually repair all the cells in the body. The old cells have to die off and be replaced by new ones that are better nourished. The natural life span of cells varies throughout the body. Some, such as blood cells, live 120 days, so you cannot really expect sudden, dramatic improvement unless the condition has come on suddenly and you have caught it early."

According to Dr. Allan Spreen, a specialist in nutrition-based medicine, anxiety disorders respond to treatment with certain natural substances. The advantages of treatment with natural substances can be numerous and substantial: by freeing people from having to take more toxic medication, the holistic approach can spare the patient the medication's side effects as well as the extra expense.

"Some amino acids, when given individually," says Dr. Spreen, "can be very effective in calming down the symptoms of anxiety disorders and panic attacks."

For example, tryptophan, which has been banned from public sale as a nutritional supplement, "was used as a sleeping agent until there was a problem with some batches of it being contaminated, which caused a syndrome that was related not to the tryptophan but to the contaminant. Some doctors use tyrosine for depression and anxiety. The 'DL' form of phenylalanine is often used on a short-term basis for depression and can be very effective if given correctly. It can lessen anxiety and depression in people by giving them more of an 'up' mood. Phenylalanine is also an appetite suppressant for many people. If they're given correctly, there seems to be no toxicity associated with amino acids, and they're much cheaper than antidepressants or antianxiety prescription medications."

Another nutritional approach is advocated by Dr. Steven Whiting, author of *The Complete Guide to Optimal Wellness.* He argues, "Once we have addressed the question of whether you are eating the proper foods, then you need to take certain supplements."

For Dr. Whiting, key supplements are calcium and magnesium. "We have been told that the B complex is centrally important. Although this is true, the importance of calcium and magnesium should not be underestimated. Remember, at periods of high stress, calcium and magnesium as well as vitamins C, B_1, B_{12}, and pantothenic acid are consumed by the body at a phenomenal rate. One recent clinical study showed that up to 1,200 milligrams of pantothenic acid can be consumed in a twenty-four-hour period of severe anxiety. With the recommended dietary intake of those nutrients well below that, we can see it is not sufficient for high-stress periods.

"So in addition to these supplements that are commonly given for stress, calcium and magnesium are probably the best weapons we have because of their action on the central nervous system. I would recommend 800 milligrams of calcium and 400 milligrams of magnesium. By accelerating that, you can create what I designate 'a natural tranquilizer replacement.' While it should be used only for short periods of time, it certainly can be used for three to five days with no side effects whatsoever."

Dr. Whiting also believes in using vitamin and mineral supplementation to replace tranquilizers. He notes, "A combination that I have used successfully to replace such harmful drugs as Valium and Librium goes as follows: calcium at 600 milligrams, magnesium at 400 milligrams, potassium at 500 milligrams, vitamin B_6 at 200 milligrams, potassium at 1,600 milligrams, and vitamin B_{12} at 500 micrograms every four hours under the tongue. This is used every four to six hours. We have had a phenomenal response with this, in terms of removing people's need for these highly habit-forming drugs."

Dr. Shapiro is also a strong proponent of magnesium. An important mineral that is in short supply in most American diets, magnesium plays a role in activating the calming part of our nervous system, the parasympathetic nervous system, which handles functions like muscle relaxation, heart rhythm, and digestion. She suggests magnesium that is bound to glycine (magnesium glycinate) or taurine (magnesium taurate).

"One other supplement I would mention is inositol, which is in the B-complex family of vitamins, and is also very helpful for helping people to calm down, and decrease repetitive thoughts, and intrusive feelings," Dr. Shapiro says.

Herbal Therapy

- Ashwagandha has antistress properties. I recommend taking 450 milligrams twice daily.
- Chamomile is a gentle yet effective remedy for anxiety and the digestive disturbances that may accompany it. I recommend taking 650 milligrams daily, preferably with food. Chamomile may also be used as a tea and is best taken in the hours before bed.
- Ginseng is an adaptogen that may help protect and strengthen the body against the damaging effects of chronic stress reactions. Do not take ginseng if you have uncontrolled blood pressure. If ginseng is safe for you to use, I recommend a dose of 200 milligrams per day.
- Ginkgo biloba increases blood circulation to the brain, protects nerve cells, and has shown promise in ameliorating mild depression and accompanying anxiety. Ginkgo can act as an anti-coagulant, and individuals taking antithrombotic drugs such as ASA, anti-inflammatories, and warfarin or Coumadin should consult with their doctors before taking ginkgo. Your daily supplement should be 300 milligrams daily, in equally divided doses.
- Indian snakeroot (Rauwolfia) is a plant that grows wild in India and Africa and is used in impacting various conditions

of the nervous system, including anxiety. Do not take Rauwolfia if you are suffering from depression. This herb is most effective when the whole herb is taken and used over an extended period of time. I recommend a dosage of 600 milligrams daily.

■ Skullcap acts as a gentle sedative for the central nervous system. Consult with your doctor if you are taking any other medications, including over-the-counter drugs such as antihistamines. If skullcap is safe for you to use, I recommend taking 350 milligrams three times daily. Skullcap is often combined with other mildly sedative herbs, including valerian, passionflower, hops, and lemon balm. If you are taking such a preparation, follow the manufacturer's instructions.

■ Valerian is effective for people who experience anxiety-related insomnia. I recommend taking 400 to 450 milligrams daily. Do not take valerian for more than two consecutive weeks. Valerian is often combined with other mildly sedative herbs, including skullcap, passionflower, hops, and lemon balm. If you are taking such a preparation, follow the manufacturer's instructions.

Other Natural Remedies

In addition to dietary modifications and nutritional supplements, anxiety may be ameliorated by relaxation techniques, yoga, massage, exercise, and stress management. An orthomolecular psychiatrist will often suggest these approaches before turning to drugs. Drugs, unlike nutrients or stress-reduction techniques, often become addictive. If you suffer from anxiety and then develop an addiction to drugs that were intended to help that problem, you will only have augmented the agony you were trying to eliminate. In addition, the direct side effects that drugs often have may leave you less capable of living a normal, healthy life than you were when you first underwent treatment.

Cognitive behavioral therapy can help people change behavior resulting from anxiety and revamp their thought processes to prevent symptoms from worsening or developing. This type of therapy is short term, lasting perhaps eight to twelve weeks. Goals of cognitive behavioral therapy include learning to identify behavior patterns and interrupt them with physical activities, such as tapping, learning breathing and other relaxation techniques to prevent some of the symptoms of anxiety from gaining hold, and gradually becoming less sensitive to situations and thoughts that provoke stress and anxiety.

Orthomolecular psychiatry puts psychotherapy on the back burner. The shortcoming of psychotherapy, according to Dr. Michael Lesser, "is that most people who suffer from anxiety have only a limited capacity to deal with it through insight psychotherapy. There is a real risk and danger that an individual, by concentrating on her pathology—phobias and anxiety—and by delving deep into her childhood and looking for trauma, will become 'fixed' on the idea of her pathology. Rather than becoming more able and competent, she will become fixed in her neurosis and in some cases will become even more anxious as a result of exploring the so-called unconscious. I have seen many cases—I am not saying this occurs in every case; perhaps I am seeing only the failed cases—of individuals who have been in psychotherapy for four, six, eight, or even twelve years with no apparent improvement. It seems to me that when a case goes on that long, someone should think about the possibility of using another approach."

Dr. Shapiro strongly recommends breathing techniques as a means of breaking a cycle of negative thinking. "Many traditional civilizations have taught breathing," she says. "I work with patients to teach heart-centered techniques that are calming and soothing, and center them in the wisdom of the heart." Deep breaths are not needed, but rather regular, easy breathing in and out focusing awareness on the center of the chest.

Walking meditations, such as walking a labyrinth or walking in nature, also help people connect with their inner sense of well-being.

In addition, essential oils can be calming, soothing, and uplifting, Dr. Shapiro says. "One real benefit is that where we process scent in the olfactory cortex is right next to where we process emotions in the brain, the limbic system. So working with scent can actually cut through a lot of our verbal chatter" and reduce anxiety. Dr. Shapiro uses ylang-ylang, clary sage, lavender, and chamomile.

According to Stephanie Marohn, a writer and editor of books on psychospirituality and alternative thought, Dr. Roger Callahan has pioneered a kind of energy therapy known as Thought Field Therapy (TFT). TFT uses acupuncture points on the body to break up energy patterns that produce anxiety. By tapping on these acupuncture points, the energy is redirected, and the pattern contributing to anxiety is broken. TFT is a self-practiced therapy that gives the individual immediate control in reducing anxiety in particular situations.

Gary Null's Protocol for Anxiety

My baseline wellness protocol can be found in Chapter 16. The following chart summarizes additional supplements I recommend for individuals who suffer from, or are specifically concerned about, anxiety. If you are concerned about conditions discussed in other chapters, consult with a health professional about how you can safely impact multiple conditions. As always, if you are taking medication—whether prescription or over-the-counter—or have any food restrictions, consult with your doctor before beginning the supplement program. Your health care provider should always be up-to-date on all vitamins, supplements, and herbal or homeopathic remedies you are taking. Supplement overdoses are rare, but possible, and certain combinations may affect individuals adversely.

SUPPLEMENT	DOSAGE	CAUTIONS
Adapton (Garum Armoricum)	4 capsules as directed daily for fifteen days; stop for one week, then continue with maintenance dose of 2 capsules daily.	
Inositol (vitamin B8)	Increase daily dosage from 250 mg to 800 mg. Do not exceed a daily supplement of 1,000 mg. Take in two divided doses.	
Magnesium	1,000 mg (for women) 1,000 mg (for men)	May take six weeks or more for effects to be felt.
Melatonin	300 mcg–1 mg at night a half hour before bed.	
Theanine	200 mg	

Research Update

An increasing body of evidence is showing the benefits of natural modalities to overall health and well-being. Following is a sample of recent peer-reviewed scientific studies in the area of anxiety.

In 2010, researchers reported in *Maturitas* that supplementing with 80 milligrams of red clover isoflavones per day for ninety days reduced anxiety in postmenopausal women. A 2010 report in *Psychopharmacology* found that supplementation with L-tryptophan increased brain serotonin levels and enhance mood and sense of well-being. A study published in the *Nutrition Journal* by French scientists found that individuals given a supplement derived from melon juice and high in the antioxidant superoxide dismutase experienced significant reductions in perceived stress after four weeks compared to a group given a placebo. A 2011 study published in the *Journal of Neuroscience* found that elevating levels of magnesium enhanced synaptic plasticity in the brain, which in turn, altered learned fear responses.

Chapter 22

Arthritis

More than 45 million Americans suffer from some form of arthritis, a large percentage of whom are women. By 2020, the number is expected to reach 60 million, or one-fifth of the population. We know the kind of discomfort this can mean: swollen joints and excruciating pain. It can be so bad it prevents a person from having a quality life.

With so many millions suffering from arthritis, maybe we should be thinking of something by way of treatment other than simply dulling the pain with drugs or performing dangerous and expensive operations. As you will see in reading this chapter, alternative medicine practitioners have been thinking this way for years with quite astounding results. Finally, over the past decade, after the *Journal of the American Medical Association* concluded that two popular nutritional supplements, glucosamine and chondroitin compounds, are safe and effective in treating osteoarthritis, there have been signs that natural therapies are starting to gain some of the recognition they so rightly deserve.

The word *arthritis* means pain and "swelling of the joints." A joint is the place where two bones meet. Cartilage covers the end of each bone and prevents the bones from rubbing together. The joint capsule surrounds and protects the joint, and special membranes cover it with a fluid that lubricates it. Muscles and ligaments around the joint provide support and make it move. When all these parts are working right, the joint moves smoothly and easily, but when something is wrong with the joint, arthritis may develop.

There are many types of arthritis. Some of the most common are described below.

OSTEOARTHRITIS

Osteoarthritis, also known as degenerative joint disease, is the most common form of chronic arthritis. It is estimated to affect more than 20 million Americans, three-quarters of whom are women. In osteoarthritis, the cartilage is worn away so that the bones rub against each other. When the cartilage breaks down, the joint may lose its shape. The ends of the bone may thicken and form spurs.

Adds Dr. Jason Theodosakis, whose treatment program is profiled later in this chapter, "At a biochemical level, the breakdown of cartilage is happening more rapidly than the buildup of cartilage. That brings up an important point. Cartilage on the end of the bones is not like a pencil eraser, which, once it is rubbed off, is gone. It is constantly breaking down and being replaced."

Osteoarthritis most often affects middle-aged and older women. Many people consider it a part of the aging process. The joints of the fingers, neck, low back, and legs are usually involved. Symptoms include joint pain, tenderness, stiffness, loss of function, and restricted mobility. Diagnosis is made by physical examination, X-rays, and ruling out other types of arthritis.

RHEUMATOID ARTHRITIS

Rheumatoid arthritis, one of the most destructive forms of arthritis, is a severe inflammatory condition that affects the joints as well as other body organs. It is an autoimmune disease in which the body attacks its own tissue. More than 60 percent of the two million Americans with rheumatoid arthritis are middle-aged women. Symptoms include pain and swelling in many joints, morning stiffness, afternoon fatigue, and low-grade fevers. Significant joint deformity and disability may occur.

Rheumatoid arthritis can be difficult to diagnose. It often begins gradually and may resemble other types of arthritis. The condition is unpredictable, marked by episodes of remission and exacerbation.

GOUT

Gout is a form of inflammatory arthritis caused by excess uric acid in the body. This excess can result from overproduction of the acid by the body itself, decreased elimination by the kidneys, or increased consumption of foods containing purines, which are metabolized into uric acid. Foods that are particularly high in purines include meats and seafood. Alcohol also increases uric acid levels. Acid crystals, which build up and congregate in the joints, are identified as invaders by the body's white blood cells. The cells attack the joints, creating painful episodes of inflammation.

Acute gouty arthritis is a sudden affliction that may last a few days to a few weeks and then disappear temporarily. Usually just one or a few joints are affected. In most cases, the big toe is the initial target. Often a person is awakened from sleep with intense pain. Gout tends to run in families, and more commonly affects overweight men in middle age. Gout may also result from blood disorders or cancers, or from the use of certain drugs. The symptoms of gout may appear following periods of excessive eating or drinking, or physical or mental stress.

Causes

A host of factors are triggers for people who are genetically susceptible to arthritis. As the late Dr. Ray Wunderlich explained, "We talk about inadequate repairs, inadequate defenses for our body. As we go along with inadequate food, digestion, metabolism, and porosity of gut, we develop increasing levels of immune disturbance, and the joints are a major place where this manifests. That may be because of their movement or because of the tremendous amount of connective tissue around them."

Joint disorders are very common in our society. Connective tissue needs high amounts of vitamin C, glucosamine, and appropriate minerals such as silica, magnesium, zinc, and pantothenic acid. "Without these," said Dr. Wunderlich, "there will be a decline of the connective tissue, which is the glue that keeps our bodies together. As the body sails along through space in our journey through life, we get bombarded with more and more toxins. Rachel Carson was right. It's a toxic planet, and it's not getting any better."

Environmental stress is central to arthritis, as it is to so many other illnesses. There has been an intellectual blind spot on our medical, health, and legislative screens. We look out there and we see herbicides, pesticides, genetically engineered foods, pollution in our water—so much new pollution that government regulators cannot even abide by the old standards, so they keep raising the allowable amount of toxins in the body.

Clinical Experience

CONVENTIONAL MEDICINE

Typically, arthritis is diagnosed on the basis of a patient's symptoms, which most commonly include pain or swelling in the joint areas or some limitation of movement. Some diagnostic tests and X-rays may show abnormalities in the joints, but often these tests are not accurate. Thus, the patient's symptoms are the central factor in determining the diagnosis.

Because medical students have been taught that there is no cure for arthritis, as doctors they look less for the cause of the disease but instead focus on alleviating the symptoms. This approach can be very dangerous because many of the drugs used to counteract pain and swelling can have serious side effects. Even aspirin, which is ordinarily considered one of the least toxic medications and normally constitutes the first line of attack in the traditional treatment of arthritis, is not without side effects. In the treatment of arthritis, aspirin is given in large doses on a constant basis. Consequently, arthritis patients have consistently high levels of aspirin in their systems; this can result in dizziness, ringing in the ears, intestinal tract bleeding, kidney damage, and death.

When aspirin does not work or when an arthritis sufferer develops adverse reactions to it, other medications called nonsteroidal anti-inflammatory drugs (NSAIDs), such as the widely advertised Motrin, are used to control inflammation. Since these drugs are nonsteroidal (i.e., do not contain cortisone), they are less toxic than some medications commonly used to combat inflammation, but they nevertheless do have side effects.

NSAIDs came onto the market as effective alternatives to aspirin, which had caused internal bleeding in many long-term users. Ironically, while the NSAIDs are less effective than aspirin as anti-inflammatories, they also have side effects that include gastrointestinal bleeding and peptic ulcers. Other side effects include dizziness, nervousness, nausea, vomiting, and ringing in the ears. If these drugs are unsuccessful, doctors often prescribe cortisone-derived drugs such as prednisone. These drugs are notorious for their severe toxicity. They interfere with the immune system, leaving the patient defenseless against infection and other diseases. Cortisone-type drugs also interfere with the body's healing ability, and it is not uncommon for a person taking these drugs to have bone fractures or wounds that do not heal for long periods.

Some rheumatologists (doctors who treat arthritis patients) use injections of gold. This method of treatment was abandoned years ago because it was considered too dangerous, but today gold treatments are finding their way back into medical practice. Another technique finding acceptance among arthritis doctors is the use of chemotherapy drugs. The theory behind this drastic measure is that when a patient's immune system is knocked out, the patient's body is no longer able to form the antibodies that may be causing the inflammation in her joints. Other techniques include radiation therapy in the area of the inflammation, again with the intent of destroying the patient's immune response, and plasmapheresis, a procedure by which a patient's blood is drained, filtered to remove antibodies, and then reinjected into the patient.

While the traditional medical approach to arthritis is undeniably becoming more sophisticated, it also appears to be missing the mark. Not only do these treatments fail to get at the cause of the disease, they are becoming more expensive, invasive, and toxic, leading to the inevitable question, Do the ends justify the means? When traditional medicine begins to turn to anticancer therapies to treat arthritis—therapies that are often cancer-causing themselves and result in side effects ranging from nausea and hair and weight loss to depletion of the immune system—this question becomes even more pressing.

ALTERNATIVE TREATMENTS

"The way I treat arthritis is probably quite different from the approach of most physicians," says Dr. Peter D'Adamo. "As a naturopath, I was taught that we should not always think about treating a disease but about treating a person. Arthritis is a very good example of a disease that is highly individualized. Not only are there different types of arthritis, but people get it and express it in different manners."

It's a good idea to try to listen to the body and realize that it has an intelligence. In other words, if you are following a certain lifestyle and your problems are the result of that lifestyle, a change in lifestyle may change the illness.

People say that as the body gets older, the most natural thing in the world is for it to get decrepit. But give the body credit for the intelligence it has. When the body tells you something, if you listen and follow what it says, you will improve.

DIET AND NUTRITION

Dr. Peter Agho of the Healing Center says, "I do diet. Not just for arthritis. The thing about the whole diet is this: Change the diet, and the arthritis—along with obesity, high blood pressure, and other problems—will get better. The diet should include fresh fruit, including fresh fruit juice, and vegetables. You should eliminate animal fats and cut high-fat foods."

Dr. Howard Robins outlines his treatment: "We use a complete vegetarian diet, including a lot of green, leafy vegetables. These are important because of all the phytochemicals and phytoestrogens that help in all the chemical processes that are necessary to getting well again. We give them juices, six to eight fresh green juices a day—the best way to take in these chemicals."

Dr. Luke Bucci, author of *Pain Free: The Definitive Guide to Healing Arthritis*, notes that part of the reason people get arthritis is the lack of essential nutrients in a highly processed, refined diet. Sure, you get plenty of calories, protein, and fat—usually the wrong kind of fat. What you do not get is just as important—the minerals: magnesium, zinc, copper, manganese, and boron. Many people are not aware of boron as a nutrient, but boron may turn out to be essential to our joints' health. These are what you do not get with the current, typical American diet. We lack the substances that enable the joints to repair themselves from the damage they sustain. That is why you want to start eating a whole-food diet that is rich in organic vegetables, fruits, and nuts.

Dr. Rich Ribner tells this story: "Recently, a woman came to the clinic with a terrible case of arthritis. She was in terrible pain and had been taking anti-inflammatory medication and tranquilizers. She was miserable. She said she thought about killing herself. I said, 'Stop this nonsense. I'm going to ask you to do something. You may not even want to do it.' She said, 'Anything.' I said, 'Between now and next week, I want you to drink six to eight glasses of water a day, but it has to be distilled or spring water. And eat nothing but brown rice, just brown rice.' 'But, but . . .' she began. 'Wait,' I said, 'you were talking about killing yourself. So listen, I'll add a few green vegetables to that.'

"You have to make sure there is a cleansing. Make sure they drink the water. Have a bowel movement daily.

"Well, this woman was so desperate that she stayed on the diet one week. When she came back, there was marked improvement. She still had a long way to go, but there was a change."

SUPPLEMENTS

Vitamins, minerals, and nutritive substances can play important roles in the treatment and prevention of arthritis. There is some evidence that the essential fatty acids furnished by substances such as cod liver oil, linoleic acid, and marine lipids, by replacing missing fatty substances in the joint-lubricating synovial fluid, can be important in treating arthritis. When the joint surfaces become irritated and undergo degeneration, some of the fat from the joint itself is lost. This fat acts as a lubricant and keeps the joint surfaces apart so that the cartilage-covered bone ends are protected and can move smoothly. When a person takes extra cod liver oil or other essential fatty acids, the oil goes to the joints and provides more lubrication.

Vitamin A, which is found in large quantities in cod liver oil, is also important for the maintenance of the mucous membranes, which manufacture mucus to cleanse the body of infectious bacteria and toxins. Without adequate supplies of vitamin A, infection and accumulation of toxic materials can set in around the joints. Furthermore, a vitamin A deficiency can lead to insufficient production of synovial fluid; when this occurs, the joints lack proper lubrication, the cartilage becomes subject to drying and cracking, and movement becomes difficult and painful.

Because lubrication is vital to the smooth functioning of the joints, vitamin E, whose primary role is to protect against the destruction of the essential fatty acids by oxidation, is also an important antiarthritic nutrient. Both vitamins E and C, which generally act as free radical scavengers within the body, can be especially important in the treatment as they can "clinch" the free radicals present at the site of inflamed or irritated joints, thereby decreasing pain, swelling, and inflammation.

Many symptoms of arthritis are alleviated by establishing a proper balance of calcium and phosphorus in the body, since these are the two minerals most responsible for bone formation and healing. This can be one of the most confusing aspects of arthritis, because X-rays of arthritic joints often show excessive calcification. Afraid of further calcification, patients mistakenly believe that they must avoid calcium-rich foods. Actually, the calcification is due not to an excess of calcium but to malabsorption of existing supplies caused by an imbalance in the ratio of calcium to phosphorus. This imbalance is caused by two major factors: (1) excessive consumption of foods containing high levels of phosphorus, such as meat, dairy products, and soft drinks; and (2) the process of joint degeneration, which releases high levels of phosphates. This excess phosphorus at the joint site binds with calcium and results in calcification. Taking extra calcium orally does not contribute to this localized calcification. Rather, by increasing calcium levels in the blood, it draws the excess phosphorus away from the joints to bind with the blood calcium so that both are eliminated; this in turn inhibits calcification around the joints.

It should be noted here that soft drinks are the number-one source of phosphorus in the American diet today. These drinks contain more phosphorus than most other foods or beverages, and the typical American consumes nearly 100 gallons of them a year. According to Dr. David Steenblock, excess phosphorus is one of the major contributing factors to the development of osteoarthritis. He says, "We see this clinically in many people, who come with osteoarthritis in their early forties who are large consumers of soft drinks, who also consume excess quantities of meats and other high-phosphorus foods, and who do not eat enough of the green, leafy vegetables which contain calcium." The other problem associated with soft drinks is that most contain citric acids, which bind calcium and cause it to be excreted. "So," says Dr. Steenblock, "not only is there extra phosphorus in the soft drinks, they contain the material that takes calcium out of the body. If you want to develop osteoarthritis, that's a very good way of doing it."

Other useful supplements include glucosamine and chondroitin. According to Dr. Luke Bucci, these substances act to "convince" your joint tissues to repair the damage caused by arthritis. (See "Specific Alternative Treatment Approaches" later in this chapter for more information on glucosamine and chondroitin.)

Several studies have shown that a small supplemental dose of boron, about 3 to 6 milligrams a day, can reverse the symptoms of osteoarthritis. Magnesium is also helpful.

AVOIDING CERTAIN FOODS AND CHEMICALS

Arthritis may be caused or exacerbated by allergies to foods and chemicals. Dr. Warren Levin says that removing offending substances from the patient's environment can produce dramatic changes.

Some doctors believe that arthritis is caused by the foods a person eats most often. Dr. Morton Teich stresses that the food the patient wants the most may be the problem. Studies have shown that milk, for example, can cause severe allergies and arthritis.

Dr. Teich also warns us about the glycoproteins in milk, wheat, corn, and cinnamon, as well as inhalants such as dust, mold, and pollen. Chemicals and food additives are also potential contributors to allergies and arthritis.

HERBS

Letha Hadady, an herbalist, tries to eliminate the toxins that result from poor digestion and poor circulation. She shares some of her herbal remedies.

In dealing with arthritis, one thing you must have every day is alfalfa. You could chew ten tablets a day with a little water to eliminate much of the uric acid that can build up to create joint pain. Rhubarb also eliminates acid. It is a laxative, but it also breaks apart the painful crystals that form around your joints.

Dandelion greens are full of vitamins and minerals. Dandelions break down pain-giving acid, too.

Star fruit is a sweet, delicious fruit you can find in the grocery store or at the vegetable stand. Juice it. Add a cup and a half of cold water per serving of six star fruits. Taken three times a day, it can eliminate inflammatory joint pain, bleeding hemorrhoids, and burning urine. It is cooling and cleansing.

It is important to realize that not everyone's arthritic pain is the same. Do you wake up in the morning with your joints feeling stiff and sore? Do they feel better after you move them around and after you exercise? If so, you need to take warming, tonic herbs that build vitality, increase circulation, and warm joints. Add a pinch of turmeric to your stews. Turmeric and cinnamon are a good combination for achy shoulders. If you have rheumatism that gets worse in cold weather, add 1/4 teaspoon of turmeric and cinnamon to a little water and drink it as a tea.

Asafetida is a spice that is available in Indian stores. A little asafetida added to cooking beans or other hard-to-digest foods will help cleanse the body and warm the joints.

Also useful is the resin myrrh; a few drops added to your tea will make your joints feel warm and your blood move, thus improving the circulation.

Hadady says that Asian medicine uses many herbs that can be added in cooking. For example, dong quai increases circulation and warms joints. Another classic Chinese remedy, one that Chinese doctors have used for generations, is du huo jisheng wan. Hadady's favorite—guan jie yan wan—is translated as "walk as smoothly as a tiger." Other Asian remedies include raw Tienchi ginseng, Efficacious Corydalis, tien ma, Three Snakes Formula, Mobility 3, Clematis 19, du zhong, leigong ten pian, and rinchen dragjor-rilnag chenmo.

CHIROPRACTIC

Many arthritis sufferers interviewed for this chapter said that of all the things they tried in their efforts to eliminate the pain, going to a chiropractor helped the most.

Dr. Mitchell Proffman, a chiropractor formerly at the Healing Center, showed me two X-rays. The first showed bones that were nice and clean and square in shape; the second showed degeneration of the bones.

He showed what arthritis looks like in the human body: thinned disks and a little lip or spur, the body's defense mechanism to heal or shore up the area so that it does not totally disintegrate. He said a woman might have a pinched nerve somewhere in the body, in the neck, for example. He administers a gentle push with his hand, which is not painful, to move the bone back into position. The nerve energy comes through, and the joint can start to heal.

RECONSTRUCTIVE THERAPY

The noted physician Dr. Arnold Blank has used reconstructive therapy to treat arthritis. Reconstructive therapy, created in the 1920s by the osteopathic physicians Gedney and Schumann, works by stimulating the body's ability to heal itself. The doctors found that by injecting substances that caused a slight irritation to tissues, they could help blood vessels grow into a region, thus bringing more oxygen, vitamins, and minerals into the cartilage and promoting tissue growth.

Dr. Blank says this therapy is most effective in patients who are in an optimal nutritional state. "Vitamin and mineral levels are important in our healing response and ability. The injection consists of a variety of different liquids. Primary liquids I use are calcium, lidocaine, and saline. They take a moment and really aren't painful. The majority of patients feel improvement after the first three or four treatments, developing some strength and feeling less pain, even increasing the range of movement.

"The nutrients we may use, natural ones, include substances that have an anti-inflammatory effect, such as vitamin C, shark cartilage, sea cucumber, glutathione, and glucosamine sulfate. All these substances are used once reconstructive therapy has begun because the new blood vessels going to the tissues will enhance healing. These nutrients may not work well when there are no blood vessels going into the area, so they should be administered after the therapy has begun its work."

ACUPUNCTURE

Acupuncture has been used by countless people throughout the world to help alleviate the pain and suffering of arthritis. Dr. Yuan Yang of the Healing Center explains briefly how this works. "We put the needle around the joint to create circulation, taking the pain away. There may be cold, blocked blood and low energy, so I apply the needle for smooth blood flow. Moving blocked energy takes the pain out."

PHYSICAL THERAPY

Shmuel Tatz typically works with people who have arthritic problems from overuse syndromes or accidents. He works directly on the joints. For example, for a pianist who has problems with the hands, he will try to move the bones, separating the joints to make more space.

As Tatz explains, "Today in physical therapy we use many modalities. One of these is magnetic pulse therapy. We know of the positive effects of magnetism on the body. Scientists have developed a machine with different programs so that we can adjust for every different situation.

"We put electrodes on the body, for example, on the hip joint, and we leave them on for fifteen to twenty minutes. Usually patients report a very mild relaxing sensation, and the pain decreases.

"Many people with pain from osteoarthritis are afraid to be touched. People with a swollen knee, for instance, can do reflex therapy. For the knee we touch an acupuncture point on the ear, which gives relief."

Once this manipulation has had an effect, they start to exercise the knee by putting the legs in slings, relieving the pressure on the joint and making it easier for the patient to move the body. Trying to open the joint and make more space around the bones allows for better circulation. Movement is very important for people with arthritis.

One patient, Lori, speaks about her improvement: "Here at Medical Arts I was able to receive physical therapy, which has enabled me to avoid surgery and has greatly improved the quality of my life. I'm still dancing."

YOGA

Molly McBride, a yoga instructor, believes you do not have to stop working on your health simply because you may have some physical limitations. Even by working with something as simple as a chair, it is easy to stay fit and help yourself with the problems of arthritis.

The basis of yoga is breath and breathing practices, she says, which help circulation and also help flush the body out by collecting toxins so that they can be exhaled. Breath is the foundation of all the yoga stretches.

"We start with just taking a simple breath; the basic beginning exercise is a three-part breath. Let the air fill the abdomen, then the rib cage, then the upper chest. Exhale, letting the breath exit the upper chest, then the rib cage, and then abdomen. Inhale, exhale."

It is important to take time every day to do these breathing exercises. A really good time to do them is first thing in the morning, when your stomach is empty; if you have eaten, wait a few hours before you start. These breathing exercises can be combined with some simple joint lubrication exercises. To regenerate the body and increase the flow of oxygen through the system, to help release all the toxins that build up in the muscles and the protective cartilage around the joints, try simple yoga exercises.

Specific Alternative Treatment Approaches

In the following pages, we discuss some specific alternative approaches to treating arthritis. Although there are many other approaches, these have had a consistently high success rate, are not toxic or expensive, and may get to the cause of the disease rather than merely masking its symptoms.

TREATMENT FOR GOUT

Traditional medicine treats gout symptoms with drugs to relieve pain and decrease uric acid levels in the body. These drugs include colchicine, corticosteroids, analgesics, uricosuric agents, and allopurinol. They may be beneficial but they do have side effects. More important, they're reactive, not proactive.

An alternative approach starts with maintaining a healthy weight, drinking adequate amounts of water, avoiding alcohol, and eliminating or limiting foods that contain high amounts of purine (beef, goose, organ meats, mussels, herring, mackerel, yeast). Moderate amounts of purine are found in other meats and fish, as well as spinach, asparagus, lentils, mushrooms, and dried peas.

Helpful nutrients include berries, vitamin C, and folic acid. Cherries, hawthorn berries, and blueberries all contain anthocyanins, a class of natural dyes that have been found to reduce inflammation and enhance the quality of collagen. They also act as antioxidants. According to Dr. Muraleedharan Nair from Michigan State University, the anthocyanins in tart cherries are ten times more effective than aspirin in reducing inflammation. As an added benefit, they don't irritate the stomach like aspirin does. Half a pound of cherries per day for two weeks has been found to lower uric acid levels and prevent episodes of gout. Also beneficial is cherry juice, 8 to 16 ounces daily.

Eight grams of vitamin C per day have been found to reduce uric acid levels in the blood. Caution must be noted, however, as gout symptoms will get worse in some people with this amount of vitamin C. In terms of folic acid, 1 to 3 milligrams daily are recommended.

A good herbal remedy for gout is bromelain, 125 to 250 milligrams three times a day during an attack. Also recommended is devil's claw, which can be taken in the following dosages: 1 to 2 grams three times daily of dried powdered root, 4 to 5 milliliters three times daily of tincture, or 400 milligrams three times daily of dry solid extract. Both bromelain and devil's claw act as anti-inflammatories.

Among the homeopathic remedies used for gout are the following:

ACONITE, recommended for burning pain, anxiety, and restlessness that comes on suddenly.

BELLADONNA, recommended for intense, throbbing pain that increases with motion and decreases with pressure.

BRYONIA, indicated for pain exacerbated by motion and decreased by pressure and heat.

COLCHICUM, suggested for pain that increases with motion and weather changes.

LEDUM, for swollen, mottled joints that respond better to cold than to heat.

In addition, hot and cold compresses and bed rest may help.

DR. JASON THEODOSAKIS: MAXIMIZING THE ARTHRITIS CURE

Dr. Theodosakis is the author of *The Arthritis Cure* and *Maximizing the Arthritis Cure*, and board-certified in preventive medicine. He is a lecturer on preventive medicine, a clinical associate professor at the University of Arizona College of Medicine, and the former director of its Preventative Medicine Residency Training Program.

"I've come up with my arthritis program out of necessity, both to treat patients and for personal use," he says. "I see a lot of patients mainly with osteoarthritis but also with the other types of arthritis.

"My program is an integrated, comprehensive approach to creating a situation that optimizes the buildup of cartilage. I will basically use anything—diet, exercise, even medicine when it's called for. We hit it from all angles, including the psychological aspects."

Nonsteroidal anti-inflammatory drugs (NSAIDs), he remarks, are part of a $37 billion worldwide market that involves such huge corporations as White-hall-Robins, which makes Advil and Motrin; other NSAIDs are Aleve, which is naproxen sodium, and aspirin. According to Dr. Theodosakis, these drugs may cause serious problems, such as bleeding ulcers, kidney dysfunction, and adverse drug interactions. "At a rheumatology conference I was at, it came out that none of these anti-inflammatories have been studied long term," he says. "Studies have suggested that they may even worsen the condition."

Dr. Theodosakis's program can be broken down into the following components: diagnosis, supplementation with glucosamine and chondroitin, a change in biomechanics, exercise, diet, and medical approaches.

DIAGNOSIS

"The very first step is getting an accurate diagnosis and working with the physician," Dr. Theodosakis explains. "Be up front with your doctor. In my book, I lay out what you should be telling your doctor and what your doctor should be asking you, the tests you should be getting for a diagnosis, and so on. Even if you are in a managed-care setting where you get only five or ten minutes with your doctor, you have to know what information to get to use that time optimally. Getting an accurate diagnosis so that you'll know what you are treating is step one."

SUPPLEMENTS: GLUCOSAMINE AND CHONDROITIN

Glucosamine and chondroitin are natural supplements from seashells and cow's cartilage, respectively. When taken orally, they improve the balance between breakdown and buildup of cartilage. Recent scientific studies support their use. "These supplements are a part of the treatment," Dr. Theodosakis cautions. "Alone, these supplements are not the answer; they need to be part of a complete program.

On his website (www.drtheo.com), Dr. Theodosakis lists the studies on glucosamine and chondroitin. Further, he states, "I also set up a national reporting center for drug side effects related to glucosamine and chondroitin to see if any negative effects have been noted. So far, although millions of people are using these supplements, I'm not aware of any side effects. And I would be the first person to be aware of them if they were occurring."

The one problem with these supplements is that there are about one hundred different brands on the market. In Dr. Theodosakis's opinion, "maybe as many as 30 percent do not meet the label claims. In other words, you are not getting what the bottle says. This is a very big concern of mine."

BIOMECHANICS

Biomechanics refers to the way the body absorbs shock from everyday movement. "You have different forces on your joint," Dr. Theodosakis says, "and if you learn to dissipate these forces throughout your body, there is likely to be less damage to your cartilage. People can learn to improve their biomechanics. They certainly do in the sports arena, which you will see if you look at athletes as well as performers in such disciplines as ballet. They have wonderful biomechanics and can absorb and dissipate tremendous shock. So my patients are taught how to alter their own biomechanics."

EXERCISE

Exercise is absolutely necessary for arthritis sufferers, but the wrong kind of exercise can worsen the condition. You need a specific program for whatever ails you, Dr. Theodosakis says. If you have a hip problem, for example, you will need to do the appropriate exercises for that.

DIET

Another component of Dr. Theodosakis's program is diet. He remarks, "The fasting in order to detoxify the body, the juicing, the vegetarian diet are all things I agree with 100 percent.

"Diet has a tremendous impact on arthritis for several reasons. One is weight control. A major risk factor for getting arthritis is being overweight. For example, women in the highest fifth of weight are eight times more likely to get arthritis of the knee than are women in the lowest fifth. Another factor is that different foods will either aggravate or alleviate arthritis. Some of the fish oils, omega-3 fatty acids, can help, while certain components of meat, such as arachidonic acid, can worsen the condition. You also need to eat a wide variety of fruits and vegetables, making sure you get a wide variety of nutrients and also taking supplements. With these nutritional elements, we are making sure your body has the optimal environment to win this cartilage battle."

MEDICAL APPROACHES

Dr. Theodosakis also incorporates medical approaches into his program. This may include prescription drugs, surgery, and treatment for depression associated with arthritis.

RESULTS

Dr. Theodosakis describes what he calls "one of my most remarkable cases," that of one of his nurses. "She is about forty years old. She had terrible arthritis, to the point where she was going to have her knee cartilage scraped off, she had so many crystals in it. She used my program for about four months and saw tremendous improvement. She was taking the supplements at that time, and then she stopped taking the supplements—that was about two years ago. Now she's become a runner; she did a half marathon. But she would have been crippled if she had had the surgery.

"I have had a number of patients who were scheduled for joint replacement therapy and after going through this program were able to avoid the surgery. Many are pain-free. It won't reverse the bony changes that occurred in the joint, but it gives them the opportunity to exercise and do some of the things they want to do."

DR. ROBERT LIEFMAN: HOLISTIC BALANCED TREATMENT

Holistic Balanced Treatment (HBT) is derived from the work of the physician Dr. Robert Liefman (1920–1973). Dr. Liefman first used this treatment in 1961, after twenty years of research. Since that time more than 30,000 arthritis sufferers have received the treatment, and many of them are living pain-free, normal lives.

HBT is based on the results of Dr. Liefman's research, which showed that many arthritis sufferers, especially those with rheumatoid arthritis, have specific hormonal imbalances. Within the body there are naturally occurring hormones called glucocorticoids whose role is to reduce inflammation and raise the level of simple sugars in the blood. One of the ways these hormones raise blood sugar levels is by converting nonglucose molecules such as protein into glucose. If unchecked, these glucocorticoids can be responsible for the collagen breakdown of cartilage in joints, which may be a contributing factor in the development of arthritis. The glucocorticoids are balanced within the body by other hormones, such as testosterone and the feminizing hormones, which include estradiol; these hormones induce tissue building and hence balance the tissue-wasting effects of the glucocorticoids. If the body is not regulating these hormones, there are therapies to correct these imbalances. Dr. Liefman developed formulas consisting of varying amounts of three basic ingredients: (1) prednisone, an anti-inflammatory steroid, (2) estradiol, an estrogenic hormone, and (3) testosterone.

According to the proponents of HBT, the anti-inflammatory property of the steroid prednisone and the healing properties of sex hormones can be used to treat arthritic conditions with minimal side effects because of the balancing action between the different components. The anabolic, or building, quality of the sex hormones acts to control the catabolic, or destructive, effects of the steroidal drug therapy (these effects include infection, decreased immunity, improper healing, suppression of pituitary and adrenal function, and fluid retention). The feminizing and androgenic activities of sex hormones are kept in check both by the catabolic nature of the glucocorticoids and by careful adjustment of the concentration of the sex hormones in accordance with the specific requirements of the individual patient during treatment.

THE SUCCESS OF HBT

Dr. Liefman developed four basic formulas to account for the different requirements of each individual using HBT: (1) White Cap, which contains prednisone, testosterone, and estradiol, (2) Black Cap, which has only prednisone and estradiol, (3) Red Cap, which contains prednisone and testosterone, and (4) Green Cap, which contains only prednisone and is used only to allow women to shed the endometrium proliferation caused by the intake of the estrogen-containing preparations. In turn, the proportions of these different compounds may vary from individual to individual and may be altered for the same person during the course of treatment.

If, for example, a female patient begins to exhibit an adverse reaction to the treatment, such as the growth of excess body hair, the testosterone level in the medication will be reduced to eliminate those reactions. Patients who exhibit some of the typical side effects of cortisone-type drugs will have the amounts of prednisone in their medication decreased, or appropriate increases in one of the sex hormones will be made to counterbalance the negative effects of the steroids. Generally, the adverse reactions to any of the elements in the compounds disappear within a short time once the proper balance among the hormones has been attained.

HBT also incorporates principles of nutrition and stresses the importance of regular exercise. The diet recommended in HBT eliminates junk foods such as sugar and sugar products, and salty and processed foods such as luncheon meats and canned goods, fried foods, and refined foods. The diet is essentially moderate in protein and emphasizes high-fiber complex carbohydrates in the form of fresh fruits and vegetables, whole grains, and legumes. Vitamin and mineral supplements are used to bolster the patient's immune system and enhance the body's natural healing abilities. For instance, vitamin D is important for strong and healthy bones because it regulates the absorption of calcium from the stomach into the bloodstream, which carries it to bone tissue. Vitamins C and A are important for the maintenance and repair of collagen, the gluelike substance that holds the tissues together and is essential for joint and muscle stability. Vitamin E and the B-complex vitamins are important for bone growth. Among the minerals, adequate supply and absorption of calcium, phosphorous, and magnesium are essential for the formation of healthy bones, while zinc and selenium are important immune system nutrients.

Exercise is also an important adjunct to HBT and is recommended to restore joint and muscle mobility and function as well as muscle mass lost during periods of inactivity. However, patients generally are told not to exercise until they are free of pain, swelling, and stiffness and feel confident enough to engage in it.

Walking may be the first exercise; then, as patients improve, they can be given specialized exercises for the hands, knees, fingers, shoulders, and other areas that may have been affected by arthritis.

The medical establishment has basically ignored, attacked, or criticized HBT therapy even though its basis is drugs already widely used by physicians. All Dr. Liefman did was combine certain commonly prescribed drugs to maximize the benefits and minimize the side effects of each component drug. The balanced hormonal approach to arthritis did, however, do one unorthodox thing: it challenged the rigidly held position of the medical establishment that arthritis is an incurable disease.

PATIENT STORIES

Here are some of the results arthritis patients have had over the years from using HBT:

At age nineteen, Cynthia began to experience the symptoms of rheumatoid arthritis. Initially the arthritis was confined to her jaw and elbows, but over a period of two and a half years, while she was undergoing treatment by a traditional physician, the arthritis spread to nearly every part of her body. Five years later Cynthia was so crippled with pain and stiffness that it took her a half hour to get out of bed in the morning. The morning after she started HBT, her pain had almost disappeared except for some stiffness and soreness, which also went away during the following three days.

About her condition and her subsequent treatment at the Arthritis Medical Center in Fort Lauderdale, which administers HBT, Cynthia says, "I was getting worse and worse. When I first went to my doctor, I had it just in my jaw and elbows. After two and a half years, I had it in just about every place except my hips and knees. I couldn't turn my head at all.

"The doctor actually told me once that he felt really bad, that he had tried everything and didn't know what else to do, and that I had better go to the crippled children's center in Palm Beach. To tell a young woman that . . . I just wanted to drive off a bridge. But I thank him for saying it because if he hadn't, I don't think I ever would have tried this place. I did it in desperation."

At the time Cynthia started HBT she was taking thirty aspirin tablets a day, which were causing headaches, ringing in her ears, and ulcers. She was spending approximately $1,000 a month on painkillers alone. While Cynthia found that she bruised and bled more easily after starting HBT, she notes that she had the same symptoms while taking large doses of aspirin. However, while the aspirin and other treatments did nothing to arrest the progression of Cynthia's arthritis, a day after she started treatment with HBT, her pain virtually disappeared, and it returned only when she forgot to take her medication. At present Cynthia is pain-free and works out three times a week at a health spa. She continues on her medication, but in much smaller doses than when she started treatment with HBT.

■ ■ ■

June suffered from severe crippling arthritis for two years before starting treatment with HBT. Over that two-year period June received almost every form of traditional arthritis treatment available: gold injections, penicillamine, Butazolidin (phenylbutazone), small doses of prednisone, and 16 aspirins daily. June says that she was spending more than $100 a week for medication alone. In the meantime she kept getting worse, and when she started HBT, she says, "I was immobile in my hands and shoulders. It was at that point that I thought, What's the use of living? I couldn't even turn my head." Additionally, her liver, stomach, and kidneys were damaged by the large doses of medication. She was forced to give up her business because she was too weak and in too much pain to work. Her medical bills were ruining her financially. The second day after June received HBT, her pain disappeared. June says about her progress with HBT:

"I woke up and I could move my ankles, I could move my hands and my feet. When I stood up, the pain wasn't there. I said to [my husband], 'My God, there's been a miracle.' It got better and better, and I guess within two months I didn't even know I had rheumatoid arthritis. I got a bicycle, and I started dancing again and going to the beach again. It used to be if I lay on the sand, I couldn't get up again."

June continues to be pain-free, leading a normal life, and her medication has been reduced by more than half the initial amount.

DR. THERON RANDOLPH AND DR. MARSHALL MANDELL: ENVIRONMENTAL ALLERGIES

Environmental medicine, also called clinical ecology, was developed by Dr.

Theron Randolph in the 1940s and 1950s when he observed early in his medical career that food allergies and sensitivities to environmental chemicals were a major contributing factor in a wide range of diseases, including arthritis. Dr. Randolph also noted that the causal relationship of allergy to disease was a very individualized phenomenon: One person could eat beef every day and never have an adverse reaction, while another person could develop a food allergy to beef even when consuming it only on rare occasions. Similarly, people with an allergy to the same product did not necessarily manifest the same symptoms. One might break out with hives, while another developed depression, and still another became arthritic. Dr. Randolph also found that seemingly innocuous chemicals found in the home, workplace, or school could in certain individuals trigger symptoms ranging from mental problems to aching joints to chronic fatigue.

The work of Dr. Randolph was applied to arthritis by the late Dr. Marshall Mandell, a physician from Connecticut and one of the country's leading environmental medical specialists. He found that a considerable number of patients who come to him with arthritis or arthritislike symptoms are in fact suffering from a form of environmental allergy such as the ones outlined by Dr. Randolph. According to Dr. Mandell, "The basic process that underlies many cases of arthritis is a completely unrecognized or unsuspected allergy or allergylike sensitivity to substances that are part of daily life, including the food we eat, the liquids we drink, including the water supply, the chemicals that are deliberately or accidentally introduced into a diet, and the various forms of chemical pollutants in the indoor and outdoor air that get into our bodies." From his clinical experience, Dr. Mandell found that more than half the patients he treats who would be confirmed arthritics by standard medical diagnostic techniques can be helped by means of simple dietary or environmental changes.

THE TREATMENT

"My approach and that of my colleagues in the field of environmental medicine and clinical ecology, supplemented by the benefits of nutritional therapy, begins by looking at the person who is predisposed to having arthritis to see if there are identifiable substances in the diet and environment that can trigger or cause the episode of illness," said Dr. Mandell. "We deal with demonstrable cause-and-effect relationships. What we do is study the patient.

"First, we take a carefully formulated history that is designed to help identify people who have problems with foods, with various chemicals, with pollutants, and perhaps with seasonal airborne substances. From this, we are able to get a fairly good idea of what we're dealing with."

Before patients are tested for food or environmental allergies, Dr. Mandell often had them fast or go on a restricted diet for four to seven days to rid the body of any residue of substances suspected to be responsible for the symptoms.

"Next," said Dr. Mandell, "we test these people using a technique known as 'provocative testing' to determine their response to extracts prepared from all the foods in their diet. The most commonly ingested foods are often the culprits, so it shouldn't come as any surprise that wheat, corn products, milk, beef, tomatoes, and potatoes are leading offenders.

"The most common technique used for provocative testing is to place a few drops of the test substance under the tongue of the patient, where it is almost immediately absorbed. This is called 'sublingual' provocative testing. When we test in this manner, only small doses are used, so the effect is brief, but since the solution enters the bloodstream, the entire body is exposed. Symptoms can show up in the joints, muscles, brain, skin, or any other part of the body.

"If we are able to produce joint pain, stiffness or swelling, or redness within a few minutes after placing the solution under the tongue for absorption into the bloodstream, we know that we've found something that must be important, because we have flared up the patient's familiar symptoms—we have actually precipitated an attack of the patient's own illness.

"Many people will have what we call 'polysymptomatic illness,' meaning that many bodily structures, organs, or systems can be involved at the same time. The arthritic person's whole body may be sensitive, and this is why such patients may have a headache or fatigue or asthma or colitis, although they may not actually have any of the well-known allergies such as hay fever, eczema, or hives.

"We also find that many people react to chemicals. We have some people whose arthritis may be due in part or exclusively to the chlorine that is in the water supply, or perhaps to an artificial flavoring or coloring which is used very frequently, or perhaps to a preservative. We have people who have trouble because they are inhaling fumes such as tobacco smoke. We have people who in heavy traffic have trouble because the exhaust fumes will travel, along with the oxygen, through the walls of the lung into the circulation; once again, the whole body is exposed."

After Dr. Mandell determined the substances in the patient's overall environment that he suspects are responsible for arthritic symptoms, he double-checked with test meals of the specific substances.

He explained, "If we're able to reproduce that patient's specific symptoms, if we can actually turn the symptoms on and off like a switch, we know that we have nailed it down, because we have demonstrated a cause-and-effect relationship that can't be questioned. Should food be the primary causative factor, we will design a diet that eliminates all of those foods. Then, depending on how well they follow the diet, the patients will be either well or sick."

PATIENT STORIES

Sarah was a rabbi's wife who began to have arthritis in her hands, but the flare-ups would take place only on Saturday mornings and then disappear during the course of the day. Using Saturday as a starting point, Dr. Mandell began to explore the possible sources of Sarah's "Saturday arthritis."

"Since she woke up with the arthritis in the morning," Dr. Mandell explained, "we knew it was not caused by something she was doing in the morning. So we went back twenty-four hours to explore Friday. What did she do on Friday? What did she eat? Drink? Breathe? What came into her system? Could it be, perhaps, the paraffin fumes from the candles on the table that were lit ceremonially every Friday night? Or could it be something they ate? Was it caused by something she was exposed to when she went to temple on Friday night, perhaps from clothing just taken out of the dry cleaners? Or was it hair spray, perfume, cologne, or men with aftershave lotion? Was it that the temple had had the rug shampooed the day before the services or that the furniture was polished? I had no way of knowing, but I retraced all her activities, and then I tested her systematically.

"This actually turned out to be an easy one, and it was humorous, because the great 'Jewish penicillin,' chicken soup, was the thing that was undoing her. When I placed a few drops of chicken extract under her tongue, within minutes the knuckles that were affected by arthritis swelled up and became painful and red. I did this on a few occasions, so we were able to demonstrate this. It is rare to find a patient in whom a single substance is the factor, but it does happen now and then. So here is a rabbi's wife with chicken-and-chicken-soup arthritis—Friday-night ingestion, Saturday-morning appearance of arthritis."

■   ■   ■

This example not only documents the dramatic effects that can be achieved by eliminating an offending food from an arthritic person's diet, it also shows the degree of resistance orthodox arthritis doctors have to accepting this even when it has been unequivocally demonstrated.

Back in the mid-1970s Dr. Mandell sent out a mailing to rheumatologists in the northeastern part of the country, indicating that he was studying the relationship between food allergies and arthritis and was interested in studying some of their patients free of charge. Out of ninety letters, he received six responses, of which three said yes and three said no. Through one of the doctors who agreed to send patients, Janet eventually saw Dr. Mandell. He discussed her testing and the results:

"I want to emphasize that we never tell the patient what the test material is, so we completely eliminate suggestion. When we tested her with pork, she had pain almost immediately in one finger on her right hand, and this was her arthritis joint. We caused the joint to swell up and become red and painful.

"This test was repeated three times, once a week, and after the last test I told her to stay off pork for at least a week and then have a large portion of it one morning as a feeding test. Once again the same thing happened. However, when she told her rheumatologist, the man who was willing to have her come to me, he said he didn't believe it because we didn't have any controls. This is . . . more than pathetic, it's almost a medical crime! Here the patient had her symptom reproduced . . . and the doctor says he doesn't believe what has happened to her."

The ironic thing about this skepticism on the part of the orthodox medical establishment is that many of the treatments it prescribes for arthritis have never been proved either safe or effective. Gold injections are a good example. This treatment is extremely costly, has very high toxicity, and is only rarely of benefit to arthritis sufferers. Furthermore, in cases where gold does provide some relief, rheumatologists are unable to offer a scientific explanation of how it operates within the body. Nevertheless, gold continues to be endorsed by the arthritis establishment while something as simple as eliminating a food from a patient's diet, even if that food has been demonstrated to cause the patient's symptoms, is ignored or criticized as being unscientific.

DANA ULLMAN: HOMEOPATHY

Homeopathy is based on the idea that the cure for an illness is similar to its cause. As a result, treatment consists of administering small doses of a very diluted natural substance that would cause the symptoms of the condition being treated if it were taken in larger amounts.

Dana Ullman of the Foundation for Homeopathic Education and Research is the author of several books on homeopathy, including *The Consumer's Guide to Homeopathy: The Definitive Resource for Understanding Homeopathic Medicine and Making It Work for You* and *Discovering Homeopathy: Medicine for the 21st Century*. Ullman explains the homeopathic viewpoint:

"There are estimated to be two hundred types of arthritis. I'm glad that [the medical establishment has] increased that number from before. [In the past,] it's been . . . about ten or twenty. From the homeopathic point of view, every person with arthritis has his or her own species of arthritis. Homeopaths see disease as a syndrome.

"*The British Journal of Clinical Pharmacology*, a major pharmacology journal, published a double-blind, placebo-controlled study on the homeopathic treatment of rheumatoid arthritis; this was way back in 1980. This study showed that 82 percent of the patients given an individualized homeopathic medicine got some degree of relief, whereas among those given a placebo, only 21 percent got that similar degree of relief."

Ullman describes some of the homeopathic approaches: "One approach is the use of single remedies to treat the acute exacerbation of the problem. Acute exacerbation of the problem means an immediate problem of a short-term nature, like a flare-up of some sort. Homeopathy and homeopathic remedies can be used to allay and relieve some of the pain and discomfort that a person is having.

"A better approach, however, is using the single remedy prescribed by a professional homeopath. This provides what we call constitutional care. It's a more highly individualized remedy, not just for the acute flare-up but also for the person's overall genetic health and entire health history. For the homeopath to do this, it requires a detailed interview, lasting at least one to sometimes two hours. And sometimes a homeopath doesn't prescribe on that first interview but needs more information. This type of care is probably, in my estimation, one of the more profound ways to augment the body's own immune defense system, to not just relieve a person's condition but to really initiate a healing and curative process."

DR. LAURIE AESOPH'S SIX-STEP NUTRITIONAL APPROACH

Dr. Laurie Aesoph is a naturopathic physician as well as a medical writer. She has authored more than two hundred articles on topics ranging from nutrition to herbs and homeopathy.

Dr. Aesoph describes her views on the relationship between food and arthritis prevention and treatment:

RESTORATIVE FOODS

"Many, many studies tell us that what I call restorative foods, which merely are the good foods we should be eating anyway, [such as] whole grains, fruits, and vegetables, are what we need to insert into our diet. The studies show not only that good diets help out with arthritis but also that specific types of food seem to have healing qualities. For example, the oils from different fish have an anti-inflammatory and pain-relieving benefit for arthritis patients. Many fruits, vegetables, and even spices double as herbs. You can use those specifically for different arthritis symptoms.

"In an article printed in *The Lancet*, a British medical journal, researchers put their patients on a cleansing diet. But eventually what they did is switch them over to a lacto-ovo-vegetarian diet in different stages, and they had a group that was their control, their placebo, that just ate as normal. They found that even on the lacto-ovo, where people are eating vegetarian diets but also eating eggs and dairy, the benefits continued throughout that year and at the end of the year. So here's evidence where we know that diet is helping.

"There are enough studies that they are taking notice. They have always said that of course, if you're overweight, there is stress on the joints, so if you have something like osteoarthritis or what we call degenerative joint disease, that's going to aggravate and wear out your joints. But they are also looking at studies involving food allergies and cleansing and fish oil, and of course the purines are involved with gout. And diet has always been a large part of treating gout." The diet should be 100 percent plant-based organic, eliminate all meat, wheat, dairy, processed sugar, coffee, alcohol, refined foods, and fried foods.

STRESSOR FOODS

Dr. Aesoph asserts that it is equally important to minimize what she calls stressor foods from the diet: "Basically, the stressor foods are what set the stage for joint degeneration and breakdown to occur. And just to give you an example of what these foods are, look at the fat category. I want to remind [people] that fats per se are not bad. In fact they're essential, and there's something called essential fatty acids that we need to have—the fish oils fit into that category. But the transfatty acids—hydrogenated vegetable oils, for example, and margarine—[contain] too much saturated fat. Those are the sorts of things that are stressor foods and that we should be avoiding. Alcohol doesn't do us any good, nor does caffeine. Refined carbohydrates, such as sugars, flour, white rice, the different sweeteners, the artificial sweeteners such as aspartame and saccharine, processed foods, of course, and the additives and chemicals that are added to our foods are other things that we should also be avoiding.

"When you eat stressor foods, a lot of them really deplete the different nutrients: vitamins, minerals, and all the other phytochemicals and nutrients that we're discovering are in our foods. These, of course, are essential for general body function. Now, arthritis isn't just restricted to the joints. We've discovered that there is a link between the joints and different body systems, and so the immune system is involved. Rheumatoid arthritis is actually what we call an autoimmune disease, where the immune or defense system of your body is attacking yourself. So if you don't have the vitamins and minerals, your immune system isn't going to function as well as it can. Also, with regard to the intestinal tract, it's also vital that it function properly for all sorts of different conditions. When that isn't functioning right, it will aggravate an arthritic condition. I mentioned that if you are overweight, that will stress the joints. If you tend to eat stressor-type foods, that tends to play into or add to conditions of obesity. Also, we talk about stress in our lives, and I really believe that foods that are not complete in nutrition and aren't as whole as they should be are a stress on the body. So that doesn't help your body function any better.

"Also, if you are eating a lot of cooked or processed foods, they tend to be lower in the enzymes that help us digest our foods. There have been numerous studies done where when people eat a diet that is largely composed of cooked foods, their digestive systems, the pancreas, different organs that contribute digestive enzymes to the gut, have to work a little harder, which makes it harder to digest, and then that adds to your gut being a little thicker than it should be, and then that aggravates the arthritis down the road. So, you can see that there are direct and indirect effects that these stressor foods have.

"When you use natural medicine and conventional medicine, it doesn't need to be an either-or situation. You can also use nutrition to cut back on the medication that you're using. You can think of it as a compromise and perhaps gradually get away from the drugs. Also, if you happen to be on steroids, [such as] prednisone, if you plan to cut back and use nutrition, you need to work with your doctor on that. That's something you don't want to cut out cold turkey. The non-steroidal anti-inflammatory drugs are not as much of a problem. But when going off any prescription drug or steroids, talk to your doctor first."

THE PROGRAM

Dr. Aesoph outlines her nutritional program:

1. Cut out all the stressor foods. You want to eliminate anything that is harming your body or undermining your body's functions and really setting the stage for joint problems to develop. These foods not only weaken the joints but impinge on their ability to repair themselves as well. These are also the foods that add to excess weight, which can overburden the joints. Some of these foods are also high in purines, which tend to aggravate gout.

2. Cleanse the body with a real whole-foods diet and start to add the restorative foods. This helps repair the gastrointestinal tract, which is an imperative part of healing arthritis. At this point you should be starting to learn how to incorporate healthy eating habits and what foods to choose.

3. Test for and then begin to cut out allergy foods.

4. Rebuild damaged joints and overall health by refining your choice of restorative foods. Sea cucumber at 1,000 milligrams may help, as can manganese at 25 milligrams and the bioflavonoid complex at 500 milligrams. Glucosamine sulfate and chondroitin sulfate, both at 500 milligrams, can also produce phenomenal results. Flax at 1,000 milligrams from the omega-3 fatty acid group reestablishes normal fluid and osmotic pressure, the synovial fluid in those joints. Taking an alpha lipoic acid, the best all-around intracellular antioxidant, actually fights free radical damage inside the cell. Then you have a very powerful healing mechanism to get your joints circulating nutrients and oxygen and expelling carbon dioxide and waste products as they should. There are many supplements: minerals, vitamins, and herbs. Other ones that you can add are ginger,

cumin, and cayenne. Cayenne cream can be rubbed on arthritic joints because it depletes substance p, which in turn decreases pain.

5. Decrease weight, if that's a problem, because it is a stress on the joints.

6. Eliminate any stress by learning to eat properly, such as by chewing your food properly and eating in a relaxed way.

DR. DAVID STEENBLOCK: ARTHRITIS AND ATHEROSCLEROSIS

Because of the susceptibility of the joints to the accumulation of toxic material that can scratch and irritate the inner linings, leading to the pain and inflammation that characterize arthritis, an analogy has been made between arthritis and atherosclerosis (degeneration of the arteries). In both diseases corrosive substances scratch the inner linings of the body part involved, causing irritation that can lead to degeneration. These substances can come from toxic material in the bowel that gets into the bloodstream. They can also come from food. In the case of atherosclerosis, these foods include cholesterol, fats, and fried foods, which, when they get into the blood, scratch and irritate the very sensitive inner linings of the blood vessels. The same substances can also pass from the blood into the joint space and irritate the inner linings of the joints.

According to Dr. David Steenblock, this correlation between arthritis and atherosclerosis is one of the reasons why a low-fat, low-cholesterol, high-fiber diet has been useful in treating arthritis. "Many patients on this type of diet," he says, "show substantial improvement because the fiber cleanses the colon and removes many of the toxic bacterial waste products, which frees up the blood system and makes it more pure. This in turn allows the toxic materials to be eliminated from the joints, and so the joints themselves can begin to heal."

HIGH-FIBER DIET

Dr. Steenblock also explains how a diet that eliminates processed foods and focuses on the consumption of high-fiber natural grains, fruits, and vegetables works specifically in the treatment of arthritis:

"We want to eliminate white sugar and white flour products and processed foods and foods which contain food additives because these processed foods cause abnormalities in the state of health of the intestine. When you eat processed foods with little fiber, the bacterial content of the colon changes from the so-called good bacteria, which are Lactobacillus bifidus and L. acidophilus, to organisms that are anaerobic such as anerococci and streptococci and organisms that generally are not healthy and produce many toxic substances themselves. When these toxic substances are present as a result of eating a diet high in refined food and lacking fiber, these toxins pass through the bowel into the blood. Also, refined foods, because they are so easily digestible and do not require work by the intestine, cause the muscle wall of the intestine to atrophy, or become thinner. This thinness of the wall allows more toxic material to pass through the bowel into the blood. Once it is in the blood, it can pass easily into the joints and cause more problems.

"The use of the high-fiber natural diet counteracts this trend because the fiber changes the bacterial content of the colon back to normal, and this eliminates many of the toxic materials, the carcinogens, and the mutagens that are formed otherwise, which are well-documented causes not only of osteoarthritis but also of cancer of the colon and atherosclerosis. The fiber also strengthens the bowel wall, making it thicker and healthier, and this creates more of a mucosal barrier between the colon's interior and the blood. Thus the diet should be more of a natural- and raw-foods diet if you want to get a good result."

Dr. Steenblock does warn, however, that people who have spent an entire lifetime eating refined, fiberless foods must approach a change to a raw, high-fiber diet with caution (excess dietary fiber can, for instance, cause calcium and zinc to be washed through the system so that calcium and zinc deficiencies result) in order to give their intestinal tract time to strengthen. A good physician with a solid background in nutritional therapy should be consulted before any drastic dietary changes are made.

CHELATION THERAPY

While atherosclerosis and arthritis often exacerbate each other, treatments other than diet that are directed at one condition often are beneficial in treating the other. For example, Dr. Steenblock discusses how chelation therapy, an intravenous chemical treatment commonly used for atherosclerosis and heart disease, can also benefit arthritic patients:

"One of the problems with osteoarthritis is that the capillaries of the synovium have become rigidified, or more rigid than they should be, as a consequence of the aging process and of atherosclerosis. This limits the blood flow through these joints; therefore, the heat that is produced when the joint is put in motion cannot be taken away because the circulation is poor. As a result, pain occurs when you exercise, and conversely, when you are resting, the blood flow through that tissue is poor and toxic materials accumulate and can cause pain. Anything that increases the diameter and the blood flow through these capillaries will aid in the restoration process. This is where chelation therapy is very valuable because it actually gets into these small blood vessels and capillaries and removes the cross-linkage of the collagen and elastin. This makes these small blood vessels more pliable and elastic, gives them more diameter so that more blood can pass through them, and thus helps in the healing process."

CHONDROITIN SULFATE

Dr. Steenblock also uses chondroitin sulfate as part of his treatment. "Chondroitin sulfate appears to be one of the best treatments for both arthritis and vascular disease," he says. "When you take it orally, it actually enters into the body through the intestinal tract and will selectively go to the joints and all the areas of damage in the blood vessels. It not only acts preventively but also will help reverse the diseases that are present."

Dr. Steenblock says that while chondroitin is a promising treatment, it is not a miracle cure. "The treatment is not the sort of miracle-drug type of treatment where you give the person one pill and get immediate results. What we are dealing with is a natural substance, and it takes time for these natural substances to create the result we are looking for, namely, healing of the injured areas." He says that it may take from two to four months to see results.

Dr. Steenblock adds, "There is another substance, which is derived from the New Zealand green lip mussel. There are a number of trade names for it. This substance is also a mucopolysaccharide, and it is effective in treating osteoarthritis as well as rheumatoid arthritis. It is available in most health food stores.

"These mucopolysaccharides can also be used preventively to heal the small nicks and irritations that occur routinely in the blood vessels and joints. They immediately seal these little cracks and crevices so that they do not get larger. Our bodies are not really capable of doing that on their own, and we need to help them along."

Gary Null's Protocol for Arthritis

PLANT-BASED DIET

Start with an overall dietary cleanse, and eliminate all allergens. Drink filtered water. Get tested for candida, food allergies, and heavy metal toxicity, as any of these may contribute to arthritic pain.

Salads, beans, nuts seeds, vegetables	
Grapefruit, lemon lime aloe (3 oz.), a capsule of cayenne, and wasabi mustard in a juice	
Pure grape juice (blue, black, or red)	
Fish oil	1 tbsp. per week
Flax seed	1 tsp per day
Garlic	all day
Raw sweet onion (Vidalia) in juice or in salad	
Avocado	
Olive oil	
Olives	1 cup daily
Tempeh, tofu, seaweeds	
Vegetable juices	4 glasses daily
Berry juice	1 glass daily
Cabbage juice	

SUPPLEMENTS

Take the following daily in divided doses:

N-acetyl-D-glucosamine	1,000 mg
Chondroitin sulfate	1,000 mg
Nettle leaf extract	500 mg
NAD glucosamine	500 mg
Ginger	100 mg
Fish oil (EPA/DHA)	1,000 mg
Boron	5 mg
Vitamin B complex	50 mg twice a day

Vitamin E	600 IU
Calcium citrate	1,200 mg
Magnesium citrate	1,200 mg
Coenzyme Q10	200 mg
DMG	150 mg
TMG	150 mg
SOD	500 mg
Beta-carotene	25,000 IU
Folic acid	1,000 mcg
DLPA (pain relief)	250 mg
Zinc	25 mg
Digestive enzymes	individualized dose
MGN 3	1,500 mg
GLA	1,000 mg
Vitamin C	5,000–20,000 mg daily
MSM	1,000 mg daily
Green-lipped mussel	individualized dose
Garlic	individualized dose
Cayenne	individualized dose
Turmeric	individualized dose
Cat's claw	individualized dose
Pomegranate juice concentrate	1 tbsp.
Bone set	individualized dose
Boswellia	individualized dose
Burdock	individualized dose
Devil's claw	individualized dose
Yucca	individualized dose
Vitamin B5	individualized dose
Grapeseed extract	100 mg
MSM	500 BID
Vitamin K	individualized dose
Silica	50 mg
Manganese	25 mg
SAMe	400 mg
L-cysteine	500 mg
L-glutamic acid	200 mg

L-taurine	200 mg
Proprietary and patented blend of natural citrus and palm fruit extract containing nobiletin and tangeretin	300 mg
Bromelain proteolytic enzyme extract from pineapple (*Ananas comosus*) (stem)	500 mg [2,000 GDU per gram/5,000 FIP per gram activity]
Vitamin D3 (as cholecalciferol)	3,000 IU
Silicon (from horsetail herb, Equisetum arvense)	5 mg
Curcumin	900 mg daily, with 5 mg of piperine
Green tea extract	725 mg daily of green tea powder, yielding at least 246 mg of EGCG
NAC	600 mg daily
Black cumin seed oil	1 tsp twice daily
Naturleaf (enzyme-enhanced) / Plant-Sprout sterols / sitosterolins (go to www.LEF.org)	500 mg four times per day

ADDITIONAL THERAPIES

Acupuncture or AMMA™ therapy with Chinese herbs

Hot Epsom salt baths

Hot castor oil packs

Massage therapy

Sauna

Chiropractic adjustments

Hyaluronic acid. A number of studies have examined the benefits of intra-articular injections of hyaluronic acid. This treatment is effective in treating osteoarthritis of major joints. Discuss hyaluronic acid therapy with your physician.

Research Update

An increasing body of evidence is showing the benefits of natural modalities to overall health and well-being. Following is a sample of recent peer-reviewed scientific studies in the area of arthritis.

In a 2015 report published in *Inflammation*, pyrroloquinoline quinone (PQQ) was shown to slow the progression of osteoarthritis by inhibiting nitric oxide production and metalloproteinase synthesis. The investigators noted that PQQ is expected to be a new pharmacological application in the near future. The Chinese herbal remedy *Tripterygium wilfordii* Hook F (TwHF) was found to be comparable with methotrexate in treating rheumatoid arthritis, according to a 2015 study in *Annals of the Rheumatic Diseases*. A 2011 *Life Extension Magazine* report cited evidence from the scientific literature that 40 milligrams per day of undenatured type II collagen, derived from chicken cartilage, can decrease the immune response to exposed collagen, and therefore alleviate pain and loss of function related to arthritis. At Harvard's Beth Israel Hospital in Boston, researchers reported a drop in joint swelling and tenderness in people with rheumatoid arthritis who supplemented with a proprietary form of the collagen for three months, and complete remission in 14 percent of the sample. Eight out of ten patients with juvenile rheumatoid arthritis who supplemented for twelve weeks had reductions in numbers of swollen and tender joints, with no adverse effects noted.

Chapter 23

Birth Control

According to a 2015 CNN report, a growing number of women, concerned about the side effects of the Pill, are turning to fertility awareness as their main method of birth control. Aided with technology from apps such as Kindra, Glow, and Ovuline, which help monitor primary fertility signs by tracking basal body temperature and cervical fluid, these women still represent a small portion of the population. However, a 2009 study published the *Journal of the American Board of Family Medicine* found that when given positive information about fertility awareness, more than one in five women expressed interest in using it. This research follows a 2007 article in *Human Reproduction Today* revealing that fertility awareness remains equally as effective as oral contraceptives, with none of the side effects.

No currently available form of birth control is 100 percent effective and risk-free, and no single method is right for everyone. A woman's fertility is a highly personal matter, so the more you are able to feel in sync with your menstrual cycle and fertility, the better able you will be to make the right decisions about birth control for you and your partner. Despite scientific research, myths and misconceptions continue to abound. My goal in this chapter is not to join the debate but to make sure that the information already available to some in the alternative health community is available to everyone.

Fertility Awareness

Fertility awareness, also called natural family planning, the Billings method (named after John and Evelyn Billings, two Australian researchers who helped popularize it), and mucus observation, among other names, is an underrated but extremely effective method of pregnancy prevention. This is not the old rhythm method promoted by the Catholic Church in the past, which was notoriously ineffective; each woman has her own "rhythm" that may change from time to time and may not fit into an established pattern.

Actually, fertility awareness can be characterized not as a method of birth control but as a way of life. That is, if you have a more accurate understanding of the dynamic physiological changes that occur during your menstrual cycles, you will be more aware of exactly when you are likely to get pregnant and will be better able to take preventive measures or, if you are trying to become pregnant, enhance your chances.

Some years ago researchers at Princeton University reanalyzed a mountain of data that had been collected by the World Health Organization (WHO) on couples who used fertility awareness. They found that this method was 97 percent effective in preventing pregnancy for those who understood its principles and used it as their sole method of contraception. This research should have put to rest the widely held myth that fertility awareness isn't very effective.

Two myths that prevent many people from using fertility awareness as their main method of birth control are that it is difficult to learn and that women have to take their temperature every day and laboriously chart their menstrual cycles for the rest of their lives. This is definitely not the case. You can learn the basic principles of fertility awareness over a few months, and by knowing what to look for, you can learn to identify your fertile period intuitively with a high degree of accuracy without having to deal with charts and thermometers on a daily basis.

Essentially, a number of specific bodily changes signal the onset of a woman's fertile time. These include changes in cervical mucus, body temperature, sexual desire, and an ovulatory pain called mittelschmerz (middle pain).

Getting pregnant requires three factors: sperm, alkaline fertile mucus to nurture and transport the sperm, and a ripe egg in one of the fallopian tubes. The menstrual cycle begins on the first day of menstrual bleeding, and the average cycle lasts twenty-seven to thirty days, although cycles as short as twenty-one days or as long as three to nine months are common. A viscous, "stretchy" mucous secretion manufactured in the glands of the cervical canal begins to ooze from the cervical opening at about day 10 of the average cycle and increases daily, peaking at days 14 to 16. Using a plastic speculum, you can actually see the clear mucus, which looks a lot like egg white, oozing from the cervical opening.

As production increases, the stretchy mucus seeps from the vagina and makes a sort of crusty secretion on your underpants or can be picked up by toilet paper.

At the same time that fertile mucus is beginning to develop, a ripe egg pops through the side of one of your ovaries and begins its trip of three to five days down the egg tube. As you approach ovulation, your temperature rises gradually and then, in most women, drops sharply on the day of actual ovulation. If fertile mucus is present and you have unprotected intercourse, the sperm slip easily along the liquid highway of mucus into the cervical canal, where they are kept alive for several days to regroup, as it were, and swim up through the uterus in search of an unfertilized egg.

The idea in using fertility awareness for contraception is to avoid having any sperm in the vagina at times when fertile mucus might be present. By carefully looking for the signs of ovulation (fertile mucus, a drop in temperature, mittelschmerz), you can identify pretty specifically when that time is. The first part of the cycle (including menstruation) is considered the "unsafe" time because fertile mucus can appear early or at low levels, but any fertile mucus presents the possibility of pregnancy. Couples who use fertility awareness as a form of birth control avoid vaginal intercourse at this time but may enjoy other forms of sexual activity. Others use a barrier method of contraception until they are sure that ovulation has occurred. After ovulation, however, another egg will not appear, so this is considered the "safe" time. After that time, according to researchers, it is perfectly safe to have vaginal intercourse without getting pregnant.

You can learn the tenets of fertility awareness from a number of excellent books, but many women and their partners find that taking a workshop with several sessions is the easiest and best way to learn. There is now a wide array of fertility detection devices that can be fun to use and are quite accurate.

The Pill

Most birth control pills contain two types of synthetic female hormones, progestin (synthetic progesterone) and estrogen. In the first part of the menstrual cycle, higher-than-normal estrogen levels prevent the release of follicle-stimulating hormone (FSH). The absence of this hormone, which is manufactured in the pituitary gland, prevents an egg from developing inside the ovary. In the second part of the cycle, higher levels of progesterone thicken cervical mucus and inhibit the cyclic buildup of the uterine lining. If an egg were to be released or sperm were to get through the cervical mucus, the uterine lining would be too thin to support an implanted fertilized egg. The combination pills interfere with ovulation, thicken cervical mucus, and interfere with the buildup of the uterine lining.

Other varieties of pills also are available. Progestin-only pills, which are called minipills, are different in that they only thicken cervical mucus and interfere with the buildup of the uterine lining. Among the newer pills are Yaz, which contains a synthetic estrogen and drospirenone, a newer form of progestin; Seasonale, which contains progestin and estrogen and is taken for twelve weeks, followed by one week of placebo tablets, thereby causing menstruation only once every three months; and Lybel, the first continuous use birth control pill, which eliminates menstruation altogether.

In theory, the Pill is an elegant solution to the age-old problem of preventing unwanted pregnancies, and it has some positive aspects. Many women like the Pill because its use can be completely separated from sex and there is no mechanical barrier to be aware of during sexual activity. Because the Pill suppresses the menstrual cycle, its users often experience less painful menstrual cramps, fewer premenstrual syndrome (PMS) symptoms, and a lowered risk of anemia. Women with endometriosis may experience a decrease in pain and other symptoms, and those who have a tendency to develop ovarian cysts are less likely to do so. Studies also show a lower incidence of pelvic inflammatory disease caused by gonorrhea as well as cancer of the uterine lining (endometrial cancer) and ovarian cancer.

However, the Pill, even in its current lower-dose formulations, has some significant drawbacks. Higher-than-normal levels of hormones not only have the desired effect of preventing pregnancy but also travel through the bloodstream and affect other organs that have nothing to do with contraception, often precipitating or exacerbating serious underlying conditions. In addition, synthetic hormones can affect mood or exacerbate a tendency toward depression. They may decrease the desire for sex or cause hair loss or fatigue, a bloated feeling, and weight gain over time. Some women don't experience any of these symptoms and enjoy the freedom from contraceptive jellies and devices, but others say that they simply don't feel like themselves.

The Pill also interferes with the way vitamins are absorbed and utilized by the body. Dr. Sherrill Sellman, a naturopath, leading women's health educator and writer, and author of *Hormone Heresy*, explains that it causes major nutritional deficiencies of the B vitamins and vitamins C and E, as well as mineral imbalances.

"The B vitamins are necessary to protect a woman's immune system, her fertility, her emotional well-being," she says. "The side effects from deficiency of these vitamins are fatigue, weakness, insomnia, aches and pains, weight loss, depression, irritability, lack of initiative, constipation, oversensitivity to noise, loss of appetite, circulatory problems, skin problems, gum disease, dizziness, depression, eye problems. Folic acid is an essential vitamin to help with the development of a healthy fetus. Women taking the Pill become deficient in folic acid. This compromises not just their own health and immunity, but also the health of their fetuses."

Vitamins C and E are key nutrients for the immune system and the heart. They help detoxify heavy metals out of the body. "These are also seriously depleted in women who take the Pill," Dr. Sellman says.

Mineral imbalances are not uncommon. "Copper goes way up and that causes migraine and hair loss and high blood pressure," Dr. Sellman explains. "Zinc goes way down, which causes poor resistance to infection, diabetes, and infertility problems. The low-density lipids, the LDLs, go way up and the triglyceride levels also go up. So we are looking at serious, serious compromising of a woman's health and her ability to function."

One of the biggest problems that women have today with the Pill is fear that it may promote the growth of cancer. Medical studies on this issue are conflicting, but too many studies show an increased cancer risk to dismiss this issue. The National Cancer Institute reported in 2012 that while oral contraceptives appear to be associated with lower risks of endometrial and ovarian cancer, they appear to be linked with higher risks of breast, cervical, and liver cancer. In 2015, a study published in the *British Journal of Clinical Pharmacology* reported higher rates of a rare brain tumor in women using the contraceptive.

In addition to cancer, the Pill has been linked to other medical conditions. In 2015, research published in the *BMJ* (formerly the *British Medical Journal*) found that women taking newer forms of the Pill, brands such as Yaz, Yasmin, and Desogen, had triple the risk for blood clots than women not taking the medication. In 2014, a study presented at the American Academy of Neurology found that women who take the Pill may be as much as 50 percent more likely to develop multiple sclerosis.

About 10 million women in the United States use the Pill at any one time, but from 30 to 50 percent stop using it within a year because of undesirable side effects.

In the 1960s and 1970s high-dose pills caused serious problems for many women and are known to have caused a small number of deaths as well, but high doses equaled high effectiveness. The Pill got a reputation for being 98 percent effective. Today most women take the progesterone-only minipill, which is only about 96 percent effective in normal use. This is still quite acceptable in terms of effectiveness, but it's not really much better than condoms, the cervical cap, or the diaphragm when those barrier methods are used consistently. Failures with minipills occur when women forget to take them or decide not to take them because they cease to be sexually active for a time. You can't just take one pill and be protected; it takes several weeks for the hormones to build up in your system.

Other failures occur because of normal fluctuations in women's hormone levels. You must take the minipill at the same time each day to get maximum protection. If you miss a day or two, double up on pills for at least two days. If you miss more than two days, you need to use another method, such as condoms or VCF.

There are numerous caveats you need to be aware of if you take birth control pills. You absolutely should not take the Pill if you have heart disease, severe varicose veins, serious circulatory problems, liver disease, or breast cancer. You should seriously consider using another method if you have diabetes, hypertension, gallbladder disease, depression, epilepsy, migraines, irregular periods, or sickle cell anemia—the trait or the disease. A woman with these conditions may take the minipill safely but should do so only after a consultation with her doctor. You should stop taking the Pill if you are planning surgery or must have your leg in a cast. The Pill may interfere with the absorption of certain vitamins—including vitamins B_1, B_2, B_6, B_{12}, C, and E and folic acid—and may alter carbohydrate metabolism. If you smoke, the Pill becomes far more risky for you.

Contraceptive Technology, a leading family-planning handbook, has devised an easily remembered acronym, ACHES, to help make you aware of the danger signs of the Pill:

A—abdominal pain (severe)
C—chest pain (severe), cough, shortness of breath
H—headache (severe), dizziness, weakness, numbness
E—eye problems (vision loss or blurring), speech problems
S—severe leg pain (calf or thigh)

If you experience any of these signs, call your doctor immediately.

In an article in the magazine *Alternative Medicine*, Dr. Jesse Hanley reminds women that being in touch with the natural monthly cycle of hormones supports their intuition and creativity, yet women's lives today make it difficult for them to fully live out their female biological cycle. Taking birth control pills regulates their cycle to the point where they hardly notice that they're having a period. As Dr. Hanley puts it, "Many women become almost addicted to not being a woman, to not understanding the natural cycling of hormones and the feelings, increased sensitivity, intuition, and creativity this evokes." She sees this as a self-destructive tendency that will create health problems in the future. "Chinese medicine describes the uterus as the place where a woman's energy and essence reside, so we need to rethink our approach to uterine health," Dr. Hanley concludes.

Male Condom

Many people, both men and women, are reluctant to use condoms because direct skin-to-skin contact feels better. However, that thin rubber membrane may be all that stands between you and pregnancy or a variety of diseases. These latex rubber sheaths that unroll to cover the penis are 90 to 98 percent effective in preventing pregnancy. The effectiveness can be raised to nearly 100 percent by combining them with the cervical cap, diaphragm, vaginal contraceptive film (VCF), or fertility awareness.

Condoms also provide the best protection from sexually transmitted diseases (STDs). According to the US Food and Drug Administration, they are "highly effective" in preventing infection from HIV, gonorrhea, Chlamydia, trichomoniasis, and hepatitis B. They are less effective against genital herpes, human papillomavirus, syphilis, and chancroid.

Condoms are often thought of as a "male-controlled" method, but actually, the effective use of condoms requires the interest and willingness of both partners. Today both men and women buy condoms and keep them in their backpacks or at the bedside for ready use. Because of low cost and wide availability, condoms are the most commonly used barrier method in the world. They come in a variety of styles, in different sizes, and with various aesthetic embellishments, with or without lubricants and/or spermicide.

To be effective, condoms must be used correctly. They should be unrolled along the shaft of the penis with a little space left at the tip to collect the ejaculate. Condoms may be lubricated or can be used with a variety of water-based lubricants (read the label), but they should not be used with petroleum-based lubricants such as Vaseline. Removal must be done carefully to avoid spillage.

Because of rumors about a high breakage rate, many people believe that condoms are not all that effective. To counter those fears, the US Food and Drug Administration (FDA) has instituted more rigorous standards of testing, so breakage rarely occurs. Condoms that are old or have been exposed to heat are more likely to break. If you are worried about breakage, use two condoms at a time. Also, try to buy them in small quantities and at places where turnover is high, such as large discount drug stores.

Female Condom

The female condom somewhat resembles the standard male condom and can be bought over the counter. It is a soft pouch that is inserted into the vagina like a lining. It has two rings. One is fitted around the cervix like a diaphragm, and the other remains outside the body and covers the labia. If always used correctly, 5 out of 100 women will become pregnant each year. If not always used correctly, 21 out of 100 will become pregnant. It takes some learning to use properly, since it can get twisted if it is not inserted correctly. It may also reduce sexual sensation and the feeling of spontaneity.

The female condom is said to provide effective protection against STDs. It can be more effective in preventing pregnancy and disease if used with a spermicide. However, it has recently been found that spermicides have certain risks. In 2007, the FDA issued a warning that nonoxynol-9, the chemical ingredient in many spermicides, may irritate tissue and actually increase the risk of HIV infection and other STDs in certain individuals.

Diaphragm

The diaphragm is considered a barrier method of birth control, but the spermicidal cream or jelly used with it is actually what kills the sperm and prevents them from entering the cervix. A diaphragm is a shallow cup made of soft latex rubber with a flexible rim that fits neatly into the palm of your hand. Once very popular, the diaphragm was overtaken in the early 1960s by the heavy promotion and the flood of research dollars behind the Pill. The diaphragm is made in a variety of sizes, ranging from about two to four inches (fifty to one hundred millimeters) so that it may be fitted in accordance with the length of the vagina. When it is in place, one part of the rim is lodged behind the pubic bone, while the opposite part cups underneath the cervix in the back of the vagina.

A diaphragm with spermicide can be inserted up to six hours before vagina-penis contact. It should stay in place for at least six hours after intercourse to ensure that most of the sperm are killed. The maximum amount of time the diaphragm should be left in is twenty-four hours. If you have repeated inter-course, it is necessary to insert more spermicidal jelly or cream with an appli-cator each time, leaving the diaphragm in place.

The diaphragm has few health risks. There is effectively no risk of it going far-ther inside than its correct position; if it pushes back against the rectum, it may be the wrong size. However, in addition to killing sperm, spermicide may kill off the lactobacilli in the vagina that keep yeast under control. To help counteract this, between diaphragm uses you can bathe with a solution of water and *Lactobacillus acidophilus* (available at most health food stores) by using a douche nozzle, a squirt bottle, or a plastic speculum.

About 20 percent of diaphragm users have occasional or recurrent bladder infections. This may occur because the rim bruises the urethra and makes it more susceptible to infection or because the spermicide alters the normal environment of the vagina and allows harmful bacteria to grow. If you are using the diaphragm and begin having recurrent bladder infections, you should look for a different method. If you have a prolapsed or otherwise displaced uterus, vaginal fistulas, or a protrusion of the bladder through the vaginal wall, the diaphragm is not an option for you.

As with other barrier methods, the diaphragm is effective only if you use it consistently and correctly. Studies have shown that the diaphragm is between 89 and 98 percent effective for women who use it during every session of intercourse (except during the menstrual period). However, the effectiveness of the diaphragm can be increased to nearly 100 percent by combining it with condoms or fertility awareness.

Your partner should not be able to feel the diaphragm, but if he does, it is usu-ally only an awareness that something is there. Of course, using the diaphragm in no way compromises your fertility, and all you have to do if you choose to become pregnant is stop using it.

Cervical Cap

According to women's health and sexuality advocate Rebecca Chalker, the existence of the cervical cap is one of the best-kept secrets of modern times. This is an approach to birth control that is as safe and effective as the diaphragm but offers a good measure of spontaneity and the convenience of the Pill.

The cervical cap is a small, silicone cup that is placed over the cervix in order to block the uterine opening. It is smaller and more compact than a diaphragm, and can be left in place for a longer time, up to forty-eight hours. As Chalker explains in *The Complete Cervical Cap Guide*, "a dollop of spermicide is placed in the dome. Then the cap rim is folded in half, tipped into the opening of the vagina, and guided with a finger to the back of the vaginal canal, where it readily slips over the cervix (the neck of the uterus). The cap stays firmly in place by gripping the cervix and forming a strong suction and provides a physical barrier to the sperm, while the spermicide affords an additional chemical barrier."

Vaginal Contraceptive Film

Another well-kept contraceptive secret is vaginal contraceptive film (VCF). This square inch of material that looks like plastic but turns into a viscous liquid after five to fifteen minutes in the vagina is 28 percent nonoxynol-9, the sperm-killing ingredient in commercial spermicides. The film was designed to be used alone and seems to be about 85 to 90 percent effective when used that way, but most practitioners recommend that it be used with a cervical cap, diaphragm, or condom. Combining VCF with these barriers should increase their effectiveness to nearly 100 percent.

Some people find the higher dose of nonoxynol-9—about three times as strong as regular spermicide—irritating. If this happens to you, you will probably have to stop using it. The other disadvantage of VCF is that it is somewhat expensive and not widely available in the United States. However, it is less messy than normal spermicidal cream or jelly and provides a stronger dose of spermicide.

Implants, Patches, and Shots

Implanon, approved by the FDA for use in the United States in 2006, is a matchstick-sized contraceptive implant that is inserted under the skin of the upper arm.

It protects against pregnancy for up to three years by releasing a form of progestin that blocks ovulation. Implanon is similar to Norplant, which was taken off the US market in 2002. However, it has only a single rod instead of six.

The birth control patch (Ortho Evra) is a thin, plastic patch that sticks to the skin. It is placed on the skin once a week for three weeks in a row, and then removed for one week. The patch contains both estrogen and progestin. Some reports have linked the patch with an increased risk of breast cancer, among other adverse effects. In 2006, Johnson and Johnson recalled its patch after users were found to have three times more strokes and blood clots than the general population.

The birth control shot, also known as Depo-Provera, releases progestin into the body. Each shot prevents pregnancy for three months.

Dr. Hanley states that the synthetic hormones in these products can negatively interfere with women's hormonal balance: "Some patients tell me that using this form of contraception makes them feel as if a black cloud has settled over them." Other side effects may include irregular bleeding, weight gain, water retention, and depression. In addition, they may disrupt thyroid function and increase the risk of blood clots and cardiovascular disease.

Intrauterine Devices (IUDs)

According to the 2015 data from the National Center for Health Statistics, the use of IUDs in the US increased nearly five-fold in the last decade, becoming the contraceptive method of choice for 7 percent of women ages 15 to 44. IUDs are small, plastic T-shaped devices that are inserted into the uterus for varying periods of time. The ParaGard IUD, which contains copper, is effective for twelve years. The Mirena, Skyla, and newer Liletta IUDs, which release a small amount of progestin, are effective for five years. They work by blocking the passage of sperm, with the latter also blocking ovulation. There are benefits as well as risks and side effects associated with IUDs.

Sterilization

Many people are surprised to learn that surgical sterilization—tying, clipping, or cutting the fallopian tubes in women or cutting the vas deferens in men—is the most widely used form of contraception both in the United States and in the rest of the world. About 15 million women and men use this method.

Although it involves surgically altering parts of the body through snips and sutures, sterilization is the ultimate in "hands-off" birth control. Once the snips have healed, you never have to think about birth control again—unless, that is, you want to have a baby. Reversal rates for surgical sterilization are around 25 percent, depending on the type of procedure. This is a relatively low rate of success, and studies have found that regret is not uncommon among women and men who have had this procedure. Moreover, the surgery, which may not be covered by insurance, may cost thousands of dollars. Once again, no available form of birth control is without its drawbacks.

In women the surgery is most often done through a small incision below the navel. The abdominal cavity is inflated with carbon or nitrous oxide, and a laparoscope is inserted through the incision to allow the surgeon to see and manipulate the egg tubes with various instruments. This surgery is usually done on an outpatient basis, and a light general anesthesia or spinal block is commonly used. Most women have some abdominal discomfort for one to three days and feel fully recovered within a week.

Chapter 24

Breast Cancer and Other Breast Diseases

Breast cancer remains the most commonly diagnosed cancer among women in the United States, other than skin cancer. According to the National Cancer Institute, there were an estimated 232,000 new cases in 2015, and 40,000 deaths from the disease. The number of survivors has risen dramatically over the years, and now stands at nearly three million. Despite tens of millions of dollars invested into research each year, little progress has been made in the fight against breast cancer. Not only are mainstream treatments like chemotherapy, radiation, and surgery generally not very effective, they also come with a host of dangerous, and sometimes deadly, side effects. Life-saving solutions don't start with toxic drugs and risky treatments but prevention. It's critical to note that prevention involves more than just exercising or purchasing a supplement. Like any inflammatory condition, a whole-body approach is needed in overcoming breast cancer.

Causes

There are a number of risk factors in the development of the disease. While some of these are out of our control, others clearly are not.

DIET

Dr. Susan Silberstein, health educator and author of *Hungry for Health*, shares some of the well-established facts regarding diet and cancer. "We know from the National Academy of Sciences and the World Health Organization that 70 to 80 percent of all cancers are diet related. We know from the National Cancer Institute that 70 percent of all breast cancer deaths are avoidable through dietary change. Much of the information we have comes from studies of Asian women, who have much lower rates of breast cancer when they are in their native countries and they are consuming their native diets. But as soon as they move to the United States and they adopt our Western diet high in meat and fat and dairy, their breast cancer rates go up 400 percent and meet the breast cancer rates of women in this country, and that happens in only one or two generations."

Dr. Charles Simone, director of the Protective Cancer Institute in Lawrenceville, New Jersey, explains the association between fats and disease: "We know that fatty foods actually convert normal cells into problematic cells. Consuming high-fat foods, particularly unsaturated fats, increases free radical production, damaging the cell membrane. At this point the damaged cell has two choices. It can die. That's fine, because if it dies, you make another one. Or it can repair itself. In the repair process, a cell can go awry and metamorphose into a cancer cell. So fats cause free radicals, which damage cells, which in turn try to repair themselves and transform themselves into cancer cells."

Robin Keuneke, a natural food counselor and the author of *Total Breast Health*, points to another diet-related factor: essential fatty acid deficiencies. These fatty acids are found, for example, in extra-virgin olive oil. Many studies have linked Italian diets, which contain lots of extra-virgin olive oil, to lower rates of breast cancer. Other diet choices that seem connected to higher rates of cancer are cooked meat and fried foods. Keuneke notes, "One of the theses of my book is that burned meat and fried foods are linked to breast cancer. I found four studies linking burned meat, such as bacon, to cancer. Yet the so-called experts said there was not enough information to recommend changes in cooking."

This is not true. The first study was published more than forty years ago. It was a population study looking at Seventh-Day Adventist women, who have a relatively clean diet. It found that women who ate the greatest amount of fried potatoes had the highest rate of breast cancer.

Hot, spicy foods, oily foods, and stimulants, such as coffee, black tea, and drugs, should also be avoided. Water should be pure, free from fluoride, chlorine, pesticides, and other synthetic chemicals.

TOBACCO AND ALCOHOL

Tobacco and alcohol are leading contributors to cancer. "We know that tobacco is the number-two cause of cancer in our country and the number-two cause of breast cancer as well," Dr. Simone says. "Regarding alcohol, we know that two to three drinks per week is enough to confer a twofold to threefold risk of getting cancer of the breast independently of everything else. So the number one, two, and three causes of breast cancer—a high-fat diet, smoking, and alcohol consumption—are totally within our control."

Dr. Lise Alschuler, author of *The Definitive Guide to Cancer*, a manual on alternative and integrative approaches to preventing, treating, and healing cancer, tells us that there is a linear relationship between the amount of alcohol that a woman consumes and her risk of breast cancer. With every drink added on a daily basis, a woman's risk of breast cancer will increase proportional to that added alcohol. However, there is a way to mitigate the increased risk.

"There have been some interesting studies to show that if a woman drinks, let's say, more than one and a half drinks a day, her risk of breast cancer goes up by about 30 percent," Dr. Alschuler says. "If, however, she consumes folic acid in the form of a multivitamin or as some sort of supplement, her risk of breast cancer with that one and a half drinks only goes up 5 percent. So the folic acid clearly has a way to reduce some of the damage from alcohol. This is good news for the women out there who enjoy a glass of wine in the evening, because it's possible to drink some alcohol as long as you're consuming some folic acid as a supplement in the same day as well. Without the folic acid, alcohol is a clear and very strong risk factor for breast cancer, and most likely cervical and ovarian cancer as well."

INHERITED GENE MUTATIONS

About 5 to 10 percent of breast cancers are believed to be hereditary. Certain inherited gene mutations can cause normal cells to become cancerous. Specific mutations in the tumor-suppressor genes BRCA1 and BRCA2 are known to be associated with increased risk of breast and ovarian cancers. According to the National Cancer Institute, BRCA mutations account for 20 to 25 percent of all hereditary breast cancers.

Although certain genes carry high risks for cancer and other diseases, caution is urged in how we respond. The actress Angelina Jolie had a double mastectomy and removal of her ovaries after learning that a mutation in the BRCA1 gene gave her an 87 percent risk of developing breast cancer and a 50 percent risk of ovarian cancer. She determined that this was the right course of action in her particular situation and correctly implores other women to get advice and consider all of their options before making any of their own decisions. In a *New York Times* commentary in March 2015, she stated, "A positive BRCA test does not mean a leap to surgery. . . . There is more than one way to deal with any health issue. The most important thing is to learn about the options and choose what is right for you personally."

This case raises an urgent question regarding invasive surgery as a preventive medical procedure due to certain genes associated with disease. This risk model used is a mathematical model that does not take into account what if we changed the circumstances of our lives.

Dr. Christiane Northrup, a board-certified OB-GYN physician and author of several bestselling books including *Women's Bodies, Women's Wisdom* and *Women and Menopause*, offers her comments. "I agree that everyone has a right to whatever they choose to do with their bodies, and if your conventional doctor tells you that you have an 87 percent risk of breast cancer and you don't know anything about [alternatives], which I've spent my whole life teaching, then her decision makes absolute sense.

"The whole flap around the Angelina Jolie decision is, unfortunately, going to get women in this huge state of anxiety. Ms. Jolie has the right to do what she did, and I completely understand it. The problem is that when you are a celebrity of that fame—she is a world citizen—your decisions influence unduly other people, and you have to take some responsibility for that. Her decision is fine. The article that she wrote, the op-ed piece was beautifully written and everyone can understand it."

With epigenetics, people have been led to believe that if you have the gene you inevitably get the disease, Dr. Northrup says, adding that research proves otherwise. (See chapter 15 for a discussion of epigenetics.) She cites several recent studies as examples. One found a 50 percent reduction of all cancer risks, including breast cancer, once vitamin D levels were in the optimal range. A 2013 article in the *New England Journal of Medicine* reported that since 1980, 1.3 million women "were overdiagnosed and overtreated for cancers they would possibly die with but never die from."

Another study, published in the *Archives of Internal Medicine*, followed 200,000 Norwegian women between the ages of fifty and sixty-four over two consecutive six-year periods. Half received regular periodic breast exams or regular mammograms. The others had no regular breast screenings. "The study reported that those women receiving regular screenings had a 22 percent increase in breast cancer just because the screenings showed things that then were treated in the conventional way," Dr. Northrup explains. "The authors said chances are good that what happened in the others is they might have had exactly the same incidence of things we pick up on screening, but that the body healed those early cancers.

"What you and I want women to know is there are so many other choices fully backed by science. Just the vitamin D thing alone or the *New England Journal* thing alone makes so much sense to me, and having been on the frontlines of women's health for so many years, I can tell you that women are tortured. They're tortured by this conventional approach."

Dr. Siberstein adds her thoughts on this issue. "In my experience, and I've worked with about 12,000 breast cancer patients, we also find that only 20 percent of the women have conventional risk factors. We tried to figure out where the rest of this breast cancer came from. And what we found is lifestyle factors. Now this is empowerment. This is empowering because you can't do anything about the conventional classical risk factors. You can't change your sex or what family you were born to or your menstrual history or the history of having given birth or not. You have no control over that, but we have tons of control over our lifestyle factors. And research shows that changing our lifestyle choices can be the difference between just having a loaded gun and pulling the trigger. In other words, we can be dealt a crappy set of a hand of cards, but it's the lifestyle factors that influence how that deck of cards plays out. As I say, genes impel but they don't compel."

HORMONES

Exposure to estrogen plays a critical role in breast cancer. Dr. Michael Schachter, a complementary physician from New York, explains. "Women whose menstrual periods start when they are relatively young have an increased risk for developing breast cancer, as do women who have a late menopause," explains Dr. Schachter. "This suggests that a woman who has a longer exposure to female sex hormones during her lifetime is at greater risk for developing breast cancer and that estrogen, the female sex hormone that stimulates cell growth, may play a role in its formation. Women who have no children and women who have children but do not breast-feed also have an increased risk. This suggests that the other female sex hormone, progesterone, may have a protective effect."

Estrogen and progesterone tend to balance each other in the body. "Excessive estrogen or reduced progesterone may lead to a condition known as estrogen dominance," Dr. Schachter says. "The symptoms of estrogen dominance include water retention, breast swelling, fibrocystic breasts, premenstrual mood swings and depression, loss of sex drive, heavy or irregular periods, uterine fibroids, craving for sweets, and fat deposition in the hips and thighs.

"Estrogen tends to be transformed into two major metabolites in the body. They can be called the good and the bad estrogen, just as there are the so-called good and bad cholesterol. The bad estrogen, known as 16-alphahydroxyestrone, favors the development of breast cancer, whereas 2-hydroxyestrone seems to protect against it. Certain chemicals stimulate the formation of one or the other."

XENOESTROGENS

Xenoestrogens are chemical substances that are foreign to the body but behave like estrogens. "These substances mimic estrogen's actions," Dr. Schachter says. "Some xenoestrogens can reduce estrogen's effects. These varieties, which are rapidly degraded in the body, usually occur in plant foods such as soy, cauliflower, and broccoli. They protect against the development of breast cancer. Other xenoestrogens, typically synthetic ones, appear to stimulate cancer growth.

The amount of synthetic chemicals produced annually has jumped into the billions. "We are living in the petrochemical era," Dr. Schachter says. "Many of these compounds are toxic, mutagenic, and carcinogenic," he warns, adding, "the majority have not been adequately tested for toxicity, let alone for their environmental and ecological effects.

"Many synthetic chemicals behave as bad xenoestrogens, particularly pesticides, fuels, and plastics. They do so in various ways. Some enhance the production of the so-called bad estrogens, and others bind to estrogen receptors, inducing them to issue unneeded signals to increase cellular growth. Xenoestrogens may enter the body through animal fat, since they tend to accumulate in fatty tissue and tend to concentrate as you go up in the food chain.

"Xenoestrogens tend to be synergistic so that a mixture of tiny amounts of many chemicals may have dire effects."

POOR LYMPHATIC DRAINAGE

Another possible cause of breast cancer is poor lymphatic drainage. Dr. Sidney Ross Singer, a medical anthropoplogist who did graduate work at Duke University, specializing in biochemistry, has championed this point in his book *Dressed to Kill: The Link between Bras and Breast Cancer*. Dr. Singer explains: "The lymphatic system is so underemphasized by modern medicine. When I was in medical school, there was not even ten minutes' discussion of it. Yet it is a critical part of the body."

The lymphatic system is the circulatory part of the immune system. It consists of tiny vessels, like capillaries, microscopic in size and originating in all the tissues of the body. They drain the tissue of fluid, toxins, debris, cancer cells, bacteria, and so forth. The blood flowing through the blood vessels delivers oxygen and nutrition through capillaries under pressure. The fluid in the blood oozes out to bathe the tissues. This fluid is called lymph fluid. It is the medium of exchange through which nutrients are delivered to the cells.

As the cells take in oxygen and food and give off their waste, some of the cell debris is flushed out through this other channel, the lymphatic system. For the breast, most of the lymph nodes are located in the armpits. These nodes are tiny factories for white blood cell production in response to infection. They filter out the lymph fluid, which then goes back to the bloodstream and through the heart.

This pattern of flow is how the body works normally, Dr. Singer says. However, "when you wear a constrictive garment, the pressure of the garment, such as the elastic of a bra, presses on these tiny vessels, shutting them off and preventing them from draining. They have no internal pressure; they are passive drains. They are not like the blood capillaries, which are under pressure from the heart. As soon as they are constricted because the bra lifts the breasts and gives them a different shape—which requires pressure—there is a backup of fluid in the breast, which is a condition called lymphedema, or edema for short." This pressure and backup can cause pain and tenderness in the breasts.

Before a woman has her period, her estrogen level is very high, and this causes generalized body fluid retention. The condition goes away after the hormones drop and the woman starts having her period. But during that time of elevated fluids she has typically been wearing the same size bra she wore all month, even though her breasts have been a little bigger. As a result of the constriction from the bra, which has become like a tourniquet, the breast cannot drain the fluid, and it backs up, causing congestion in the breast tissue.

The end result, Dr. Singer explains, is that "the cells are sitting in their own waste and debris. The pressure builds, there's tenderness, and cysts form. That's why women get cysts in their breasts. These cysts, which are filled with lymph fluid, eventually become hard. This condition is called fibrocystic breast disease. Eighty percent of American women have it, and it's because of the bra."

X-RAYS

The late Dr. John Gofman, professor emeritus of molecular and cell biology at the University of California, Berkeley, sounded the alarm on the harmful effects of X-rays in his book *Preventing Breast Cancer*.

The effects of X-rays take years, even decades, to manifest, which is why orthodox medicine does not pay attention to this danger. Indeed, X-rays are standard practice for medical diagnosis and treatment. "The incubation time is what has led organized medicine exactly in the wrong direction," he said.

"In the first half of the twentieth century, medicine looked at treatments in this way: If you gave someone poison, the effects would be seen in weeks or months. They did not think in terms of years or decades. What we have learned about X-ray–induced cancer is that a very small proportion occurs in the first few years after the X-rays are administered. But most of them take ten, twenty, even fifty years. Women with breast cancer who are forty-five, fifty, or sixty are thinking, 'Why me? I haven't done anything wrong.' What these women are not thinking about is what they were exposed to early in life."

It is not the radiation itself that persists but chromosomal damage, Dr. Gofman said. "Inside the nucleus of every one of our cells is a string of DNA organized into forty-six chromosomes. That's a treasure. Damage to your chromosomes is going to be there for the rest of your life.

"A couple of years ago, I tried to answer this question—not whether X-rays cause breast cancer but what part of all breast cancers are being caused by X-rays? My estimate was about 75 percent. Everybody said, 'Oh, that's too high. It must be much lower.' Since that time I've done much more extensive work, and I have changed my numbers from 75 percent to more than 90 percent. Moreover, I now have enough data on a variety of other cancers to say that most cancers, not just breast cancer, are caused by medical X-rays."

Whether Dr. Gofman was 100 percent right or just partly right—whether medical X-rays are a primary cause of breast cancer and other types of cancer or merely an important secondary factor that until now has been ignored by our government and the medical establishment—women need to recognize the seriousness of the problem and insist that radiation exposures be as minimal as possible.

Symptoms

The initial symptoms of breast cancer include thickening, a lump in the breast, and dimpled skin. Later on there may be nipple discharge, pain, ulcers, and swollen lymph glands under the arms.

Once breast cancer is diagnosed, the prognosis depends on the course of the disease. The staging of breast cancer involves the size of the cancer in the breast, whether it has spread or metastasized to regional lymph nodes, and whether it has metastasized to distant organs. The more lymph nodes involved and the greater the size of the tumor, the worse the prognosis. Stage zero is limited to the topmost layer, and the five-year survival rate is about 100 percent. In stage four, in which cancer has metastasized to lymph nodes above the collarbone or has distant metastases to organs such as the liver, lungs, and brain, the five-year survival rate drops to 22 percent.

The Tamoxifen Debate

The use of tamoxifen is highly touted by conventional medicine. It has been used for nearly forty years as a treatment to prevent a recurrence of breast cancer. While it may benefit some women, it is also a highly toxic drug with serious side effects. We saw earlier that excessive estrogen production is held responsible by some for breast cancer. This is the rationale for prescribing tamoxifen. However, this treatment is far from the panacea it is claimed to be.

Tamoxifen is in a class of drugs collectively known as SERMs, serum estrogen receptor modulators. Although the way these drugs work is not totally understood, it is believed that SERMs block the action of estrogen on the breast tissue, which in turn inhibits the growth of tumors. Many but not all breast cancers require estrogen to grow. These types of tumors have a site on the cell called an estrogen receptor. Tamoxifen competes with estrogen to reach these receptors, where it creates a barrier that prevents estrogen from binding to the cell.

In theory, then, tamoxifen acts like a phytoestrogen, although it has contradictory effects. In the breast it seems to reduce the effects of estrogen on tumor growth, yet in other parts of the body it acts like one of these estrogens, stimulating growth, for example in the uterus, where it can cause endometrial cancer. According to Dr. Sherrill Sellman, naturopath, psychotherapist, and author of the best-selling book *Hormone Heresy*, "It's unpredictable in the sense that we don't really know what are going to be the consequences in a woman's body."

In the early 1980s American researchers began to speculate about whether tamoxifen might actually prevent breast cancer in women who had never had the disease. So in 1992 the National Cancer Institute initiated a $60 million clinical trial to test tamoxifen as a cancer preventive. Thirteen thousand healthy women who were at higher than average risk for breast cancer were enrolled in the trial. Half the women took tamoxifen (20 milligrams a day); the other half received a placebo.

From the beginning, the Breast Cancer Prevention Trial was controversial. Critics of the trial were outraged that healthy women would be exposed to the health risks associated with tamoxifen.

Results of the trial were made public in April 1998. At first glance, the trial results seem impressive. Women in the trial who took tamoxifen had a 44 percent reduction in breast cancers compared with the placebo group. But these results are misleading; tamoxifen also caused uterine cancer, blood clots, and cataracts. In fact, women who got tamoxifen had almost three times the rate of endometrial cancers and blood clots. Two prominent health groups, the National Women's Health Network and Public Citizen, have calculated that for every thousand women who take tamoxifen, there will be 2.9 fewer cases of breast cancer, but 2.8 more cases of extremely serious health problems. Even more important, results of the trial show there is no difference in overall survival rates or in the number of women who died of breast cancer.

In addition to cancers, blood clots, and cataracts, tamoxifen also caused strokes, hot flashes, vaginal discharge, mood changes, menstrual irregularities, and skin rashes.

In October 1998, the Food and Drug Administration (FDA) approved the use of tamoxifen to reduce the risk of breast cancer in healthy women. But even members of the FDA's own advisory committee voiced concerns about giving tamoxifen to healthy women. One committee member noted that every woman who took tamoxifen was exposed to the health risks, but only a few women would benefit from the drug.

Critics of the FDA say that approval of tamoxifen as an anticancer drug is premature. Two European studies found tamoxifen provided no benefit as a preventive measure. Still other criticism focuses on the statistical model (known as the Gail model) used to assess breast cancer risk for women considering taking tamoxifen as a cancer preventative. Opponents say this model greatly overstates risk, putting large numbers of women into a high-risk category and therefore eligible to take the drug.

In addition to tamoxifen, raloxifene has also been approved by the FDA to reduce the chances of breast cancer in high-risk postmenopausal women. According to a 2012 National Cancer Institute fact sheet, the common side effects of tamoxifen and raloxifene include hot flashes, night sweats, vaginal dryness, and disruptions in menstrual cycle. Less common but serious side effects of tamoxifen are blood clots, strokes, bone loss, mood swings, endometrial and uterine cancers, and cataracts. Side effects of raloxifene include blood clots and stroke. Animal studies found a link between tamoxifen and liver cancer in rats, but the results of human studies have been less conclusive. A Swedish study looked at 1,327 breast cancer patients who took 40 milligrams of tamoxifen a day for two to five years. Comparing this group to one of the same size that didn't take the drug, it was found the tamoxifen users upped their chances for getting uterine cancer sixfold.

Strangely enough, many women's groups are supporting and advocating this treatment. Most of the time, however, these are groups that take money from the pharmaceutical industry. But other women's groups have been the primary activists opposing tamoxifen, the lead group being the National Women's Health Network. And there have been so many false reports and so much misinformation that unless you really investigate the issue thoroughly, you will very seldom get access to truthful data. As Dr. Sellman says, "It's very easy to play with results, stats, and studies to make it look like something wonderful is occurring when in fact it is a scam. This drug has the potential to be such a big money spinner. It is already the number-one drug given to women with breast cancer. The industry will stop at nothing to get its drug out there. Health is not their primary concern."

Mammography Mendacity

We have a health care system in the US that emphasizes early diagnosis and treatment. On face value this sounds like a logical and prudent approach. But coercing healthy individuals to subject themselves to tests searching for microscopic signs of illness is far from merely an overzealous waste of time and money because these tests are frequently not benign—they can be invasive, harmful, and even fatal. There is perhaps no better example of this than the $5 billion American women spend annually on mammograms. Lauded as a tool that saves lives, mammograms are starting to come under attack by a host of critics and consumers and for good reason.

A mammogram is an expensive test that requires a slew of health care professionals: a skilled technician to do the procedure, one or two board-certified radiologists to interpret the results, and more time by the primary care physician to discuss the results. If there is a suspicious finding, then usually there is a repeat mammogram, possibly a surgeon, a surgery suite, a nurse, and an anesthesiologist to do a biopsy, then a pathologist to interpret those results, then back to the primary care physician. How many thousands of dollars does this add up to so far? And how much stress and anxiety does it create for the woman who worries about the outcome? Studies show that women experience severe psychological distress for up to a year or more as a result of a breast cancer scare.

Nowhere in this scenario are women warned that there is a dark side to mammograms. They actually are a crude and inaccurate diagnostic test for breast cancer. There are large numbers of both false positives and false negatives, meaning that women will be told they have cancer when they don't, and told they don't have cancer when they do. A large Swedish study concluded that an incredible 70 to 80 percent of all women with a positive mammographic diagnosis of cancer were found not to have cancer on biopsy. A 2015 editorial in *JAMA Internal Medicine* warned of the dangers of overdiagnosis: "Overdiagnosis is the diagnosis of a tumor that would not have become clinically apparent in the absence of screening. Treatment of an overdiagnosed tumor cannot provide benefit, but it can lead to harm." This editorial referenced a recent study that found that more mammograms did not equal reduced detection of larger cancers or lower death rates. Over the course of the next decade, American women are expected to spend as much as $70 billion on unnecessary surgeries stemming from false positive mammogram results.

It is estimated that for 2,000 women who receive mammograms regularly over a ten-year period, one life will be saved but ten more will undergo needless and harmful treatment for cancer that they don't have—including chemotherapy, radiation, and even breast removal. Conversely, a supposed clean bill of health from a normal mammogram result is not something that should cause any woman to breathe a sigh of relief. Many women have a negative mammogram only to discover a suspicious lump on their own a few weeks or months later, and it is estimated that a full 40 percent of women between age 40 and 49 will have breast cancer that goes undetected by mammography.

Far worse than the fact that mammograms do not provide reliable results is the fact that they are dangerous, due to the extreme amount of ionizing radiation emitted from the machine directly to vulnerable breast tissue. According to Dr. Samuel Epstein, the amount of radiation from a mammogram is 200 times that from a chest X-ray. Research presented at the Radiological Society of North America's Scientific Assembly incriminated low dose radiation as a key factor in the development of breast cancer. The research demonstrated that women were 2.5 times more likely to develop breast cancer if they had received either a mammogram or chest X-ray before the age of 20.

Mainstream medicine tells us that more women have breast cancer than ever before but the survival rate has increased because of mammograms and early treatment. They don't tell us that a significant percentage of the increase in breast cancer is due to the fact that mammograms are finding cancer that isn't there, which would possibly explain the improved cure rate. They likewise don't tell us that the definition of breast cancer has changed significantly since the advent of mammograms. A frequently overlooked statistic shows that the rate of one type of breast cancer, ductal carcinoma in situ (DCIS), has skyrocketed by 328 percent since mammograms were first introduced in the 1970s. DCIS is a condition that can only be found by mammography because these lesions are too small to be picked up by physical examination. DCIS is currently the most common diagnosis resulting from breast tissue biopsy, but is DCIS even breast cancer at all? Ductal carcinoma in situ is actually a precursor lesion for breast cancer. Rather than cancer itself, a precursor lesion is a collection of cells that could grow into breast cancer, but also might not; we simply cannot know and have no way to predict the outcome. DCIS has been called the poster child for uncertainty because we really can't say whether it is even a serious threat to women's health: studies of DCIS that were missed at biopsy suggest that the lifetime risk of progression to cancer if untreated is very low.

The mammography industry is very lucrative and powerful, and has worked effectively to prevent other means of breast cancer identification from being developed. In fact, studies show that MRI would likely be more effective at identifying breast cancer, and thermography also shows promise as a technology that is non-invasive and does not emit radiation. While a mammogram begins to detect cancer clumps of about 4 billion cells, thermographic imaging may be even more sensitive, picking up abnormal growth as small as 256 cells. However, we must keep in mind that so-called early detection is a dangerously misleading term because finding cells that are a variation from normal is not the same thing as identifying cancer. There are many abnormal cells that never progress to malignancy and we truly cannot tell the difference in most cases. Thermograms, like mammograms, hold the potential for disease mongering by finding abnormal cells that will not develop into cancer, thus bringing women into a destructive treatment regimen they have no need for.

There is an enormous conflict of interest between our cancer authorities and promoters of mammography; no fewer than five American Cancer Society presidents have been radiologists specializing in mammography. In light of such industry influence, it should come as no surprise that the ACS has consistently adopted policies favorable to the companies that make mammogram machines, such as DuPont, Siemens, and General Electric. DuPont, in fact, was a major sponsor for the group's ACS Breast Health Awareness Program, an initiative that encouraged women to receive a mammography screening while failing to publicize the scientifically established methods of prevention that would help them avoid the disease altogether. Another disturbing conflict of interest lies in the fact that the ACS actually contracts with the mammography industry to conduct cancer research, calling the results of such research into question.

A well-funded campaign of fear prompts women to undergo regular mammograms believing that they are being responsible and taking the best possible action for their health based on science. But as the *Cochrane Review* has concluded in their meta-analyses from both 2001 and 2011, the currently available reliable evidence does not show a survival benefit of mass screening for breast cancer. A Canadian study published in *The Lancet* went farther, stating that "since the benefit achieved is marginal, the harm caused is substantial, and the costs incurred are enormous, we suggest that public funding for breast cancer screening in any age group is not justifiable."

The National Cancer Institute nevertheless continues to recommend that all women should submit to mammograms every two years beginning at age 40. Our current promotion of "breast cancer awareness" leading to widespread mammography is simply drawing more healthy women into the patient pool rather than saving lives. Women would be better served by learning what they can do to improve their chances of never developing breast cancer: eating a healthy plant-based diet free from processed foods and animal products, exercising, losing weight, and avoiding the toxic materials in our surroundings that are known to cause breast cancer.

Natural Approach to Prevention and Treatment

DIET AND NUTRITION

Dr. Tori Hudson, a naturopathic physician in Portland, Oregon, is among the many practitioners who claim that breast cancer is a preventable disease. "Just look around the world," she says. "Women in our culture have one of the highest—if not the highest—incidences of breast cancer, while women in Asia have the lowest. The reason is diet. To make a big story simple to understand, cultures that have a vegetarian diet or are closest to a vegetarian diet have the least breast cancer. That's how it all pans out no matter how you look at it. This implies that cultures that eat less fat, especially less animal fat, have the least breast cancer. So the big picture is really clear. Eat a lot of vegetables, fruits, and whole grains and beans. Those foods provide protection."

Quite a few large epidemiological studies have looked at the relationship between a person's lifelong eating pattern and the development of cancer. Those studies have shown that the more vegetables and fruits a person eats, the less likely they are to develop cancer. People who eat five to six servings of vegetables a day plus another couple of servings of fruit have the lowest risk.

"A serving usually refers to a cup of raw vegetables or a half cup of cooked vegetables," says Dr. Alschuler. "So getting six servings, while that may sound a little intimidating, is actually quite doable. If you eat a big salad at lunch you've probably got almost five servings right there. Add another vegetable to your dinner plate and you're done for the day."

Letha Hadady, an herbalist and educator in New York City, visited China to learn why Chinese women have such a low incidence of breast cancer compared with American women and those in other Western nations. She found that Asians build immunity through diet and cleansing herbs, as well as the avoidance of pollution, stress, negative emotions, smoking, alcohol, and radiation.

In addition, Hadady made this important discovery. "I found it quite interesting that breast cancer is considered a disease of melancholy in China. That feeling of heaviness in the chest leads to poor circulation and excess phlegm. This leads to two conclusions: Increase circulation and you have a better chance of prevention, and reduce phlegm. The easiest way to reduce phlegm is to stay away from foods such as cheese, chocolate, fried foods, and milk. You will not find dairy in the diet in China. Their diet tends to consist of grains and greens."

Certain foods are medicinal in their ability to protect against breast cancer. They include soybeans, soy products, and lima beans. Isoflavones and phytoestrogens found in soybeans, soy products, and lima beans protect against cancer. The low incidence of breast cancer among Japanese women is largely attributed to the widespread eating of soybeans. Other cancer-fighting foods include flax, fish that is high in omega-3 fatty acids (salmon, tuna, sardines, mackerel, and herring), cruciferous vegetables (broccoli, cauliflower, and brussels sprouts), mushrooms (reishi, shiitake, and maitake), and onions.

VITAMINS AND MINERALS

Vitamins and minerals are important in breast cancer prevention as well as after diagnosis and treatment. Among the vitamins recommended are vitamin A, beta-carotene, vitamin B_1, vitamin B_6, vitamin C, and folic acid. Dr. Schachter states that trace minerals play a vital role in the prevention of free radical damage that can contribute to breast cancer. "The body contains certain antioxidant proteins, such as SOD (superoxide dismutase), which help neutralize oxidatively induced free radicals. SOD requires three minerals—zinc, copper, and manganese—to function properly. Deficiencies of any one of these minerals may predispose to oxidation damage, with a resulting increase of susceptibility to breast cancer. Adequate amounts of calcium, magnesium, selenium, chromium, and molybdenum also are important."

Dr. Schachter says he uses the whole range of trace minerals in colloidal form as a supplement. "That's a liquid form where the minerals are bound to organic chemicals. We use about seventy different minerals. Many of these minerals are in trace amounts, have already been shown to be essential, and are probably lacking in our synthetically fertilized soil. I believe these colloidal trace minerals will play an important role in bolstering the immune system."

HERBS

Natural herbal substances are a veritable gold mine for treating as well as preventing breast cancer. Some herbs to know about are listed below:

CARNIVORA (VENUS FLYTRAP)—This powerful herb is popular in Europe but less known in the United States. In Germany it is even used to wipe out cancer that already exists.

ESSIAC—Essiac is a Native American herbal combination that has a synergistic effect in putting an end to cancer and aiding in its prevention.

CAT'S CLAW—A cat's claw formula is used by the Peruvian Indians for the prevention and treatment of cancer.

EVENING PRIMROSE, BORAGE, AND BLACK CURRANT SEED OILS— All these herbs supply gamma-linoleic acid, which is known for its strong anticancer activity.

XIAO YAO WAN—This combination of digestive herbs increases circulation, builds blood, and breaks apart fibroids. The Chinese say it prevents breast cancer caused by phlegm and feelings of melancholy, which impede circulation to the chest. Xiao yao wan is available in Chinatowns throughout America.

DANDELION—Dandelion helps prevent cancer by breaking up phlegm and eliminating it from the system. Excess phlegm can turn into tumors.

ASTRAGALUS—Astragalus is a wonderful immune-system-strengthening herb that can be used in cancer prevention or as an adjunct to cancer treatments. Add a teaspoon of astragalus powder to some pure water and drink once or twice a day. Or try Astra-8, a combination of astragalus and other immune-system-strengthening remedies in capsule form that is found in health food stores.

ROSEMARY—Rosemary has been highly researched and is recommended even more than soy for its breast-protecting qualities. According to Keuneke, "Use rosemary in a vinaigrette or to marinate fish. Try to buy rosemary on a regular basis. Perhaps make a salad dressing with rosemary and garlic, fresh lemon, and extra virgin olive oil. All those ingredients are wonderful foods that are eaten throughout the Mediterranean."

MINT—Include mint in your diet on a regular basis. Mint has a phytochemical in it called limonene, which is effective in fighting breast cancer. In one study, it was found to reduce mammary tumors in animals up to 80 percent. The foods containing limonene are mint, dill, sage, celery seed, caraway, and organic citrus peel. The last item is also found in the Thai diet, which frequently uses lime peel.

TURMERIC—Turmeric also contains a vital phytochemical that has been found to prevent mammary tumors in animals.

ENZYMES

Enzymes are organic substances that help create reactions in the body, such as breaking down fats. They are linked to breathing and all the bodily functions we need to live and stay well. There are 3,000 enzymes in the body. A healthy person can produce enough enzymes to fight off cancer cells, but substances such as free radicals from smoke, pollutants, junk foods, and medications interfere with enzyme production.

"So, as you can imagine," Robin Keuneke says, "there are many people who are low on enzymes. To combat this, people can increase the amount of raw foods in their diet and increase fresh juice—juice all kinds of fruits and vegetables."

Numerous studies, she recounts, link enzymes and breast health. More than 90 were conducted by universities throughout the world regarding the beneficial effects of enzymes. Much of this work has been done in Germany.

OTHER THERAPIES

Activities that detoxify the body can further reduce the chance of acquiring breast cancer. For instance, aerobic exercise assists in lymphatic drainage and induces sweating, which is a natural way for the body to eliminate waste products. And exercise has been shown by studies to be correlated with a lowered breast cancer risk.

Lymphatic detoxification is aided by manual lymphatic drainage (MLD), a simple method of massage that uses light, slow rhythmic movements to stimulate the flow of lymph in the body. Massage therapist James Kresse notes that this is especially important for women suffering from lymphedema, a condition that often occurs after a mastectomy: "When our lymph nodes are not functioning properly or have been irradiated or removed, an excessive accumulation of stagnant waste occurs. The lymph system becomes overloaded, thus forming lymphedema.

"MLD should be applied directly after surgery rather than when a massive edema has formed. This will guard against any possibility of a blockage in the system or alleviate any that exists. Studies in Europe show that severed lymph vessels regenerate with constant MLD therapy. The therapy makes the scars from the mastectomy more subtle, which increases the mobility of the arm. It also lessens pain from surgery and the uncomfortable sensitivity that occurs."

Increasing melatonin may also help in the prevention of breast cancer. "Melatonin is a hormone that is produced at night," Dr. Alschuler explains. "It helps us to fall asleep, and it helps us to stay asleep. It's produced throughout our body, particularly in our brain and in our intestinal tract, and it's been shown that women who have lower levels of melatonin have a higher rate of breast cancer.

"In addition to helping us fall asleep, melatonin has very strong immune regulating or stimulating properties. At the same time, it reduces the amount and the influence of estrogen on cancer cells. It actually blocks estrogen binding to estrogen receptors, and it blocks the production of estrogen. And then finally, melatonin literally helps to put the cells to sleep. It slows down cellular division. It slows down cellular growth enough so that some of the reparative mechanisms that our body innately has have time to work and repair the cells."

To get more melatonin, Dr. Alschuler recommends sleeping at night in a dark room without alarm clocks with bright lights, night lights, or the glow of the television. "All of that light at night reduces our production of melatonin, so it's really important to sleep in a very dark room."

In the 1950s Dr. Lawrence Burton and a team of researchers discovered Immuno-Augmentative Therapy (IAT), a nontoxic, noninvasive method of controlling cancer by restoring the patient's own immune system. Although the therapy was successful, Dr. Burton left the United States after medical politics prohibited him from practicing here. In 1977 he opened the Immunology Research Center in Freeport in the Grand Bahama Islands, where thousands received treatment for the disease.

Since Dr. Burton's death, Dr. John Clement, an internationally respected cancer specialist who studied with Dr. Burton, heads the center, now called the Immuno-Technologies Cancer Clinic. Dr. Clement gives an overview of the treatment: "The intellectual basis of the treatment is that many cancers can be controlled by restoring the competence of the patient's immune system, as the body's complex immune-fighting system may well be the first, best, and last line of defense against many cancers.

"The method we use is similar in any type of cancer we treat, although each patient has her treatment tailored to the results of her own blood test. We do not deal with toxic chemicals in any way. We assay the blood for the factors we believe are aiding the patient's cancer. By identifying these factors, we are able to control them, put them back into balance, and hopefully destroy the patient's cancer."

Regarding breast cancer, Dr. Clement says, "We have had patients with breast cancer who have had no other treatment but IAT for upward of twenty years who have no recurrence of disease. While we are still claiming only to control their cancer, you will see that to all intents and purposes, by any kind of medical description, they have been cured."

Dr. Clement reports less success with patients who come to him after extremely arduous chemotherapy and those with advanced cancer where there is a loss of bone marrow and fluid collection in the abdomen or pleural effusions in the lungs.

The late Dr. O. Carl Simonton, medical director of the Simonton Cancer Center in California and coauthor of *Getting Well Again* and *The Healing Journey*, firmly believed that emotions drive healing systems and that the imagination and standard counseling can be used to increase a patient's will to live. "I would like to give an example of a patient I have worked with for more than twenty years," he said. "This thirty-six-year-old woman came to me with metastatic breast cancer that had spread to her ribs and spine. Her father was a physician, and her husband's family had run a retail store for three generations. She was involved in helping her husband run the family business.

"Her religious and spiritual life was important to her. It was a great source of strength. She wanted more time to be involved in religious administration and spiritual counseling. As she began to pursue these areas, her beliefs about how she should be the good daughter, the good wife, and the good mother came into play. These beliefs were all quite rigid, allowing virtually no freedom for her own creativity. Over time we helped her make a shift in these beliefs and behaviors that was central to her recovery.

"She has been free of disease for fifteen years. Currently, she is weller than well and runs marathons. The family store burned down about ten years ago.

Now she works primarily in church administration, doing religious and spiritual counseling, which is what she always wanted to do."

SAMPLE DAILY PROTOCOL

The following daily protocol of vitamins and minerals is recommended by Dr. Steven Rachlin, an internist in Long Island, New York.

Emulsified vitamin A (up to 50,000 IU)

Beta-carotene (up to 100 mg)

Vitamin B1 (100 mg)

Vitamin B6 (100 mg)

Folic acid (3,200 mcg)

Vitamin C (up to 5 g)

Coenzyme Q10 (400 mg)

Flaxseed oil (1 tbsp)

Cat's claw (300 mg)

Melatonin (up to 10 mg)

Pycnogenol (150 mg)

Pancreatic digestive enzymes (up to 40 g)

Aloe vera juice (9–12 oz)

Minerals

NK Cell Activator (500 mg)

Cytokine Supress with EGCG (300 mg)

Modified Citrus Pectin, as directed

Vitamin C to bowel tolerance (8x day)

medically supervised IV Vitamin C (35,000–150,000mg)

probiotics (5 billion, 3x day)

Fibrocystic Breast Disease

Fibrocystic breast disease is caused by overcongestion from foods that clog the system, such as wheat, dairy products, refined foods, and fats. Caffeinated products such as coffee, tea, chocolate, and soft drinks are hard on the body and add to the problem, as does a sluggish thyroid gland, which makes metabolism more difficult and leads to constipation, causing a buildup of toxins. Toxic accumulations worsen congestion and can manifest as breast lumps (cysts). Stress worsens the condition.

SYMPTOMS

Fibrocystic breast disease shows up as single or multiple breast lumps. Cysts are usually harmless but are related to a higher than normal chance of contracting breast cancer later. Mammograms determine whether breast lumps are benign.

Drs. Ruth Bar-Shalom and John Soileau, naturopaths from Fairbanks, Alaska, add that the symptoms may also include tenderness and pain in the breast. In an article on the American Association of Naturopathic Physicians website (www.naturopathic.org) they stress the importance of learning breast self-examination and performing it every month, a week to ten days after the menstrual period starts. This enables you to recognize the cystic areas. If you are not sure whether a lump is a cyst or something else or if there is a discharge from the nipples, consult a physician.

CLINICAL EXPERIENCE

DIET AND NUTRITION

A diet high in complex carbohydrates can make a difference; fruits, vegetables, grains, beans, and some fish are recommended. Red-hot peppers, cayenne pepper, and regular or daikon radishes cut through mucus and help eliminate breast lumps.

According to Drs. Bar-Shalom and Soileau, the most important dietary measure for reducing cysts is to eliminate from the diet all forms of caffeine, including coffee, tea, chocolate, and soda. Meat, especially the hormone-containing commercial type, should be avoided as much as possible. Finally, since constipation can aggravate fibrocystic breast disease, it is important to eat more vegetables, fruits, and whole grains and drink eight to ten glasses of water a day.

SUPPLEMENTS

The following nutrients offer extra help when combined with a cleansing diet: selenium, vitamins A, C, and E, magnesium, and iodine drops. Iodine speeds the metabolism of the thyroid gland. As the metabolism perks up, breast lumps tend to disappear. Iodine drops from seaweed can be obtained in the drugstore in a saturated solution of potassium iodide or Lugol's solution. There is also an Edgar Cayce remedy called Atomodine. In addition, health food stores sell iodine drops in the form of liquid kelp. Before you use iodine, a thyroid blood test should be done to check for thyroid antibodies. This ensures that there is no thyroiditis, an inflammation of the thyroid gland. Drs. Bar-Shalom and Soileau suggest the following supplements:

- Multivitamin
- Vitamin B complex—50 mg twice a day
- Vitamin B$_6$—100 mg twice a day
- Vitamin E—600 IU a day
- Flaxseed oil—2 capsules or 1 tbsp a day
- Beta-carotene—25,000 IU a day (if you are pregnant or of childbearing age, take no more than 15,000 IU a day)
- Vitamin D3—5,000 units daily
- Black cumin seed oil—2 teaspoons daily
- Curcumin—3,000 mgs daily
- Amino acids—1,000 mg each of choline and methionine a day to remedy the hormonal imbalance that is said to result in formation of cysts

HERBS

Herbalist Letha Hadady recommends the following plant remedies to break up congestion in the chest and release phlegm and mucus from the system before they lead to more serious problems:

XIAO YAO WAN—This formula is a combination of digestive herbs that increase circulation, build blood, and break apart fibroids. Xiao yao wan is available in Chinatowns throughout America.

DANDELION—Dandelion tea or capsules can be taken every day to break apart fibroids.

Drs. Bar-Shalom and Soileau recommend in addition poke root and iris versicolor taken as tinctures. Take 5 drops of each three times daily for up to three months. Do not take these herbs if you are pregnant.

EXTERNAL TREATMENTS

CASTOR OIL PACKS—According to the medical psychic Edgar Cayce, stimulating liver circulation ends constipation. Substances that clog the body and form breast lumps are then eliminated. To do this, rub castor oil on the skin over the liver. Cover this area with a towel and place a heating pad over it. Do this for twenty minutes each day.

PEPPERMINT OIL—Rubbing peppermint oil on breast lumps diminishes them by stimulating the circulation.

PHYTOLACCA OIL AND HYDROTHERAPY—Dr. Joseph Pizzorno has found success with this combination treatment: "We have a woman put a hot compress on her breast so that it gets real warm. She then covers the area with phytolacca oil. After the application, she covers it with a cold pack. We combine herbal medicine with hydrotherapy to help the cysts drain out of the breasts. I use that treatment with a lot of women and have had quite a good response."

HOMEOPATHY

Drs. Bar-Shalom and Soileau suggest the following homeopathic remedies. Choose one based on how well it matches your symptoms and then take it under the tongue three times a day, stopping when the symptoms are relieved.

PHYTOLACCA—Use 6c potency for hard, sensitive breasts or when you have multiple nodules.

CONIUM MACULATUM—Take 12c potency for sharp pain in the nipples and for breast swelling.

SEPIA—Take 6c potency when irritability accompanies breast swelling.

YOGA

Dr. Gary Ross, a family physician and certified yoga instructor from San Francisco, recommends yoga poses, meditation, and breathing exercises to alleviate fibrocystic breast disease brought on by stress and a sluggish thyroid. These three postures increase blood flow to the thyroid and chest area:

SHOULDER STAND—On a mat or thick blanket, lie flat on your back. You may place a rolled towel under your neck. Raise your legs over your head so that your body is in a U formation. Rest the elbows firmly on the floor and support the back with both hands. Adjust your body so that it is completely vertical. Then press the chin against the chest. Hold still as you breathe slowly, concentrating on the thyroid gland. You may be able to do this for only several seconds at first, but then you will be able to work up to one minute. To come down, lower the legs slowly toward the head. Then lower the back to the floor one vertebra at a time. When the back is on the floor, continue to lower the legs gradually until you are once again flat on your back. Do this once in the morning and once in the evening. To get the full benefit, follow with the fish pose.

FISH POSE—Lie on your back with the legs straight or folded. If the legs are straight, place the hands under the buttocks with the palms down. Otherwise, hold on to the crossed feet. Resting on the elbow, arch the chest and neck back. The head should be on the floor, but do not apply pressure there. Support should come from the elbows. Do not bend the neck too far back as that can impede circulation. Focusing on the thyroid, breathe deeply in this position, holding for thirty seconds.

COBRA—Lie facedown with the elbows and palms down on the floor or mat and the palms beneath the shoulders. With a smooth, gradual motion, raise the eyes upward, then the head, neck, and spine, one vertebra at a time. Allow the area below the hips to remain on the blanket. Hold the pose and then come out of it using reverse motions that are equally slow and gradual. Breathe in as you come into the posture, hold the breath while in the cobra, and breathe out when coming down.

In addition, Dr. Ross advocates deep-breathing exercises to bring more energy into the chest area. Visualization creates a mindset that helps make lumps disappear. Further, meditation creates spiritual and mental tranquility that is conducive to healing.

Lymphedema

Lymphedema, a swelling of the limbs caused by an accumulation of lymph fluid, affects 1 percent of the US population. Health practitioner James Kresse explains: "There are two types of lymphedema. The first is primary lymphostatic lymphedema, a condition that predominantly affects women in their mid-thirties but can manifest at birth or during adolescence. The second is more common and frequently occurs in patients who have had mastectomies or the removal of malignant tumors. The large increase in the incidence of breast cancer and subsequent mastectomy operations is one of the major reasons for the rise in lymphedema today. Secondary lymphostatic lymphedema can occur from six months to three years after the initial surgery."

SYMPTOMS

Lymphedema appears as a swelling or skin thickening in a limb. It is important to detect the condition early, and this can be done in several ways. Kresse advises, "Notice any jewelry becoming tighter on the affected limb over a short period of time. Or squeeze the affected limb for ten seconds. If an indentation is noticed, notify your surgeon immediately or measure your arm with a cloth tape measure around your wrist and forearm. If you notice an increase in the circumference of your arm, call your surgeon right away."

MANUAL LYMPHATIC DRAINAGE

Lymphatic detoxification is aided by manual lymphatic drainage (MLD), a simple method of massage that uses light, slow rhythmic movements to stimulate the flow of lymph in the body. "This type of therapy is very, very light," says Kresse. "It's almost featherlike. We're working on the parasympathetic nervous system. A regular massage stimulates the sympathetic nervous system. That is our fight-or-flight nerve. The parasympathetic nervous system is our night nerve, our rest and relax nerve. This is the nerve that lymph drainage affects in order to calm the patient down."

COMPRESSION BANDAGING

In addition to MLD, compression bandaging is used to apply pressure around the affected limb. Exercises performed with the bandage enhance muscular contractions that help with lymph flow.

LIFESTYLE CHANGES

Kresse has several lifestyle recommendations. "The person needs to practice meticulous skin care with the use of pH-balanced lotions and creams to protect the skin. Following a good nutritional program consisting of lots of fruits and vegetables is helpful. Salt and fatty foods should be eliminated, and protein intake should be limited. It is important to maintain an optimum weight, as obesity contributes to lymphedema. Exercise such as swimming, walking, and stretching is excellent. Incorporating deep diaphragmatic breathing techniques, along with specific exercises taught by an MLD therapist, is good. While sleeping, the patient can elevate the limb by tilting the mattress or by placing pillows under the arm. Antibiotic solutions should be carried at all times for incidental cuts, scratches, or bites. Infection should be treated at the first sign."

Kresse also lists a variety of safety measures. "Precautions to take include not subjecting oneself to extreme temperature changes such as hot tubs, saunas, steam baths, and other thermal treatments. Care must be taken when using instruments on the affected limb, such as the instruments used in manicures and pedicures. Pets must be watched to see that they don't scratch or bite. Blood pressure readings, injections, vaccinations, and acupuncture should be avoided on the infected arm. Constrictive clothing and jewelry should not be worn. Heavy prostheses can cause excess pressure on the affected limb. Care must be taken when cooking, gardening, and doing daily chores. Finally, heavy objects must not be lifted. This can cause a lymphedema right away or somewhere down the line."

Other therapies that help lymphatic conditions include rebound exercise, ozone therapy, enzyme therapy, colon hydrotherapy, deep breathing exercises, and a good vitamin and herbal program.

Research Update

An increasing body of evidence is showing the benefits of natural modalities to overall health and well-being. Following is a sample of recent peer-reviewed scientific studies in the area of cancer and more specifically, breast cancer.

A 2015 article in *Life Extension Magazine* cited many research studies showing the anticancer properties of the spice saffron. Saffron was shown to slow and reverse cancer growth in 2012 reports in *Current Pharmaceutical Biotechnology* and *European Journal of Biological Science*, and a 2014 report in *Biochemistry and Cell Biology*. Saffron was also found to help reduce the harmful effects produced by chemotherapy drugs. A 2011 article in *Life Extension Magazine* discussed evidence that citrus pectin can disrupt inter-cellular communication, slow metastasis, and improve quality of life in cancer patients. In 2015, the magazine reported on research showing that curcumin can be used against certain cancers by blocking the inflammatory master molecule nuclear factor-kappaB (or NF-kB).

A 2014 report in *World Journal of Clinical Oncology* summarized the epidemiological research indicating that diet plays an important role in breast cancer. Beneficial results were found with intake of probiotics in combination with a balance of fatty acids, fruits and vegetables, dietary fiber, and vitamin supplements. Consumption of probiotics with fermented products containing lactic acid bacteria was linked in some studies with decreased breast cancer risk.

Soy was found in a 2013 *PLoS One* literature review to be nonestrogenic and safe for women with breast cancer when consumed in amounts similar to that of a traditional Japanese diet (two to three 25–50 mg servings per day). Use of soy remains controversial, however, as reported in a 2012 *Nutrition and Cancer* study, which found that high intake of soy isoflavones increased the risk of cancer recurrence in HER2-positive breast cancer patients.

In a 2014 report in *Townsend Letter*, Dr. Barbara MacDonald summarized recent scientific evidence regarding the effects of exercise and diet on breast cancer prognosis. Although many studies have shown the benefits of moderately strenuous, regular physical activity, as noted in *Cancer Epidemiology, Biomarkers & Prevention* in 2013, most survivors fail to meet the recommended guidelines, with only 21 percent saying that they exercise the suggested three hours weekly. As reported in *Cancer Diagnosis & Control* in 2011, African American and Hispanic women with early-stage breast cancer who ate a diet consisting of fewer calories, added sugar, alcohol, and saturated fat, decreased their risks of mortality related to breast cancer by 88 percent. A 2010 meta-analysis in *Breast Cancer Research and Treatment* confirmed the positive effects of green tea.

Chapter 25

Cervical Dysplasia, Fibroids, and Reproductive System Cancers

Cervical Dysplasia

Cervical dysplasia is a precancerous change to the cells of the cervix caused most often by the sexually transmitted human papillomavirus (HPV), the same virus that is responsible for cervicitis, genital warts, and cervical cancer. Approximately 20 million people in the United States are currently infected with HPV, with more than 6 million new cases expected annually.

CAUSES

The likelihood of a woman developing cervical dysplasia increases with intercourse at an early age, unprotected sex with several male partners, smoking, birth control pills, and weak immunity. Naturopathic physician Dr. Tori Hudson explains: "Women who have intercourse at an early age are more vulnerable to getting genital warts and cervical dysplasia because the cells of the cervix at that age are more susceptible to being infected by the virus.

"If you smoke, and you are exposed to the virus, you are much more likely to develop dysplasia, and you are much more likely to develop cervical cancer from your dysplasia," Dr. Hudson says. "We know that nicotine actually lodges in the glands of the cells of the cervix. When exposed to the virus, the DNA can change to take on more abnormal features. If you have genital warts and you smoke, it is much more likely that they will turn cancerous as well.

"Oral contraceptives are known for creating a folic acid deficiency, and folic acid deficiency is associated with acquiring cervical dysplasia and having the disease progress to cancer."

SYMPTOMS

Dr. Hudson describes cervical dysplasia as a progressive syndrome that develops over time. "After initial exposure to the virus, there is no indication that anything has changed. Later, immune changes may occur. Warty tissue may develop, then mild dysplasia, moderate dysplasia, severe dysplasia, carcinoma in situ, and then invasive cancer." These symptoms are not evident upon physical examination, so Pap smears are necessary.

PREVENTION

Since HPV is sexually transmitted, the conditions associated with it are preventable. Notes Dr. Hudson, "Cervical dysplasia, genital warts, and cervical cancer are all sexually transmitted diseases. That should make an impression on all of us, because it really dictates how we should protect ourselves.

"Obviously, we shouldn't smoke. We should protect ourselves by having safe sex and a healthy immune system. If you take birth control pills, it is advisable to take folic acid. A good maintenance dose would be 800 micrograms daily. Those are the main ways to protect against cervical dysplasia and genital warts." Additional preventive daily supplementation may include 5,000 milligrams of vitamin C and 25,000 units of beta-carotene.

To detect the condition early, Dr. Hudson stresses yearly Pap smear exams. Statistics show that the longer women wait between Pap smears, the higher the incidence of cervical dysplasia and cervical cancer.

DIAGNOSIS

Before treatment, it is essential to get fully diagnosed to determine the stage of the illness. If a woman has an abnormal Pap smear, her partner needs to be examined by a urologist for warty tissue. Otherwise, they will pass the virus back and forth, reinfecting each other. Diagnosis by a licensed, well-trained alternative practitioner will determine whether a woman is a candidate for natural treatments only or needs to integrate these approaches with conventional methods.

CONVENTIONAL TREATMENTS

Conventional medicine usually does nothing to treat mild dysplasia and genital warts. "Basically, they wait to see if it gets worse," says Dr. Hudson. "Often the body can reverse mildly abnormal states to normal on its own, as the body has an extraordinary ability to heal itself. But when it can't, then the disease progresses, and the downside of waiting becomes apparent."

In the later stages, aggressive measures may be taken. The preferred conventional treatment is known as LEEP (loop excisional electrosurgical procedure), which uses an electrical wire to cut out abnormal tissue. This is less expensive and less traumatic than the older method, cone biopsy. Cryosurgery, cauterization, and laser vaporization are other options. In advanced disease states, a hysterectomy may be needed to save a woman's life.

ALTERNATIVE TREATMENTS

NATUROPATHIC APPROACH

Women with cervical dysplasia often achieve excellent results using naturopathic approaches. Dr. Hudson notes, "In the results of a research study that I conducted at the College of Naturopathic Medicine in Portland, we treated forty-three women with varying degrees of cervical dysplasia. Through my treatment protocol, thirty-eight of the forty-three reverted to normal, three partially improved, and two had no change, meaning that they didn't get better and they didn't get worse."

Dr. Hudson's protocol consists of three parts: systemic, local, and constitutional treatment. She stresses that after a woman follows the protocol for three months, it is important for her to once again be examined by a health practitioner and to obtain another Pap smear. Sometimes a biopsy is also needed.

SYSTEMIC TREATMENT

- Beta-carotene—25,000 IU daily
- Vitamin C—10,000 mg in divided doses daily
- Folic acid—1–3 mg daily (Note: High doses of folic acid must be prescribed by a naturopathic physician. After three months, the amount of folic acid is decreased.)
- Immune herbal formulation

LOCAL TREATMENT

- Vitamin A suppositories
- Herbal suppositories

CONSTITUTIONAL TREATMENT

- Diet: An optimal immunity diet is low in fat and high in whole grains, vegetables, and fruits. Immune system inhibitors such as coffee, sugar, alcohol, and fat are omitted.
- Use of condoms
- Avoidance of smoking

HERBAL TREATMENT

Amanda McQuade Crawford, a medical herbalist, uses herbal infusions to treat cervical dysplasia. In her book *Herbal Remedies for Women*, Crawford also recommends herbal douches. Her favorite douche uses 1 ounce of wheatgrass juice for every 6 ounces of sterile water. If wheatgrass is not available, she recommends the following douche solution:

- 1 ounce marshmallow root
- 1 ounce goldenseal root as directed
- 1 ounce gotu kola herb

Grind the herbs and mix with 4 ounces boiling water. Strain, and allow the mixture to cool to room temperature before using.

Here's another one:

- 1 cup warm, but not hot, sterilized water
- 15 drops thuja oil
- 1 ounce calendula oil
- 15 drops vitamin E oil

You can also add:

- 4–6 drops blue chamomile oil
- 4–6 drops geranium oil

Dilute the oils in water and mix together well.

IMMUNO-AUGMENTATIVE THERAPY (IAT)

Treating cervical cancer by restoring the patient's own immune system has also proved successful at Dr. John Clement's Immuno-Technologies Cancer Clinic in Freeport in the Bahamas. Dr. Clement specifies that success can occur if the treatment is begun early, even after surgery. (See chapter 24 for more information.)

Fibroids and Uterine Bleeding

Fibroids are growths composed of muscle tissue that are usually benign. They attach themselves to the inner or outer wall of the uterus. One in five women over thirty-five has them, with the majority being African American. Fibroids grow in response to estrogen levels. Medically, they are also referred to as fibromyoma uteri and leiomyoma uteri.

Complementary physician Dr. Robert Sorge says that fibroids are nature's way of encapsulating toxins that result from an unhealthy diet and lifestyle: "Most of our patients with this condition consume tremendous amounts of coffee . . . Every person concerned about their health must stop drinking coffee. Diet sodas, greasy fries, pizza, potato chips, doughnuts and danishes, and other devitalized foods add to the problem."

Registered nurse and licensed acupuncturist Abigail Rist-Podrecca adds that Asian medicine sees fibroids as the result of blockage to the uterine area. "This can be caused by anger, emotional upset, or a history of problems with menstruation, where it is either late or prolonged. Sometimes, after an abortion, the endometrial wall will still have some cells from that particular pregnancy. Further down the line, that can develop into fibroids."

SYMPTOMS

Small fibroids are symptomless, but when they grow, they may result in painful periods, bladder infections, and infertility. Uterine bleeding is another common symptom. Explains Rist-Podrecca: "If the fibroid is located on the inside of the uterus lining, then you will have this uterine bleeding, which usually sends women to the gynecologist, where she opts for hysterectomy. If the fibroid is located on the muscle wall, there is not so much bleeding, but the fibroid will continue to grow."

Dr. Sorge adds that bleeding is the body's attempt to restore balance, according to naturopathic medicine: "Circulation and oxygenation of the uterine muscles and blood vessels are diminished, and metabolic waste products begin to build up. Bleeding is the sign of a highly toxic condition attempting to correct itself."

CONVENTIONAL APPROACH

Small fibroids that do not cause problems may be left alone or removed by a procedure known as a myomectomy. This procedure removes the fibroid only and does not interfere with a woman's ability to have children.

For larger tumors or fibroids that cause heavy bleeding, hysterectomies are the standard treatment. Dr. Herbert Goldfarb, a gynecologist and assistant clinical professor at New York University's School of Medicine, reports that the majority of these operations are unnecessary, as well as dangerous. In addition, hysterectomies can be psychologically destructive.

"A laser procedure, called myoma coagulation, has the potential to end the use of hysterectomies for fibroids once and for all, but most people don't know about it," Dr. Goldfarb says. "My book, *The No Hysterectomy Option*, was written in response to my frustration at having a technology to help women avoid hysterectomies but women not knowing about it. Sometimes women need hysterectomies but often they are told they need them for frivolous reasons. My book is designed to help women understand when a hysterectomy is needed and when other options are available. I always like to say that a hysterectomy may be indicated, but may not be *necessary*. Our best patient is an informed patient."

According to Dr. Tori Hudson, one alternative to hysterectomy is hysteroscopic surgery, which is used when a fibroid is protruding into the uterus. The surgeon inserts a hysteroscope, a tubular instrument that allows the surgeon to visualize the interior of the uterus, through the cervix and shaves away the fibroid with instruments passed through the hysteroscope. The hysteroscope is also used to shrink larger fibroids with lasers or electric currents.

An alternative for relatively small fibroids on the outside of the uterus is laparoscopic surgery. The laparoscope, an instrument used to visualize the interior of the abdomen, is inserted through an incision in the abdomen, and the fibroid is vaporized by an electric current or removed surgically, using instruments passed through the tube.

ALTERNATIVE THERAPIES

MYOMA COAGULATION

Dr. Goldfarb lectures extensively to doctors on this technology, which has enabled him to prevent hysterectomies in hundreds of women with fibroids and uterine bleeding. The typical candidate is a woman uninterested in reproduction, since the uterine wall may become too weak to support a pregnancy. Also, the size of the tumor must be 10 centimeters or less (approximately six inches). If the fibroid exceeds this size, it can be reduced with the medication Lupron. "Lupron reduces estrogen levels in the body, and temporarily reduces the size of fibroids," Dr. Goldfarb says. "With Lupron, we get a 30 to 50 percent reduction in size."

Once the tumor has become smaller, coagulation can be performed, which shrinks it another 50 to 75 percent and puts an end to the problem. "When we do this procedure, we literally undermine the tumor by destroying its blood supply. As we put needles around the fibroid, it turns blue, showing that the blood supply has been interrupted. Fluid and blood go out, and the tumor shrinks. It becomes stringy tissue and just sits there, becoming very small, eliminating the need for removal. The patient has no symptoms and can go about her life without the need for further surgery."

DIET AND EXERCISE

Fibroids grow in response to estrogen, so nutritionist Gracia Perlstein advocates the natural lowering of estrogen through diet and exercise as a first-line defense. As Perlstein explains, "Research shows that an overfatty diet increases estrogen in the diet, and we know overweight women produce more estrogen. So the first approach would be dietary.

"The best diet for a woman attempting to decrease the size of her fibroids, or at the very least keep them from getting any larger, consists of whole foods and is semivegetarian or vegetarian. The best protein sources are from vegetables and include whole grains, especially millet, amaranth, quinoa, buckwheat, whole oats, and brown rice.

"Eat small quantities of legumes daily. Soybeans and foods made from soy, in particular, contain isoflavones that discourage tumor growth. Foods made from soy include tofu, fortified soy milk, miso, and tempeh. A variety of other beans can be used to make wonderful ethnic dishes: black beans, adzukis, pinto beans, chickpeas, mung beans, lentils, and lima beans. Grains and beans are your best source of proteins.

"The liver detoxifies excess estrogen, so you want to support liver function by avoiding all recreational drugs, alcohol, fried foods, coffee, and any processed or refined foods. Be sure to drink at least two quarts of pure water a day to help your bowels and kidneys. You are trying to remove excess estrogen from the system, and this is supported when your organs of elimination work properly."

Exercise is also very important, says Perlstein. "Regular exercise will reduce excessive estrogen levels. Most people are familiar with the fact that hard-training women athletes sometimes reduce their estrogen levels to the point where they stop menstruating. We are not after that kind of effect, but regular exercise is very beneficial."

For further uterine support, Perlstein recommends the following supplements and herbs:

- Balanced oil supplement (a mixture of flax, borage, and other unrefined, natural, organic oils), 1 tbsp daily
- Multiple vitamin/mineral supplement
- Iron and herb supplement (This should be taken if there is anemia from heavy bleeding. Avoid high doses of iron as they are implicated in cancer and heart disease.)
- Vitamin E, 400 IU, twice daily
- Silica supplement
- Vitamin C with bioflavonoids, 1,000 mg five times daily, divided over the course of the day
- Evening primrose oil, 100 mg three times daily
- False unicorn root tincture, 15 drops in a small amount of water, taken every hour, for acute uterine problems
- Shepherd's purse tincture, 15 drops in a small amount of water three times a day (may stop excessive bleeding)
- White ash (may reduce size of fibroids)

Perlstein asserts that such a comprehensive program of diet and lifestyle changes, geared toward reducing excess estrogen, gives the body the tools it needs to shrink fibroids or keep them from growing any larger.

NATUROPATHIC TREATMENTS

Dr. Joseph Pizzorno, past president of John Bastyr College of Naturopathic Medicine, recommends oil-soluble liquid chlorophyll. He says this old natural therapy can quite effectively put an end to abnormal uterine bleeding. Oil-soluble liquid chlorophyll is available in capsules. Two to three are usually taken two to three times a day. Dr. Pizzorno says that for some reason, the chlorophyll seems to relieve this condition. "Many people think this works because it improves clotting, but it turns out that women with abnormal uterine bleeding do not have clotting abnormalities. So why it works is not clear, but the bottom line is, it works quite well."

HERBS

According to Judy Griffin, an herbalist from Texas and author of *The Woman's Herbal*, as quoted in *Positive Health* magazine, treating fibroids involves decongesting the liver by using safe herbs that can be taken over an extended period of time, including dandelion and vitex berries. Vitex is particularly beneficial for fibrocystic disease because it lowers estrogen levels.

Abigail Rist-Podrecca says the following herbs are good for stopping dysfunctional uterine bleeding when taken under the supervision of a Chinese herbal practitioner:

POO WHA—Made from bee pollen.

ER JOW—Made from the hide of an animal.

CHUAN XIONG (LIGUSTICUM WALLICHI)—Regulates bleeding by the amount taken. Too much causes uterine bleeding, and too little stops it.

HAN LIAN CAO (WARRIOR'S GRASS)—Helps tone the spleen and uterus and stops intense uterine bleeding.

ACUPUNCTURE

Acupuncture points that relate to the uterus are found on the ankle. Rist-Podrecca explains how electrical acupuncture to this area helps reduce fibroids: "We use a small electrical current. This makes the uterus contract and expand. It palpates the area slightly to get the body to recognize that the fibroids are there, increase circulation, and start vibrating the fibroids so that they are released."

HOMEOPATHY

Beth MacEoin, a homeopath and the author of *Homeopathy for Women*, as quoted in *Positive Health* magazine, says that since fibroids are a chronic condition, they are best treated by a practitioner. For acute symptoms, however, a number of remedies may be effective; these must be chosen based on the specific symptoms a woman is experiencing at a given moment. "The idea is that for a remedy to be active, the remedy chosen must match the symptoms as closely as possible. So it would be very important to select that remedy with the help of either a practitioner's support or a very good, solid self-help manual."

With that in mind, consider the following remedies for uterine bleeding and fibroids:

IPECAC—Dr. Marjorie Ordene, , a gynecologist from Brooklyn, recommends this remedy to stop acute hemorrhaging with bright red blood. "When given in the 200 potency, every fifteen minutes, Ipecac slows down the bleeding. That's two pellets under the tongue until the bleeding actually stops. I have had success with a number of patients, and other physicians have reported this as well."

SHINA AND SABINA—The late Dr. Ken Korins said the two remedies to think of first for heavy bleeding are Shina and Sabina. Shina is for heavy, dark blood that forms clots and leads to debility and exhaustion. Sabina is also for clots, but here the blood is bright red. When large clots are being expelled, there is a laborlike pain that radiates from the sacrum to the pubis.

SECALE—Women who need Secale have dark blood that is almost black. Periods are profuse and prolonged.

PHOSPHORUS—Phosphorus is indicated when there is bright red blood with no clots.

TRILLIUM—Trillium is indicated when bleeding is very heavy and bright red. The person characteristically feels faint and dizzy after bleeding. Periods occur biweekly, and the woman feels worse with even slight movement.

AURUM MURIATICUM—This remedy may reduce the size of fibroids. It should be used when there are no other symptoms, such as heavy bleeding, and there is no particular discomfort.

HYDRASTINUM MURIATICUM—This remedy has been known to cure large fibroids, especially when they seem to be on the anterior wall of the uterus, pushing on the bladder and causing symptoms of urinary frequency and pain.

Reproductive System Cancers

Among the reproductive system cancers are those involving the ovaries, uterus or endometrium, and cervix. Of the three, ovarian cancer occurs most often and is increasing in frequency. Uterine cancers are easier to detect in the beginning stages and tend to be more treatable, whereas ovarian cancers are rarely discovered early, and are terribly damaging to the woman's quality of life.

OVARIAN CANCER

Women who are sedentary and don't exercise have an increased risk of ovarian cancer, explains Dr. Susanna Reid, a naturopathic physician in Connecticut. Dr. Reid also believes that being overweight, smoking—especially if you are postmenopausal—consuming alcohol and milk, eating meat (especially fried meat), and eating a diet lacking in fruits, vegetables, and fiber also increase the risk of ovarian cancer. The drug tamoxifen is associated with ovarian cancer, and hormone replacement therapy may also increase the risk.

Ovarian cancer usually manifests after menopause, especially in women who have few or no children, were unable to conceive, or gave birth later than the average age. Other factors that place women at risk include a past history of spontaneous abortions, endometriosis, type A blood, radiation to the pelvic region, and exposure to cancer-causing chemicals, such as asbestos.

Women should look for the following early indications of ovarian carcinomas: abnormal vaginal bleeding, weight loss, and changes in patterns of urination and bowel movements. While a Pap smear will not detect ovarian cancer in the beginning stages, ovarian cancer can be diagnosed through annual pelvic exams.

Dr. Reid emphasizes therapies to help prevent reproductive cancers or help heal the body after surgery. "I focus a lot on lifestyle. Fruits and vegetables have been shown in epidemiologic studies to protect against ovarian cancer, so I suggest that people put a lot of fruit and vegetables in their diet. Carotenoid-containing foods appear to specifically protect against ovarian cancer, carrot consumption in particular. Vegetable fiber is also important. Green vegetables and carrots seem to have a particular affinity for the ovaries and help protect them from reproductive cancers. Cruciferous vegetables in particular are very important in increasing natural killer-cell toxicity. Whole grains also provide protection."

One of Dr. Reid's guiding principles is to have people return to natural or raw foods as much as possible. She says that animal products have a strong association with ovarian cancer and recommends eliminating animal products from the diet. "That even includes yogurt, which many people think is one of the best dairy products to eat. I don't think a person can be too careful. Ovarian cancer doesn't have a very positive prognosis, so if anything, a person should do too many things rather than not enough.

"Legumes seem to help as well, and the woman should also help eliminate alcohol; wine consumption is associated with an increased risk of ovarian cancer. Although green tea isn't specific for ovarian cancer, it does act specifically on breast cancer, so that might be something a woman would want to add to her diet. Also, moderate exercise increases immune function and is an important aspect of treatment."

Dr. Reid says that women with ovarian cancer seem to have a problem with the antioxidative mechanism in their bodies, and suggests using antioxidants like vitamin E and selenium to help deal with oxidative conditions in the body. Indole-3-carbonyl may also be useful.

Camptotheca acuminata, native to China and Tibet, contains an anticancer ingredient that has been modified to create topotecan, which has been approved by the FDA for ovarian cancer therapy.

UTERINE AND ENDOMETRIAL CANCER

The uterus, or womb, is where the baby grows during pregnancy. The endometrium is the lining of the uterus. Cancer of the endometrium is the most common type of uterine cancer.

Endometrial cancer is associated with hormones, including hormone replacement therapy with or without progesterone, a history of infertility, failure to ovulate, the use of drugs containing estrogen, and uterine growths. Tamoxifen is one drug that significantly increases the risk for endometrial cancer.

According to Dr. Reid, other risks include not having given birth to any children, beginning menopause after age fifty-five, being overweight, consuming alcohol, and eating a diet high in calories, especially when you are post-menopausal. Eating meat and saturated fats—even fat from fish, especially processed fish—and low consumption of vegetables, fruit, fiber, and legumes are also risk factors. Other poor dietary habits that increase risk are drinking soft drinks and consuming sugar.

The symptoms of endometrial cancer are abnormal bleeding in the vaginal area, especially after menopause, and pain in the lower abdomen or back. A Pap smear does not always catch endometrial cancer early, but the cancer can be detected with a surgical examination of the uterus.

As with other reproductive cancers, Dr. Reid believes that endometrial cancer has to be surgically treated. "It's not something that we would ever treat in natural medicine."

Dr. Reid says that natural treatment is focused on helping the patient heal from surgery. She uses therapies that facilitate healing, such as zinc and antioxidants and anti-inflammatories such as bioflavonoids and quercetin and bromelain. The specific therapy depends on how the surgery was done. "If it was done vaginally, you can use hydrotherapy treatments on the abdomen. There is a time during which you have to be quiescent because clots are setting, so you don't want to encourage bleeding. Patients should drink lots of fluids and eat very light foods so that their bowels are minimally taxed and their digestive systems can rest as the abdomen is healing."

CERVICAL CANCER

Cervical cancer is associated with cervical dysplasia, as discussed earlier in this chapter. Although not all cases of cervical dysplasia result in cancer, it can be the first stage of a malignancy. According to the American Cancer Society, an estimated 13,000 new cases of invasive cervical cancer will be diagnosed in 2015.

Oral contraceptives and DES (diethylstilbestrol), reduced physical activity, multiple sexual partners or having the first intercourse at a young age, smoking, frequent douching, genital herpes, and multiple pregnancies are all associated with cervical cancer.

In the early stages of cervical cancer, symptoms are usually absent, although there may be a watery vaginal discharge or spotty bleeding. Signs of advanced cervical cancer include dark, odorous vaginal discharges; fistulas; weight loss; and back and leg pain. One's chance of survival increases with early discovery through yearly Pap tests.

Dr. Reid warns that a chronic inflammation left untreated can become cervical dysplasia and eventually cervical cancer. She says that cervical conditions may be related to a virus. "Natural medicine has a really good track record in treating cervical dysplasia before it gets to cancer. I would not treat cervical cancer with natural remedies. A woman would normally have the cervix removed surgically.

"To treat cervical dysplasia, we use a diet high in fiber as well as flax seeds, olives, and avocados. There is some recent research that shows that olives contain immune-enhancing substances. And of course, I recommend a lot of fruits and vegetables."

Dr. Reid also recommends using supplements and botanicals. These include folic acid, beta-carotene, and vitamins E and C with bioflavonoids. She also has a six-week set protocol that utilizes suppositories. It begins with mild herbal suppositories, which she alternates with more intense herbal suppositories followed by a healing herbal suppository. In one study, thirty-eight out of forty-three patients with cervical dysplasia using this treatment had their Pap smears revert to normal.

COMBINATION TREATMENTS

Gar Hildebrand, formerly of the Gerson Research Organization in San Diego, California, says that more patients would triumph over reproductive system cancers if a combination of approaches was employed. This is the case because contemporary treatments for ovarian cancer are disappointing. While they can make cancers disappear for weeks or months at a time, they fail in the end, as the cancer returns with a vengeance to finish the job. In fact, orthodox survival rates for ovarian cancer patients are only between 5 and 10 percent.

Cancers of the uterine cervix initially exhibit higher success rates with surgery, which may involve the removal of the uterus (hysterectomy), as well as both ovaries and the fallopian tubes (salpingo-oophorectomy), in addition to X-ray and hormone therapies. But there is no guarantee that the cancer will not return. He states, "No one should be treated by a single specialty, and then watched in hopes that the cancer will not come back. It's not scientifically justifiable, nor is it acceptable to the patient. Sitting and waiting just causes horrible, immune-suppressing anxiety."

Among the multiple modalities that work best for patients with ovarian and uterine cancer are nutrition, coffee enemas, hyperbaric oxygen, and Coley's toxins.

NUTRITION

"Let's say a woman with an ovarian cancer has just been admitted to Memorial Sloan Kettering Cancer Center," Hildebrand says. "The first thing the doctors will do is a laparotomy. She will be opened up, and a surgeon will get the bulk of the tumor out. I have no problem with that.

"But the second step would be to use drugs that kill tumors. Tissue damage always accompanies cancer; unless it is addressed, the cancer is sure to reappear. In other words, throughout the body tumor toxins cause cells to lose potassium and swell with extra salt and water. This state is worse around the tumor itself. Often a treatment that goes into the bloodstream fails to penetrate to a tumor effectively because the tissue next to the tumor has no immunity. What's really needed, then, is for the patient to be stabilized physiologically. The ideal treatment would be for the person to receive nutritional salt and water management, a diet that nourishes and corrects the water retention in the cells. We're going to feed the whole body to try to get the tissues back to normal functioning."

Hildebrand recommends a diet that detoxifies and stimulates cells back to health. "Doctors have long been aware that most cancer patients have an aversion to meat. They'll smell it and gag; that's a self-defense mechanism. It's absolutely essential for these people to stop taking in heavy proteins—animal proteins and sometimes even heavy vegetable proteins like legumes—for a while, just to clear up. The tumor is converting that stuff into caustic chemicals, related to the ammonia we use in our laundry machines. It's those chemicals that create damage systemwide.

"We can also detoxify the body by supplying oodles of plant chemicals, called phytochemicals. These foods can be eaten cooked or raw, and should include vegetables of all sorts, fruits, and a few whole grains. Fruit and vegetable juices are especially important. You have to flood the system with nutritious fluids such as carrot and green leaf juices. Apple juice should always be added because apples contain a material that is very good for cellular energy. If you put those juiced phytochemicals into the body every hour, these cancer patients will have their cellular enzyme systems speeded up so that the individual cells can spit up toxins.

"Eating an excess of empty calories and proteins creates toxicity that causes the immune system to overproduce white blood cells that aren't very adept at what they do. Once you restrict protein and calories and get the nutrient level up, these patients' immune systems become intelligent again. They stop making excess stupid white cells and create more lymphocytes that are interested in more types of challenges. In other words, you get a very lean, mean immune system."

COFFEE ENEMAS

Coffee enemas have been used by thousands of cancer patients outside the realm of traditional medical care. Hildebrand explains: "Coffee in retention enemas stimulates the liver's enzyme system, which in turn causes great relief from pain in cancer patients. The liver has more than a thousand documented medical functions. When we help it work better and faster, a cancer patient's overall physiological condition changes, sometimes within hours and certainly within the first several weeks of treatment. You have a whole different person. People come off gurneys and out of beds, excruciating chronic pain is eased, and addiction to morphine is broken.

"Every three minutes, all the blood in our bodies goes through the liver. Our livers and small intestine walls have an enzyme system with a fancy name that we will call GST for short [GST refers to the glutathione S-transferases]. This enzyme system naturally responds to cancer in the body by going up, and coffee enemas have been shown in laboratory experiments with rats, and in later experiments with humans, to produce increased liver bile flow and to stimulate the GST enzyme system. In fact, it's raised to 700 percent of normal levels of activity. When the GST system is running that fast, it can effectively remove tumor toxins from the bloodstream. And it doesn't take very long. The effects of these coffee enemas will last for sometimes four, six, or eight hours before a feeling of discomfort and pain around the tumor returns. They're that effective."

HYPERBARIC OXYGEN

Hildebrand also looks at increasing circulation with full-body-immersion oxygen therapy. "Hyperbaric oxygen treatment is given in a diving chamber that used to be used to treat the bends," he says. "There's been a lot of fascination with ozone in cancer treatment in the alternative field. But what we found is that ozone applications raise tissue oxygen only by 25 to 50 percent, whereas hyperbaric oxygen can predictably raise oxygenation much higher. This means that tissue around the tumor, which doesn't have enough oxygen to function, can get sufficient oxygen for energy production. This will also allow the tissue to repair itself by producing a high-potassium, low-sodium environment, so that this edema can come out of the tissue."

COLEY'S TOXINS

Hildebrand states that this treatment has the best record of any treatment in the cancer literature, especially when combined with the Gerson diet program. "I am hopeful that much interest will be sparked in this therapy because right now the only reports I've seen of long-term survival for ovarian cancer patients have been from a combination of these approaches.

"The word *toxin* is a little confusing, because Coley's toxins are not really poison. It refers to a bacterial endotoxin that is an immune stimulant. I would put that directly into the abdominal cavity once the tissue around the tumor has been stabilized."

Coley's toxins have an interesting history. "Coley was a physician who searched the literature for cancer treatments after a heartbreaking experience of losing a child patient to the disease," Hildebrand says. "Much to his surprise, he found a skin infection called erysipelas. Erysipelas is caused by a streptococcus that causes a skin fever of 105 to 106 degrees Fahrenheit. This fever causes an inflammatory infection which interferes with tumor action.

"Coley constructed a live erysipelas vaccine, which was too toxic at first. Some patients died, but others experienced a tumor regression. He went through a lot of trial and error and eventually settled on something that we now call Serratia marsecens. He mixed the Serratia and the strep in a ratio of 1,500 cells to one, and then crushed the mixture through a microfilter to liberate the internal toxins of the bacteria. This liberated antigens, which in turn caused the immune system of the patient to respond as if there were a chronic infection that had to be fought."

Hildebrand explains why Coley's toxins work so well. "The effectiveness of Coley's toxins seem to be due to the fact that the immune system, when turned on, can cause a lot of dust to rise. These patients need to be put into an intensive care unit and hooked up to monitors in case there is a problem, although there have never been any heart attacks or kidney failures reported in the 900 cases that have been thoroughly studied. Then a tiny amount of toxins was administered intravenously for four hours through a drip. About two hours into the process, the immune response begins. The patient will develop chills and shaking that last for about thirty to ninety minutes, followed by a rise in temperature of about a degree every ten minutes. Once that temperature hits 105 or 106, the ICU staff lays the patient down or puts in a suppository of Tylenol to stop it.

"The reaction is the immune system's response. This is not a poison. This is not a toxin. It's not like chemotherapy, which makes your hair fall out or causes bone marrow suppression. The Coley's toxins are much more like what happens when your immune system decides to cure you of an infection. So the symptoms are more flulike, without the nausea and vomiting. After the second or third IV application, patients usually get sleepy and actually nod off. The fever lessens progressively. In other words, there's a honeymoon period.

"Coley himself said that if you don't keep these up for at least three or four months, in booster dosages, you won't get a permanent response. The literature reveals that gains are lost when Coley's toxins are given in lower concentrations or for shorter durations. But when they are properly used, there is an extraordinary 50 percent cure rate in advanced, inoperable uterine and ovarian cancers."

THE BENEFITS OF A COMBINATION APPROACH

Hildebrand reemphasizes the importance of utilizing any and every cancer protocol that works. "We believe that it's time we stopped living in an either/or world where orthodoxy is over on one side and the marginalized alternative professions are in the trenches and foxholes, and nobody talks. We believe it's time to get the doors and windows of communication open so that we can find the context for each of these treatments and the way they fit together.

"Our own experience reveals that using the nutritional approach takes a toxic load off the immune system and speeds up intracellular enzymes so that they can repel toxins and pull them from the blood rapidly. Calorie and protein restrictions and a diet high in nutrients can lead to the sensitization of a tumor. Years of experience show that diet therapy alone can produce monthly fevers, and tumors may or may not regress through those fevers. But if you stimulate the immune system when those fevers are hitting, you have a much greater chance of tumor reduction. That's why we suggest the marriage of these disciplines and the respectful recognition of the role of every aspect of anticancer medicine that's ever been developed."

PATIENT STORY

I still have cervical cancer, but I am working on overcoming it through a number of approaches. I watch my diet very carefully. I feel that my condition is in an early enough stage where I can handle it nutritionally. But it's not just nutrition that I have to deal with. I have to deal with all the emotions that help to create disease in the body. It's also a matter of detoxing. I do colonics and a lot of juicing. I take supplements. And I do meditation and exercise.

The major reason I started to see a nutritionist was, of course, the wake-up call, the cervical cancer, which was just diagnosed three months ago. But I had also had ulcerative colitis for almost twenty years.

I feel like I now have energy again. I exercise at least several times a week, which was literally impossible before. I even had trouble getting up a flight of subway steps without feeling exhausted at the top. So I have several different things that I am working with: nutrition, meditation, and detoxification. I'm working on it.

Now I have to find a gynecologist who is holistically oriented because my primary care physician dropped me after I refused to have a hysterectomy. I feel very lucky. I feel that someone else trying to deal with this would have followed the recommended course of action and would have given up her reproductive rights, allowing herself to be mutilated while always being fearful of having the cancer reappear.

Also, I feel that the cancer is nothing more than a wake-up call. Your body is saying, "Hey, something is wrong here. You're out of balance. You need to address this and this and this." If you don't, disease is the end result. Now I am vegetarian and doing a lot of things differently. If I didn't, I might not be alive now.

I might be at a higher risk for the cancer to spread throughout more of the body. This doesn't mean that I am 100 percent there. I still have a lot of work to do. But I feel very hopeful.

—Morgan

Research Update

An increasing body of evidence is showing the benefits of natural modalities to overall health and well-being. Following is a sample of recent peer-reviewed scientific studies on cervical dysplasia, fibroids, and reproductive system cancers.

According to a 2015 study published in *Cancer Epidemiology, Biomarkers & Prevention*, women who drank about four cups of coffee daily had an 18 percent lower risk of developing endometrial cancer than those who drank less than a cup a day. A 2014 report in *Cancer Prevention Research* found that folate and vitamin B_{12} may benefit women with human papillomavirus (HPV) by maintaining a high degree of methylation at specific sites. In 2010, a report in *Fertility and Sterility* showed that epigallocatechin gallate (EGCG), a component in green tea, and vitamin D inhibit the proliferation of cultured human leiomyoma (HuLM) cells and induce apoptosis (programmed cell death). A 2013 study published in the *International Journal of Women's Health* showed similar results.

Chapter 26

Chronic Fatigue Syndrome

Chronic fatigue syndrome poses a major problem for traditional medicine. The medical establishment has fumbled in its treatment to the point of sometimes claiming that the illness does not exist, but chronic fatigue is a major problem in the United States, particularly among women. According to 2013 data from the Centers for Disease Control and Prevention (CDC), between one and four million Americans are afflicted with the syndrome, including four times as many women than men.

Chronic fatigue syndrome is the term used to describe a state of constant exhaustion. A syndrome is a disorder that includes a collection of symptoms but is not necessarily a disease entity. Although not labeled as such until the late 1980s, chronic fatigue syndrome is quite similar to other disorders that have been known for centuries. In the nineteenth century, for example, a common complaint of middle-class women was neurasthenia, which was characterized by chronic exhaustion and a variety of other physical symptoms.

Why is it that for years Americans with a debilitating illness were not recognized as having a disease? They were simply told that chronic fatigue syndrome does not exist. Dr. Dean Black says, "If you go back to the last century, you can read about women suffering from nervous disorders—so many of them that clinics had to be set up to care for them. There was always the search for a cause, but one couldn't be found, so doctors wouldn't say it was a disease. It had to be in the patient's mind. This is not a new way of sweeping things under the carpet.

"Medicine's power base is the idea of its basis in certainty, which hinges on the concept of a single linear cause-and-effect relationship. That's why medicine is always looking for a single causal factor. This is called the theory of specific etiology."

Dr. Black compares the situation of chronic fatigue syndrome to that of the Epstein-Barr (EB) virus, which was initially thought to cause chronic fatigue syndrome, although later this theory was challenged. "That is why they were so happy to discover this EB virus," he explains. "It seemed marvelous to them because it served to justify the single-cause idea. Yet, as has been frequently pointed out, everyone may have Epstein-Barr [because it is so widely distributed]. Chronic fatigue syndrome is caused by many factors operating together. But this idea has been excluded by traditional medicine, which refuses to come to grips with multifactorially generated disease. Medicine is reluctant to accept this multifactorial explanation because it holds to this idea of absolute truth, which requires simplicity and must have one cause and one effect."

Dr. Andrew Gentile stresses that we need to differentiate chronic fatigue syndrome from other health problems: "Since chronic fatigue syndrome has no known cause, we need to rule out other disorders whose cause we do know. The working definition provided by the government for this disease says there is no other illness at the root of it. Differentiating it calls for great care, since fatigue is ubiquitous as a symptom of many diseases, such as anemia, low thyroid, hypoglycemia, and a variety of other illnesses. These other illnesses must be clearly ruled out."

Potential Causes

VIRAL INFECTION

A number of studies have looked at viruses in connection with this syndrome. One theory posits a single viral agent. Dr. Gentile states, "I have heard chronic fatigue syndrome being called a number of things from Epstein-Barr to mononucleosis.

"Epstein-Barr was brought into the discussion by way of a lab in Philadelphia that exclusively studies this virus. One of the lab assistants was negative for current and acute Epstein-Barr virus, but during the course of the study developed the symptoms of chronic fatigue syndrome. He was treated and found to be positive for Epstein-Barr virus. So we had the first studied case in which a person went from Epstein-Barr-negative to Epstein-Barr-positive at the same time that he had all the symptomatology for chronic fatigue syndrome. That began a flurry of studies investigating the Epstein-Barr connection. We now know there is not a high degree of correlation between the symptoms of chronic fatigue syndrome and Epstein-Barr serological titers. So Epstein-Barr is probably not the cause of chronic fatigue syndrome."

Dr. Gentile goes on to note that the Epstein-Barr virus is widely distributed in the populace. Most people have it by age eight. Thus, there is no clear distinction between those who have it and those who do not. We would expect many more people to be ill with chronic fatigue if it were indeed Epstein-Barr that was causing it. Several other candidates have presented themselves, including human herpes virus 6 (HHV-6), a B-lymphocyte virus that was studied by the National Institutes of Health, and human T-cell lymphotropic virus (HTLV-2).

Dr. Neenyah Ostrom, author of *America's Biggest Cover-Up*, believes that HHV-6 may be involved. "What is interesting is that there are two types of this virus. One form is found very widely in the general population, and the other is found in people with cancer, AIDS, chronic fatigue syndrome, and other immunological problems. This virus can attack the immune system very effectively, and I believe it will eventually be found to be instrumental in causing chronic fatigue syndrome, AIDS, and some forms of cancer."

Other viruses that have been thought to contribute to chronic fatigue syndrome are Coxsackie virus, adenovirus, enterovirus, and the hepatitis virus, among others. Dr. Gentile states, "The consensus among practitioners is that a single virus probably does not cause this illness. We have to carefully distinguish between cause and trigger. Clearly, a virus may trigger a cascading set of events in various body systems: neural, endocrine, cognitive, and hormonal. A variety of abnormalities may be found in these systems, but if viruses do trigger these imbalances, then they quickly hide within the normal cells—which is usually how viruses behave—while their effects wreak havoc in the body system."

It is as if the virus triggered something in the immune system that makes the system unable to self-regulate and find its way back to homeostasis. Thus, each time the immune system is stressed by a toxic load from the environment or from food allergies, or when infections are reactivated, there is a breakdown. The flare-ups and relapses occur and recur frequently, reproducing all the symptoms. These relapses then compound themselves. If a patient is not sleeping every night, symptoms such as exhaustion and lowered immunity crop up.

"We know, by the way," Dr. Gentile adds, "that the rhythms of this illness dovetail nicely with ninety-minute circadian rhythms. In sleep, we have a REM [rapid eye movement] cycle that occurs every ninety minutes, and this is the cycle by which our immune system is synthesizing proteins. The immune system works lock and key with this cycle. But if one has a sleep disturbance caused by a virus or a set of viruses from this disorder, one's sleep will be off and therefore the immune system will be off."

Environmental Factors, Nutrition, and Allergies

Dr. Majid Ali sees the surrounding environment and lifestyle as playing causal roles. He says that the immune system becomes injured by environmental pollutants such as mold, formaldehyde, and pesticides as well as by allergenic foods, poor nutrition, stress, and lack of physical fitness.

The late Dr. Shari Lieberman, a professor of nutrition, expanded on this point. She published articles and several books, including *The Real Vitamin and Mineral Book*. "We as a country are not healthy. We have all these discussions, lectures, books, and so on, concerning a healthy lifestyle. We have the information, but we are not actualizing it. I don't think people understand how all of the body's circumstances are impacted by the immune system.

Dr. Michele Galante also believes that allergies are important: "The patients I have seen have been very allergic not only to pollens and airborne agents but especially to foods and chemicals. These people are so sensitive and so debilitated that a short exposure to perfume, nail polish, gas fumes, carbon monoxide, or even just paint, such as from a freshly painted room, will give them headaches, make them weak, even make them emotionally upset. Chronic fatigue syndrome is closely connected to allergy."

Unfortunately, Dr. Ostrom adds, "some of these allergy-causing substances are unavoidable. Chemicals in our environment, aside from those in our foods (coloring, preservatives, and so on), are everywhere. There is chlorine in our water; the air is filled with pollutants—things that were not in our ecological system fifty or sixty years ago. Recent phenomena that accompany technological advances, such as the mercury in silver amalgam dental work, are weakening our systems. Each of these chemicals in itself does not necessarily have so strong an impact, but exposure to all of them together, day after day, for many years, overloads the liver and immune system. Electromagnetic influences, previously ignored, are now also under discussion. Many believe the cathode rays from computers affect the electromagnetic fields of the body, for instance, as does the electromagnetism of cellular phones, radio waves, and television waves—things relatively new to our environment."

METABOLIC REGULATION

Chronic fatigue syndrome can also be explained in terms of immune system depression related to a failure in metabolic regulation. When glucose production is up, it brings on hypoglycemia, with a high degree of glucose in the blood causing an increased level of insulin, which lowers the glucose level excessively. Because of poor utilization of glucose, fatty acids increase in the blood to provide a sufficient level of energy. A high level of triglycerides will occur, and the immune system will be depressed because it needs a new army of T lymphocytes, which are not being produced because of derangement in lipid metabolism.

VITAMIN, MINERAL, AND HORMONAL DEFICIENCY

Dr. Neil Block explains that lack of necessary vitamins, including C, E, and beta-carotene, can affect the immune system, as can a lack of minerals, particularly calcium, vanadium, copper, magnesium, potassium, molybdenum, boron, iodine, selenium, and chromium. The trace minerals are especially important for organ function.

Dr. Block also points to hormonal imbalances, particularly thyroid imbalance (especially hypothyroidism), which affects women six times as often as men. It tends to develop spontaneously between the ages of twenty and fifty, although it can come at any time, often from unknown causes. The rare causes, which are the ones known for this disease, involve either a superabundance or a deficiency of iodine in the body, although the latter is unlikely in our society, where we have iodized salt and other sources. Another rare cause is consuming too many of certain vegetables, such as cauliflower, broccoli, and brussels sprouts, which tend to bind the active ingredient and inhibit thyroxin production.

Other hormones frequently out of the normal range include the adrenal hormones and the gender hormones. It is not unusual to have imbalances in the estrogen that governs the ovarian function or in other governors, such as LH [luteinizing hormone] from the pituitary gland or progesterone." In fact, women frequently come to Dr. Block with lack of menstruation, milky discharge from the breast, breast tenderness, or more menstrual cramps than usual.

DRUG USE

Dr. Galante remarks, "The allopathic drugs, conventional drugs, antibiotics, and steroids are major influences. The use and abuse of these drugs in childhood, for example, sets up chronically weakened conditions that will extend into adulthood and contribute to a predisposition for chronic fatigue. These drugs are suppressive in nature, not curative. They themselves impose an illness on the system. This may be one of the largest of the causal factors."

Dr. Ali talks about a young person suffering from chronic fatigue syndrome who went to a medical clinic and was given a prescription for steroids. We know steroids suppress the immune system, so why would anyone give these drugs to someone with this disorder? Steroids can create a sense of well-being and euphoria for a couple of days, but it is false.

PSYCHOLOGICAL FACTORS

Dr. Gentile tells us that chronic fatigue seems to reduce a person's tolerance to stress. He has had patients who were marathoners before contracting the illness. They report that they had been working hard and then got sick with fever and chills. The illness waxed and waned. They would feel better at times and go back to running but then quickly relapse. These patients cannot tolerate stress in either the physical or the psychological form. Stress will exacerbate the illness again and again.

According to Dr. Paul Epstein, a key tenet of naturopathic medicine is to treat the underlying cause. "A person diagnosed with chronic fatigue syndrome has a suppressed immune system, which can be documented by blood tests and other measures. But what caused this? It may be improper diet; then the patient will need to eat properly. But we also need to ask why she adopted that diet in the first place. If the answer is stress, we can then ask what caused the person to follow certain patterns of reaction to stress. As we treat the patient, going through all the different problems layered one on top of the other, we eventually get in contact with the person's core self.

"One way to make this contact is through the inner child. Many people have been influenced by John Bradshaw's work on recovering and healing the inner child and on seeing how the wounds and scars of childhood may have led us to create lifestyles that are addictive. Thus, even as I help the person medically by giving advice on diet, stress reduction, and so on, I remember this. If we do not touch deeper problems, healing may not occur."

Symptoms

Chronic fatigue syndrome causes fatigue and usually begins after the onset of flulike symptoms. The fatigue is not a simple tiredness; it is an exhaustion accompanied by feelings of being unwell. Many people have difficulty getting out of bed and may become weakened to the point of needing to lie down all the time. Often patients are bedridden for months; extreme tiredness can last for years.

Chronic fatigue syndrome may be accompanied by depression, irritability, headaches, low-grade fever, infection, confusion, focusing difficulties, diarrhea, sharp muscle pain and weakness, swollen glands, and sleep disorders. The woman is not able to fall asleep or stay asleep and does not feel refreshed or restored even after much sleep.

According to Dr. Martin Feldman, "Immune system difficulty somehow pulls down hormonal function. Almost all patients with this syndrome have low adrenal function, and many have low thyroid function. So we have a hormonal mix-up causing fatigue, but behind this is the viral disease pulling down the immune system."

Dr. Michael Vesselago uses laboratory tests to diagnose his patients and then treats them accordingly. He looks for viruses as well as allergies and stress. "I test the person for allergies with an IgE RAST [radioallergosorbent test] and get back a report showing how the body responds to more than one hundred tested foods. We adjust the diet so that the person is no longer eating allergy-causing foods, and that alone brings about a significant improvement in over 70 percent of individuals.

"If someone collapses unduly fast or wakes up tired and requires several cups of coffee to get going, then I will focus on the adrenals first. I do a test for adrenal function that involves checking cortisol, which is one of the main adrenal hormones. From that I get a picture of how well the adrenal glands are coping with stress during the day."

Dr. Martin Feldman says that the first step in the analysis of any woman who comes to him with fatigue, whether mild, moderate, or severe, is to profile the patient to see how she fits with the five major problems associated with the syndrome:

- Immune viral breakdown, leading to low adrenal function
- Thyroid imbalance

- Vitamin B deficiency
- Hypoglycemia
- Cerebral allergies

Dr. Feldman also tests the thymus, spleen, and lymphatic system. "You could test the T- and B-cell counts. That's easy to do, but it's very expensive, so in daily practice it's easier to test thymus electrical energy. You can also do this for the spleen. When we find a weak thymus circuit, we can try any aspect of therapy within the weakened circuit to obtain a resonance that will help strengthen that circuit."

Dr. Gentile is more concerned with self-diagnosis. "If you feel you have chronic fatigue syndrome, ask yourself these questions: Have I had debilitating fatigue for six months? Do I have flulike symptoms? Have I not found any phys-iological cause? Do I have pronounced sleeplessness? Do I have low stress toler-ance so that if I take a short walk or try any sport, I feel vaguely ill and tired?"

Dr. Majid Ali states that most physicians have a tendency to focus narrowly on a problem. But, he says, "I don't think trying to find a diagnosis for one or two symptoms is terribly important. What is important is how the patient describes his or her suffering. We need to think of what we can do at a molecular and ener-getic level to relieve his or her suffering and restore his or her health.

"I've seen patients whose lives have been devastated by chronic fatigue syn-drome. They've gone through all these drugs, antivirals, steroids. With each drug, they get better initially and then nose-dive. What do we do?"

Clinical Experience

ALTERNATIVE THERAPIES

The key to finding treatment for chronic fatigue syndrome, according to Dr. Gentile, is choosing the right expert. "It has reached the level of scientific respectability, and most practitioners and medical examiners believe it exists. It is important to have someone who is up to date on the literature and who has seen a minimum of fifty to one hundred patients, someone who understands the ups and downs of the disease and is aware of the number of different treatments that have developed."

He points out several ways to locate a credible expert. For one thing, there are chronic fatigue syndrome support groups in every major town in our country, and now worldwide, that have lists of physicians who have specialized in the disorder. There are national groups, such as the Chronic Fatigue and Immune Dysfunction Syndrome Association. They maintain a list of doctors who understand the disease, have treated it, and are sympathetic.

"This last trait is so important," Dr. Galante explains, "because many sufferers have gone through scores of doctors. We're treating a woman now who has already seen seventy-five physicians all over the world. She was ready to give up because she feels people do not believe her. So a critical part of treating this illness is belief. A second thing to bear in mind is that because this is a chronic illness with a wide range of symptoms, it will tend to fall between the cracks of all the medical subspecializations. With this disease, it will not be adequate to go to a single physician. It would be worth considering putting together a team, which would include a GP/internist, one who works both with traditional and alternative therapies; an allergist/infectious-disease specialist; and a psychologist/psychiatrist. This team could coordinate to work out a treatment plan so that the client understands what is coming next. And if these treatments don't work, the team could determine why that might be and what would be worth trying next."

THE SPIRITUAL ELEMENT

Dr. Ali tells us that in dealing with a chronic, devastating illness like this, hope and the spiritual element are essential for long-term success. He has had cases that truly stretch the bounds of credulity. "Creating hope is very easy to do; sustaining hope is difficult, but it is central to healing. By the time I see patients, they have each seen at least seven specialists. They've had biopsies, CAT scans. When they come to me, it's not that easy to simply reassure them, after they've seen the previous failures, that they'll get better. But fortunately, by the time they get to me, they've listened to some of our tapes, read our books, and, most important, talked to some of the other patients who have gotten better. So when they come in and they meet our nursing staff, our ancillary staff, they realize we are all serious. If they ask how my program differs, we say this: They do not have the option to remain sick."

VITAMIN SUPPLEMENTS

Another component of treatment is supplements. The intention is not only to repair damage and stabilize the weakened immune system, but also to overboost the system.

At Dr. Ali's clinic I watched a nurse making up an intravenous chronic fatigue syndrome protocol with vitamins and minerals. She said that patients who come in are very tired and have joint pains, headaches, and memory loss, and that these IVs help repair cell membranes and boost the immune system. About 90 percent of the patients have responded well. Dr. Ali will usually order a set of five to begin with, she says, and after that he can measure the patient's response, see how deep the problem is, and whether she requires further treatment.

"I see these drips as jump-starting the cellular enzymes," Dr. Ali says. "The enzymes, which are detoxification enzymes, are dependent on minerals and vitamins. If I feel there is enough time, when the patient is not acutely ill or has been chronically ill for a number of years, I will try to use a more conservative approach. But when I see people with severe, incapacitating fatigue, I use the IV. In fact, in one of our studies where we compared one group that had the IV and one group that didn't, we saw that the IV speeds up the recovery process.

"We have fourteen different formulations or protocols to manage different clinical problems in our IV drips. For chronic fatigue syndrome, we use vitamin C, magnesium, calcium, pyridoxine, pantethine, zinc, B vitamins, molybdenum, potassium, copper, and selenium. Most of our protocols have fifteen to eighteen items, and we change their quantities depending on the individual's state."

Dr. Feldman has found that chronic fatigue sufferers are lacking in vitamins A, B_5, B_{12}, and E; bioflavonoids; the essential fatty acids; zinc; selenium; and GLA (gamma-linoleic acid).

Dr. Neil Block discusses his treatment: "If proteins or amino acids are low, we can try to individually supplement the amino acids. If minerals are lacking, they can be given individually or in tandem, trying to operate by an economy of scale so that a patient doesn't have to take from more than ten to fifteen bottles at a time.

"As for hormonal imbalance, I have 20 to 25 percent of my chronic fatigue syndrome patients on thyroid hormone. I prefer to use the more natural brands of thyroid hormone. Again, I believe in giving both the male and female hormones. We also have to try to adjust the pancreas and adrenals. For the pancreas I use chromium or chromium picolinate. For adrenals, the glandulars or homeopathics, and sometimes things such as licorice, tend to help multiple hormones. If we are working on the pituitary, we use glandulars, the homeopathics, and on rare occasions I use a lot of the amino acids to try to build neurotransmitter activity. The amino acids to be used are arginine, tyrosine, and phenylalanine. Tryptophan was also once useful to me until they took it off the market. I'm also not afraid to use, correctly and in small doses, items obtained from the pharmacy. What I tend to shy away from are the tranquilizers, such as Valium and Librium. I do make use of antidepressants on occasion."

Often his patients have seen other physicians and holistic healers and may need only one or two things to turn the body around on multiple levels. "With neurotransmitters being easily adjusted nowadays, with items like the antidepressants such as Paxil and Zoloft, which lack drastic side effects and have a response beginning in two to four weeks, they're worthwhile. It's nice for a patient who has suffered two, four, or six years to take these new agents and within two to four weeks get at least some indication of the direction in which he or she is going."

ENZYMES

Dr. Steven Whiting, author of *The Complete Guide to Optimal Wellness*, tells us about enzyme supplementation. There are two forms of supplementation, he says, and it is important to understand the difference between them. One type of product you can get at health food stores consists of whole enzymes and actually contains such things as pepsin and trypsin, the real enzymes. They have their place, and they have their drawbacks. Their primary use is for chronic disease and for people who are very debilitated. The big problem with using them is that the body can grow dependent on them quite rapidly. When they are taken orally in the form of supplements, the body is not always encouraged to make them on its own.

"The second group of supplements," Dr. Whiting says, "is called enzyme precursors. These are substances that not only contain the raw materials for the body to build its own enzymes but frequently contain the vital stomach acid hydrochloric acid, which helps the body build many of the protein digestants. Remember, proteins are digested in the stomach, and carbohydrates and starches are digested in the intestinal tract. This is why a very unique enzyme system has been created and needs to be maintained."

He continues: "For the average person looking for a good enzyme product, I recommend one that would contain at least the following things. First, hydrochloric acid. After years of eating junk foods and dead, lifeless foods, we need it to help with stomach digestion. According to a survey by the University of California at Berkeley, only 9 percent of the population eats the recommended number of fresh fruits and vegetables per day. This product should also contain protein digestants, which should include papain and pepsin. There should be fat digestants, ox bile and pancreatin. Also a starch digestant, which would be bromelain."

"The bulk of the five years of research I have done for my book is about what I call whole-spectrum nutrition. We have been able to isolate about 102 nutrients that the body needs every day. These include the sixteen vitamins, the three fatty acids, eight to twelve amino acids, and about seventy-two minerals.

"What we found out in working with patients such as those with chronic fatigue syndrome in a clinical environment is that the concept that has developed in the last twenty years of using potency to address chronic diseases may have been only part of the picture. In reality, we are finding that the ratio of nutrients to each other is as important as, if not more important than, potency alone."

HERBAL THERAPIES

Many herbs can help to heal the immune system and thus play a role in chronic fatigue syndrome. Herbalist Letha Hadady offers some recommendations. Strengthening agents include Chinese ginseng, dandelion, false ginseng, Andrographis, Eclipta alba, and honeysuckle. Honeysuckle flower, Andrographis, and dandelion may also help destroy germs. Chinese blood tonics include han lien tsao, which is called Eclipta alba in Latin and grows wild in the American Southwest. It builds blood without any side effects, such as inflammation. You can take it every day in powdered form. Hadady also mentions fo ti, which builds blood while it keeps us cool.

There are three types of ginseng: American, Chinese, and false. The American type provides more moisture and more saliva and is good after a fever. Chinese ginseng, called ren shen, gives us energy. Dang shen, or false ginseng, makes us feel stronger without feeling hotter. All can be used in soups. When dang shen and astragalus are used together, the first lifts our energy and the second sends our defenses to the surface. Cayenne pepper increases circulation and makes us feel stronger.

There are also herbs for relaxing the nervous system. Siberian ginseng can be taken as an extract or in capsule form. Valerian, taken in capsules, can quiet the nervous system: "For people who are depressed," Hadady says, "we need to bring them to their center as a way to be grounded and to feel more whole. Use ginger and mint. Mint helps bring the worries out of the head, and ginger helps burn them away because it is digestive and heating, so it brings us warmly to our centers. They make a good combination."

High Energy preparation is an herb mixture that uses Western and Eastern ingredients: gotu kola, American ginseng, damiana, red clover, peppermint, and cloves. It strengthens the adrenals and lungs.

Hadady adds that cloves and hot water will increase your energy and make you breathe more deeply.

Dr. Lieberman looked at American plants to find ones that can strengthen the debilitated immune system that accompanies chronic fatigue syndrome. "I'd say hands down that about the most important herb in this area is licorice root," she said. "A specific valuable compound found in this root is glycyrrhizin, available in health food stores as a supplement. It's not the easiest thing to find, but a few companies make it. Glycyrrhizin is just remarkable at boosting the lymphatic and immune systems, the white blood cells, and the thymus gland."

Glycyrrhizin can actually be therapeutic in relation to some of the viruses implicated in chronic fatigue syndrome. Glycyrrhizin stimulates the production of interferon naturally. It supports the thyroid gland and boosts natural killer cells and other aspects of immune functioning. A therapeutic dose ranges from 75 to 300 milligrams per day. It's important to monitor your blood pressure while taking this supplement. "I haven't seen many patients' blood pressure go up when taking this, but it will occasionally happen," Dr. Lieberman noted.

Another antiviral is echinacea. Dr. Lieberman believed that it is not used nearly enough for chronic disease and immune dysfunction. Many people use it for influenza, but it can be useful for other viruses as well. Echinacea has a remarkable ability to naturally stimulate interferon, natural killer cells, and phagocytes.

The liquid extracts of echinacea work best, Dr. Lieberman said. Use 50 drops once or twice a day, depending on the severity of your symptoms. "It's been recommended that you use echinacea four days on, four days off. There is some concern that if you use it all the time, you may adapt to it and it may stop boosting certain aspects of immune function. We don't know that for sure, but to be on the safe side, that's my recommendation. But I keep my patients on glycyrrhizin long term, though I gradually cut the dose down and maybe eventually have them on 75 milligrams per day as a prophylactic."

DIETARY CHANGES

Gracia Perlstein, an alternative health care practitioner with a private practice in New York, says that for chronic fatigue, food is the best medicine. "We really don't have any existing drugs on the market to help this condition. In fact, most drugs will weaken immunity and delay recovery further. It is best to approach this with natural supports to inherent healing processes." While there are no quick fixes, she makes the following recommendations to speed up recovery.

A diet of pure, nutrient-rich whole foods is imperative. "You want to include plenty of fresh organic vegetables. Cruciferous vegetables such as broccoli, cauliflower, and brussels sprouts are very important for their immune-enhancing properties. You want onions and garlic, the poor man's cure-all.

"Choose from a wide assortment of whole foods. Don't eat the same few over and over again. In this weakened state you can develop allergic responses to foods consumed repeatedly in large amounts. Eating different foods will ensure that you get a variety of nutrients and will keep you from developing allergic responses. Amaranth, quinoa, and other grains not commonly eaten by Americans are good to include. Really emphasize the green foods. Have a dark green salad daily. Super green powders are very helpful as well. Add them to juices, but do not emphasize sweet fruit and carrot juice."

Proteins should also be emphasized. "The best sources." Perlstein says, "are vegetarian because of the low toxicity and ease of digestion. Good vegetarian proteins are tofu, tempeh, fortified soy milk, and legumes. You can benefit from small amounts of fresh fish because fish is high in omega-3 fatty acids. But there are some precautions you must take. Be sure to find a market that gets fish from clean, unpolluted waters and make sure they do not dip it in chlorine, which is a common practice. If you eat farm-raised fish, it should be organically raised. If you eat poultry, it should be naturally raised as well, free of hormones and pesticide residues. Consume only small amounts of animal protein, no more than three to four ounces a day.

"The best way to have protein is in a soup. An excellent old Chinese recipe for an immune-enhancing soup combines a whole astragalus root with onions, garlic, ginger, and free-range chicken, fish, tofu, or tempeh. Some fresh green vegetables and a handful of brown rice are added to that. The soup is brought to a boil and then simmered. Some miso is added for flavor. This is highly nourishing, easy to digest, and excellent for helping a weakened individual regain strength."

Don't forget your liquids. "Drink plenty of pure water daily," Perlstein says. "In colder seasons unsweetened herb tea, such as immune-supportive echinacea tea, is a very good source of liquid. Cold water is a little shocking to the digestive system for people with chronic fatigue syndrome, so you want warm liquids and plenty of them."

HOMEOPATHY

Homeopathy is Dr. Galante's specialty; it has been very effective against chronic fatigue syndrome. Homeopathic remedies, all made from natural substances, are given in microdoses. The essence of homeopathy is to select for each individual a remedy based on her or his unique physical constitution and manifestation of symptoms.

ACUPUNCTURE

Registered nurse and acupuncturist Abigail Rist-Podrecca points out that the chi, or bioelectrical energy, flows through pathways called meridians in the body. Disease, she says, is associated with an energy blockage. Acupuncture needles inserted in some of the 365 points can open the blockages so that the energy can flow smoothly through the meridians. In addition, the needles dilate the blood vessels so that more blood flows through the area, bringing more oxygen and nutrients, which aid all aspects of health.

TAI CHI

A benefit of tai chi is that it increases one's awareness both internally and environmentally. "Then you can choose which to work on, whether there is something physically wrong or something in the environment that needs to be corrected," says practitioner and educator Eric Schneider.

According to Schneider, you have to cultivate a part of your body that can observe phenomena dispassionately without having to grab on to every experience and run with it, so that when you find yourself in stressful situations, you can say quietly, "Oh, so this is what is happening now. What can I do about it? What are my options, and how am I feeling?"

However, it takes ten years to achieve what is called the gung chi, which means that the body is able to contain energy. This is not a quick fix.

IMAGERY AND HEALING

Imagery is a therapeutic technique that helps people explore themselves through words and symbols so that they can understand the language of the subconscious. According to Dr. Paul Epstein, "Usually what comes up is the issue that is at the core of what will be the healing. People may get in touch with childhood wounds or abuse from the past that needs healing. Perhaps they'll get in touch with the fact that the work they are doing is not real work.

"In one such case, with a person suffering from chronic fatigue syndrome, we found that the illness was a case of a person trying to get love. She had not let go of trying to get love from her mom and dad. She was still stuck at that place. And the pain and grief of not having that love were not only weakening her immune system but keeping her stuck in the unhealthy way she was living her life.

Dr. Majid Ali reiterates some of Dr. Epstein's message: "What I demonstrate to my patients is that the way you look at the world around you determines the biology under your skin. If you can be in a self-regulatory, healing mode, your brain activity, heart activity, muscle energy, skin energy will all be functioning positively. Or you can be trying to figure things out, think everything through in an overly intellectual way, and your biology will be as up and down as the New York skyline. This is the stress mode, and it causes disease. Another mode is an even, steady-state mode, a resting mode.

"Our goal is to perceive the energy in these modes and understand how the energy profoundly affects the electrophysiological profile. Can we allow this energy to guide us into the healing mode? We want a transition from an ordinary, thinking, nervous, stressful mode that causes disease to a nonthinking, meditative, deep-breathing mode that makes us well. That is our goal."

AYURVEDA

Dr. Nancy Lonsdorf, who has 25 years of experience in Ayurvedic medicine and co-wrote *A Woman's Best Medicine*, defines fatigue as an imbalance in the body's rest-activity cycle. According to Ayurvedic principles, the natural structures of rest cycles allow the body to recover from activity cycles: "A state of chronic fatigue means that the body has not fully rejuvenated itself."

Dr. Lonsdorf reports that many of her clients overcome fatigue by adhering to the basic rules of Maharishi Ayurveda, which address rest, activity, digestion, cleansing, and meditation.

THE NOTION OF SELF-HEALING

Dr. Epstein wants to help patients listen, explore, and understand the message of their disease, which is the key that unlocks the door to recovery. "After the diagnosis and medications, natural or other, there still has to be an exploration of healing for this person," he says. "We might have conditioned immune-suppressant responses built into our attitudes, beliefs, the way we live our life, the way we think, and the way we eat. An illness cannot be fixed from the outside; there is no magic bullet for chronic fatigue syndrome.

"People heal themselves by engaging in a self-healing process, by looking at their life and its meaning. It may seem rather complicated, but it is not. It is based on the knowledge that we do not get sick overnight. The condition may manifest suddenly in certain symptoms, but it took years and years to arrive. And it was not from one virus, not just from Epstein-Barr or herpes or parasites, low blood sugar, or electromagnetic pulsations. It was a combination of all of them.

"What is needed in treating chronic fatigue syndrome or AIDS and similar problems is a new approach. We should be looking not for the quick fix or what will work for everybody but for an approach that is individualized and holistic and empowers the patient to get involved in the cure and gives that patient belief and hope that healing is possible.

"There are two points in my treatment that I've been told by patients have helped them most: that I have given them hope and belief that healing is possible and that I have shown them that there are things they could do to help themselves. I don't heal anybody. Doctors don't heal anybody. They support people as they heal themselves."

Research Update

An increasing body of evidence is showing the benefits of natural modalities to overall health and well-being. Following is a sample of recent peer-reviewed scientific studies on chronic fatigue syndrome.

A 2014 report in *Panminerva Medicine* determined that a proprietary form of French oak wood extract administered to people with chronic fatigue syndrome in supplements of 200 mg/day for at least six months yielded notable improvements in mood with no side effects. Chinese researchers reported in a 2015 issue of *Evidence-Based Complementary and Alternative Medicine* that Cistanches Herba and Schisandrae Fructus may be useful for the treatment of CFS with Yang deficiency. The astringent and immunomodulatory actions of the latter may also be beneficial to CFS patients with Yin deficient symptoms such as increased sweating, dry mouth, and immune dysfunction.

Chapter 27

Dementia

Dementia (from the Latin for "irrationality") describes a group of symptoms that are caused by changes in the way the brain functions. Senile dementia refers to the onset of these symptoms in older people. Dementia can strike anyone at any age. However, the most common conditions with dementia as a symptom include Alzheimer's disease and vascular disease, both of which are specific to older individuals.

Symptoms

People with senile dementia have impaired memory as well as changes in other areas of cognition, such as language, vision, and abstract thinking, which prevent them from functioning properly on a daily basis. The signs and symptoms occur primarily in the absence of delirium and may be associated with an organic cause. The classic indicators of dementia are short-term memory loss, inability to think through problems or to finish complex tasks, difficulty concentrating, confusion, and abnormal behavior. While some types of dementia, such as that caused by Alzheimer's disease, cause a steady and progressive decline in patients, other types of dementia can be prevented, treated, or reversed by addressing the underlying conditions. Reactions to medications, emotional stress, metabolic imbalances, problems in optical or auditory processing, nutritional deficiencies, hormone imbalances, diabetes, AIDS, Huntington's disease, head trauma, brain tumors, or inflammation or infection can all trigger symptoms of dementia. (See chapter 19 for a full discussion of Alzheimer's disease, including diagnosis and natural therapies.)

By providing an optimal environment for brain health, and through a healthful lifestyle, attention to nutrition, and proper supplementation, you can preserve your mental abilities as you age.

Types of Dementia

Vascular dementia is the second most common type of dementia after that caused by Alzheimer's disease. Vascular problems in the brain or body are the main causes. In general, vascular dementia occurs suddenly, frequently after a stroke. It usually does not progress steadily, however, like Alzheimer's-related dementia. The patient may have long periods of stability or even improvement, but quickly develops new symptoms if more strokes occur.

Lewy body dementia (LBD) resembles Alzheimer's disease, but the abnormal brain cells, called cortical Lewy bodies, that are characteristic of this disease are found in the cortex and substantia nigra regions of the brain. Lewy body disease produces symptoms similar to Alzheimer's but may progress more rapidly.

Pick's disease affects the frontal and temporal lobes of the brain and is some-times referred to as frontotemporal dementia (FTD). This illness is also similar in symptoms to Alzheimer's and generally affects individuals between ages forty and sixty. It is characterized by a gradual loss of social skills and personality alteration, as well as damage to the memory and language functions. Pick's disease is characterized in the brain by swollen neurons.

Some elderly people may suffer anxiety and fear that their mental abilities and memory are declining. These feelings may trigger a severe depression called pseudodementia. Cognitive changes, memory loss, and slowed motor movements are typical of this condition. Pseudodementia may also trigger other symptoms, like those of senile dementia, including apathy, inability to answer simple questions correctly, poor eye contact, or little spontaneous movement. Treatment of the underlying depression will cause the dementia-like symptoms to disappear.

Natural Therapies

Lifestyle changes, environmental changes, exercise, memory boosters, weight management, and coping strategies can help prevent the onset of dementia or slow the progression of symptoms. In addition, certain foods, vitamins, minerals, and herbs are important. A full discussion of natural therapies for dementia is provided in chapter 19.

Gary Null's Protocol for Senile Dementia

The following chart summarizes the supplements I recommend adding to the protocol for overall brain health from chapter 16. In some cases, I recommend increasing the dose of a particular vitamin or supplement to specifically impact senile dementia. In these cases, you should increase the daily dosage from chapter 16 to the level recommended for this specific condition.

This protocol is designed for individuals who suffer from, or are specifically concerned about, senile dementia. If you are concerned about additional conditions discussed in other chapters, consult with a health professional about how you can safely impact multiple conditions.

If you are taking medications, whether prescription or over-the-counter, or have any food restrictions, consult with your doctor before beginning any supplement program. Your health care provider should always be up-to-date on all vitamins, supplements, and herbal or homeopathic remedies you are taking. Supplement overdoses are rare, but possible, and certain combinations may affect individuals adversely.

SUPPLEMENT	DOSAGE	CAUTIONS
acetyl-L-carnitine (ACL)	Increase daily dosage from 2,000 mg to 3,000 mg, taken in three equal doses. Do not exceed a daily supplement of 3,000 mg.	
calcium	1,000 mg daily, in four equal doses after meals and at bedtime	
intravenous vitamin B-complex	Discuss with your health care provider whether you might benefit from injected vitamin B.	
L-glutamine	500 mg, taken three times daily	

magnesium	500–1,000 mg, in two equal doses	May take up to six weeks for for effects to be felt.
Potassium	300 mg daily	Do not take potassium supplements if you are taking medication for high blood pressure or heart disease or if you have a kidney disorder. Consuming-foods rich in potassium is okay. Do not exceed a supplementary dose of 500 mg daily without consulting your doctor.
N-acetylcysteine (NAC)	500 mg, three times daily	Daily supplementation increases urinary output of copper. If supplementing with NAC for an extended period, add 2 mg of copper and 30 mg of zinc to your daily supplement regimen.
phosphatidylserine (PS)	Increase daily dosage from 300 mg to 400 mg	Do not exceed a daily supplement of 40 mg.
S-adenosylmethionine (SAMe)	Dosage range of 400–1,600 mg	Raise the dose gradually from 200 mg twice a day to 400 mg twice a day, to 400 mg three times a day, to 400 mg four times

		a day, over a period of twenty days.
vitamin C	Increase daily dosage from 500–1,000 mg to 3,000 mg	
vitamin E	400 IU twice daily	Vitamin E may cause increased risk of bleeding and may have adverse interactions with other medications. Consult with your doctor before beginning high-dose supplementation with vitamin E.
zinc	Up to 30 mg daily	Large doses (50 mg or more) can interfere with the body's absorption of essential minerals, impair blood cell function, and depress the immune system.

Research Update

An increasing body of evidence is showing the benefits of natural modalities to overall health and well-being. Following is a sample of recent peer-reviewed scientific studies on dementia.

A 2013 report in the Swiss journal *Revue Medicale Suisse* concluded that lifestyle factors such as nutrition and physical exercise are the cornerstones for dementia prevention because no efficient pharmacological treatments exist. In 2011, a study published in the *Journal of Traditional Chinese Medicine* found that directional ability, living ability, and short-term memory were significantly enhanced after treatment with Chinese medicine plus rehabilitation or acupuncture. A 2011 report in *Phytotherapy Research* described the herbal extracts and compounds that have been shown to reverse or halt neurodegeneration when tested against known pathogenic markers related to dementia, including Panax ginseng, Polygala tenuifolia, Acorus gramineus, and Huperzia serrate. A systematic literature search of all randomized placebo-controlled clinical trials of Ginkgo biloba led researchers to report in *Pharmacopsychiatry* (2010) that the extract was effective on cognitive symptoms of dementia with a treatment period of approximately six months.

Chapter 28

Depression

Depression is a major health problem that can leave an otherwise healthy woman unable to cope with the even the simplest of everyday situations. It affects nearly 10 percent of Americans, including twice as many women as men. This does not include the many individuals who function normally for the most part despite frequently finding themselves in low moods. Two-thirds of those who suffer from true depression are never treated and live their lives in misery without being recognized as sufferers of a mental illness. The American Psychiatric Association estimates that 80 percent of depressed people will recover with appropriate diagnosis and treatment.

Types of Depression

Several types of clinical depression have been identified:

MAJOR DEPRESSION interferes with normal, everyday life. It is characterized by sleep disturbances, agitation, appetite and weight changes, feelings of guilt and worthlessness, and an inability to work and concentrate. Suicidal thoughts may occur. These symptoms may last several months or more. The National Institute of Mental Health reported that in 2012, about 16 million adults had at least one major depressive episode in the past year.

DYSTHYMIA is milder than major depression, but it lasts longer. It prevents people from functioning at their full capacity. Some people with dysthymia also have major depressive episodes.

BIPOLAR DISORDER or MANIC DEPRESSION, which affects about 1 percent of Americans who are depressed, manifests as serious cycles of depression and mania. In the depressed phase, the person may be sluggish, sad, hopeless, and withdrawn. In the manic phase, the person swings to the opposite extreme: hyperactive, energetic, impatient, easily distracted, and too "busy" to sleep. Most often the changes are gradual, but some people, known as "rapid cyclers," may change moods several times a day. Bipolar disorder is usually chronic and generally begins in the teenage and young adult years.

Causes

BIOCHEMICAL FACTORS

For the past four decades, psychiatry has been aware that certain biochemical changes that take place in the brain can both influence and reflect fluctuations in mood. A change in the delicate biochemistry of the brain is capable of governing how a person feels at any given moment. A deficiency in any of the chemicals responsible for maintaining "good moods" may lead to depression, just as a psychologically stressing factor in a person's life may manifest itself in the body by altering the sensitive chemical balance in the brain, also causing depression or low moods.

While psychiatry has recognized this mind-body connection in general terms, it is only in the last twenty years or so that it has actually isolated some of the specific brain chemicals involved. Especially important among these chemicals are substances called neurotransmitters, which are released at nerve endings in the brain and allow messages to be relayed throughout the rest of the brain and the body. Perhaps the most commonly known neurotransmitters are the endorphins. They are responsible for pain relief within the body and are thought to be responsible for the "high" that runners experience after exercise.

Mood swings can be traced to a similar mind-body relationship. Scientists have found that a large number of depressed people have significant deficiencies of the neurotransmitters norepinephrine and serotonin. These neurotransmitters belong to a chemical group called the amines, which are responsible for the control of emotions, sleep, pain, and involuntary bodily functions such as digestion. Almost 90 percent of these amines are found deep in the brain; because of their importance, the normally functioning body has developed a recycling system, called reuptake, by which the nerve cell takes back 85 percent of a neurotransmitter for future use once the chemical reaction has been completed. Only the remaining 15 percent is destroyed by enzymes.

The metabolism of the neurotransmitters is intricate, and deficiencies can occur for many reasons. Dr. Priscilla Slagle, a board-certified orthomolecular psychiatrist who practices in Southern California, states that age or genetics may cause one person to use up amines more rapidly than someone else. She also points out that a defective receiving cell or reuptake mechanism, or a deficiency of the amino acids, vitamins, and minerals that make up amines may be the culprit here. The nutrient deficiencies involved may result from excessive intake of caffeine, sugar, alcohol, or tobacco. Sugar and coffee can destroy the B vitamins and the minerals magnesium and iron, all of which figure significantly in neurotransmitter formation. Alcohol and tobacco also deplete almost all the B vitamins, vitamin C, zinc, magnesium, manganese, and tyrosine. These nutrients are essential to maintaining a good mood.

STRESS

Stress is another factor that can contribute to depression. Most people tend to associate depression with what are called major stressors, such as the loss of a loved one, being fired from a job, or another circumstance that upsets one's life in a significant way. However, even the stress associated with everyday living can directly deplete the vitamins, minerals, and amino acids that are so important in maintaining a good mood.

Dr. Slagle explains, "We have found very high levels of the hormone cortisol, which is secreted by the adrenal glands, in severely depressed patients. Indeed, scientists have devised a test that measures the levels of this hormone in the body to determine the degree of depression. When people are depressed and highly stressed, their adrenal glands may secrete higher levels of cortisol, triggering certain enzymes in the body that destroy tyrosine and tryptophan. One would think that under extreme stress the body would compensate for this breakdown by facilitating the survival of these important amino acids. Instead, for whatever reason, these amino acids are used up. I believe that high cortisol levels induce depression in certain people."

SIDE EFFECTS OF MEDICATIONS

Dr. Slagle also points out that depression is a common side effect of many prescription medications. The list of medications that can cause depression is quite extensive; it includes antibiotics, antiarthritis pills, antihistamines, blood pressure medication, birth control pills, tranquilizers, and even aspirin. When people are given these medications, they are often not warned that they may experience depression as a side effect. Most orthomolecular psychiatrists believe that drugs for which the Physician's Desk Reference (PDR) lists depression as a side effect should include a nutritional program with the prescription in order to replenish the vitamins and amino acids that may be depleted by the medication.

ENVIRONMENTAL FACTORS

It is common for depressed people to have a family history of depression. In addition to the genetic factor, such family histories may also be due to common environmental factors, shared experiences in depressed families, and poor eating habits that are passed on from one generation to the next.

Environmental factors may play multiple roles as causes of depression. For example, being raised in a family in which one or more people are depressed may often be associated with poor nutrition. As the late Dr. William J. Goldwag reminded us, "Just being exposed to depressed people can be an influence, since children learn how to behave by imitation. Also, family members are eating the same food, and if, for instance, the mother is depressed and is cooking for and serving her family, that food is apt to be sparse in nutrients since she is interested in just getting the meal over with and has difficulty finding enough energy to prepare it."

The children of depressed parents may be abused physically or verbally. As a way of handling abuse, a child may withdraw and become depressed and inactive as a defense against harsh treatment from the parent.

Dr. Doris Rapp, a board-certified pediatric allergist and specialist in environmental medicine, adds that mood disorders often lead to battering of family members and intimates: "Husbands batter wives, wives batter husbands, they both batter the children, and boyfriends batter their girlfriends. Mother battering, I might add, is very common. Many of the children I treat beat, kick, bruise, bite, and pinch their mothers. When some individuals have typical allergies and environmental illness, if they have a mood problem, they can become nasty and irritable and angry. All I ask is, 'What did you eat, touch, and smell?'

"To help find the cause, I try to discover whether the change in behavior occurs inside or outside, after eating, or after smelling a chemical. It might be a food, dust, mold, pollens, or chemicals, which affect not only the brain as a whole but also discrete areas of the brain. As a result, the allergen or food or chemical exposure may make you tired or, if it affects the frontal lobes, make you behave in an inappropriate way. It could affect the speech center of the brain so that you speak too rapidly or unclearly, or stutter, or don't speak intelligently. It's just potluck as to what area of the brain or body will be affected when you are exposed to something to which you are allergic."

MAGNESIUM DEFICIENCY

According to Dr. Lendon Smith, a specialist in nutrition-based therapies and the author of many books on that topic, including *Feed Your Body Right: Understanding Your Individual Body Chemistry for Proper Nutrition Without Guesswork*, craving chocolate may also be a sign of depression. It usually means that people need magnesium, because there's magnesium in chocolate.

"I often had the delightful experience of giving an intravenous mixture of vitamin C, calcium, magnesium, and B vitamins," Dr. Smith says. "Usually it has more magnesium than calcium. Afterward I asked patients whether they would like some chocolate and they told me they didn't need it. It really is connected."

Dr. Smith explains that once food has been processed, magnesium is one of the first minerals to disappear. "Magnesium is also one of the first minerals to leave the body when there is stress, which accounts for how many women behave a day or so before their periods. They feel stressed because they're losing their magnesium.

"We need to supply magnesium to these people. We can determine who needs it by a blood test and by the sense of smell. If people smell a bottle of pure magnesium salt—magnesium chloride is a good one—and it smells good or if there's no smell, then the person needs it. The blood test we usually use is the 24-chem. screen, the standard blood test.

"Many symptoms of depression, hyperactivity, headaches, loss of weight, and other conditions are related to genetic tendencies. If there is a tendency to be depressed in the family, a magnesium deficiency will allow that tendency to show up. If there's alcoholism, diabetes, or obesity in the family, low magnesium may allow those things to show up in a person. There are reasons for all these things, and nutrition is basic. These patients don't have an antidepressant pill deficiency; they usually have a magnesium deficiency."

TOBACCO

The late orthomolecular psychiatrist Dr. Abram Hoffer told the story of a classic case of a misdiagnosis corrected, enabling one man to start anew after his life had seemingly been ruined. "A high school teacher and principal about forty-five years old developed a severe depression. In fact, I believe he was misdiagnosed as a schizophrenic. He exhibited what we call a straightforward, deep-seated, endogenous depression. He was in a mental hospital for about a year or two and was then discharged. He was so depressed that no one could live with him. His wife divorced him and eventually he was living with his aunt, who looked after him as if he were a child. As a last resort, he was referred to me.

"When he came to see me, which was many years ago, I had just started looking into the question of allergies. At that time, I wasn't very familiar with food allergies, but I thought he was a very interesting case and I said to myself, 'He is a classic case of a depression, maybe schizophrenic. He'd be the last person in the world who would respond to this anti-allergy approach.' At that time I was using—and I still do—a four-day water fast. This is a way of determining whether or not these allergies are present. He agreed that he would do the fast, which also involved refraining from any smoking or consuming of alcohol; he had to drink about eight glasses of water a day and nothing else. His aunt said she would help make sure he complied. When he came back to see me two weeks later, he and his aunt explained that at the end of the four-day fast, he was normal. All the depression was gone.

"This man then began to get tested for food allergies, and he found that not a single food made him sick. But now he began to smoke again. Within a day after he resumed smoking, he was back in his deep depression. The ironic thing was that he had a brother who was a tobacco company executive, who kept sending him free cartons of cigarettes. When we made the connection to his cigarette smoking, he stopped smoking. Thirty days later, after he had been depressed for four years and hadn't been able to work, he was back in school teaching. I remember this clearly because the insurance company that was paying his monthly pension was so astounded at this dramatic response that it sent one of its agents to see me, to find out what the magic wand was that I had waved to get this patient off their rolls. This is a classic case of an allergy to tobacco that was causing this man's depression."

Clinical Experience

DIAGNOSIS

Traditional psychiatrists diagnose depression according to the criteria set forth in the DSM-V (Diagnostic and Statistical Manual of Mental Disorders, 5th edition), which essentially defines major depression as a condition that includes at least five of the following symptoms during the same two-week period nearly every day, with at least one symptom either depressed mood or loss of interest or pleasure.

1. Depressed mood
2. Markedly diminished interest or pleasure in all or almost all activities
3. Significant weight loss or gain (when not dieting)
4. Insomnia (a constant inability to sleep) or hypersomnia
5. Psychomotor agitation (a hyperanxious state) or retardation
6. Fatigue or loss of energy
7. Feelings of worthlessness or excessive or inappropriate guilt
8. Diminished ability to think or concentrate or indecisiveness
9. Recurrent thoughts of death

While orthomolecular psychiatrists may use this definition as a starting point, they do not confine the diagnosis to these criteria. Orthomolecular psychiatry views depression or any other illness as a unique and individual condition. While there may be certain guidelines, such as those set forth in the DSM-V, a diagnosis that rigidly adheres to these criteria can arrive at a wrong conclusion either by missing the diagnosis altogether, because the person's symptoms are not those normally associated with depression, or by falsely diagnosing a person as being depressed simply because he or she has the textbook symptoms.

Often a depressed patient is not aware of the condition, especially when it is complicated by associated physical symptoms. If you suffered from chronic back pain, indigestion, or neck stiffness, would you immediately think that you might be manifesting symptoms of depression? Probably not. You might go to several doctors in search of relief, and there would be a very good chance that none of them would ever consider depression as the root of your problem. Even if someone were to ask whether you were depressed, you might quickly protest if, as Dr. Priscilla Slagle puts it, you "have 'somatized,' that is, put [your] emotional feelings into the body, thereby inducing bodily symptoms."

Sometimes a patient may develop responses to medication that are misinterpreted as purely physical. "For example," Dr. Slagle says, "an acquaintance of mine who lost her daughter through death a year ago became so anxious that her doctor started her on tranquilizers. Although she was on tranquilizers for six months, she got worse and worse. When I visited her, it was readily apparent to me that she had severe depression. It was difficult to convince her of this because she could relate only to the anxiety and the insomnia she was having. I started her on a nutrient program, and she improved dramatically in two to three weeks. Of course, I tapered her off the tranquilizers, because if they are stopped abruptly, one can have withdrawal symptoms that can aggravate the anxiety."

TRADITIONAL TREATMENTS

Orthodox treatments for depression include counseling, psychotherapy, and electroshock therapy. However, when a traditional psychiatrist arrives at a diagnosis of depression, more likely than not the next step will be to put the patient on antidepressant medication. Some of the most common of these medications are the selective serotonin reuptake inhibitors (SSRIs) such as Prozac (fluoxetine), Zoloft (sertraline), Paxil (paroxetine), and Luvox (fluvoxamine). They are all designed to increase the concentration of the neurotransmitter serotonin, which is not necessarily a good thing. In fact, some neurologists and psychiatrists believe that an excess of serotonin can cause mania or hyperactivity. Other types of antidepressants include the older tricyclics, monoamine oxidase inhibitors, and newer inhibitors that act on the brain chemicals norepinephrine and dopamine.

For bipolar disorder, lithium, Depakote (divalproex), and Tegretol (carbamazepine) are used to stabilize moods. If the mania is severe, antipsychotic drugs such as Risperdal (risperidone) may be prescribed. In the depressive phase Wellbutrin (bupropion) and the SSRIs are often used. Some patients receive monoamine oxidase inhibitors or tricyclic antidepressants.

Although the manufacturers claim that there is no evidence of addiction to most of these drugs, they are not without side effects. The Physician's Desk Reference (PDR) entry for the monamine oxidase inhibitor Elavil (amitriptyline), for instance, mentions many contraindications, warnings, precautions, and adverse reactions, including severe convulsions and possibly death if this drug is used improperly with other drugs, complications in patients with impaired liver function, hypertension, stroke, disorientation, delusions, hallucinations, excitement, tremors, seizures, blurred vision, dizziness, fatigue, baldness, and elevation and lowering of blood sugar levels.

Because suicidal tendencies are a common characteristic of depression, perhaps one of the most serious problems associated with antidepressants is the potential for drug overdose. The potential for suicide caused by the very medication prescribed to prevent it is further enhanced by the synergistic interaction of antidepressants with alcohol, barbiturates, and other central nervous system depressants. A glance through the PDR indicates that the quantity and magnitude of the dangers associated with Elavil are equally present with the other antidepressants.

The dangers and abuses of these drugs have provoked public outcry in recent years. This has come in the form of research studies, newspaper articles, legal actions, and congressional investigations. There is increasing concern about the repression of information about the side effects of commonly prescribed drugs. Among the actions have been a 2004 lawsuit against the makers of Paxil for concealing information about the antidepressant's safety and efficacy in children, and a 2006 study published in the *New England Journal of Medicine*, which determined that women taking SSRIs during the second half of pregnancy were more likely to deliver children with birth defects. In addition, there is the FDA's 2005 requirement for drug companies to add black box warnings to antidepressant labels about the risk of suicidal thinking and behavior in children and adolescents, as well as its 2007 extension of that warning to young adults. The number one cause of death in ten- to fourteen-year-old boys in the United States is suicide. Many psychiatrists and health care professionals believe these suicides are directly related to the high incidence of these same teenagers being on SSRIs. In April of 2016, an English study showed that most depression does as well with a placebo sugar pill as with any drug.

Alternative Therapies

DIET AND NUTRITION
It is surprising how often diet and nutrition are factors in depression and how effective enhanced or improved nutrition can be in helping someone suffering from depression to improve her mood. According to the late Dr. William J. Goldwag, "Often the quality of the diet suffers in depressed people. If the depression is

profound, the individual doesn't even feel like eating. Depressed people who live alone or who are major providers or cooks in the home may not feel like preparing meals or even shopping. They're apt to restrict their nutrition to fast food or anything just to get eating over with." In many cases, weight loss is a symptom of severe depression. In others, there is substantial weight gain.

Dr. Goldwag noted that significant weight loss is likely to bring about "marked deprivation of the essential nutrients, including the amino acids needed to manufacture the proper proteins, as well as a deficiency in many vitamins and minerals. That in itself can aggravate the depression."

Dr. Goldwag suggested straightforward solutions to at least some of the challenges associated with depression. "There are some simple ways to prepare food in advance so that the food has to be prepared less often. I recommend preparing a raw salad once a week. Certain fresh vegetables keep well for quite a while in a refrigerator. There is a whole variety to choose from: carrots, celery, radishes, cauliflower, broccoli, peppers, red cabbage, green onions, snow peas, string beans. They can all be cut up and mixed together. They can be stored in a plastic bag or sealed container. When mealtime comes, a person can take a handful of these vegetables and then perhaps add some other ones that don't keep as well, such as tomatoes and sprouts. You then have a fresh salad that is already prepared with a lot of important nutrients. This is just one way of having food prepared in advance. It's good for people who are depressed and don't have the energy to make a whole meal."

Dr. Goldwag believed that the B-complex vitamins are especially important. "One of the major groups of vitamins to incorporate is the B-complex family. Years and years ago, when people suffered from severe vitamin deficiencies, some of the resultant diseases, such as pellagra, were characterized by accompanying psychotic reactions. That is, the thinking process was the most obvious one to be affected by the vitamin deficiency. Simply providing the proper vitamin, in this case vitamin B_3, or niacin, was the treatment. It cleared up the psychosis.

"There's no doubt that brain function is very dependent on nutrients such niacin and others, because when they're absent there is apt to be some very disturbed thinking. Depression is one of the symptoms that can occur with this."

All of the B-complex vitamins are important, but niacin is especially so. As Dr. Goldwag explained, "Niacin is often used in much higher doses than the others to accomplish some of these changes. Niacin is a ubiquitous vitamin. It is being used to improve cholesterol levels, to increase the good cholesterol and reduce the bad. The doses being used are much greater than those used to simply overcome a deficiency."

At the same time, there are plenty of foods that should be avoided. Fast foods can affect mental symptoms by causing blood sugar abnormalities. Women who have tendencies toward hypoglycemia, or low blood sugar, should avoid eating too many simple carbohydrates, such as candy bars, which are converted very rapidly to sugar in the blood. As Dr. Goldwag said, "Simple carbohydrate foods temporarily raise the blood sugar, but then they drop it to a very low level several hours later, resulting in depression. This encourages the individual to repeat the cycle of taking sugar or some simple carbohydrate that's converted to sugar in order to feel that high again. This constant seesaw from a high to a low mood can account for many episodes of depression in individuals."

Both alcoholics and chronic dieters often have depressive tendencies. Alcoholics often suffer from symptoms of low mood. Although alcohol may appear at first as a stimulant and mood enhancer, it is in fact a depressant and substantially decreases the ability of the body to extract nutrients from the food we eat. Dieters tend to eat very few B-complex-containing foods, and they often suffer from depression as well.

AMINO ACIDS: TYROSINE AND TRYPTOPHAN

A leading authority on the treatment of depression with amino acids and nutritional therapy, Dr. Priscilla Slagle became interested in the treatment of mood disorders as a result of her own depression, which lasted for many years and did not respond to traditional psychoanalysis or psychotherapeutic treatment. Disinclined to use antidepressant medications because of the adverse reactions that so commonly accompany them, Dr. Slagle discovered that "there are natural food substances that will create the same end effects, that is, elevate mood in the same way without causing side effects or toxicity. I started myself on [a program using certain single amino acids to control mood] and achieved very dramatic results. Although I have had tremendous stress over the past ten years, particularly the past year, I have not had one day of a low mood. This has been a marvelous reprieve, since I have had, and therefore understand, the pain that low moods can create for many people."

In her book *The Way Up from Down*, Dr. Slagle outlines a safe and easily implemented program of treatment for depression using amino acids and other precursors required for the production of norepinephrine and serotonin. She is careful to emphasize that people should follow the program under the supervision of a physician. For those already on antidepressant medication, it is not advisable to stop abruptly because of the potential for withdrawal symptoms.

Dr. Slagle explains the basis of the program: "It consists of taking an amino acid called tyrosine, which in the presence of certain B-complex vitamins, minerals, and vitamin C will convert into norepinephrine in the brain. This neurotransmitter not only sustains positive moods but also helps our concentration, learning, memory, drive, ambition, motivation, and other equally important qualities. Additionally, it helps to regulate food and sexual appetite functions. Thus it is a very important chemical. The other amino acid used in the program is tryptophan, which forms serotonin in the brain if the requisite cofactors–the B vitamins, minerals, and vitamin C—are present. In addition to sustaining mood, tryptophan has other functions, such as controlling sleep and levels of aggression. People who are quite aggressive, irritable, or angry are often suffering from a marked deficiency in serotonin. Indeed, very low levels of serotonin have been found in the brain of suicide victims at autopsy.

"With these two amino acids, a good multivitamin-mineral preparation is taken to provide all the nutrients necessary to catalyze or promote the conversion of the amino acids into the neurotransmitters."

Dr. Slagle suggests the following dosages for the two amino acids: about 500 to 3,000 milligrams of tyrosine taken twice daily and about 500 to 2,000 milligrams of tryptophan. Public sale of tryptophan was banned by the Food and Drug Administration in 1990, but the supplement is now available through most compounding pharmacies. Dr. Slagle recommends that tyrosine be taken first thing in the morning on an empty stomach and then also sometime in the midmorning or midafternoon. Tryptophan, because of its sleep-inducing effects, is taken before bed. Any amino acids used therapeutically must be taken separately from other protein foods, because protein interferes with their utilization. Dr. Slagle also specifies that the amino acids be taken in capsules (tablets can pass through the body undigested) or in the "free form," a preparation in which the amino acids are ready for immediate absorption by the body.

OTHER SUPPLEMENTS

Other nutrients that can improve mental and emotional states are listed below:

OMEGA-3 FATTY ACIDS—A study from Harvard Medical School published in the *Archives of General Psychiatry* found that omega-3 (fish oil-type) fatty acids may be important mood stabilizers. Thirty people with bipolar disorder received either fish oil or a placebo (olive oil) along with their standard medications for four months. Sixty-five percent of those who got the omega-3s improved during this period, compared with only 19 percent of the placebo group. The omega-3s were associated with longer remissions and fewer symptoms.

SAME—S-adenosyl-l-methionine (SAMe), available commercially in Europe since 1975, more recently became available in the United States. The SAMe molecule is a methionine, an amino acid.

ACETYL L-CARNITINE—This nutrient crosses the blood-brain barrier and provides the brain with more energy. The energy it provides is a gentle, not jittery, type of energy, and it is especially important for older people, who tend to lose brain cells due to a lack of energy. Between 500 and 1,500 milligrams should be taken on an empty stomach.

LIQUID ZINC—Dr. Alexander Schauss, clinical psychologist, certified eating-disorder specialist, and author of *Anorexia & Bulimia*, describes his studies with liquid zinc: "In our eating-disorder studies, we used a multidimensional design and evaluated the affective or mood state of our patients for five years. One of the first things to improve in patients treated with liquid zinc was the degree of depression that they were experiencing based on psychometric instruments such as the Beck Depression Scale, the Profile of Mood Scales, and other indexes of depression. This suggests that we might consider using zinc as an antidepressant. There is a growing concern among many patients, and even therapists, that antidepressant drugs, such as Prozac, may not be safe, and we are looking at viable alternatives. We have discovered this antidepressive effect and have documented it in patients under blind conditions."

PHOSPHATIDYL SERINE—This nutrient is produced by the body but lessens with age. Taking 200 to 500 milligrams improves the ability of brain cell membranes to receive signals and improves their function. That, in turn, can elevate mood levels, help overcome winter depression, and enhance short-term memory.

HERBS

ST. JOHN'S WORT (HYPERICUM) is very popular in Europe, where double-blind, placebo-controlled studies exist to support its efficacy in alleviating depression. I recommend taking 450 milligrams once daily.

GINKGO BILOBA is an extract of the ginkgo plant, increases blood circulation to the brain and protects nerve cells, and has shown promise in impacting mild depression. One study revealed that elderly people suffering from depression who showed no improvement on antidepressant drugs did respond when a ginkgo biloba extract was added. Your daily supplement should be 300 milligrams in two divided doses.

CHINESE SCHISANDRA BERRY is an adaptogen that redirects energy, calms nerves, and can act as a mild sedative. I recommend taking 100 milligrams twice daily.

CALAMUS ROOT can be used externally by adding it to a bath to induce a state of tranquility. It should be avoided during pregnancy.

HOMEOPATHY

Homeopathic remedies can be quite effective in lifting depression. Dr. Gennaro Locurcio, a homeopathic physician, says that while money does not create happiness, the king of remedies for treating depression is gold, also known as Aurum metallicum. Here he describes this and other remedies for treating depression in women; men can benefit as well.

AURUM METALLICUM—Gold is for a perfectionist woman who has set high goals for herself but is unable to meet them. At first she will become irritable, a state that can last for several months. She feels as if she has lost the love of those around her and that it is her fault. This leads to feelings of frustration, accompanied by a strong sense of guilt, which may push her to suicide in extreme cases. Dr. Locurcio observes, "At first sight, this woman appears perfect and polished. When we start talking to her, we get the idea that there is an abnormal focus on career and achievement. Being a workaholic just covers up the emptiness inside."

ARSENICUM—This remedy is for depression accompanied by anxiety. The woman is restless day and night. She fears being alone and is constantly calling her friends. She wakes up at night and walks around the room thinking about her fears and anxieties. She is afraid of a poverty-filled future and of death. "Arsenicum is from arsenic," says Dr. Locurcio. "If we give that to a person, the person dies. But giving homeopathic arsenic to a person is completely safe and better than Xanax."

IGNATIA—This helps depression associated with grief. A woman has lost her child or her mother, or has been disappointed by a romantic relationship. The patient may exhibit physical characteristics such as a tic on the face, numbness, a lump in the throat, and sighing. "According to the homeopathic literature, if the patient says that she gets aggravated when she eats sweets and she improves by traveling, these are signs that Ignatia is indicated," notes Dr. Locurcio.

SEPIA—Sepia is a good example of how homeopathic healing uses substances that relate to a person's symptoms. According to Dr. Locurcio, "This remedy is made from a black mollusk that emits a black ink. Black is the ink from which the remedy is prepared, and black is the color the depressed woman sees around herself. She sees black in her future. This little sea creature, at some point in its life, will deposit about three hundred eggs, which are incredibly big for the size of this little animal, and then it will die. This is the housewife who has had a job and has also had to come home and prepare dinner for the husband and children. For years, she has given the best of her energy to her family and children. Now she is forty, forty-five, or fifty. The children are gone, and she feels as if her mission in life is over. She sees no purpose in her life anymore. She does not hate her husband, but feels indifferent toward him. She does not want to be touched sexually, and cries many times during the day without knowing why. Inside she feels despair and isolation. Physically, she has a dull, inexpressive face, and the muscles of the body have lost their tone. The woman has varicose veins; she is constipated. Sepia is a remedy for the exhausted housewife."

ACUPUNCTURE

Acupuncture frees blocked energy, and in so doing naturally lifts depression. Look at what one woman has to say about her experience: "When I was in my twenties, just after finishing college, I would go into a depression whenever I was about to get my period. It came on so suddenly that it was frightening. I went to see a doctor about it and was given a referral to an acupuncturist.

"After I was in treatment for six months, my practitioner and I sat down to talk about how I was feeling. I realized then that the depression was gone.

"That was twelve years ago. I've stayed in treatment, although not as regularly as when I first started. It's my primary form of health care. My eating habits and sleeping patterns have become totally regulated. I have been able to lose forty pounds and maintain my weight without dieting. I also quit smoking without ever trying. I never get sick anymore. I never get colds or flus. In general, I'm much more balanced.

"The whole experience of being brought into harmony keeps me from going to extremes. I don't work too hard, I don't play too hard, I don't rest too hard. I manage to stay pretty much in the center of my life. It's a huge improvement. I often wonder how people live without going through a treatment process like I did."

EXERCISE

Physical exercise is another key to lifting depression, especially when accompanied by a nutritious diet, meditation, and vitamin and mineral supplementation. According to the late Dr. William J. Goldwag, exercise is one of the most profound aids in the treatment of depression: "One of the major errors in the thinking of patients and therapists is the notion that in order to be active, you have to feel better. This is exactly contrary to our approach.

"We recommend that you do first, and the feeling comes later. In other words, you must do what you have to do regardless of how you feel. This aids in feeling better. You can't wait until you feel good to do something, because in depression that may take days, weeks, months, or even years. You want to accelerate the process."

Then Dr. Goldwag explained that people who exercise regularly will have days when they just don't feel like doing it. "That's the way depressed people feel about everything. They just don't feel like it. They don't have the energy, the motivation, the stimulation to do even the ordinary things. When it's severe, you may not even have the will or desire to get out of bed in the morning.

"The exercise may consist of very, very simple things, such as just getting out and walking, getting up and doing some simple movements, some mild calisthenics, any kind of physical movement that gets the body in action. For some people just getting out of bed and getting dressed is a big accomplishment. That may be the first step."

Exercise has many benefits. Dr. Goldwag added, "Even doing a little bit of exercise will make you feel more energized later on. Finishing an exercise routine, even one that's fatiguing, after a brief period of rest will give you a feeling of revitalization, energy, and a psychological feeling of accomplishment. It gives a feeling of 'I've done it. It's completed.'"

YOGA AND MEDITATION

Dr. Michele Galante, a complementary physician in Suffern, New York, overcame depression in adolescence by learning how to center energy with yoga and meditation. "When I was in my late teens, I went through a period of depression where my energy was low. My whole being was unhappy. My parents and others I loved thought I should try seeing a psychiatrist for a while. I went a few times, but that wasn't satisfying to me. I thought nutrition might help, so I started drinking raw vegetable juices and became a vegetarian. I started eating to detoxify myself and to get myself back to feeling stronger again.

"Then I got into meditation and kundalini yoga. I learned about energy centers and started to learn how inner energy flows through the system. I began to sense blockages and to identify emotions and limiting thoughts that were holding me back. Through practice, I was able to center energy into the emotional center in the chest and abdomen, where stabilizing rootedness can occur. That started to awaken inner energies and to strengthen me."

Dr. Galante says that depression is not limited to the mind. "The important thing is to not get too hung up in the head, where we have all these conflicts. Our center is the lower abdomen, where a baby grows in a woman. The Japanese call this the hara. In Zen we concentrate the mind and the whole being there. That's the hub of the wheel. The mind can be clearer when you do that, and you don't get hung up living in the realm of thought.

"Set aside ten to twenty minutes daily to quiet the mind, let tensions drain, open up, and resonate with the environment. Everyone does it in a different way. You can do it with meditation or biofeedback. You can do it with music, yoga, a hobby, it doesn't matter what. Anything that takes you to a creative, quiet place and allows you to recharge. Learn to take the time to express your inner needs.

"I like to ask my patients the question, 'Why do we have a physical body?' My answer is always that we exist as a physical entity to carry around our minds and our hearts, in a sense our spirits, so that we can fulfill ourselves. We can then learn and grow and do what we need to do in life. We are nothing without our emotions. Yet we neglect and suppress our feelings. We don't consider nourishing ourselves in a spiritual way. We need some sort of daily practice."

Dr. Galante adds, "We have a lot of outward pressures. We have rules made by corporations that are fulfilling needs for profits and ruining resources. There is a huge lack of wisdom across the board. The only thing that can make you happy is looking inward. Bring your mind and energies inside. Sometimes, when you start out, all you see is unhappiness and tension. But if you keep at it, sitting down, breathing quietly, not moving, and slowly bringing the mind inside, you will start to feel a sense of peace, relaxation, and buoyancy. That is recharging your battery. That is the most profound thing you can do to bring your energy up."

Gary Null's Depression Protocol

In chapter 16, you will find my Baseline Wellness Protocol. The following chart summarizes additional supplements I recommend for individuals who suffer from, or are specifically concerned about, depression. If you are concerned about other brain conditions discussed in other chapters, consult with a health professional about how you can safely impact multiple conditions. As always, if you are taking medication—whether prescription or over-the-counter—or have any food restrictions, consult with your doctor before beginning the supplement program. Your health care provider should always be up-to-date on all vitamins, supplements, and herbal or homeopathic remedies you are taking. Supplement overdoses are rare, but possible, and certain combinations may affect individuals adversely.

SUPPLEMENT	DOSAGE	CAUTIONS
5-HTP (5-hydroxytryptophan)	50–100 mg three times daily	Several months of treatment may be needed for maximum benefit. Nausea is the main side effect, but if it occurs, it usually dissipates within several days. Do not combine with prescription antidepressants. If

		you are taking prescription medication for depression, you should consult your doctor before taking 5-HTP. Excess levels of serotonin in the blood can be dangerous in case of coronary artery disease.
Adapton (Garum Armoricum)	4 capsules as directed daily for fifteen days; stop for one week, then continue with maintenance dose of 2 capsules daily.	
DHEA hormone	Follow doctor's directions for dosage.	Must be prescribed by your health practitioner. Individuals with hormone-related cancers should not take DHEA.
DLPA (DL-phenylalanine)	1,000–1,500 mg	Do not combine DLPA with prescription antidepressants or stimulants unless specifically directed to do so by your doctor. Do not take DLPA if you have high blood pressure, or are prone to panic attacks, are taking levodopa for treatment of Parkinson's disease, are pregnant, have melanoma, or have PKU (a rare,

		inherited metabolism disorder).
DMAE (dimethylaminoethanol)	Increase daily dosage from 150 mg to 250 mg.	May be overstimulating for some people. Headaches, muscle tension, and irritability may occur. Do not take if you have epilepsy, a history of convulsions, or bipolar disease. If you have kidney or liver disease, consult your doctor before taking this supplement.
Inositol	Increase daily dosage from 250 mg to 1,000 mg. Do not exceed a daily supplement of 1,500 mg. Take in two divided doses.	
Magnesium	320 mg (for women) 420 mg (for men)	May take six weeks or more for effect to be felt.
Potassium	500 mg	Do not take potassium supplements if you are taking medication for high blood pressure or heart disease, or if you have a kidney disorder. Consuming foods rich in potassium is okay. Do not exceed a supplementary dose of 3.5 g daily without consulting with your doctor.

Pregnenolone	Increase daily dosage from 10 mg to 20–	Individuals with hormone-related cancers should not take pregnenolone.
SAMe (S-adenosylmethionine)	Dosage range of 400–1,600 mg	Raise the dose gradually from 200 mg two times a day to 400 mg two times a day, to 400 mg three times a day, to 400 mg four times a day, over a period of twenty days.
Vitamin D	1,000–3,000 IU daily	Do not exceed 3,000 IU daily.

Research Update

An increasing body of evidence is showing the benefits of natural modalities to overall health and well-being. Following is a sample of recent peer-reviewed scientific studies on depression.

In a 2015 article in *Townsend Letter*, vitamin C, B complex vitamins, and omega-3 fatty acids were among the substances noted to have proven effectiveness against depression. A study published in 2011 in *Human Psychopharmacology* found notable reductions in personal strain, confusion and depressed/dejected mood following a twelve-week course of treatment that included B-complex vitamins plus vitamin C, vitamin E, calcium, magnesium, potassium, lecithin, choline bitartrate, inositol, Avena sativa, and Passiflora incarnate. In 2013, researchers reported in *ISRN Psychiatry* that thirty participants taking a B-complex supplement had significant improvement in depressive and anxiety symptoms.

A long-term study appearing in *Public Health Nutrition* in 2011 observed that people who commonly ate fast food and processed baked foods were 51 percent more likely to suffer from depression than those people who rarely or never indulged in these foods. These findings are consistent with a 2009 analysis by British researchers that produced a clear link between diet and depression. Published in the *British Journal of Psychiatry*, the study concluded that people who consumed a diet high in fried food, processed meat, refined grains, and sweets were 58 percent more likely to experience depression compared to those who consumed a diet rich in fruits, vegetables, and fish.

The millennia-old practice of tai chi was shown to effectively combat major depression in seniors in a recent study by scientists at UCLA. The findings, which were published in the *American Journal of Geriatric Psychiatry*, indicate that elderly patients diagnosed with the condition saw remarkable improvements after practicing a Westernized version of the Chinese martial art. The study compared the outcomes of two groups of seniors receiving standard depression treatment. One group engaged in two hours of tai chi classes weekly over the course of ten weeks, while the other group spent the same amount of time attending a health education class. Both groups realized notable improvements, but the tai chi group experienced significantly better improvements in memory, cognition, and quality of life and had reduced levels of depression.

Chapter 29

Diabetes

A September 15, 2014, report shows that 50 percent of all adults in America have pre-diabetes or full-blown diabetes. This is indicative of a pandemic situation.

According to the *National Diabetes Statistics Report, 2014*, the number of Americans with diabetes skyrocketed to 29 million in 2012, with women comprising more than half of the cases. Researchers estimate that the diabetes population and related costs are expected to double in the next twenty-five years. Study after study has confirmed what many of us in the alternative medicine community have known for years: moderate exercise and changes in diet can significantly reduce the risk of this serious disease.

Causes

Diabetes is closely associated with heart disease, and the incidence of both conditions increased when Americans began to change their dietary patterns. *The Saccharine Disease*, written more than four decades ago by Dr. T. L. Cleave, provided some observations that are relevant today. Among them, said the late Dr. Robert Atkins, is the law of twenty years, "which says that after you introduce refined carbohydrates into a culture, two illnesses emerge two decades later, diabetes and heart disease. We know that a Third World diet without refined carbohydrates leads to no heart disease and no diabetes. When one illness emerges, so does the other. Studies of this sort have linked diabetes with heart disease."

Under normal circumstances, insulin is released by the pancreas in response to elevated levels of sugar in the blood. It promotes the transport and entry of glucose to muscle cells and various tissues, thus lowering blood sugar levels. In a diabetic, part of the process is interrupted as a result of a deficiency in, resistance to, or insensitivity to insulin.

Insulin Deficiency

For many years, it was thought that diabetes was purely and simply a deficiency syndrome in which the body did not produce sufficient quantities of insulin for proper glucose metabolism and assimilation. More recently, it has been learned that many diabetics do produce enough insulin, but their cells do not take it in. The problem, then, is due to insulin insensitivity or resistance.

Insulin Insensitivity

Insulin enters cells at points known as receptor sites. When the receptor sites are plugged because of fat, cholesterol, inactivity, and obesity, insulin cannot enter. As a result, glucose stays in the blood and creates hyperglycemia, or high blood sugar. This excess sugar is diagnosed as diabetes. In such cases, there is no need to increase insulin production but rather a need to enhance insulin sensitivity. A person with diabetes needs to work at making his or her own insulin more efficient, and simply increasing the amount of insulin will not do that.

Insulin Resistance

Insulin resistance is a phenomenon that is closely related to insulin insensitivity. With insulin resistance, there is also a sufficient or even overabundant supply of insulin, but allergic responses prevent insulin from doing its job. Usually allergies to specific foods suppress the activity and efficiency of insulin. Different factors may be responsible for a disordered carbohydrate metabolism in different people. Wheat, for instance, may create symptoms of high blood sugar in one woman, whereas corn may affect another. Offending substances can be determined on an individual basis with food allergy tests.

Types of Diabetes

Type 1 diabetes is the most serious form of the disease. It used to be called juvenile diabetes, because for many years it was believed that it only occurred in the childhood or teenage years. This form of diabetes is characterized by a true insulin deficiency. It results when the pancreas is damaged from some exotic viral infection or even a highly toxic state. The disease may also be a genetic condition. In type 1 diabetes the beta cells in the pancreas that produce insulin are destroyed. Since type 1 diabetics have an insulin deficiency, they have to take insulin by injection daily, and generally for life.

Type 2 diabetes, also known as non-insulin-dependent or adult-onset diabetes, is more of an acquired disease. It is often precipitated by chronic excess weight from poor diet and/or lack of exercise. It may also be brought on by overconsumption of stressor foods or other allergens that are insulin resistors.

Type 2 diabetes accounts for some 90 percent of all diabetes cases in the United States. It occurs most frequently in adults over age 40, and more often in women than men. In type 2 diabetes, the beta cells in the pancreas still produce insulin, but for a variety of reasons there may be insufficient production or the body may not be adequately using the insulin that is produced. Thus this form of the disease is characterized by complications of insulin resistance and insulin sensitivity rather than, in most cases, a true deficiency of insulin.

Type 2 in children was practically unheard of until recently. Now, nearly 4,000 children are diagnosed every year. Research reported at the 2012 annual meeting of the American Diabetes Association showed that from 2001 to 2009, the incidence of type 2 diabetes among American children and teens rose by an alarming 21 percent.

Some nondiabetic women develop a type of diabetes called gestational diabetes during pregnancy, usually in the last trimester.

Symptoms

Often there are no symptoms present, especially in the beginning stages of type 2 diabetes. Obesity is sometimes a sign of a prediabetic state, especially when the excess weight is concentrated at the waistline and just above the waistline. Classic diabetic symptoms are more often experienced by type 1 diabetics and include frequent urination, especially at night, great thirst and hunger, fatigue, weight loss, irritability, and restlessness. Progressively, the eyes, kidneys, nervous system, and skin become affected. Infections and hardening of the arteries commonly develop. In type 1 diabetes, coma from a lack of insulin is a constant danger.

Clinical Experience

MEDICATIONS

Before the development of insulin in the 1920s, diabetic patients had a bleak prognosis. Sufferers saw the condition rapidly go from bad to worse as complications such as blindness, gout, and gangrene developed. Overall life span was drastically shortened.

Initially, insulin appeared to be a miraculous drug, and it probably was. The life span of diabetic children was extended from months to decades. Today, many of these children live normal, productive lives.

Insulin is still the primary therapy for type 1 diabetes. Type 1 diabetics generally take insulin at least once a day, frequently several times a day.

While some type 2 diabetics require injections of insulin, many are given oral hypoglycemic medications. Many type 2 diabetics incorrectly believe that these pills are simply a form of insulin, but that is not the case. None of the oral medications used to treat type 2 diabetes contain insulin. They are designed to help your body use the insulin that is in your pancreas more effectively, or to stimulate better insulin production. Consequently, oral medications can only be used by diabetics whose pancreas still makes some insulin. In addition, some type 2 diabetics can control their diabetes entirely through diet and exercise.

In recent years, a number of new drugs have been introduced to treat type 2 diabetes. Some of these drugs are being rushed through the approval process without adequate review of their safety. The popular drug Avandia has been linked to several side effects, including heart attacks, and its use was severely restricted by the Food and Drug Administration (FDA) in 2010. (The restrictions were lifted in 2013.) Actos has been linked to an increased risk of heart failure and bladder cancer. Rezulin, another diabetes drug, was pulled from the market in early 2000. Some 500,000 Americans had been using the medication, which was approved for use by the FDA in 1997. The FDA asked the manufacturer to withdraw Rezulin after it was linked to eighty-nine confirmed reports of liver failure, including sixty-one deaths.

COMPLICATIONS AND BLOOD SUGAR CONTROL

Although diabetes can cause a wide variety of complications, from kidney and eye problems to nerve damage, some can be reduced considerably by controlling blood sugar. For many years doctors assumed that diabetics whose blood glucose levels were as close to normal ranges as possible reduced their risk of serious complications. About twenty years ago, the Diabetes Control and Complications Trial (DCCT), one of the largest studies ever conducted, confirmed that diabetics in the intensive control group, with glycohumaglobin rates that averaged 7.1, reduced their risk of eye disease by 76 percent compared with the less aggressively managed group, with glycohumaglobin rates of 8.9 percent. Across the board, diabetics in the intensive control group had a 50 percent reduction in all serious diabetic complications. Although the trial was conducted only on type 1 diabetics, experts believe that the findings of the study apply to all diabetics.

DIETARY RECOMMENDATIONS

Eating the right foods can help maintain proper blood sugar levels, as well as helping to boost your immune system. In the past there was one standard diet prescribed for all people with diabetes. Now the American Diabetes Association recommends that people work with experts in diet and nutrition to individualize their plans.

Complex carbohydrates are not the problem they were once thought to be. Emphasis is now put on the total amount of carbohydrates in a meal, rather than the source. People with diabetes are frequently taught to count carbohydrates and to match medication requirements to carbohydrate intake. This is especially true for insulin-dependent cases.

Unlike simple sugars, complex carbohydrates are beneficial. Although both are broken down into glucose, the latter do not go directly into the bloodstream. While simple sugars immediately enter the blood, complex carbohydrates go through a long process of digestion and only very gradually release sugar into the blood. Therefore, they do not contribute to the high blood sugar levels, as do simple carbohydrates. Instead, they stabilize and improve health.

Fat and protein are carefully monitored. Overweight people are told to keep fat intake to no more than 20 to 25 percent of total calories. Large amounts of protein may be related to accelerated kidney damage. This is because protein must be immediately processed by the body; it cannot be stored. This puts a great stress on the nephron cells, which filter the body's toxins. Many people suffer from kidney deterioration as a result and must receive dialysis or a kidney transplant. Studies show that the elimination of meat from the diet is often enough to reverse kidney damage.

THE NATURAL APPROACH

Despite its severity, diabetes need not be as debilitating as it usually is. While there is currently no cure, there are ways of enhancing the body's natural defenses through nutrition, avoidance of allergy-producing substances, and exercise. A healthy lifestyle and alternative approaches to treatment can decrease the amount of insulin or oral medications needed by some people, although type 1 diabetics will need to continue taking insulin for life.

The goal of treatment can and should be to build up the body's ability to function as independently as possible. When changing to a more holistic approach it is important not to immediately discontinue any of your medications. Instead, a preventive-medicine physician should assist in the gradual transition. With a doctor's guidance, medication may be reduced or eliminated over time. Complete elimination, however, is not always possible.

While type 2 cases respond most dramatically, even people with type 1 diabetes may be able to reduce their insulin dependency. More important, they may alleviate many of the insidious complications that have come to be thought of as intrinsic to diabetes.

DIET

Years ago, Dean Ornish laid out a heart-right diet that was targeted at eliminating the foods that make one liable to develop heart disease. Since diabetes and heart disease are closely related, many physicians have recommended that people with diabetes follow this Ornish program. The central tenet of Ornish's diet is to cut down on dietary fats. For him, the best diet would be one that emphasizes high-fiber vegetables, eaten raw, steamed, baked, or stir-fried with little or no oil.

Other recommendations include chlorophyll drinks, lentils, peas, quinoa, steel-cut oatmeal, whole grain pasta, brown rice, soy, and fish. Bean pod tea tonifies the kidneys and adrenal glands.

People who have a true insulin disorder will not fare well on a high-carbohydrate diet. "It is important to know who needs carbohydrate restriction versus who needs fat restriction," the late Dr. Robert Atkins said. "To determine that, there are a variety of tests, including a cholesterol profile in which we look at the ratio between the triglycerides and the HDL [high-density lipoprotein]. When a person has a blood sugar disorder leading to a lipid disorder, the ratio is extremely high. To be really safe, the number should be approximately the same, or the

HDL should be higher than the triglycerides. It is perfectly appropriate to spend five or six weeks on one diet and then get all of your parameters checked again, and then spend five or six weeks on the other diet and get them checked again. In that way, you can make an intelligent decision."

EXERCISE

An exercise regimen is crucial for burning calories and normalizing metabolism, and is especially important for overweight adults, who are often inactive. Exercise also heightens the body's sensitivity to insulin. By lowering cholesterol, it lowers triglyceride levels in the blood, making cells more available for glucose assimilation. This is why the insulin requirements of diabetic athletes always drop while they're engaged in swimming, soccer, and other sports. Athletes also notice an increase in their insulin requirements when they cease doing their physical activities for an extended period of time.

Athletes are not the only ones who benefit from exercise. Ten to twenty minutes of light exercise after each meal helps reduce the amount of insulin necessary to keep blood sugar levels under control. A brisk walk gets the body's metabolism working a little faster so that food is more easily absorbed. That prevents blood sugar from rising too high.

An exception to the rule involves patients with diabetes and heart disease. In these cases, exercising after eating may precipitate an angina attack because of the transfer of blood from the intestines to the legs and other parts of the body.

ALLERGY TESTING

Testing for food allergies can determine which foods are responsible for insulin resistance. Clinical experience has shown that this approach to treatment is the most useful way to get to the root of adult-onset diabetes and reverse the condition. Patients can usually be weaned from insulin, since an insulin deficiency is not the cause of the problem. Eliminating allergy-producing foods may also foster weight loss. This occurs because people crave foods when they are allergic to them. When these foods are taken out of the diet, the desire for them eventually stops.

To determine whether a specific food is causing hyperglycemia, a doctor can monitor a patient's blood sugar before and after that food is eaten. Foods that raise the blood sugar cause allergic reactions and should be eliminated.

SUPPLEMENTS

In addition to diet and exercise, the following supplements may be helpful, among others: alpha-lipoic acid (ALA), chromium, zinc, omega-3 fatty acids, polyphenols, garlic, magnesium, ginseng, and vanadium. Enzymes useful in controlling insulin-dependent diabetes are digestive protylase, amylase, and lipase.

HERBS

Plants containing phytochemicals with antidiabetic properties include chicory, Indian snakeroot, thyme, safflower, Indian fig, dandelion, rice paper plant, jack bean, flax, barley, evening primrose, oats, and alfalfa. Plants containing phytochemicals with insulin-sparing properties include coconut and the common plantain. Also helpful may be prickly pear cactus, aloe vera, fenugreek, and bitter melon.

TOPICAL TREATMENT FOR DIABETIC ULCERS

Ulceration at various locations plagues many patients with diabetes and causes a condition that is often serious enough to warrant amputation. This tragedy may be averted with a simple solution. According to clinical studies, raw, unprocessed honey is an ideal dressing agent for almost every type of wound or ulcer. It sterilizes the ulcerated area, and often works even after antibiotics fail.

OTHER APPROACHES

Mucokehl (made from the fungus Mucor recemosus), which was originally developed in Germany, may actually reverse diabetic neuropathy. People using this remedy get feeling back in their extremities, and their eyesight improves. Many practitioners also recommend chelation therapy for reducing diabetic retinopathy and healing foot ulcers.

MONITORING AND PREVENTING DIABETES

People with diabetes and those who wish to prevent diabetes can do a great deal to monitor themselves. It's important to look for the presence of antibodies that attack some of the body to defend against an ingested allergen. This is easy to see if the symptoms are blatant, but not if they are subtle. The thing to look for is a general lowering of the body's immune response.

The best way to see this is to go five days without eating the food (or any of its relatives) you wish to test. If you want to test milk, abstain from cheese, ice cream, and all other dairy items or processed foods that contain milk as an ingredient. After five days, eat a meal consisting of just milk and eat generous amounts of it. Then tune in to your body's response. If you experience headaches, stomachaches, pulse rate changes, increased heartbeat or blood sugar, depression, lethargy, dizziness, or even delusions, you can see that your body has reacted negatively to this substance. In other words, you have an allergic response to it. You will have to back off from it. Leave it alone for twelve weeks initially. When it is reintroduced into the diet, it must be rotated with other foods. Eat it in modest amounts no more often than once every four days.

"Of course, there are a lot of good things about that four-day basis," says Dr. William Philpott, a prominent diabetes researcher and clinician. "You will eat thirty or forty kinds of foods instead of the half dozen you've been eating. This is a very wholesome thing. To have the necessary nutrition you will have a wide range of foods." It is a good idea to try introducing new foods into your diet, ones that you have never thought to eat. Try not to eat any foods more frequently than twice a week.

Dr. Philpott recommends that you invest in some diabetic equipment so that you can monitor your blood sugar an hour after each meal. "At least 90 percent is optimum," he says, "and 140 or beyond is high blood sugar. Before the next meal, test your blood sugar again to make sure it is at least 120 before starting your next meal. If it is not, wait and exercise. Get it down before your next meal. Monitor your pH from saliva; it should be 6.4. If it is below 6.4, you are having a reaction to the food. Measure your pulse; if it varies drastically, you are reacting to the food. Blood pressure is more significant. Physical symptoms, mental symptoms, and blood sugar are the most important. They are absolutely essential. It will take about thirty days to do this."

Gestational Diabetes

Out of every 100 pregnant women in the United States, three to eight develop gestational diabetes, usually in the last trimester. Gestational diabetes is diagnosed with an oral glucose tolerance test. In many cases this type of diabetes can be controlled with diet and exercise. Although gestational diabetes disappears after delivery, as many as 50 percent of women with gestational diabetes will develop diabetes later.

Dr. Susanna Reid, a naturopathic physician at the Center for Natural Medicine in Connecticut, says that diet and exercise are key to controlling gestational diabetes.

DIET

Dr. Reid advises women with gestational diabetes to learn how to eat on the low end of the glycemic index. The glycemic index was developed some thirty years ago by Dr. Sullivan, who gave people glucose and then measured the rise in blood sugar levels. He then established that level as 100 percent of the glycemic index. He repeated the experiment by giving people various foods and measuring how high their blood sugar would go just as he had with glucose, and then assigned each food a percentage.

Dr. Reid says that foods we don't normally associate with sugar may still be high on the glycemic index. "A baked potato and puffed rice are both 100 percent on the glycemic index, which means that they raise your blood sugar significantly. This is bad for your body; it goes into a state of alarm when your blood sugar rises so quickly and significantly, and it produces more insulin. Since the rate of rise is so rapid, the body tends to overproduce insulin, and people get what is called reactive hypoglycemia (low blood sugar). Then they have to eat sugar to get their blood sugars back up again. Therefore you need to eat foods low on the glycemic index to avoid either hypoglycemia or reactive hypoglycemia."

She explains that the position of some foods on the glycemic index may seem counterintuitive. These include fruits, nuts, and legumes. For example, peaches, plums, grapefruit, and cherries are between 20 and 29 percent on the glycemic index. But potatoes and even carrots and parsnips and rice are at the top level. She says, "When you eat foods that are high on the glycemic index, you need to have a healthy fat with them. Doing this seems to prevent the rapid rise in blood sugar. If you had a baked potato, for example, you'd want to have olive oil in it."

Foods you may think would be low on the glycemic index, such as vegetables, are often among the highest. "Peas are between 50 and 59 percent on the index and corn is between 60 and 69 percent. Yams are very high, but sweet potatoes are much lower on the index than yams. Brown rice and all the grains tend to be very high."

EXERCISE

Dr. Reid also tells her patients about the importance of exercise. By exercising regularly, we can often keep our blood sugar levels within the normal range. "When a person exercises, it improves insulin's ability to remove glucose from the blood and also decreases insulin resistance. If you exercise sixty minutes a day at 60 to 70 percent of the maximum heart rate, then usually after just one week of exercise you'll see an improvement in the glucose tolerance test. But be careful not to overdo it and cause your blood sugars to drop too low."

Dr. Reid warns that a woman should not attempt to become a world-class athlete while pregnant. "But she should continue and enhance her current exercise program. There are some things she needs to be careful about. She should not lie supine and attempt to lift weights, she shouldn't get too warm, she should maintain adequate hydration, and she probably shouldn't take up a new sport in which balance is a main requirement because she is having to adjust daily to changes in the shape of her body and her orientation in space. She wouldn't want to do anything where she might fall, such as inline skating at top speed."

Dr. Reid's favored exercises are running and walking. "Women need to feel free to move when they are pregnant. It is not a pathological state. They are not ill."

NUTRITIONAL SUPPLEMENTS

Dr. Reid cautions against using some herbal supplements during pregnancy. "Most of the herbs are contraindicated in pregnancy, so one has to be cautious in treating gestational diabetes. For example, traditional herbs we would use to treat non-insulin-dependent diabetes, which gestational diabetes usually is, are bitter melon (Mamordica charantia), fenugreek, elecampane (Inula helenium), and garlic and onion supplements. All those are contraindicated in a pregnant woman. Ginkgo and Jerusalem artichoke are not contraindicated, and in all of the research that I've done I can't find a contraindication for Gymnema sylvestre, which is an herb that seems to increase the pancreas's ability to produce insulin, which would be advantageous in patients with gestational diabetes."

Gary Null's Protocol for Diabetes

My baseline wellness protocol can be found in Chapter 16. The following chart summarizes additional supplements I recommend for individuals who suffer from, or are specifically concerned about, diabetes. If you are concerned about conditions discussed in other chapters, consult with a health professional about how you can safely impact multiple conditions. As always, if you are taking medication—whether prescription or over-the-counter—or have any food restrictions, consult with your doctor before beginning the supplement program. Your health care provider should always be up-to-date on all vitamins, supplements, and herbal or homeopathic remedies you are taking. Supplement overdoses are rare, but possible, and certain combinations may affect individuals adversely.

Supplement	Dose
Chromium picolinate	200 mcg 2–3x/day
Vitamin C	1,000 mg 5x/day
Biotin	500 mcg
Vitamin B6	100 mg
Vitamin B12	1,000 mcg
Vitamin E	400 mg gamma tocopherol 2x/day
Calcium citrate	1,000 mg
Magnesium citrate	1,000 mg
Potassium	200 mg
Manganese	15 mg
Zinc	30 mg
Selenium	200 mcg
Quercetin	1,000 mg 2x/day
EFAs	3,000 mg/day
GLA	500 mg 2x/day
L-Carnitine	500 mg 2x/day
Inositol	500 mg
L-Glutamine	follow directions
Vanadyl sulfate	follow directions
B Complex	50 mg
Garlic	1,000 mg 2x/day
Bitter melon	100 mg
Gymnema sylvestre	follow directions
Ginseng	100 mg
Aloe vera	3 tsp/day
Alpha lipoic acid	600 mg
Grape seed extract	200 mg 3x/day

NAC	500 mg 2x/day
Coenzyme Q 10	300 mg 3x/day
Turmeric	100 mg
Dandelion extract	follow directions
Evening primrose oil	1,000 mcg
Sea vegetable powder	follow directions
Maitake complex	follow directions
Proteolytic enzymes	follow directions
Fiber Complex	Your diet should have 30–50 g of fiber a day; if not, have 15 grams with a beverage at night
R-Lipoic acid	210–420 mg daily
Carnosine	500 mg 2x/day
DHEA	15–75 mg early in the day, followed by blood testing after 3–6 weeks to ensure optimal levels
EPA/DHA	1,400 mg EPA and 1000 mg DHA daily silymarin containing 900 mg silybum marianum standardized to 80 percent silymarin, 30 percent silibinin, and 4.5 percent isosilybin b
Green tea extract	725 mg decaffeinated green tea extract (minimum 93 percent polyphenols)
Ginkgo biloba	120 mg daily
Bilberry extract	100 mg daily
Cinnamon extract	125 mg Cinnamomum cassia standardized to .95 percent trimeric and tetrameric a-type polymers (1.2 mg) 3x/day
Black cumin seed oil	2 teaspoons daily

Research Update

An increasing body of evidence is showing the benefits of natural modalities to overall health and well-being. Following is a sample of recent peer-reviewed scientific studies relating to diabetes.

In the *Townsend Letter* (2014), Dr. Mona Morstein described numerous studies in which micronutrients and botanical agents, including zinc, cinnamon, chromium polynicotinate, *gymnema sylvestre*, berberine HCL, and resveratrol, were found to offer the best chances of meeting treatment goals in diabetic patients without the side effects of hypoglycemia from overmedication of glucose-lowering agents. A 2014 report in *Nutrition Journal* reviewed clinical trials of the effect of fenugreek on markers of glucose homeostasis. Significant effects on fasting and two hour glucose were found in studies that administered medium or high doses of seed from the plant in people with diabetes. According to a 2010 study published in *BMC Complementary and Alternative Medicine*, curcumin supplementation may improve diabetes-induced endothelial dysfunction associated with decreased vascular superoxide production and PKC inhibition. Another 2010 study, in the *Journal of Nutrition*, reported that dietary bilberry extract (BBE) given to type 2 diabetic mice significantly reduced the blood glucose concentration and enhanced insulin sensitivity.

Chapter 30

Digestive Disorders

According to 2012 data from the Centers for Disease Control and Prevention (CDC), digestive problems account for 51 million doctor's office and emergency room visits annually in the United States. In examining digestive disorders, one must realize that there are few special clinics where research and treatment focus exclusively on these disorders and that there are few particular pioneers in the field of digestion. One reason for this is that digestive disorders are not often clearly diagnosed as such. A determination may be made that a person has cancer, arthritis, or renal failure, for example, but not that the condition is related to a chronic digestive disorder that has gone undetected for a long time. While you may be undergoing extensive, costly, and perhaps toxic treatment for a diagnosed disease, it is possible that only the symptoms of your disease are being treated, not the underlying cause.

Furthermore, many people go through life with a chronic digestive problem and assume that it is a normal state of affairs. Any complications that result again are rarely understood as being connected to an underlying problem with the digestive mechanism. Some disturbances that obviously are related to digestion—diarrhea, constipation, and the like—are handled by taking over-the-counter drugs such as laxatives and antacids. Some people think they have a "weak" stomach or that these problems are just part of getting older, and so end up taking drugs habitually, unaware that they are likely exacerbating the real problem.

Causes

If any of the systems involved in digestion are faulty in any way, the efficiency of the absorptive process will diminish and the body will not be receiving the nutrients it needs.

Insufficient or suboptimal production of stomach acid, which is not an illness but a sluggish stomach, is the most common digestive problem, especially in people over forty. In the presence of low stomach acid, food digestion in the stomach is impaired and thus protein and minerals are not digested efficiently. Many people with this problem burp and belch after meals.

The pancreas is a gland that produces enzymes for digesting protein, carbohydrates, and fats. The enzymes neutralize the acidity of partially digested food (chyme). If the enzymes are inefficient, difficulties will result. Very often, when a patient complains of digestive problems two to three hours after eating, the pancreas is the culprit.

The liver produces bile, which is stored in the gallbladder and sent into the small intestine through the bile duct. This alkaline fluid is partly responsible for fat absorption, as it emulsifies or breaks down fats into smaller particles. The liver is a major workhorse of both digestion and the detoxification of the body, and it can be overtaxed by a poor diet or by any inefficiency in the digestive process. If production of stomach acid or pancreatic enzymes is sluggish, this sub-par functioning can be a major stressor on the liver.

The pancreatic enzymes described above come into play when partially digested food moves from the stomach to the duodenum, which is the first part of the small intestine. The digested food then moves farther down the small intestine into the jejunum, where food absorption takes place. The nutrients are then carried through the bloodstream to various parts of the body. A malfunction in this part of the process, or anything leading up to it, can impair nutrient absorption.

The ileocecal valve is located between the small and large intestines. Diarrhea and constipation are often associated with malfunctions of this valve. The valve's job is to open when the contents of the small intestines are ready to pass through, to let a certain amount through, and then to close. However, if the valve stays open too long, or is too tight or closed, problems can occur.

If the ileocecal valve remains in the open position it can enhance diarrhea, because everything is flushing through too quickly. Food passes through the digestive apparatus so rapidly that the absorptive process is impaired. In addition to the rapid transit due to the open valve, the movement of food may reverse, as the contents of the colon backflush. The colon is the "garbage disposal" area, whereas the small intestine is the "kitchen" area. Therefore, a backflush of waste material puts biochemical stress on the small intestine and irritates the liver as well.

In short, the waste material makes a mess in the kitchen. The material may be absorbed into the bloodstream, causing various toxic reactions.

If the ileocecal valve is too tight or too closed, this can cause constipation. The tight valve, by not facilitating the passage of the small intestine contents into the colon, retards the entire digestive flow, which leads to infrequent bowel movements, or constipation.

When the stomach acid and pancreatic enzyme systems do not work properly, undigested particles of food or actual pieces of food may reach the colon, also called the large intestine. This not only irritates the colon but also leads to flatulence because the undigested food will be fermented by the friendly and not-so-friendly bacteria residing in the colon.

Finally, the colon may be irritated throughout its entire length or in any of its anatomical parts: the ascending colon, the transverse colon, or the descending colon. Often, the most common pattern is that all three parts are out of balance. In this case, the patient should consider how she handles stress because the colon may be the organ in which various stress elements are manifesting themselves.

There has been found to be a high correlation between food intolerances or allergies and irritation in the descending colon (see below). It's always a good idea to keep a careful food diary to identify frequently eaten foods and those you may suspect are culprits in allergic reactions. Foods that commonly prompt allergic reactions include gluten foods (wheat, barley, oats, and rye), sugar, peanuts, citrus fruits, dairy products, soybeans, corn, and caffeine.

Irritation of the ascending colon alone means that its ecology is off balance. For example, there may be an overgrowth of yeast because the ascending colon becomes a fermentation factory of sorts when undigested food particles reach it. The unfriendly bacteria that live in the small and large intestines may be especially likely to overgrow if the production of stomach acid is so low that the digestive system becomes underacidified or excessively alkaline. A highly alkaline environment favors the growth of yeast, which may then exceed the usual niche it maintains within the ecological population of the colon.

Symptoms

Digestive system disorders can be placed into two main categories: those that are clearly and directly related to digestion, and those that are a step or two removed from the digestive process and therefore more difficult to connect with digestion.

Symptoms of disorders in the first category are more easily recognized. The most common include burping, belching, flatulence, a feeling of indigestion, undigested food in the stool, or a feeling of food "just sitting there." When such symptoms are present, it is relatively easy to connect the problem to some malfunction in the digestive process.

Problems that occur over time and are related to the long-term inefficient absorption of nutrients and/or an insufficiency of nutrients in the food to begin with are often not directly connected to digestive difficulties. Insufficient stomach acid production can result in malabsorption of calcium, leading to osteoporosis and osteoarthritis, for example. Periodontal problems may be caused by a deficiency of calcium and other nutrients. Anemia may be linked to low stomach acid levels, because iron is not absorbed efficiently. Poorly nourished skin is another common result of malabsorption due to digestive problems. The skin may show minor symptoms, such as blemishes, dryness, scaling, or a tendency toward irritation. These are often due to dietary deficiencies and/or poor absorption of calcium, zinc, vitamins A and E, and essential fatty acids.

Clinical Experience

TRADITIONAL VS. ALTERNATIVE APPROACHES

The differences between traditional and alternative medicine are particularly evident in the treatment of digestive disorders. In the traditional paradigm, a person is generally deemed healthy unless she has a major breakdown in the digestive apparatus or a major disease. In essence, the paradigm says that health is the absence of disease.

Traditional physicians are more used to treating symptoms than correcting causes. For this reason, one of the most common problems in digestion—a "cause" rather than a "symptom"—is one that is rarely considered in traditional medical practice. This is the malabsorption syndrome, or the failure of the body to absorb the nutrients that have been ingested. The problem here is that even though a food is eaten and goes through the digestive system, the nutrients, minerals, and vitamins do not get into the blood and hence do not penetrate the body at the cellular level.

Traditionally trained physicians are skilled at identifying and treating conditions when they have reached a disease state. Their approach to diagnosis and treatment is anatomical in nature. They use sophisticated technologies to evaluate the anatomy of the digestive tract—the stomach, pancreas, small intestine, colon, and liver—and look for evidence of tumors, polyps, ulcers, and other problems. They are less likely to search out or treat conditions such as underactivity, sluggishness, or suboptimal function. Even when such conditions are detected, they are often not considered significant.

The digestive process, like all body systems, produces a wide spectrum of symptoms when it is not functioning properly. Complementary physicians, who combine traditional medicine with alternative practices, consider mild or moderate symptoms to be signs of suboptimal functioning that should be addressed as such. These symptoms include burping, indigestion, and constipation. Complementary physicians often analyze the body biochemistry using sophisticated blood laboratory testing that goes beyond traditional medicine's use of the standard SMA-24 profile to identify major digestive disorders. They are very interested in the foods a person eats, and whether any specific foods cause irritation or other reactions. Thus they tend to test for food sensitivity as part of a complete analysis of body function.

In terms of treatment, complementary physicians tend to use natural substances such as foods, herbs, and homeopathic preparations. Supplements that contain concentrated forms of vitamins and minerals are fundamental elements of body rebalancing. Complementary physicians tend to be attuned to the concept of even the mildest malabsorption since they frequently see the end product of this condition, namely deficiencies of nutrients.

DR. MARTIN FELDMAN'S APPROACH TO DIGESTIVE WELLNESS

Dr. Martin Feldman, whose ulcer protocol is described below, is a traditionally trained physician who practices complementary medicine. Over many years of practice, he has found that a surprisingly large number of health disorders are related to suboptimal digestion, which, as mentioned earlier, reduces the body's ability to absorb the vital nutrients needed for proper functioning. Rather than taking the traditional approach of waiting for symptoms to develop into full-blown disease states, Dr. Feldman strongly believes in treating sluggish conditions before they progress. By identifying and treating digestive system disorders when they first begin, he believes that many degenerative diseases can be avoided.

DIAGNOSIS

This approach makes use of standard medical procedures and tests. A complete medical history is taken, and comprehensive blood and laboratory analyses are conducted. Dr. Feldman looks for indicators of suboptimal functioning in the digestive system, such as a slight elevation of SGOT enzymes on an SMA-24 blood test. The SGOT, an enzyme found in liver cells, can double or triple in the presence of hepatitis. Traditional physicians will generally look for such extremely elevated levels and tend to disregard slightly elevated levels. Dr. Feldman, however, considers that even a small increase in the level of this enzyme can indicate that the liver, while not diseased, is off balance and in need of attention. As he explains, "I'm looking for the early evaluation of an imbalanced or a suboptimal liver, not a very diseased liver."

Lab tests can also disclose other indicators of malabsorption. These include low levels of minerals such as calcium, magnesium, zinc, manganese, chromium, and selenium, and deficiencies of fat-soluble vitamins such as vitamins A, D, and E. The water-soluble vitamins, including B complex and C, are generally less affected because they are more easily absorbed. Dr. Feldman also may test for bacteria and parasites.

In addition, Dr. Feldman uses a noninvasive technique, based on acupuncture pressure points, to test the strength of various internal organs and mechanisms. This technique can determine which components of a patient's digestion are sluggish by testing the level of electrical activity in their specific meridians. If the flow of energy in a given meridian field is deficient, that aspect of digestion is often suboptimal.

Dr. Feldman explains: "Acupuncture theory has taught us that there are many energy flows throughout the body. The energy flow is quite specific along anatomical pathways. A deficient electrical flow often reflects an organ weakness. Traditional acupuncture intervenes by inserting needles into specific acupuncture points to either improve the flow of electrical energy through that flow channel or meridian or to reduce the flow." Because he uses acupuncture theory only for diagnosis and not for treatment, Dr. Feldman has no need for needles. Instead, he uses meridians to profile the component parts of the digestive apparatus and pinpoint areas that are underactive or suboptimal in strength. In this way he can determine the energy flow or lack of flow and thus assess the body's function.

Once the areas of weakness are identified, Dr. Feldman may consult with a gastroenterologist to see if additional testing is needed, such as X-rays or colonoscopy.

TREATMENT

Dr. Feldman then begins to formulate a plan to soothe, replace, repair, and rebuild faulty mechanisms. Treatment decisions are based on area of dysfunction, whether and where irritation is present, and whether any pathogens are present, such as parasites or unfriendly, harmful bacteria. To correct any of these problems, Dr. Feldman's treatment relies heavily on natural substances, including vitamins, minerals, herbs, and occasional homeopathic preparations.

The first step in this process is to soothe any parts of the digestive system that are irritated, whether the stomach, the small intestine, or the colon. Various herbal preparations, such as marshmallow, slippery elm, and aloe vera, may be used for this purpose. Aloe vera, in particular, can help soothe the ileocecal valve, the ascending or descending colon, or the entire digestive tract when it is irritated.

Next, it is important to replace whatever is insufficient or suboptimal. When deficiencies of stomach acid are determined, oral acid tablets (such as betaine hydrochloride or glutamic acid) may be prescribed in order to optimize the stomach-acid phase of digestion. Dr. Feldman warns that this therapy must be supervised by a knowledgeable practitioner. Other natural substances, including zinc, folic acid, intrinsic factor, and duodenal substance, can help get the stomach back on track to produce its own acid.

The most crucial step in Dr. Feldman's treatment is repair. The focus is on (1) eliminating negative influences on the organ in question, including foods that provoke allergic reactions, irritants such as caffeine, and poor food choices (such as fatty and denatured foods) that stress the digestive system; and (2) using natural therapies to rebuild the suboptimal or sluggish components of digestion. For example, the following substances may be used:

STOMACH—Cabbage juice, vitamin D3, black cumin seed oil, vitamin C, licorice, zinc, vitamin A, n-acetyl-glucosamine, marshmallow, ginger, and cayenne. Natural therapies such as goldenseal and a citrate bismuth can help to combat an infection of Helicobacter pylori, although an antibiotic may be needed as well to eliminate the bacteria.

ILEOCECAL VALVE—Lipid-soluble chlorophyll, aloe vera, slippery elm bark, and echinacea. Increased consumption of water can also help in the case of a closed valve.

COLON—For an imbalance of the ascending colon: bifido bacteria (which can help rebalance the ecology of the colon), fructooligosaccharides (FOS), insoluble fiber, and calendula. For a parasitic infection of the descending colon: grapefruit seed extract, black walnut herb, artemesia, and homeopathic antiparasite remedies. For a general irritation of the colon: aloe vera, lipid-soluble chlorophyll, butyric acid, Jerusalem artichoke flour, 1-glutamine, a mix of soluble and insoluble fiber, calcium, and magnesium.

LIVER—Choline, methionine, inositol, milk thistle, combination herbal formulas, and homeopathic solutions.

Food Allergy and Digestion

Foods to which a person is allergic or sensitive are considered invaders by the body's immune system. Thus, they irritate and weaken the digestive apparatus. It is quite common to find that people consume large amounts of foods to which they are allergic. Reading food labels and choosing food correctly is a critical part of treatment.

Digestive malfunctioning can cause complications when allergens are present. If there is a deficiency of the gastric juices or pancreatic enzymes, for instance, a food will be in the system for a much longer time than it would if there were adequate amounts of acids and enzymes to break it down. If the food is one to which the body is sensitive, that sensitivity will be heightened by the delayed action of the digestive mechanism. Furthermore, if protein molecules are not broken down into small enough particles because of faulty digestive processes, the larger units entering the bloodstream will be treated like foreign invaders by the body's immune system, and an allergic reaction will ensue.

HIGH-PROTEIN DIETS

High-protein diets pose a special problem with respect to food allergies. People who consume a lot of protein usually tend to have it in their systems around the clock. This is because it takes at least four to seven hours for proteins to be digested, and if the protein is fried, deep-fried, or charcoal-broiled, it can take even longer. Consider the person who starts the day with bacon and eggs, has a sandwich of cold cuts and cheese at lunch, eats more meat and drinks milk at dinner, and tops it off with a late-night snack of ice cream. This person will have protein in his or her system all the time.

If any substance—in this case, protein—sits in the digestive system virtually all the time, two things will occur. First, the person will almost certainly develop an allergy to it because of overexposure. Second, the person will probably not be aware of the allergy because her system will never be without the substance long enough for her to notice changes due to its presence or absence. The negative symptoms then become cumulative and chronic, and are manifested as disease states. Digestion is usually strained, and the disorders that appear are generally regarded as signs of poor health, which becomes tolerated as unavoidable or is attributed to genetics or age.

FOOD ROTATION

Food rotation is one way to help alleviate this problem. It can be combined with medical care. Don't eat the same foods day after day, because no matter how healthy and nutritious they are, you will not benefit from them if your body rejects or reacts negatively to them. Wheat, for example, is nutritious, but because it is found in practically every processed food, it is also a very common allergen. Therefore, it must be rotated in the diet with other grains. Eat it no more frequently than every fourth day and in no more than a 4-ounce portion at each meal. Then there is a good chance it can be eaten without causing an allergic reaction.

All foods should be rotated in this manner. Even if your body is not responding negatively in an overt way, you may be having hidden reactions to many different foods. Even if you are not, by overusing a food—eating it too frequently and in oversized portions—you may eventually develop an allergy to it. Try to make a routine of rotating all foods and avoid eating processed foods as much as possible because certain foods, such as corn and wheat, are ingredients in many of them.

Lactose Intolerance

Lactose intolerance is a common digestive disorder. Probably two-thirds of the world's adults cannot tolerate lactose, which is found in milk and all milk products. When lactose-sensitive people continue to eat dairy products, they begin to suffer from a wide range of symptoms, which include abdominal cramping and bloating, chronic nasal discharge or postnasal drip, puffiness under the eyes, gas, and diarrhea.

Lactose intolerance is a malabsorption of lactose caused by a deficiency of lactase, the enzyme responsible for milk digestion. Lactase breaks lactose down into the readily digestible forms glucose and galactose. If it is absent or deficient, lactose remains undigested in the system. Some passes through the blood and is excreted in the urine, but most ends up in the large intestine. The lactose molecules draw water out of the tissues and into the intestinal cavity, while the undigested glucose is fermented by intestinal bacteria. Carbon dioxide is given off during this process, and diarrhea, bloating, flatulence, and belching may result.

The lactase deficiency can be caused by damage to the intestinal mucosa; this damage may be brought on by acute infectious diarrhea in infants. Malnutrition, cystic fibrosis, and colitis also have been known to cause lactase deficiency. Even in the absence of these traumas, lactose deficiency is very common.

The most obvious remedy for lactose intolerance is to stay away from milk and all milk products. Also, keep in mind that lactose is found in many vitamins and most processed foods, so it is best to avoid processed foods and request from vitamin manufacturers a full disclosure of their exact ingredients. It is important to eliminate lactose from the system completely in order to recover from its ravages. Another option may be to purchase a commercially prepared lactase supplement that boosts your supply of lactase and enables you to better digest the lactose. Some lactase-deficient people, however, can still eat a few fermented milk and dairy products without negative consequences. These items—primarily yogurt, buttermilk, and cottage cheese—must be tested on an individual basis to determine one's reaction to them.

Gastritis

Gastritis, another common digestive disorder, involves an inflammation of the mucosa lining the inner wall of the stomach. The inflammation is accompanied by symptoms such as nausea, vomiting, and loss of appetite. In the acute form, gastritis can be caused by infections and/or the ingestion of corrosive agents such as alcohol and aspirin. In the chronic form, gastritis is a serious condition that may be the cornerstone of degenerative diseases such as ulcers.

The treatment of gastritis should include the elimination of any substance (an allergen or anything else that is difficult to digest) known to be causing or aggravating the condition. The diet should include lots of liquids. Vegetables should be steamed to maximize their digestibility and reduce their acidity. A blood chemistry test should be performed to determine what, if any, vitamin deficiencies exist, since they often play an important role in this disorder. Vitamin deficiency related to gastritis is responsible for many complications, among which are a prickly sensation in the skin, loss of memory, depression, and general weakness.

Pressure Diseases

Another group of disorders associated with the digestive system have been termed pressure diseases because they are caused by a pressure buildup that results from failure to eliminate waste efficiently. They include diverticulitis, hemorrhoids, hiatus hernia, and appendicitis, among others.

DIVERTICULITIS

Diverticular disease is the most troublesome and widespread of the pressure conditions. It occurs when the muscle rings encircling the colon, which move along bulk matter, become clogged. Try clenching your fist and then imagine that mud is stuck in the creases of your hand. The creases can be thought of as diverticula, and the mud in them is food being trapped in the digestive organs. When bulk and fiber are lacking in the diet, the colon must deal with a mass of food too dry to be pushed along with ease, and so it becomes overworked, overstressed, and overstrained. Its membranes eventually herniate, or rupture, and it is these ruptures that are called diverticula. When there are many diverticula—and there can be hundreds—they tend to become inflamed and cause more acute symptoms. This condition is known as diverticulitis. Approximately one in four people with diverticular disease develop these acute symptoms.

Diverticulitis barely existed before the twentieth century, but now is said to affect one-third of all adults middle-aged or older, half the population over fifty, and two-thirds of the population over eighty. It is the most common digestive disorder of senior citizens.

Research on the genesis and development of diverticular disease has shown that it results from a gross lack of fiber in the diet. The refining of carbohydrates seems to be the main culprit here, since this condition is almost wholly absent in cultures where whole grains, legumes, vegetables, and such are the mainstays of the diet and where processed foods are not used.

The traditional treatment for diverticular disease has been to give the patient stool softeners to help the stool pass through the system and expanders to force it out. Antibiotics are also used. The patient is placed on a fibrous diet that helps the colon begin processing waste more efficiently and with less strain. Bran is usually prescribed, and patients are often told to avoid milk products and spicy foods, since these tend to produce abdominal pain, pressure, and gas.

Alternative treatments for diverticular disease may include the above suggestions but will add to the patient's diet other abdominal and intestinal cleansers taken orally. These include cellulose, hemicellulose, pectin, and noncarbohydrate lignin. Celery, brussels sprouts, broccoli, and especially beet juice will also help the condition. Bran should be unprocessed because this type has a shorter intestinal transit time and helps increase stool weight. The diverticula pockets may be cleansed with dietary supplements of chlorophyll, chamomile, garlic, vitamin C, aloe vera concentrate, zinc, nondairy acidophilus, pectin, and psyllium. Instead of medicinal antibiotics, natural antibiotics such as garlic may be used.

HEMORRHOIDS

Constantly straining to push dry, compacted stools out of the system causes the veins in the rectal and anal passages to become distended and engorged with blood. The veins become weakened, lose their elasticity, and can no longer carry blood properly. This causes the blood to pool instead, creating a ballooning effect known as a hemorrhoid.

When the hemorrhoids are internal, they can become obstructive to stool passage. With constant pressure being exerted against them, they may rupture and bleed and, in severe cases, hemorrhage. External hemorrhoids, also called piles, are very sensitive and may grow to the size of golf balls.

It is estimated that half of all Americans over fifty years of age have hemorrhoids and that hemorrhoidal treatment is a $50 million a year industry. Most of the profit comes from sales of suppositories. Suppositories are given to shrink and lubricate hemorrhoids to prevent them from rupturing. Alternative treatments for hemorrhoids center on hygiene, diet, and exercise. Warm tub or sitz baths and ice packs may help. If you increase your intake of water, vitamin C, and fiber, and exercise regularly, the blood trapped in the hemorrhoidal veins will be reabsorbed into the body and the problem will be cleared up. However, it will recur unless you integrate these changes into a new, more healthful lifestyle.

Prevention of the recurrence of hemorrhoids is aimed at changing conditions associated with the pressure and straining of constipation. Doctors will often recommend increasing fiber and fluids in the diet. Eating the right amount of fiber and drinking six to eight glasses of fluid (not alcohol) result in softer, bulkier stools. A softer stool makes emptying the bowels easier and lessens the pressure on hemorrhoids caused by straining.

Eliminating straining also helps prevent the hemorrhoids from protruding. Good sources of fiber are fruits, vegetables, and whole grains. In addition, doctors may suggest a bulk stool softener or a fiber supplement such as psyllium (Metamucil) or methylcellulose (Citrucel).

In some cases, hemorrhoids must be treated surgically. These methods are used to shrink and destroy the hemorrhoidal tissue and are performed under anesthesia. The doctor will perform the surgery during an office or hospital visit.

HIATUS HERNIA

Hiatus hernia is another condition related to constipation and low-fiber dietary regimens. Like the other pressure diseases, it is essentially a modern-day Western disorder affecting primarily middle-aged and older people. There are no warning symptoms until it causes a sharp pain just below the breastbone. It is a condition in which part of the stomach wall becomes distended and pushes up against the diaphragm and the skeletal system. Obesity may contribute to the condition, which also sometimes develops during pregnancy.

The traditional treatment for hiatus hernia usually includes antacids, a bland diet, and sometimes surgery. These steps are adequate to relieve the pain, and you certainly should follow the suggestions of your physician. The alternative (or even complementary) approach is aimed at going beyond alleviation of the painful symptoms by establishing a dietary regimen that can reverse the condition while ameliorating the source of discomfort. Since constipation due to a low-fiber diet is frequently the cause of this condition, make sure to get plenty of high-fiber bulk foods. Losing weight may also help.

APPENDICITIS

Appendicitis is an inflammation of the appendix, a small pouch that extends from the first part of the large intestine. The appendix has no known function. It can become diseased as a result of infection or obstructed from contents moving through the intestinal tract.

Appendicitis is caused mainly by troublesome elimination. The most common abdominal emergency in the Western world, it is often brought on by continuous constipation, straining during stool elimination, and anal retention—failing to evacuate solid waste when the body tells you to. By delaying your bowel movements, perhaps because you are too busy to be inconvenienced, you confuse your body. The water from fecal matter begins to be reabsorbed, and the dry, hard stool that is left will pass only with great pain and difficulty. In the meantime, you strain the muscles that must retain this mass and eventually train them to delay normal elimination.

Some people learn to have a bowel movement only once a day or even once every two or three days. You should have two or three bowel movements a day, depending, of course, on what and how often you eat. When there is not enough dietary fiber to move food and waste readily through the digestive system, pressure builds up and blocks the passage of stool. Bacteria accumulate and back up into the three- to six-inch-long appendix, which is attached to the large intestine. The appendix becomes inflamed and infected, and an appendectomy must be performed.

To see how critical the issue of fiber is here, consider the 6,000 appendectomies performed in the United States each week compared with only a handful per year in rural Africa, where processed fiber-depleted food is virtually nonexistent. This again is a pressure disease that can be avoided or even treated with a high-fiber diet consisting of complex carbohydrates.

ULCERS

Ulcers of the digestive tract afflict about one in twenty women. Digestive-system ulcers occur most often in the duodenum, which is the upper portion of the small intestine. The duodenal ulcer is usually found in the first few inches of the duodenum. The second most common type is the peptic or gastric ulcer, which affects the stomach.

Some ulcers are slight abrasions of the internal mucosal lining; others advance to the stage where they totally perforate the stomach or intestinal wall. Their three stages of development are known as perforation, penetration, and obstruction. In acute perforation, the ulcer eats through the wall of the abdomen. This is the most serious state and causes the greatest number of deaths. Surgery to close the perforation is virtually unavoidable.

Penetration is the stage where the patient usually awakens at night with severe pain in adjacent areas of the body—the back, liver, and so forth—not just the stomach. This transfer of effect to other organs makes the ulcer hard to diagnose. Obstruction is the stage in which swelling caused by inflammation affects the stomach and the opening to the small intestine.

The vast majority of ulcers are caused by the Helicobacter pylori bacteria. These bacteria take up residence in the lining of the digestive tract and then contribute to the breakdown of that lining, resulting in a lesion or crater. Doctors used to think that ulcers were caused by stress or the production of too much hydrochloric acid.

TRADITIONAL TREATMENT

Traditional physicians generally limit their treatment to the use of antibiotics to combat the bacteria, and acid-production blockers such as Tagamet and Zantac to prevent the stomach acid from irritating the broken-down tissues in the mucosal lining. The heavy reliance on acid-production blockers is troublesome for two reasons: The drugs do not address the real issue, which is why the bacteria have proliferated in the digestive wall; and since the natural stomach acid opposes the bacteria, the blockers may reduce the body's ammunition against the infection. In the process, these drugs may also lessen the effectiveness of the overall digestive process. The stomach's role in digestion is to produce acids that help to digest foods. When that mechanism is suppressed by acid-production blockers, the body may not digest foods efficiently and absorb nutrients. Thus, a patient may suffer from malabsorption.

ALTERNATIVE APPROACH

As a complementary physician, Dr. Martin Feldman advocates a much more comprehensive approach to the treatment of ulcers. In addition to eliminating the bacteria, he says, the treatment should accomplish three goals: helping the stomach to heal the erosion; rebalancing the stomach acid production so that it works properly; and optimizing the immune system so that the body can protect against reinfection.

DIAGNOSIS

The mainstream medical community uses endoscopes and upper-GI X-rays to determine if an ulcer actually exists. Dr. Feldman may call on these diagnostic techniques as well to obtain as much scientific data as possible on the status of an ulcer. He also uses tests performed by specialty laboratories to identify the presence of Helicobacter pylori. Dr. Feldman also draws on his clinical judgment in the diagnostic process. If the laboratory blood test is negative but his clinical experience suggests the presence of Helicobacter pylori, he may conduct a therapeutic trial by having the patient take some natural substances that combat the bacteria. He can use this technique because the substances are safe and well tolerated, producing very few side effects. Dr. Feldman then monitors the patient to determine if the therapy reduces the symptoms.

OPPOSING THE BACTERIA

Both antibiotics and natural substances can be used to fight the Helicobacter pylori infection. For antibiotic treatments, Dr. Feldman favors the use of amoxicillin because it is usually effective and well tolerated by most patients.

In addition, he may combat the bacteria at a second level with natural therapies. These include goldenseal, an herb that has antibacterial properties, the mineral bismuth in a citrate form, and various combinations of homeopathic solutions. Because homeopathic solutions function primarily as transmitters of energy, Dr. Feldman can test the effect of specific homeopathic products on the body's acupuncture-meridian energy fields.

HEALING THE ULCER

In addition to removing the bacteria, it's important to help the body heal the ulcer irritation or erosion. Dr. Feldman uses a variety of natural treatments to heal the digestive lining. These include cabbage juice, aloe vera, licorice herb, buffered black cumin seed oil, curcumin, vitamin D3, vitamin B-complex, vitamin C, and n-acetyl-glucosamine, a nutrient complex. Other substances that soothe the irritation and thus promote the healing process are marshmallow, ginger, cayenne, and an herbal combination called Robert's Formula.

TESTING FOR FOOD ALLERGIES

Food allergens tend to irritate the stomach, making it harder to heal an ulcer or any other irritation of the stomach or intestines. Therefore, any foods to which a patient is allergic should be eliminated from the diet. To identify such offenders, Dr. Feldman will test a patient's reaction to various food substances by placing them upon the taste portion of the tongue. The brain-taste mechanism, which is very highly developed, has the ability to ascertain if a given food substance is a danger to the body.

REBALANCING THE ACID-PRODUCTION MECHANISM

Paradoxically, many patients with ulcers have a low production of stomach acid. As Dr. Feldman notes, the low-acid environment allows the Helicobacter pylori bacteria to get a foothold in the mucosal lining, while a normal acid level would tend to provide some antibacterial protection.

In addition to allowing the bacteria to grow, a low acid production can cause other problems. One is that food will sit in the stomach for a long period of time and ferment abnormally due to the lack of sufficient stomach acid. This fermentation then produces abnormal acids that irritate the stomach and the ulcer. The result: People with low stomach acid experience the symptoms of a high acid production. They may take antacids to suppress the symptoms, but that remedy doesn't correct the true problem. The stomach must work efficiently so that food does not ferment abnormally.

Dr. Feldman has found that many patients suffer from this problem, so he puts a strong emphasis on reoptimizing the stomach's acid mechanism. Again, he uses a variety of natural therapies to get the acid-production system back on track. These remedies include zinc, folic acid, intrinsic factor, and duodenal substance. In some cases, he also prescribes oral acid supplements, which may assist the acid mechanism in strengthening itself. This latter treatment requires careful supervision to ensure that a patient takes the proper form of acid in the proper doses.

REPAIRING THE IMMUNE SYSTEM

As a final phase in his treatment of ulcers, Dr. Feldman focuses on rebuilding the immune system. The logic here, of course, is that the immune system must be working at its maximum level to fight the bacteria that cause most ulcers in the first place. This part of the treatment consists of nutrients that serve as the building blocks of the immune system. They include vitamins A, E, D, and C, bioflavonoids, gamma linolenic acid (GLA), essential fatty acids, zinc, and selenium.

FOODS TO AVOID

As a final note, people who suffer from ulcers should avoid ingesting substances that exacerbate the condition. These include alcohol, nicotine, aspirin, coffee, soft drinks, salt, high-oil nuts, and even raw fruit (except bananas). Foods that are excessively spicy and difficult to digest should be avoided as well.

You don't want to eat a lot of high-protein foods, especially those that are high in fat. Animal foods require more gastric involvement and should be avoided if possible. If you do eat meat, at least trim off the fat; also avoid overcooking, deep frying, and charcoal broiling since these processes make the molecules bond more tightly so that more digestive effort is required to break them down.

Carbohydrate foods have their own protective buffer in the natural state (brown rice and whole grain and vegetables), but once they are refined (white flour and white rice, cakes and pastries) the buffer is stripped away. Therefore, avoid denatured, processed carbohydrates. Vegetables are usually quite acidic, so avoid those causing gas (turnips, cucumbers, brussels sprouts, broccoli, radishes, and cauliflower), especially in the raw state. Vegetables will be less acidic if you cook them, preferably by steaming since it does not destroy their fibrous structure.

Irritable Bowel Syndrome

According to a 2015 fact sheet from the International Foundation for Functional Gastrointestinal Disorders, irritable bowel syndrome affects 10 to 15 percent of all adults in the US, two-thirds of whom are women. Signs and symptoms include bowel irregularity, constipation, diarrhea, alternating constipation and diarrhea, a sense of bloatedness and cramping in the intestinal area, and generalized gastrointestinal discomfort. Most people who consult a traditional medical doctor are given the diagnosis but not much in the way of treatment. Typically, says Dr. Elizabeth Lipski, a certified clinical nutritionist and author of *Digestive Wellness*, "you're told to eat more fiber, go home, and not worry about it."

That advice might be easy for a doctor to give, but not for those affected to take. "A study was done not too long ago comparing people who have different chronic health issues and different health issues and diseases," Dr. Lipski says. "What they discovered was that people who have irritable bowel syndrome have the quality of life of people who are undergoing chemotherapy for cancer treatment. People who are undergoing chemo, it's a bad thing, but it's short. Maybe they have to do that for two months or three months or maybe even a horrible year; but for people with irritable bowel syndrome having constipation, diarrhea, cramping can affect them lifelong. The sad thing is that there is so much that can be done and physicians don't really know how to help everybody to do that."

CAUSES

Among the causes of irritable syndrome are food sensitivities and intolerances, infection, and stress.

Dr. Lipski explains how to determine whether food is the culprit. First, eat your regular diet and keep a chart of symptoms, ranking them from one to ten in terms of severity. Then, for two weeks eat only these specific foods: all the rice that you want (any type); all the fruits and vegetables that you want, either cooked or raw; poultry, organic if possible; fish; oil such as olive oil on a salad for a salad dressing to make your food taste good; salt, pepper, herbs and spices. Chart your symptoms after following this regimen, and compare them with the earlier readings.

"What I find," Dr. Lipski says, "is that probably eight out of ten people with irritable bowel syndrome and many other mystery illnesses are feeling remarkably better within two weeks."

Food intolerance is another common cause of irritable bowel syndrome. "Seventy percent of the world's population is lactose intolerant, and for many people just taking dairy out of their diets for a couple of weeks also can give them remarkable results," Dr. Lipski says.

Stress can cause problems because we have neurotransmitters in our digestive system that cause us to feel our emotions in the gut. "I have one client who every time she had to speak at a meeting would get diarrhea before she went in," Dr. Lipski says. "It can be very important to learn stress modification techniques," such as abdominal breathing, positive self-talk, meditation, prayer, hypnotherapy, and biofeedback.

NATURAL APPROACH TO TREATMENT

Dr. Lipski has seen good results with probiotic supplements, increased fiber, and herbs that nourish the digestive system.

"Personally," she says, "I feel like all of us should take a probiotic every single day. What we know about probiotic supplements is that they help balance the immune system. They can help lower and normalize serum cholesterol and triglycerides levels. They make vitamins, most of our B vitamins and vitamin K. They help protect us against food poisoning. They make little bits of antibiotics. They're very soothing to the digestive system, and they also make little bits of anti-cancer-causing substances. They're very important. They also help with bowel regularity: whether we have too many bowel movements in a day and diarrhea or whether we have too few, probiotics can be really useful.

"There is one specific type of probiotic that's been very well researched for people who have diarrhea type irritable bowel syndrome. It is an unusual probiotic because it's not a bacterium like most of them are. It's actually a yeast. It's a cousin to bread baking yeast, and it's called Saccharomyces boulardii. A French pharmaceutical company has been doing research on this particular yeast for over fifty years, and finds that it's very useful for helping with diarrhea from all causes. It's widely available in health food stores."

Fiber can best be obtained from food. Dr. Lipski recommends that people eat a lot of fruits, vegetables and whole grains, and small amounts of nuts, seeds and legumes. "I prefer that to fiber supplements, but fiber supplements also can be useful if people just for some reason can't make those changes to their diet," she says.

Among the herbs that can soothe and nourish the digestive system are basil, rosemary, nutmeg, ginger, aloe vera, turmeric, cumin, and coriander. Dr. Lipski also recommends peppermint tea, valerian tea, and lemon balm, as well as slippery elm and marshmallow root.

Another helpful herb is chamomile. "Think about Little Peter Rabbit when he came in with a bad tummy," Dr. Lipski says. "What did his mom give him? It was chamomile."

Celiac Disease

Celiac disease is an inherited autoimmune disorder that damages the small intestine and prevents adequate absorption of nutrients from food. The damage is caused by a toxic reaction of the immune system to the ingestion of gluten, a protein found in wheat, rye, and barley. According to 2015 data from the National Foundation for Celiac Awareness, the disease affects about 1 percent of the population in the US. Unfortunately, some 83 percent of people with Celiac are undiagnosed, and therefore not aware of the many successful ways to manage this potentially disabling condition. When left untreated, Celiac disease can cause complications such as other autoimmune disorders, osteoporosis, infertility, and neurological disorders.

SYMPTOMS

Symptoms can arise throughout the lifespan. They may include bloating, gas, or abdominal pain; chronic diarrhea or constipation or both; pale, foul-smelling stool; bone or joint pain; behavior changes, depression, and/or irritability; vitamin K deficiency; skin problems; fatigue; weakness; and delayed growth or onset of puberty. Some people do not experience any symptoms; however, they still may be at risk for future complications.

Naturopathic physician Dr. Christine Doherty says that women with Celiac disease may have osteoporosis, irregular menstruation, miscarriage, and infertility. It can be a cause of heavy periods and anemia. Celiac can cause early menopause, as early as age thirty, or late onset of the first period.

DIAGNOSIS

Diagnosis can be difficult because the symptoms are so varied and similar to those of other diseases. Screening for Celiac disease is done with blood tests that measure levels of certain antibodies. The next step would be a small bowel biopsy and possibly testing for specific human leukocyte antigen (HLA) genes.

TREATMENT

"Celiac is one of the classic malabsorption diseases," Dr. Doherty says. "The good news is that once you know what you're dealing with and you take the gluten out of the diet, the body's ability to absorb nutrients bounces back."

Treatment for Celiac disease is always dietary. A gluten-free diet must be followed. People with Celiac should not eat foods that contain wheat, rye, or barley. Gluten is found in breads, pastas, and cookies, and is "hidden" in many other foods. Dr. Doherty says she recommends a version of the Mediterranean diet. "Basically," she says, "meat is only a condiment maybe once a month. Sweets, eggs, poultry, fish maybe once a week. Of course fruits, legumes, nuts, beans and vegetables." Fortunately there have been an increasing number of gluten-free products on the market in recent years, and many support groups and websites to help people sort through what they can and cannot eat.

"I make sure people are eating a good quality diet and not just replacing their donuts with gluten-free donuts," Dr. Doherty says. "You actually want to be focusing on the fruits and the vegetables and the gluten-free whole grains."

Supplements are often beneficial. Many people with Celiac have vitamin D deficiency, Dr. Doherty says. "It's very difficult to get enough from foods. So I usually give between 2,000 and 4,000 IUs a day of Vitamin D3. I personally like a drop version. It's very hard to find a multivitamin that has that level of vitamin D in it."

Vitamin K, calcium, and magnesium also may be recommended. "I look at how well the gut is functioning," says Dr. Doherty. "Calcium and magnesium are both fairly difficult for the gut to manage. Calcium tends to be very constipating on its own, and magnesium tends to have a laxative effect. So you have to see what the individual system will tolerate. The standard dose is two times more calcium than magnesium. So if you're taking 1,000 milligrams of calcium, you're taking 500 milligrams of magnesium. Food sources are better when it comes to calcium, but sometimes, especially initially, we need supplemental calcium."

Dr. Doherty says that a broad spectrum B vitamin is important for improving fatigue and mood. Vitamin A is also used, 10,000 to 50,000 IU's daily. "I use the fat soluble version of vitamin A because people with Celiac often can't convert beta-carotene into vitamin A efficiently. So you'll see frequent infections, night vision problems, skin problems, acne, and that 'chicken skin' on the back of their arms. That can be a sign of vitamin A deficiency." Vitamin A must be used cautiously because it can be toxic during pregnancy and over the long term, Dr. Doherty says.

One of the symptoms of Celiac also can be elevated liver enzymes, which means something is basically destroying liver cells. "My favorite herb for that is milk thistle, and I like to use about 600 milligrams a day," Dr. Doherty says. "The liver is the key to metabolism and hormone balance and health. So it's important to look at what's going on there.

"I've seen a number of kids in my practice who were on the verge of being diagnosed bipolar at seven or eight years of age and it turned out that they were Celiac," says Dr. Doherty. "And once they got gluten out of their diet and got their B vitamin levels and their essential fatty acid levels up, they were entirely different, happy-go-lucky children. And that's true for adults, too."

Research Update

An increasing body of evidence is showing the benefits of natural modalities to overall health and well-being. Following is a sample of recent peer-reviewed scientific studies relating to digestive disorders.

According to a 2013 report in *Life Extension Magazine*, research has shown that chewing on tablets composed of marine alginate and bicarbonate can be used to block acid reflux and thereby reduce the risk of accompanying esophageal problems including cancer. As described in a 2011 report in *Digestion*, colonoscopy performed after one year revealed that a combination of the probiotic Bifidobacterium breve (1 gram three times a day) and the prebiotic galacto-oligosaccharide (5.5 grams one time a day) improved the clinical status of people with ulcerative colitis. Supplementation with the probiotic Saccharomyces boulardii has also proven effective against acute infectious diarrhea, as evidenced in a study published in 2012 in *Expert Opinion on Biological Therapy*.

Chapter 31

Eating Disorders

Eating disorders have plagued women in Western societies. According to the National Association of Anorexia Nervosa and Associated Disorders, up to 30 million Americans have an eating disorder, with women affected at a much greater rate than men. Among the most common eating disorders are anorexia nervosa and bulimia nervosa. Anorexia involves compulsive dieting to the point where the woman eats so little that she becomes malnourished and may actually starve to death. It is marked by muscle wasting, loss of menstrual periods, body image problems, and an exaggerated fear of becoming fat. Bulimia is compulsive eating and forced vomiting or the use of laxatives or diuretics to eliminate the calories that are consumed during binge episodes.

Causes

Particularly among women, disordered body images and destructive eating behavior came "out of the closet" about thirty years ago, spurred in part by the revelation that popular singer Karen Carpenter had died of anorexia. Social critics and psychologists have looked to media pressure—and the more available surgeries for re-shaping the human body—as some causes of the dissatisfaction women often feel about "normal" bodies.

Most experts agree that a spectrum of factors contributes to these diseases—individual, family, interpersonal, biological and cultural. Treatment, often multidisciplinary, addresses both the physical and psychological components of the eating disorder. Among the interventions being used are individual and family therapy, support groups, medical treatment and medications to treat associated depression or anxiety. Nutrition has been recognized as part of the problem and part of the cure.

Carolyn Costin, author of *The Dieting Daughter* and other books, came to the study of eating disorders through her own experience: "I had anorexia myself when I was about sixteen years old. I had a pretty severe case, was seventy-nine pounds for a few years." In Costin's opinion, a number of seemingly benign factors, such as the emphasis on exercising and dieting in our culture, as well as interpersonal family pressures may cause a person to fall into any of these negative eating practices.

EATING BEHAVIORS

The problem with diets is that they often disappoint their users. Costin explains, "The main thing I say to people about any kind of diet program is, 'Don't do anything to lose weight that you're not prepared to do for the rest of your life, because going on a diet certainly implies that you'll ultimately go off it.'"

So what happens when you go off it? This will lead to disillusionment and weight disorders, such as constantly going on and off trendy diets, unless a person realizes that a healthy lifestyle, not a temporary eating change, is the only answer to maintaining proper weight.

Another problem is that a healthy desire to exercise can be developed in the wrong way. This, Costin says, is "a little bit like an activity disorder. They can't not do it. There's an addictive component that makes them have to do more and more. Things in their life get put on hold in order to do the activity. They will continue to do it even if they've been injured or are in pain or it's snowing outside. And the way the eating disorders correlate with activity disorders, there are certainly a lot of anorexics and bulimics who also have activity disorder."

In Costin's view, eating disorders are also caused by the way people obsessively codify rules of eating, what she calls "the Thin Commandments." She notes, "Over the years I started to come up with these rules that people with eating disorders have, such as 'If I eat anything, then I have to exercise and burn it off,' or 'I have to wear clothes to make myself look thinner. I have to punish myself if I've eaten anything fattening.'"

INTERPERSONAL RELATIONSHIPS

Delving deeper, one finds that eating disorders in women are often rooted in relationships they had with their parents, particularly their mothers, though not the type of relationship that's commonly assumed to be at fault. "In the beginning,"

Costin explains, "anorexia nervosa was often blamed on overcontrolling mothers. But that's way too simplistic." Rather, the problem is the type of role models that mothers sometimes provide for their daughters. Costin asks, "What are little girls learning from these role models about their bodies and about weight and about food?"

Not only those who actually end up with eating disorders but almost all young women and girls are influenced by these role models. Costin says, "When you have statistics that 80 percent of fourth-grade girls report that they're dieting and 10 or 11 percent of those girls report that they're vomiting on these diets, you've got to look at what's happening with their role models."

Costin describes a six-year-old girl in her waiting room who said she was really excited at having chicken pox. Asked why, she said it meant going to bed without any dinner. "I said, 'Well, what's so good about that?' And she said, 'Because it means I didn't have any calories.' The thing is, she's six. Her mother was a binge eater seeing me for treatment. But kids are little sponges. And she hears her mother saying that calories are bad, so she just learns that part of being female is trying not to have too many calories."

Fathers can also have a negative influence. "I talk to fathers a lot," Costin comments, "about being conscious about what they say about female bodies when they're reading magazines or watching television or things like that. I talk to them about not just praising their daughters for the way they look, which is a very common thing that fathers do with their little girls. A lot of praise and attention focus on appearance as opposed to internal validation. I also encourage them to pay attention to who their daughter is, and to do things with their daughter."

GENETICS

There is mounting evidence that eating disorders have some basis in genetics. Costin states, "It's pretty clear from twin studies that we're going to learn more and more in the next few years about genes that predispose people to inherit this. It's probably going to turn out that there's a biological predisposition. And then maybe a cultural trigger sets it off. Thus, there's a swing back to a more biological basis of these illnesses and not as much of a focus on the big, bad culture. But I think there's no doubt that the culture plays a big role in it, which is why we see over the years an increasing incidence of anorexia and bulimia. But I think it's a combination of someone who has a predisposition and dieting, which is certainly a risk factor. So if more of the population is dieting, more people who have the biological predisposition are exposed to this trigger."

ZINC DEFICIENCY

Some research has shown that anorexia nervosa, bulimia, and obesity may be the result of a zinc deficiency. Dr. Alexander Schauss, a clinical psychologist and eating-disorders specialist from Tacoma, Washington, reports that science has long been aware of this connection: "We've known since at least the 1930s that when animals were experimentally placed on diets deficient in zinc, those animals would develop anorexia. Our interest in eating disorders in relationship to zinc has to do with the observation that when humans are placed on zinc-deficient diets, they, too, develop eating disorders."

"By characterizing three of the most common eating disorders," Dr. Schauss continues, "you can see how vital zinc is. In morbid obesity, when people are significantly overweight in such a way that it could shorten their life span or increase their risk of disease, we know that there is an inverse relationship between the level of obesity and the level of zinc, meaning that the more obese they are, the less zinc they have in the body. We don't know yet whether this is cause or effect, but it is a very important observation because at the other end of the continuum, with anorexia nervosa, self-induced starvation, we also have individuals who are generally always zinc-deficient. We believe there is strong evidence today . . . that the lower the zinc status is, the more likely it is that the patient will not recover from any treatment plan to resolve the anorexia."

Stress is commonly associated with the onset and continuation of eating disorders and can also be understood in terms of zinc loss, since constant mental stress results in the depletion of this mineral. Women are more prone to stress-related zinc loss than men and therefore more likely to have eating disorders. Dr. Schauss explains: "The answer may lie in the fact that males have prostate glands and women do not. Zinc is highly concentrated in the prostate in males; it provides a mineral that is essential for the development, motility, viability, and quantity of sperm. If a male is under psychological stress, he can catabolize or seek out stores of zinc in the prostate. Since women don't have a prostate, they will catabolize the zinc from other tissue.

"In women, the richest source of zinc is found in muscle tissue and bone. A common feature of anorexia is muscle wasting and an increased risk of osteoporosis. Anorexics actually catabolize or eat their own tissue as a way of releasing nutrients they are not getting in the diet. The last muscle, and one that contains only about 1 percent zinc, is the heart muscle. When the body starts to scavenge zinc out of heart muscle tissue, it can interfere with the heart's function, which contributes to bradycardia, tachycardia, arrhythmia, and eventual heart failure. It is particularly dangerous when patients with damaged hearts are in recovery. As they put on weight, they add extra pressure to the heart. That is what killed the singer Karen Carpenter, for example."

Clinical Experience

NUTRITIONAL TREATMENT

Carolyn Costin outlines some of the basic approaches to nutritional therapy. "There are many ways to do nutritional therapy with eating-disorder patients," she notes. "One is educational. A dietitian will do some educational sessions. The patients have a lot of myths about food, such as 'If I eat anything with sugar, it's going to turn into fat,' or 'If I eat anything at night, it's going to turn into fat.' So you send them just to be educated."

Costin may also combine education with therapy. This is needed because "patients' food fears are related to some very deeply rooted psychological stuff. So you combine nutrition therapy and nutrition education."

There are various ways to do this. "For example," Costin explains, "I can send someone to a dietitian, and they get a food plan set up. They get some help, and they go for a few weeks, and then they continue with their therapy, but they don't go back for more nutritional sessions until they're ready to take the next step."

PSYCHOLOGICAL COUNSELING

The first step in counseling is to help the person analyze why she has this problem. Costin starts off by asking, "Why do you have this disorder? What's good about it? How has it helped you? Let's talk about the advantages of it." The person needs to understand how the eating disorder has come to serve a purpose. And that's the whole psychological aspect of it.

"Getting to the emotional aspect is really, really important, and if you don't deal with that, I think you don't really deal with the illness."

SUPPLEMENTS

Costin finds supplements helpful in treating eating disorders: "We're using amino acids in some cases with patients instead of medication, and it's working. It's pretty interesting. We use tyrosine and tryptophan and glutamine."

More specifically she recommends "the use of tryptophan, particularly with bulimia nervosa. We use it for people who have trouble sleeping as well. Phenylalanine also, for depression. Tyrosine for depression. For people who are often given medications such as Ritalin, we use a combination of tyrosine, glutamine, and phenylalanine together."

Dr. Schauss adds that liquid zinc may have a positive effect in the treatment of eating disorders, as it is directly absorbed into the blood. Powders, tablets, and capsules, which must first be broken down by the stomach and absorbed by the small intestine, do not work as well because many eating-disorder patients are unable to digest nutrients properly. Once the patient shows marked improvement, a good zinc supplement will do unless deterioration occurs, in which case the more expensive Zinc Status is needed.

While results are not usually immediate, taking from several days to weeks, once liquid zinc takes effect, its benefits are long-lasting. According to Dr. Schauss, "In fifteen years I worked with hundreds of eating-disorder patients. Until I saw this treatment, my colleagues and I felt that the best we could expect in long-term outcome in treating patients with either bulimia or anorexia was maybe a 20 to 30 percent recovery. In our five-year study, we found that bulimics had a 64.1 percent success rate after recovery on the liquid zinc treatment. In anorexic patients, our five-year follow-up study found an 85 percent recovery rate. These are extraordinarily high recovery rates for a condition that is considered difficult to treat and insidious."

Another favorable finding is that liquid zinc can lift the depression that is usually associated with eating disorders. Dr. Schauss reports, "In our eating-disorder studies, we used a multidimensional design and evaluated the mood state of our patients. One of the first things to improve was the degree of depression they were experiencing based on psychometric instruments such as the Beck Depression Scale and the Profile of Mood Scales, among other depressive indexes. The fact that we have discovered this antidepressive effect and could document it in patients under blind conditions is of great value."

REFEEDING

People recovering from bulimia and anorexia need to return to normal eating patterns gradually. Carolyn Costin explains: "In fact, a lot of the deaths that happened early on with anorexia occurred during the refeeding process, because the heart just can't take the volume that you start giving it if you do the refeeding too fast."

In her practice, "We slowly raise the patients' calories. We get lab tests two to three times a week. We take their pulse in the morning and sometimes even during the day and after meals just to make sure their bodies are handling the stress that comes from refeeding. You can't just take someone who's emaciated and say okay, start eating."

COGNITIVE THERAPY

Dr. José Yaryura-Tobias, an orthomolecular psychiatrist, also finds that because of the life-threatening severity of a condition such as anorexia nervosa, any nutritional approach must be preceded by a program of cognitive therapy. "Anorexia nervosa, from our perspective, is an obsessive-compulsive disorder that is related to self-image, the way that we perceive ourselves. Basically, anorexia nervosa is the process by which a human being self-starves. Thirty percent of the population who self-starve eventually die.

"In the vast majority of cases, when patients come for a consultation, they are already very emaciated. The chemistry we can measure is very altered. From the biochemical viewpoint, we know that there is a groove related to an area of the brain called the limbic system. This is the hypothalamic area, which regulates sugar, thirst, appetite, and so forth. This information can help us classify some of these patients but does not tell us how to manage and eventually cure the problem. The rest of the problem, we feel, has to do with body-image perception, the way these patients see their own bodies. They feel too fat. They have different perspectives than the rest of us do.

"How do we treat this condition? Basically, we use a nutritional approach after the patient has undertaken a behavioral program with cognitive therapy. Cognitive therapy is important because the idea is to educate the person about her problems and to discuss with her the many false beliefs she has about who she is, why she thinks this way, why her body looks the way it does for her, and so forth. So false-belief modification is an important part of treatment."

BREAKING THE CYCLE OF FOOD ADDICTION

Dr. Hyla Cass, a holistic psychiatrist who integrates psychotherapy and nutritional medicine, describes her experience as follows: "Some time ago, a psychologist who specializes in eating disorders began to send her clients to me because she had heard that antidepressant medications work for these patients. I had shifted to a more holistic way of looking at things, so I told the psychologist that before I did anything with antidepressants I would try some other things. With certain eating disorders, such as food cravings, the underlying problem is a food allergy. We often crave the very foods to which we are allergic. Typically, it's the very things we want to eat that are the most damaging, that create the symptoms. In fact, it's like an addiction to alcohol: as you abstain from the foods you're addicted to, you begin to have withdrawal symptoms and crave those foods even more.

"In order to break the cycle in cases of food addiction, just as in breaking the cycle with drinking (alcoholics are actually allergic to alcohol), you need to supply the body with the appropriate nutrients. When we correct the deficiencies and restore body balance, the food cravings and allergy symptoms will often be relieved. Rather than having to rely strictly on 'willpower,' it is possible for individuals to break addictive cycles by achieving metabolic balance through avoiding the offending foods and supporting the body with a balanced nutritional program of vitamins, minerals, and amino acids. Often the cravings will then simply go away. It's quite remarkable: with a good vitamin and mineral product, you can often put a stop to the food allergy and its accompanying symptoms."

Amino acids may a play a role. "I may order a plasma amino acid analysis, a blood test to determine which amino acids—especially among the essential ones the body cannot synthesize by itself—are low," Dr. Cass says. "The amino acid glutamine, in a dose of 500 to 1,000 milligrams, is particularly useful for reducing cravings, including alcohol cravings. Dr. Cass also recommends magnesium supplements, acupuncture and acupressure.

"As we can see," Dr. Cass concludes, "there are many ways, other than psychotherapy and medication, to approach what at first seems like a psychological problem."

Carolyn Costin, however, disagrees with those who say that eating disorders such as bulimia are an addiction like alcoholism. "It's really, really important that you can be recovered from conditions such as anorexia and bulimia. With alcoholism, you have it and your body responds to alcohol differently. For your whole life you can't have a drink because you are then going to be off the wagon and compulsively drink." This is distinct from eating disorders: "For example, the approach to bulimia shouldn't be, well, okay, if you eat chocolate you binge on it, and therefore you can't eat chocolate. I think that instead we have to learn how to teach you that you can absolutely be in control of this. You have to learn how to have it without bingeing and purging it.

"The bottom line is that the new studies show that people become fully recovered from these illnesses. It takes a long time. The new research shows approximately five to eight years, but the recovery rates are high, much higher than originally thought. It's like 76 percent full recovery with anorexia nervosa. There's fewer studies on bulimia, but it's pretty good."

FOOD CRAVINGS AND EMOTIONAL STATES

Dr. Doreen Virtue, former director of a clinic and inpatient psychiatric unit specializing in eating disorders, has a Ph.D. in counseling psychiatry and is the author of several books on dieting and health, including *Constant Craving from A to Z.*

"Most nutritionists would have you believe that nutritional deficiencies are at the heart of all food cravings," Dr. Virtue says. "The problem with that approach is that it still leaves many food cravings unexplained. Food cravings tend to be so specific. For example, a person may crave a hard-boiled egg but not a soft-boiled egg. Or a person may want a chocolate candy bar but not chocolate pudding. It sounds bizarre and a little childish, but anyone who has experienced food cravings will understand how intense and specific they can be.

"Another reason why nutrient deficiencies may not be the only possible cause of these cravings is that not everyone satisfies his or her craving for food before the craving passes. Just as mysteriously as the food craving appears, it may vanish. A food craving can change as easily as a person's state of mind." Dr. Virtue has been researching food cravings for some twenty years and has found patterns that correlate with people's personalities and emotional issues. Again and again, for instance, she found that someone who craved, say, bread was very different from someone who craved ice cream. It's similar to drug-taking behavior. Someone addicted to marijuana, say, has a very different personality and style from someone addicted to another drug.

Noting this, she says, "I investigated further to look at the correlation between personality, emotional and spiritual issues, and how they are connected to food cravings. I did a great deal of research in university libraries, looking at the psychoactive, that is, mood-altering, chemicals found in different foods. I'm not talking about chemicals such as pesticides. I mean the inherent properties, such as vitamins, minerals, amino acids, and so on, that can actually increase or decrease our blood pressure and trigger the pleasure centers of the brain and other areas, chemicals that really affect our moods and energy.

"What I found is that we all tend to act as intuitive pharmacists. We tend to crave foods that will bring us to a state of homeostasis, which means balance or peace of mind. Whenever we are upset, it is normal for us to do something to fix that. If we don't want to take direct action, for instance, by making changes overtly in our lives, a more covert way of dealing with the upset is food cravings, which are cravings for a chemical that will make the body feel at peace."

From this point of view, Dr. Virtue believes that food cravings should be dealt with by trying to understand their underlying emotional sources. Instead of getting angry at yourself for having food cravings, thinking, "Oh, I'm so weak. I should have more willpower," it's better and healthier to listen to those cravings, which are a form of intuition. As Dr. Virtue puts it, "Deciphering them is almost like dream interpretation. They can give us guidance in our lives and help us in many ways."

Just as a food craving is not due to a nutritional deficiency, neither is it due to physical hunger. Dr. Virtue explains, "Let's think about the difference between emotional hunger and physical hunger. They can feel identical, and actually, this is one of the most important points in managing the appetite: to know the difference between emotional cravings and physical cravings."

She notes several underlying differences. For one thing, emotional hunger comes all of a sudden, out of the blue. As she puts it, "You feel like you are starving. Whereas physical hunger is gradual, at one moment you might just feel a little pang in your stomach, then over the course of the next hour or so it grows into a voracious hunger."

The second difference is that emotional hunger is usually for a very specific food. It has to be Rocky Road ice cream or it must be a pepperoni pizza. Physical hunger, while it may have preferences, is open to different types of food. It doesn't require an exact type of food to be satisfied.

Third, Dr. Virtue says, "Emotional hunger is always above the neck, whereas physical hunger is based in the stomach. Emotional hunger is a kind of 'mouth hunger' where you get a taste for a certain thing. It's a very cerebral type of hunger. It is also very urgent. It has to be satisfied now, whereas physical hunger says, 'I am hungry but I could wait fifteen minutes or a half hour if I needed to.'"

The demanding nature of emotional food cravings is due to the urge's misguided attempt to fill an emotional hole: "One of the reasons emotional hunger is urgent is that it really is uncomfortable with the feeling and wants to make that feeling go away. Emotional hunger is also usually paired with some upsetting emotion. And if we stop for a moment when we are experiencing this emotion and ask, 'Could there possibly be something that upset me that I wasn't acknowledging?' as we go into introspection, we usually see that a clerk was rude or a driver cut us off on the road. We are upset, not really hungry."

SPECIFIC TRIGGER FOODS

Usually, if you really look at it, Dr. Virtue notes, there are a few trigger foods that cause a voracious appetite. If you want to find out what your triggers are, you can ask a friend or someone who eats with you, "What kind of food do I seem to binge on?" If you are aware of your own food cravings, you can ask yourself, "What's going on and how do I feel?"—the same way you would about stress.

Dr. Virtue says, "What I've found is that several factors are involved that correlate the particular trigger food to the emotions. One is the texture. Is the food crunchy or soft or chewy? The next is the actual physical components and the underlying chemical properties that either increase or decrease blood pressure, elevate or lower mood, and create neurochemicals that alter mood. The last thing is the flavor or the taste, whether it's spicy, salty, sugary. All these things have to do with who we are as a personality."

Again, identifying your trigger foods is a way to understand what your underlying fears and other emotions are expressing. "Instead of getting mad at ourselves for craving these things," she counsels, "we need to see our cravings as a blessing in disguise. It's the body's way of talking to us. It's just like when a person puts his or her hand on a hot plate. Then the body talks back and says, 'Get that hand off that heat.' Our appetite is trying to do the same sort of thing and give us a message."

INSULIN REACTION AND OVEREATING

Colette Heimowitz has a master's degree in nutrition from Hunter College, is certified in health and nutrition by Pratt University, and has twenty-five years of clinical experience in weight management. The number-one biological cause of obesity in our sedentary population, she maintains, must be understood in terms of insulin resistance. "In a normal homeostasis, an individual ingests a carbohydrate and it raises the glucose levels in the blood. When someone eats protein or fat, by contrast, this doesn't happen. Once the glucose level rises in the blood, it sparks an insulin response from the pancreas. What the insulin does is take the glucose to the peripheral tissues, either to the fat cells, the liver, or to muscle as storage. As a result of years of eating refined carbohydrates, maintaining high-sugar diets, and living a sedentary life, when we age, the insulin is no longer efficient at taking the glucose to the peripheral tissue.

"One of two things happens. Either the glucose levels remain high or the insulin is constantly being produced—overproduced in a prediabetic state—and fat is constantly being stored. When we are sedentary, the process of burning glucose for energy is not happening. It will even provoke the reaction more."

Among the factors that contribute to insulin resistance, "one, of the utmost importance, is lifestyle, a sedentary lifestyle. Some research was done with retired master athletes. Glucose tolerance tests with insulin levels were studied before putting them on bed rest for only one day. The glucose tolerance factors were normal, and the glucose in the blood was normal, because they were still leading an active life, not an elite athlete life, but still one that was active. After one day of bed rest, the glucose tolerance test was repeated and the glucose levels were much higher."

Equally important, Heimowitz says, was a history of eating refined foods, which "the American public is known for—taking the bran out of food, taking the fiber out of food, and replacing the essential fatty acids with hydrogenated fats. This causes a complete stress on the insulin level. The glycemic index of foods [a measurement of the amount of glucose found in the blood as a result of eating a specific food] is much higher, provoking more of an insulin response. The pancreas eventually gets trigger-happy."

There is also a genetic component. It has been shown that people whose parents have a history of diabetes or cardiovascular disease have a weak gene that makes them susceptible to this particular condition. She says, "They have to be especially careful and have an active lifestyle and a low-saturated-fat, higher-protein, lower-carbohydrate diet."

TREATMENT

To alter this continuous fat-and-flabby syndrome, a lower-carbohydrate diet is needed to give the pancreas a rest. Heimowitz recommends eating "low-glycemic-index-type foods, that is, complex whole foods such as fruits and vegetables." She also recommends specific supplements for the insulin-resistant individual.

Alpha-lipoic acid (ALA) is the biological spark plug in converting glucose to energy. She states, "It can lower and stabilize glucose levels and stimulate insulin activity. Some research was done with diabetics being given 600 milligrams daily, and it stabilized their glucose levels without any medication. A nondiabetic or hypoglycemic person could probably use 200 to 300 milligrams a day."

The mineral vanadium, found in vanadyl sulfate, also reduces insulin resistance; 15 to 30 milligrams a day is appropriate.

Chromium is a component of the glucose tolerance factor, a molecule essential for normal insulin function in glucose metabolism. Usually 200 to 1,000 micrograms daily is the range for a beneficial effect.

Heimowitz also emphasizes "essential fatty acids, which are grossly lacking in the American diet and also improve insulin sensitivity and reduce insulin resistance. So supplementing the diet with 3,000 to 6,000 milligrams of the omega-3 fatty acids is appropriate."

Vitamin E is also important. It relieves some of the oxidative stress caused by excessive glucose, which results in free radicals. It will also reduce the risk of cardiovascular disease. Heimowitz adds, "Excessive insulin also causes a lipidation of the triglycerides, and that causes free radical pathology. The excessive insulin also thickens the aortic valve. You are at a higher risk of cardiovascular disease. The vitamin E should be anywhere between 400 and 800 international units [IU] daily."

Zinc also influences carbohydrate metabolism, increases the insulin response, improves glucose tolerance, influences the basal metabolism rate, and supports thyroid function; 50 to 100 milligrams of zinc a day is important.

Magnesium helps maintain tissue sensitivity so that insulin is more effective at taking that glucose to the peripheral tissues. Magnesium helps control glucose metabolism and also decreases sugar cravings; 500 to 1,000 milligrams a day is recommended. "Sometimes," she cautions, "when you go as high as 1,000 milligrams, it may cause diarrhea, so the dose should be determined individually. People should start at 500 and work up slowly."

Heimowitz notes that manganese has been shown in studies to be important for insulin activity: "Manganese-deficient rats showed reduced insulin activity and impaired glucose tolerance. This lack also lowered glucose oxidation and the conversion of triglycerides in the rats' adipose tissues. However, the manganese should be dosed in relation to zinc and copper because they will compete at the cell site. So as little as 35 milligrams of manganese is all you need. The proportionate amount of zinc would be 100 milligrams."

She notes further, "If someone has hypotension because of the insulin resistance, the amino acid tyrosine could also help control the hypotension; 1,500 to 3,000 milligrams daily is appropriate. Hawthorn berry, an herb, can also help control hypotension; 240 to 480 milligrams is a good range.

"When there is cardiovascular involvement, with a high risk, especially with low HDL [high-density lipoprotein] and elevated triglycerides in individuals with insulin resistance, coenzyme Q10 is also appropriate. I suggest 100 to 200 milligrams a day."

Lack of exercise also causes blood sugar problems. Thus, exercise is key. Heimowitz recommends that "for exercise, we look at the fitness level of the individual. I wouldn't tell someone who has been a couch potato to go out and exercise an hour a day. The fitness level needs to be increased slowly so that the body can adjust to the different mechanisms that are going on.

Why Popular Diets Don't Work

THE HIGH-PROTEIN, LOW-CARBOHYDRATE SCAM

The multifaceted approach to combating eating disorders presented so far combines assessing your emotional state, exercising, eating right, and taking supplements. This is in contrast to the faddish, highly touted wonder diets that appear in the media every season. These diets are more often feel-good panders to eaters' worst cravings than scientifically sound practices.

Dr. Joel Fuhrman is a board-certified physician in private practice in New Jersey who specializes in preventing and reversing diseases through nutritional methods. He is the author of *Fasting and Eating for Health*.

"High-protein, low-carbohydrate diets have become increasingly popular over the past few years," he notes, "and doctors who promote these diets list a number of reasons why people with weight problems need to get onto this type of diet. One reason they give is that these people's bodies do not metabolize carbohydrates properly, a condition popularly referred to as insulin resistance."

"In fact," Dr. Fuhrman cautions, "such diets, promoted in some of the most heavily promoted, best-selling diet books, are among the most dangerous. Among these books are *Enter the Zone* by Barry Sears, the [Dr. Robert] Atkins books, and *Protein Power* by Michael Eades."

The problem is how these books recommend breaking the habits. "All these people who read these books, wanting to lose weight by eating a high-protein, low-carbohydrate diet, remind me of people who want to lose weight by snorting cocaine and smoking cigarettes. In other words, there are lots of ways that may work to help you lose weight, but we are interested in more than just having a person temporarily lose weight. We want a diet that is going to enable us to lose weight and protect our health simultaneously, not something that will end up making us look thin in a coffin or increase our cancer risk."

These diets recommend replacing one bad food, refined carbohydrates, with another, animal fats. "You know," Dr. Fuhrman says, "some of these high-protein-diet gurus claim that they have the truth [about the value of eating meat and animal products] and that there's a conspiracy among the 1,500 scientific studies that continue to point to the association between the consumption of meat, eggs, and dairy products and cancer, heart disease, kidney failure, constipation, gall-stones, and hemorrhoids, just to name a few. They are overlooking the fact that you must pay a price with your health for eating increased animal proteins as a way to lose weight."

"Of course, there is one good point in what these people say," he adds. "It's true that refined carbohydrates such as pasta, bread, sugar, sweets, candies, bagels, croissants, potato chips, and all the junk food that Americans eat are not doing us any good. This junk now constitutes about 50 percent of the American diet. We know that this food is linked to heart attacks, cancer, obesity, and diabetes. That is absolutely true."

However, the gurus "are taking the fact that these highly refined, low-fiber carbohydrates can cause increased insulin levels, obesity, and insulin resistance, showing that those are dangerous foods and then saying that therefore the diet should be low in carbohydrates and high in animal protein.

"But that's a jump that the nutritional and scientific literature doesn't make. As a matter of fact, there are no data showing that a person on a high-carbohydrate diet rich in unrefined carbohydrates, such as mangoes, cabbage, beans, legumes, and squash, is in any danger. In fact, many studies show that a diet centered on unrefined carbohydrates—vegetables, whole grains, legumes—will not raise blood sugar or insulin levels."

What people don't realize, Dr. Fuhrman continues, is the value of plant protein. "Compare a steak to broccoli, for example. Let's look at the protein comparison for 100 calories of steak and 100 calories of broccoli. Sirloin steak has 5.4 grams of protein for 100 calories, and broccoli has 11.2 grams. In other words, green vegetables are very rich in protein. Beans are very rich in protein. We can devise a diet that is very low in animal fat or totally vegetarian, but with a good, satisfactory amount of healthy protein.

"People have to realize that there is a big biochemical difference between animal and plant protein. Plant protein lowers cholesterol; animal protein raises cholesterol. Plant protein is a protector against cancer; animal protein is a cancer promoter. Plant protein promotes bone strength; animal protein promotes bone loss. Plant protein has no effect on aging or kidney disease, and animal protein accelerates both of them. In other words, plant protein is packaged along with fiber, phytochemicals, vitamin E, and omega-3 fatty acids. Animal protein is packaged with saturated fat, cholesterol, and arachidonic acid."

Therefore, "if you are on a diet such as the Atkins diet or another high-protein diet in order to lose weight, you are paying a price with, for example, the risk of increased cancer."

In Dr. Fuhrman's opinion, after studying the food recommendations of these diets, "I suspect that a person really following one of these high-protein diets that restrict fruit and carotenoid-rich starches—found in foods such as sweet potatoes, corn, and squash—could be more than doubling her risk of colon cancer.

"There are studies that show a clear and dose-responsive relationship between increased cancers of the digestive tract and low fruit consumption. High fruit consumption has a powerful dose-response relationship to reduction of mortality from all causes of death. The only other food that even approaches this powerful effect of reducing cancer is raw vegetable consumption. So I suggest that if you are going to average 60 to 70 percent of your calories from fat and animal products with no fruit, you have to consider that diet exceedingly dangerous."

THE BLOOD-TYPE DIET

Other popular diets advocate eating according to a person's blood type. These diets have sold many books, and the authors have appeared on all the shows. The authors say, "It's your blood type. You have to eat this for your blood type." I've seen a ton of scientific evidence that could disprove that and show its lack of validity. So why is that approach not being challenged by the American public or the media?

According to Dr. Fuhrman, these diets are popular because they give free rein to people's ingrained bad habits: "I think it reinforces what people want to believe. People are addicted to their rich diets. They are looking to hang on to any reason, however irrational it may be, not to have to change.

"If you talk to smokers, you'll see the same thing. You'll hear how irrational are the reasons they give for why they must still smoke and how they have diminished in their own minds the strong reasons against smoking. The same is true with eating. People want to rationalize why it is okay to do whatever they are addicted to.

"The American addiction to such things as junk foods is such that when you stop doing it, you get uncomfortable. The problem is that the American diet is so toxic and so unhealthy that when people try to go off it, when they skip a meal and start eating fruits and vegetables, they feel sick. They get headaches and abdominal cramps. They get shakes and confusion. Then they think that it must be this new diet. It must be that eating healthily is making them sick. They must need this rich animal-fat protein and the junk food. In other words, they don't see that this is a temporary phase that lasts a week or two, when they are withdrawing from caffeine and the rich nitrogenous waste. You might feel a little ill when you change your diet. That slight resistance to change is one basis of people's addiction to harmful foods, and it makes them turn to these quack diets."

Research Update

An increasing body of evidence is showing the benefits of natural modalities to overall health and well-being. Following is a sample of recent peer-reviewed scientific studies related to eating disorders.

Publishing in *Disability and Rehabilitation* in 2014, researchers found that aerobic exercise, yoga, massage, and basic body awareness therapy significantly lowered scores of eating pathology and depressive symptoms in patients with anorexia and bulimia nervosa. A 2010 study published in the *Journal of Adolescent Health* determined that an eight week trial of individualized yoga treatment in conjunction with biweekly physician and/or dietician appointments decreased eating disorder symptoms in adolescents. Researchers concluded in *Nutrition and Clinical Practice*, also in 2010, that assessment by a nutrition professional via food intake history may be more practical than laboratory tests and more accurate than current food intake for determining potential micronutrient deficiencies in people with anorexia and bulimia.

Chapter 32

Endometriosis

Endometriosis is a condition in which the glands and tissues that line the inside of the uterus grow outside the uterine wall. Normally, cells build up in the uterus each month in preparation for pregnancy, serving as a nest for an incoming embryo. When pregnancy does not occur, the lining is shed and appears as menstrual flow. In endometriosis, endometrial-type cells may attach themselves to the fallopian tubes, ovaries, urinary bladder, intestinal surfaces, rectum, part of the colon, and other structures in the area.

Current estimates indicate that 6 to 10 percent of reproductive age women in the United States have endometriosis. This amounts to approximately five million women. A 2011 study found that 11 percent of a group of women with no symptoms actually had the condition, suggesting that the number could be even higher. Endometriosis is one of the most common causes of pelvic pain and infertility in women.

Causes

The exact cause of the condition remains a mystery, though several theories exist. Many researchers agree that endometriosis is exacerbated by estrogen. Following are some possible causal explanations:

RETROGRADE MENSTRUATION—Blood flows backward instead of downward through the cervix and out of the body. It is thought to go out the fallopian tubes and into the pelvic and abdominal cavity. Once it is there, cells from the exiting blood implant themselves outside the uterus onto other tissues.

LYMPHATIC CHANNELS—Cells of the endometrium lining pass through lymphatic channels or migrate via blood and then implant themselves outside the uterine cavity.

GENETIC PREDISPOSITION—Certain families are predisposed to the condition.

IMMUNOLOGIC DISORDER—The immune system is deficient in some way, causing tissue to proliferate in abnormal areas. The idea is that through some type of immune deficiency, hormonal and chemical influences cause endometrial tissue to become activated at different times in the cycle.

CHILDBEARING—Childbearing in combination with methods of contraception may be responsible.

Symptoms

Dian Shepperson Mills, a nutritionist and tutor at the Institute for Optimal Nutrition in London, is the author of *Endometriosis: A Key to Healing through Nutrition*. She explains that endometrial implants cause a problem "because the endometrium is designed to shed blood at the end of every month if a pregnancy has not been achieved. So these endometric implants, which are scattered around on the bowel and the bladder and so on, do likewise; they shed blood. When you are having a normal period, the blood comes out of the body down the vagina. However, with endometriosis, the implants bleed into the abdominal cavity, and the blood is trapped there because it has no exit. Thus, people with endometriosis have considerable pain.

"We also think that the reaction going on in the body, which is trying to remove the implants that the body's immune system knows should not be there, may affect people's fertility in some way, although we don't know how. It's believed that it is mainly the chemical secretions by the immune cells that are trying to remove the endometrium that are affecting the sperm or the ova."

Endometriosis can produce slight to severe pain, ranging from mild cramps to agony and dysfunction. About 70 percent of women with endometriosis have severe, chronic symptoms. Endometrial implants produce chemicals, including prostaglandins, which cause the uterus to contract, resulting in cramping. Pain also results from swelling, inflammation, and scarring of affected tissues. It is usually cyclical and most commonly occurs just before menstruation. Some women have pain during sexual intercourse any time in the month.

Where and to what degree pain is felt depend on the location of the endometrial tissue and the degree to which it has spread outside the uterus. Some women have pain during urination as a result of implants on the bladder. Some have pain during bowel movements because of colon and rectal implants. There can be ovarian pain or pain radiating to the back or buttocks or down the legs. Upon manual gynecological examination, there may be pelvic pain.

Internal bleeding may occur as well as nose bleeding or bleeding from another orifice at certain times of the month. Any cyclic bleeding is suspect for endometriosis. Other symptoms that sometimes appear include aggravated premenstrual syndrome (PMS), bladder infections, fatigue, and lower back pain.

Clinical Experience

DIAGNOSIS

Endometriosis may be suspected in the presence of one or more of the symptoms listed above, but the only real way to confirm a diagnosis is with a surgical procedure known as laparoscopy, which allows the doctor to actually see and biopsy tissue. Sonograms and magnetic resonance imaging (MRI) scans may be helpful, but they are not definitive in making the diagnosis.

The proper diagnosis is important, notes Dr. Anthony Aurigemma, because while endometriosis is considered benign, it can become malignant.

CONVENTIONAL THERAPY

Treatment usually consists of medical prescriptions for pain control and reduction of endometrial growth. Antiprostaglandin medicines such as indomethacin, ibuprofen, and naproxen are often given to reduce pain.

Another popular pharmaceutical, danazol, is also used for this purpose, but in some women it does not provide total or lasting relief. Studies show that danazol has a good effect after surgery to remove adhesions. After some of the adhesions have been removed, it may help an infertile woman become pregnant. A side effect of the drug is that it may increase cholesterol, especially the low-density lipoprotein (LDL) variety, which is implicated in accelerated arteriosclerosis. The adverse effects of all these drugs can include weight gain, edema, decreased or increased breast size, acne, excess hair growth on the face, and perhaps even in a developing fetus, and deepening of the voice.

Hormones are sometimes given to fool the body into believing it is pregnant, since pregnancy seems to retard or prevent the development of endometriosis. This method appears to have some benefit, but the side effects include depression, painful breasts, nausea, weight gain, bloating, swelling, and migraine headaches. Since the side effects can be fairly severe, this is not a popular method.

Newer drugs, called gonadotropin-releasing hormone compounds, are sometimes given by injection. These agents suppress pituitary gland release of the female hormones follicle-stimulating hormone (FSH) and luteinizing hormone (LH), causing what is called a clinical pseudomenopause. They help reduce pain in many women and decrease the size and volume of endometrial tissue after surgery.

Through the advanced surgical technique of female reconstructive surgery (FRS) developed by Dr. Vicki Hufnagel, the uterus and ovaries can be repositioned, thus reducing the deep pelvic pain that is associated with endometriosis.

ALTERNATIVE THERAPIES

PAIN RELIEF

"When I started looking at nutrition for the endocrine system," Mills says, "I came across a lot of research that suggests that if you are deficient in various nutrients, it may affect the way your body deals with pain. These nutrients would be the essential fatty acids, such as evening primrose oil, fish oil, linseed oil, safflower oil, and vitamins C, E, and K. All these are important in the body's control of pain. The B vitamins, particularly B1, seem to be important in building up the endorphins, which are the body's natural painkillers. There is also an amino acid called DLPA, which is DL-phenylalanine, which seems to help in dulling pain, and there are zinc, selenium, and magnesium."

If you are deficient in many of these nutrients, your body may not be able to cope well with pain. Mills says, "If we look at, say, magnesium, we see that it is very important in allowing muscles to relax. Calcium and magnesium balance one another. Calcium causes muscles to contract, and magnesium allows them to relax. Seeing that the uterus is one of the largest muscles in the body, it would be quite important to make sure you are getting enough magnesium-rich foods, such as green leafy vegetables, nuts, and seeds. The same is true of B vitamins.

There are lots of those in vegetables and fruits. That's also where you'll get vitamin C. Zinc is found in nuts and seeds. Selenium is in seafood."

DIGESTION AND THE REPRODUCTIVE SYSTEM

"Once I have a patient who has a major endometriosis problem," Mills says, "the first thing I look at is her digestion. If she doesn't get the nutrients from food or any supplements she takes, nothing will work. So you have to heal the digestion first. If she has constipation or diarrhea or heartburn indigestion, I will give her digestive enzymes, acidophilus, and possibly slippery elm. Then, once we've got that healed, you can try a digestive supplement, such as a multivitamin, and some magnesium, zinc, and vitamin C.

"You have to analyze what is wrong with each individual person and tailor the treatment specifically to her needs. Generally, for endometriosis, I try to ensure that the woman is taking evening primrose and fish oil. The supplements must also be wheat-, yeast-, sugar-, and dairy-free. By taking magnesium, zinc, the probiotics, and the digestive enzymes, you are working through the body system from different angles to try to relieve the pain while supporting the endocrine and immune systems."

NATUROPATHY

Dr. Tori Hudson, a naturopath from Portland, Oregon, believes there is most support for the immunological weakness theory of endometriosis because women with this condition have altered immune cells and fewer T lymphocytes. By improving immune function with supplements, diet, and botanicals, she claims to help many patients: "I've seen women with severe pelvic pain who were scheduled for surgery one month from the date I saw them. My treatment helped them recover completely without the surgery." She adds that most, but not all, women respond to her protocol, which is designed to stimulate a maximal immune response. The basic program consists of the following:

- Antioxidants
- Vitamin C—to bowel tolerance, up to 10,000 mg
- Beta-carotene—30,000 IU
- Selenium—400 mcg
- Vitamin E—400–1,200 IU

Changes in the diet are made to further stimulate the immune system. This is accomplished by lowering fat; adding whole grains, vegetables, and fruits; and eliminating immune system inhibitors such as coffee, sugar, alcohol, and high-fat foods. Foods such as cheese and meat have high amounts of estrogen and are omitted, because estrogen aggravates the disease. A mostly vegetarian diet is best for lowering estrogen and stimulating the immune system.

Two botanical formulas are included. One contains chaste tree berry, dandelion root, motherwort, and prickly ash in equal amounts. One half-teaspoon is taken three times daily. The other formula contains small doses of toxic herbs that must be carefully prescribed by a naturopathic physician.

In addition, Dr. Hudson sometimes prescribes natural progesterone made from wild yam. The wild yam extract is converted in the laboratory to natural progesterone.

OTHER NUTRITIONAL RECOMMENDATIONS

Dr. Susan M. Lark, a physician who is the author of *The Women's Health Companion: Self-Help Nutrition Guide & Cookbook*, recommends vitamins, herbs, and minerals that will decrease estrogen stimulation of the endometrial cells.

VITAMIN A—In the form of beta-carotene, a maximum daily dose of 5,000 IU to help decrease the excess menstrual bleeding that may occur with endometriosis.

VITAMIN B COMPLEX—50 to100 milligrams with an additional dose of up to 300 mg daily of vitamin B_6. These vitamins help the liver convert excess estrogen into less stimulating forms.

VITAMIN C—1000–4000 milligrams of bioflavonoids daily. Vitamin C not only regulates estrogen levels but also reduces cramps and bleeding by strengthening capillaries. You can get bioflavonoids by eating citrus fruits (including the inner peel), berries, the skins of grapes, alfalfa, buckwheat, and soybeans and taking 800 milligrams a day of vitamin C as a supplement.

VITAMIN E—400–2,000 IU daily. If you have high blood pressure, begin with 100 IU and work up to the higher levels gradually. Vitamin E helps even out the effects of high levels of estrogen.

ESSENTIAL FATTY ACIDS—Essential fatty acids (EFAs), including linoleic and linolenic acids, are the source for the manufacture of prostaglandins, which prevent cramping of muscles and blood vessels. Good sources of EFAs are raw seeds, especially flax seed, nuts, salmon, mackerel, and trout. They can also be taken as dietary supplements.

HERBS—100 milligrams daily maximum dose of fennel, anise, blessed thistle, black cohosh, and false unicorn root works to restore hormonal balance. You can also use white willow bark and meadowsweet to reduce pain, fever, cramps, and inflammation of the endometrial implants. Be sure to follow the directions on the label, since these herbs can cause an upset stomach and diarrhea.

ASIAN MEDICINE

The late Dr. Roger Hirsch, a naturopathic doctor in California who specialized in Asian medicine, said that the Chinese diagnose endometriosis by looking at the way the blood flows in the body, specifically in the pelvic cavity. This is determined by the appearance of the root of the tongue, which represents the pelvic cavity. "If a woman has endometriosis, there will be raised bumps and papillae in the back of the tongue and perhaps a greasy yellow coating," Dr. Hirsch said. "If you look at the back of your tongue in the mirror and see raised bumps that are red and fiery, especially during the time of menstruation, you may well have endometriosis."

HELLERWORK

Hellerwork is a bodywork technique derived from Rolfing. Both modalities use deep tissue work to improve body structure, but Hellerwork is different in that it is not painful. Certified Hellerwork practitioner Sarah Suatoni gives an overview of the process: "There are three components to Hellerwork. There is a hands-on part, which feels much like a massage; a movement educational aspect; and a mind-body dialogue aspect.

Suatoni describes each component. "In the hands-on process, we analyze the body much as a chiropractor would, looking at the posture, or the structure, as we call it, to determine which parts of the body are out of balance. We look to see which myofascial tissue connections are creating this misalignment. Then we work with our hands to release it.

"The second part of the work is movement education, in which we do very simple everyday movements. We look at how a person sits or stands. In the case of computer programmers, we look at how they sit at the computer and use their arms. We look at whatever it is that may be contributing to the dysfunction in the body, and then we begin to look at how we can have the person move in a way that will not create the same problem."

The third component is mind-body dialogue. "We work under the belief that our emotional patterns, memories, and attitudes are reflected in our bodies," Suatoni says. "In the same way one needs to look at a movement pattern in order to shift some sort of physical dysfunction, one needs to look at emotional patterns or beliefs in order to shift those as well.

"This work is a process where people come in for eleven sessions. Once a week for an hour and a half is ideal, although other time frames are possible. Each session touches upon a different part of the body and different aspects of the being."

Suatoni tells how she began using Hellerwork to treat endometriosis and similar chronic conditions: "I met Dr. David Kaufman, a urologist, who determined that women with interstitial cystitis had severe spasm of the pelvic muscles. He has since started working with patients with endometriosis, vulvodynia, vestibulitis, and a number of other conditions that show the same symptoms of severe spasm or contraction. Dr. Kaufman was using biofeedback and felt that he needed someone who did hands-on work to accompany the biofeedback treatments. That's how I began.

"Although this process deals with mind-body relationships, this does not imply that these diseases are imaginary. Some women have been told for years that their disease is all in their head, when there are all kinds of physical evidence for the disease. Rather, the disease is the result of a set of relationships between the mind and body. Hellerwork and other forms of bodywork help because they are process-oriented and look at relationships. Once women start understanding these relationships, they find that they have a whole lot of power to overcome disease and regain health."

HOMEOPATHY

Homeopathy is another holistic therapy that addresses underlying emotional causes. Dr. Aurigemma has been treating his patients homeopathically for ten years and claims that the therapy is completely safe and highly effective. "There is no doubt in my mind that something actually happens and that it helps people," he says. "I utilize the remedies because I see them work. What spurs me on is the continuous improvement of most of the patients I see."

PATIENT STORY

One woman came to see me who was on prescription narcotic medication for the pain. The medicine gave her no relief, and she was at the point of wanting a hysterectomy to get relief from the pain. I put this woman on a natural hygienic regimen for a couple of weeks. First she fasted for five days. Then she followed up with a nutritional plan.

Let me briefly describe a typical hygienic regimen. The patient has a breakfast consisting of a vegetable juice or a vegetable and fruit juice combination, a blended salad, a piece of fruit, perhaps some hot cereal, and a couple of soft-boiled egg yolks. Lunch is a vegetable juice or vegetable and fruit juice combination, a blended salad, a cup or a little more than that, a piece of fruit, and then some raw nuts or unsalted raw-milk cheese. For the evening meal the patient starts with juice again, blended salad, tossed salad, and steamed vegetables such as string beans, broccoli, or escarole. Then she goes on with the main course, which includes a steamed potato or yam, natural brown rice or another whole grain, and a legume. I also might supplement the meal with egg or cheese, depending on the protein needs of the woman. Of course, there are variations for individual patients.

After following this general plan, this patient was pain-free at the end of a month. That was ten years ago. Right now she is pregnant with her second child, whereas before she was infertile. Natural hygiene has tremendous implications for endometriosis. There is absolutely no reason why a woman should have pain or be infertile because of such a simple condition.

From my perusal of the literature I can see that endometriosis is plainly a condition of liver toxicity, where the liver is failing to completely break down the estrogen hormones the body is manufacturing. These breakdown products wreak havoc in the form of endometrial tissue in the pelvic cavity.

—*Dr. Anthony Penepent*

Research Update

An increasing body of evidence is showing the benefits of natural modalities to overall health and well-being. Following is a sample of recent peer-reviewed scientific studies relating to endometriosis.

In a 2013 report in *Angiogenesis*, researchers found that green tea epigallocatechin-3-gallate significantly slowed the development and growth of endometriosis in mice, indicating that it could be a powerful agent against the disease. A study in *Human Reproduction* published in 2013 concluded that resveratrol is a potent inhibitor of vascularization and cell proliferation in experimental endometriosis. In *Reproductive Sciences* (2013), the traditional Chinese medicine Wenshen Xiaozheng Tang was shown to inhibit production of proinflammatory cytokines and regulate the expression of invasion-related genes in lesions associated with endometriosis.

Chapter 33

Environmental Illness

Environmental illness was first recognized more than five decades ago, but mainstream medicine still generally disregards this syndrome. When patients come in with the symptoms of sensitivity to a toxic environment, doctors often do not know the correct protocol. Standardized blood tests appear normal, leading them to assume that no problem exists.

Another issue is that most doctors today are not trained to work with a disease that affects the whole body. Heather Millar, author of *The Toxic Labyrinth* and former sufferer of environmental illness, notes, "In the medical community we have created a world of specialists. Physicians are now neurologists, cardiologists, rheumatologists, and so on. We have gotten away from the old-fashioned approach. We no longer have a large percentage of general practitioners. Before, you would go to a doctor's office and tell him your history from start to finish. He would look at you as a whole individual, checking the psychological as well as the physical aspect of the body. Only then would he make an assessment.

"Now technology has compartmentalized the body. The neurologist looks only at the symptoms of numbness, tingling, and headaches. The rheumatologist looks only at arthritis, joint pain, and aches. The infectious disease doctor looks only for infection. What happened to me was, I would go in and give a detailed history of what was happening. The doctor, according to his specialty, would look only at one specific area. He or she did not want to hear about the other symptoms I had.

"What we are failing to realize with all this supertechnology in medicine is that the body works in harmony. You do not have one body system that works separately from something else. They all work together. So if you are having symptoms in one system, you are probably having symptoms elsewhere."

PATIENT STORY

I started becoming ill a year before I realized what was happening. At first I just thought I was tired. I was having trouble getting out of bed. I was dragging myself to work. I would come home feeling exhausted. Sometimes I had asthma like symptoms and couldn't quite catch my breath. I wondered why this started all of a sudden when I was thirty years old, because my understanding was that most people develop asthma as children. I attributed these symptoms to working and living a fast-paced lifestyle, and I ignored them. One day my wrist started to ache for no apparent reason, which made me wonder if I was getting arthritis. But I ignored that as well and thought it would go away. I had these warning signs for a year before collapsing at work.

I had woken up feeling as if I had the flu but thought I was well enough to go to work. I had gone shopping with my mom that morning and had had difficulty walking up stairs. When I arrived at work, I realized that I was feeling quite unwell and that I would be able to work only part of my nursing shift. At the end of the first hour, I needed to go home because I was too ill to walk down the corridor and deliver medications to my patients. It was then that I returned to the nursing station and collapsed. I could hear, but I couldn't move. I felt as if I were paralyzed. I couldn't communicate with the other nurses who came to attend to me.

They took me to the emergency room, but I started to feel better and went home. I decided that I had the flu and that I would be better in three days.

Three days of flu evolved into a year and a half. During this time, I experienced many difficulties. The problem with environmental illness or chemical sensitivity is that you have a wide array of symptoms that come and go. You don't really know where to start and what connections to make. These are some of the symptoms I experienced:

Flu symptoms plagued me every day and became worse with time. As time passed, I was having more difficulty getting out of bed and walking around the house. I was extremely tired. No matter how much I slept, I just could not seem to get enough sleep. Even small tasks that shouldn't take much energy overwhelmed me. Cooking a meal was too much to even think about.

I also started having disturbed sleep. Despite my fatigue, I would wake up between two and four o'clock each night with numb hands. Sometimes I would have an incredible thirst. And sometimes I would wake up shaking as if I had a very high fever.

At one point I lost sight in my right eye. This happened for a short time but was extremely frightening nonetheless. All of a sudden, the vision in my right eye became completely silver, as if I were trying to look through a piece of tinfoil.

I had headaches with stabbing pains in my temples and a burning sensation in the back of my neck that made it difficult to turn my head. If you try to drive a car or move to do something, you realize how important it is to have range of motion in your neck.

The next month, I started to experience food allergies. It started with a few things. First I wasn't tolerating wheat very well and stopped eating it. Then I noticed that I did not feel well after drinking coffee and milk, so I eliminated them also. As the months progressed, I was unable to tolerate more and more foods. By January, I was virtually down to two foods: lamb and yams. By February, I lost my tolerance for everything. I was caught in a vicious cycle. I knew I needed to get nutrition in order to turn my health around, but eating these foods would make me even sicker.

As I became increasingly ill, my sense of smell became more and more acute. All of a sudden perfumes were a problem. I absolutely hated going to the department store and passing the perfume counter. I couldn't stand the smell of car exhaust either. I even avoided the hardware store because of the strong smell in there. Going to public places became difficult, as many people wear scented products such as clothes washed in scented laundry detergents, perfumes, and aftershaves. I would walk into a room, and if someone had perfume on, I would suddenly feel like I had the worst flu. My shoulders and muscles would start to ache. I would feel short of breath. I would get a headache.

A heightened sense of smell is part of the illness. People who are not affected need to understand what is happening when individuals with environmental illness ask, "Please do not wear that fragrance because it makes me feel sick."

I also started to have ringing in my ears. That would come and go, so I never could associate it with any particular event. Sometimes it would affect one ear, sometimes both. It was bothersome trying to have a conversation with somebody and trying to hear that person over the ringing in my ears.

Additionally, I felt dizzy. I had days when it was even difficult for me to stand up and navigate my way to the bathroom. Several times I fell over.

One of the most disturbing symptoms I had was difficulty concentrating. I could no longer read something from start to finish. It would take me three to four tries to read material I should have comprehended in the first reading.

I also noticed that I was forgetful. Previously I had had an exceptional memory. All of a sudden I noticed that I couldn't remember things that were extremely important. At age thirty I was wondering if I was getting the beginning stages of Alzheimer's disease, the loss of memory was so apparent. Some days my memory was better than others, and some days my ability to concentrate was better than others.

Then there were the panic attacks. My heart would race while I was driving my car on the interstate. I did not understand why I felt better on residential streets. Later, I real-

ized that I had difficulty on the interstate because the exhaust was so much more preva-lent there. Every time I was exposed to exhaust, my heart raced; I felt anxious and had difficulty concentrating.

I also felt extremely anxious in shopping malls. I have since learned that there are extremely high levels of chemicals in shopping malls, such as formaldehyde, emitted by new building materials. These synthetics are highly toxic. What I couldn't understand was why I felt anxious at some times and not others. The reason was that some shopping malls are less toxic than others, and some stores, because of the types of merchandise they carry, are also better than others.

The day I collapsed at work was the last day I worked as a nurse. I kept assuming that within a month I would feel better and go back to my job. One month rolled into two, two months into three, and three months into a year and a half.

Being a nurse, I felt that I would receive the support I needed. After all, I was a med-ical person myself. What I experienced instead was how a patient feels when he or she is told that nothing is wrong. I had always been on the other side of things. I found this new perspective extremely alarming.

The medical community has become technologically based. Everything relies on a diag-nostic test. I would go in, and they would run a gamut of tests. As with most people with environmental illness, the standard tests would come back negative. The doctors would then tell me that there was nothing wrong. This was disturbing because I was extremely ill. I was so sick that I could hardly get up off the couch. Nor could I make myself a meal. Going to the bathroom was an effort. How, on a diagnostic test, could I look perfectly normal?

When the doctors could not diagnose me, they said that I was suffering from stress. But this was not the case. Before I got sick, my life was wonderful. I had one of the least pres-sured jobs I had ever had, and I was enjoying what I was doing. At the end of a contract I would go on vacation to Europe for a month. I was about to get married. My life couldn't have been better.

Stress is becoming the catchall diagnosis in the medical community. We must ask why so many people in our society are being told that they have stress, panic disorder, anxiety, and depression. That category is growing larger and larger. People have to ask: Why is this happening in our society? Is something chemical bringing this on? Do we need to make changes in the environment?

If you are feeling some symptoms of toxicity, it is time to take action now. Don't wait until you end up, as I did, in a wheelchair, bedridden, and completely intolerant to food.

—Heather Millar

Causes

Dr. Stephen M. Silverman of Port Washington, New York, says that thousands of poisons in our food, water, and surroundings are responsible for environmental illness: "The first thing you must realize is that what you eat can have a tremendous effect on your immune system. One of the most toxic foods that people expose themselves to unknowingly, for example, is hydrogenated oil. People don't realize how widespread that ingredient is. It's in crackers, all commercial breads, potato chips, pretzels, and cookies, and it has a very strong damaging effect on the immune system.

"Along with what you eat, you must consider what you drink. Most people are being exposed to tap water, whether directly from the sink or outside when they buy a cup of coffee or tea. Probably one of the highest exposures to carcinogens comes from this source. . . . Ralph Nader's group identified over 2,000 chemicals commonly found in people's drinking water. When water is tested over the course of the year, it is tested for approximately 120 chemicals. When you are told that the water is safe to drink, it means that it is safe with respect to what it was tested for. You have no idea about the other 1,900 chemicals. Insecticides and pesticides in the water have been associated with Long Island's high rate of breast cancer. Certainly, if they can create cancer, they can cause immune system damage."

Skin and hair care products may be another source of environmental illness. "Among the other factors that can set you up for illness are the things you put on your body," Dr. Silverman says. "I am talking about cosmetics, moisturizers, and hair sprays. We know through medical applications of the nicotine and estrogen patches that what you put on your skin will be absorbed into the bloodstream. If you were to take a look at the ingredients in your cosmetics, hair sprays, and underarm deodorants, you would see that they are loaded with chemicals. You have to realize that when you use these chemicals every day, they eventually get into the bloodstream. When you think about it, is it possible that these chemicals have no effect on your immune system? It's almost impossible."

According to the late environmental medicine specialist Dr. Marshall Mandell, "There is absolutely no question that environmental factors play a major role in many diseases; where they do not actually start the disease, they can complicate it. Anything that makes your illness worse is important for you to know about."

In the same way that cocaine goes right from the nose of the user to the nervous system in a matter of seconds, producing a wide variety of effects, toxins in food or air produce a range of effects in the systems of highly sensitive individuals. Conventional physicians and traditional allergists simply miss this phenomenon by recognizing only a very limited range of symptoms. If their patients aren't sneezing or itching, they will not recognize the possibility that an allergy may be present. But logically, once a doctor recognizes that minute flecks of animal dander or pollen in the air can produce marked symptoms, is it so difficult to see that chemical toxins in meat or milk or air pollution, among a host of other possible causes, might also have an adverse effect?

Simply put, the human race has evolved over millions of years and has adapted to most of the conditions on this planet. But many of the pollutants and toxins we are dealing with have arisen over the last thirty to fifty years. Our bodies just haven't had time to evolve in response to these changes in our environment. Unless we act sensibly by at least recognizing this discrepancy, we may cause great damage to our environment and ourselves.

Whatever you breathe in enters your body along with the oxygen. If your home, work, or school environment is polluted, the pollutants will travel through the walls of the lungs, go into the blood vessels of the lungs, and ultimately reach the heart through the pulmonary circulation. Similarly, chemicals, additives, and contaminants in our food and beverages will pass through the digestive system and reach the heart. Once there, they will be pumped through the bloodstream. Every tissue in your body is exposed to what you eat, drink, and breathe. That is why so many people are sick today.

"Research shows that women are more prone to environmental illnesses," says Heather Millar. "The reason is that many chemicals, such as formaldehyde, benzene, phenols, and chlorine, have estrogen-mimicking properties. These chemicals take the place of estrogen in the body. The body thinks it has enough estrogen and doesn't make enough. Estrogen is responsible for reproduction as well as many other vital functions in the body. Problems occur when the body calls upon the estrogen it thinks it has but doesn't.

"Silicone breast implants are making women terribly ill. They have a tendency to grow fungus inside the implant, which adds a problem to an already existing one. Fungus is extremely hard to get rid of once it starts to grow. After breast implants are removed, women do not feel better. This indicates that their immune systems have been damaged. It will probably take a very long time for them to recover, and we do not know the long-term effects."

Symptoms

Symptoms vary with a woman's constitution and may include fatigue, aching muscles, a flu-like feeling, ringing in the ears, burning eyes, headaches, migraines, disturbed sleep, shortness of breath, food allergies, a heightened sense of smell, loss of balance, inability to concentrate, memory loss, anxiety, panic attacks, depression, and irritable bowel syndrome. There is a marked progressive debilitating reaction to consumer products such as perfumes, soap, tobacco smoke, and plastics.

Clinical Experience

DIAGNOSIS

In her book, Heather Millar has a checklist to help people determine whether they may be suffering from environmental illness. These are some questions she asks people to consider:

- Do I have a toxic lifestyle?
- Does my environment contain chemicals that could be making me sick?
- Do I feel ill at work?
- Do I feel ill at home?
- Do I live in a new home?
- Have I recently painted or installed a new carpet?
- How much plastic do I have in the home?
- Does my neighborhood contain chemicals that could be making me sick?

"Discovering the cause of the problem is a detective process," Millar says. "It involves taking a close look at your home, workplace, and neighborhood.

In the home there are several factors to address. "You may ask," Millar says, "'Why didn't we have these problems before? We always painted our house and put new carpet in.' What I'd like to suggest is that technology has changed a lot of chemicals and manufacturing processes. Since the 1980s we have added more synthetics and are now seeing their effects. A lot of these products emit gas. The newness smell is a gas that is coming off. Basically, it's a chemical soup that is very hazardous to our health. Also, since we live in energy-efficient buildings, we do not have the ventilation needed to lessen the concentration of these gases.

"Plastics present further problems. They have a lot of these estrogen-mimicking properties. Softer plastics have more toxicity. We used to live with metal, wood, and glass. These are far safer alternatives. When replacing plastic with wood, consider the type of finish on it. Does it smell?"

After evaluating what's going on at home, turn your attention to the workplace. Millar says, "Ask yourself, what are you doing as an occupation? Are you working with chemicals on an ongoing basis? Or are you working in an energy-efficient office building that was recently renovated? Is it currently being renovated? Does it have no open windows? Do other people in the office frequently get colds and flu or feel unwell?"

The neighborhood should also be examined. "Where do you live?" Millar says. "Do you have chemical manufacturing in your backyard? Is there some kind of toxic incinerator nearby? What is in your water supply? What kinds of pesticide regulations does your neighborhood have?

"You may react differently to toxins in your environment than your coworkers do. For example, in my workplace, which was extremely toxic, my symptoms were mainly neurological. Other colleagues were diagnosed with chronic fatigue. Still others experienced asthma or fibromyalgia, which is an aching of the muscles. We react differently depending on our genetic predispositions."

Fortunately, there are physicians who do recognize the illness, and there are tests available to pinpoint the condition. Occupational health doctors and environmental physicians prescribe tests that look at solvent levels in the blood. They look at pesticide levels in the blood and check mineral levels, which are usually low in people who suffer from chemical exposures.

FOUR CLUES TO PROPER TREATMENT

Dr. Michael Schachter, a clinical ecologist, or environmental medicine specialist, identifies four contributing factors that he considers key in his examination and in determining a course of therapy: the quality of nutrition generally and the identification of any nutritional deficiencies, infections, psychological stresses, and toxicity. According to Dr. Schachter, the course of therapy should be determined by the condition of the patient in regard to these four criteria.

Dr. Schachter is also concerned with improving the oxygenation and energy utilization of the body at the cellular level. Anything we can do to improve that process is going to strengthen the immune system and thereby help reduce a person's tendency toward sensitivity and reactions. Thus, Dr. Schachter encourages the use of oxidant therapies, but only up to a point, since oxygen in too great quantities can have a damaging effect. The key here, as in virtually every area of health, is balance.

The first and foremost oxidant therapy must be aerobic exercise. Keeping in mind that oxygen is the main nutrient of the body, it is easy to understand that as we improve oxygenation, we improve the body's ability to detoxify and enhance the immune system. Beyond exercise, a number of new nutrients are available to enhance oxygenation, such as germanium and ubiquinone, as well as a variety of traditional oxygenation techniques.

Vitamins and minerals are another key component in Dr. Schachter's approach. He sees vitamin A as a major protective factor that guards against both chemical sensitivities and infections. Thus, cod liver oil, which parents once gave automatically to children, is indeed an excellent preventive medicine with its high concentrations of vitamins A and D. In treating children with recurrent ear infections, Dr. Schachter has found that by simply enhancing their diet, removing most of the sugar and refined foods, and adding a spoonful of cod liver oil, the ear infections can be controlled and prevented in many cases. Other useful vitamins include vitamin C, vitamin B_{12}, and vitamin E, which is an antioxidant. Selenium and beta-carotene are also important antioxidants. Vitamin B_{12} can help counteract the adverse effects in the body of pesticides in the environment. Moreover, while conventional physicians may test for vitamin B_{12} levels in the bloodstream, normal levels may be present in the blood while there are deficiencies at the cellular level.

According to Dr. Schachter, infections are a key factor in going from troubled to good health. Frequently, infections will yield to nontoxic treatments.

Take Candida, for example. Women who have repeatedly used antibiotics, include a lot of refined carbohydrates in their diet, and may have been exposed to steroids or birth control pills tend to develop a chronic overgrowth of Candida albicans, a yeastlike, funguslike organism that we all have in our bodies. In certain cases the infection will give off toxins that may impair the immune system and produce a variety of symptoms. Some of these symptoms will be the result of food and chemical sensitivities that have been aggravated by the infection.

Dr. Schachter has found that starting the patient on a special diet that excludes refined carbohydrates, especially sugars and alcohol, and includes various nutrients, especially certain fatty acids that inhibit candida growth, will go a long way toward controlling the infection in many cases. He also notes that garlic has strong anticandidal properties.

Chronic viral syndromes are another key problem. A previously healthy individual suddenly gets a flu and instead of recovering completely experiences frequent fatigue, exhaustion, swollen glands, sore throat, night sweats, anxiety, and loss of appetite. However, conventional testing shows nothing definite. More sophisticated testing may show exposure to various viruses, but the main problem here may be that the person's immune system just isn't responding as it should. Dr. Schachter has obtained excellent results in patients with this profile by using nutrients to bolster the immune system. Intravenous vitamin C may be used, along with germanium and a variety of other vitamins and minerals given orally. In cases of herpes virus, for example, he may use high doses of the amino acid lysine, which has antiviral effects for the herpes virus and certain other viruses. For short treatment periods, he may administer as much as 10 to 15 grams of lysine per day.

Psychological stress is another key factor, according to Dr. Schachter. Environmental medicine specialists, he warns, must be careful that in emphasizing the importance of the physical environment they do not underestimate the importance of psychological factors in determining the strength of an individual's immune system.

As for toxicity, Dr. Schachter feels that hydrocarbons and other chemicals are already playing a major role by damaging our immune systems, as are heavy metals. He sees chelation therapy as a valid treatment to detoxify our systems of the effects of heavy metals. Chelation therapy has also shown impressive results in patients with cardiovascular disease.

DETOXIFYING THE BODY

Without detoxifying the system, all other steps to repair the body will be of no avail. Dr. Zane Gard, an expert in toxicology, explains some methods of detoxification that have had impressive results in the reversal of environmental illness: "Heat stress detoxification includes wood saunas, hot sand packing, steam baths, and sweat lodges. The history of these approaches goes back several thousand years. Careful supervision is required. Heat stress detoxification can be effective but requires knowledge of toxins and their potential effects on the body. If it is not administered properly, there can be a lot of complications, and the patient can actually end up worse.

"The biotoxic reduction program was designed with the toxic-chemical-syndrome patient in mind. It is a comprehensive, medically managed program that addresses toxicology, psychology, neurology, pathology, and immunology. The program must be followed seven days a week, one to two hours a day, for a minimum of two weeks. It would be nice to have Saturday and Sunday off, but patients actually regress one or two days every time they take a day off during the first two weeks. So it has to be every day during that initial period."

Increasing niacin, aerobic exercise and sauna therapy also may be recommended. "With those who have neurological damage, other therapies will be needed," Dr. Gard says, "including one that stimulates the myelin sheaths of the nerves to regenerate. As a result, many peripheral neuropathies completely reverse. In more than eighty peripheral neuropathies, including multiple sclerosis (MS), we have only two patients who did not fully recover."

DETOXIFYING THE ENVIRONMENT

It is no longer enough to watch what we eat or the medicines we take; environmental toxins have become an unavoidable reality, especially for those living in densely populated urban areas. The very air we breathe on the streets or in our homes and offices can attack our health; noise pollution and artificial lighting add to the physical and mental stress of urban life.

The myth is that you should look for the big toxin. But it's the chronic, day-in, day-out exposure to small toxins that are really the concern. It may take decades—none of these environmental toxins, even asbestos, will knock you out right away—but you may pay for your lack of awareness with lung cancer, leukemia, arthritis, or heart disease down the line. Perhaps worst are the subtle symptoms of fatigue, anxiety, and minor nagging physical problems that many of us come to accept as a normal part of life.

Elimination of the unseen substances that attack your system stealthily, over time, is half of achieving good health. If you never use any supplementary vitamin, mineral, or herb but simply eliminate those factors that depreciate your health, you should be able to live to one hundred years of age in a healthy way. One group of people, nearly 70,0000 in number, in the north of Pakistan at the base of the Himalayas, often live well past ninety or even one hundred, putting in full days of work daily until they die. It may not be possible for all of us to live in the pure atmosphere of the Himalayas—not to mention emulating the diet, activities, and social structure of these people—but we can alter our environment realistically and functionally. A good place to start is where we live.

Dr. Alfred Zamm, a fellow of the American College of Allergists and the American College of Physicians, has written a book, *Why Your House May Endanger Your Health*, which explores the relationship between our homes and our well-being more thoroughly than we can here. Dr. Richard Podell also contributed to the discussion.

THE SICK BUILDING SYNDROME

The "sick house" is a relatively new development. Materials and methods used to construct houses have changed considerably since World War II; an extreme example is the energy-efficient office buildings built during the energy crisis of the 1970s, about which we'll have more to say later in this chapter. But not only are houses built with more emphasis on energy efficiency—which means heavy insulation and minimum ventilation to the outside—the construction materials themselves, as well as the furnishings (carpeting, fabrics, furniture) are new, often more convenient, cheaper, lighter synthetic compounds unheard of in prewar houses. The particleboard that is so useful in modern house and furniture construction exacts a price for this convenience; it is a silent time bomb, giving off invisible, odorless—but no less dangerous—vapors years after it is installed.

Formaldehyde is a major culprit in the modern house or office building. Particleboard, new synthetic carpets, insulation, many interior paints, and even permanent-press fabrics can give off formaldehyde. It is invisible and odorless except in high concentrations, but even quite low chronic levels can cause symptoms ranging from burning eyes and headaches to asthma and depression. New houses may be built largely of materials that vaporize formaldehyde for years; the worst culprits are mobile homes, which also are often poorly ventilated.

Another important factor in a house's potential toxicity is its source of heat. Combustion-heating appliances using natural gas, oil, coal, kerosene, or wood can all create afterburn by-products even if you can't see or smell them. Good ventilation can help, but this makes it harder to keep a house warm. Electric heat, though expensive, is the safest source.

What can be done about a toxic house? Some changes can be made in the furnishings, floor coverings, and ventilation and heating systems, but often much of the problem lies in structural components that would be expensive and difficult, if not impossible, to alter. Building your own house or having it built with attention to all the materials used is one solution if you can afford it or have the time and skill. If you are looking for a place to live, consider an older home. Prewar houses were often constructed of bricks, plaster, and hardwood, not the chemi-cally treated plywood, composite board, and other synthetic materials used almost universally now. If synthetic materials were used in an older house, they will have had years to emit their toxins. Often a house built before the energy crisis will allow more air circulation. Ceilings are often higher, allowing fumes to rise away from the inhabitants.

There may be disadvantages in an old house, however; molds and mildews may have accumulated over the years. Old carpet is a fertile ground for mold as well as accumulated dust, animal hair, and whatever toxins have been tracked in or sprayed over the years, but it can often be pulled up to reveal a hardwood floor. Outdated heating systems can usually be replaced without too much trouble.

If moving or rebuilding your house is not an option, you can still do a lot to detoxify your home. We'll identify the weak spots room by room.

THE GARAGE

An attached garage is like a toxic waste dump stuck to the side of your house. Many garages have heating and cooling systems that lead directly into the house; anything that can be absorbed through any crack or ventilation system will end up in the house. What's in the garage? The car, of course, and gasoline. Gasoline vaporizes. The afterburn fumes caused by inefficient burning of gasoline are mostly carbon dioxide, which has no odor and is invisible. Breathing these fumes results in headache, dizziness, and mood swings. (Think of people stuck in traffic jams, breathing the afterburn of all the cars around them for hours at a time.) When you park a hot car in the garage and close the door behind it, the hot oil in the engine is volatile and gets into the air. Park the car outside and wait for it to cool off before you bring it into the garage.

Other things you may keep in the garage—paint thinners and removers and turpentine—also vaporize easily and stay in the air for months at a time. If you smell a rag that was used for paint thinner three months ago, you will see that it is still giving off these fumes. Try to minimize the number of these substances in your garage. If you must keep them, use a small shed or garbage can outside the garage to store them. And the garage should be ventilated out, not into the house, with a suction fan. There should be no ducts from the garage into the house.

Your garage is probably where you keep chemicals you use on your lawn and garden: pesticides, fungicides, or herbicides, for instance. In the first place, do you really need them? Look at it this way. If it's going to kill an insect, a plant, or a mouse, it's a toxin and it can affect you, your pets, and your children. If you spray a weed killer on your lawn and then walk around on the lawn, you will repeatedly be bringing it inside on your feet. It doesn't just go away. Think of all the things you bring in on your feet and think, for instance, of your kids playing on the carpet, perhaps putting things into their mouths that have been on it.

Taken individually, none of these things is going to kill you, but be aware that everything you spray outside is likely to be in the air you breathe or will make its way back into your house and settle there. There's no real need to run this risk: We can use diatomaceous earth and natural biological controls or just weed without spraying.

THE BASEMENT

A typical basement in a private home is often damp. People like their lawns unencumbered by debris that might wash down from the gutters of the roof through the downspout, and so the downspout is kept close to the house. Thus the water runs off the roof, down the downspout, and into the ground directly by the foundation of the house. You might just as well run this water directly into the basement, since its walls are rarely waterproof. A little dampness in the basement is enough to support a healthy growth of mold, which can then permeate the house. A forced-air system of ventilation, which has ducts running to the basement, will create a vacuumlike effect that will suck particles of mold into the system, to be dispersed around the house.

Many people react to mold whether it is eaten or inhaled, a point that is obvious to anyone who begins to sneeze as soon as she walks into a damp basement. More insidiously, though, mold that is inhaled even in small quantities cross-reacts with mold that is ingested in food. This effect, known as concomitancy, means that a small quantity of inhaled mold that in itself would hardly cause a noticeable reaction will enhance sensitivity to foods that contain mold.

Any food made by fermentation can induce this reaction. Wine and vinegar are fermented fruit juice, cheese is fermented milk, yeast in bread ferments, and even mushrooms are in the mold family. Thus, it is easy to ingest mold three times a day, exacerbating our inability to tolerate the mold that has circulated upward from a damp basement. Obvious symptoms are sneezing and watering eyes, but allergic symptoms can also be systemic, making them harder to pin down to a specific source. Fatigue, headaches, depression, and even arthritis can have a basis in chronic allergic irritation.

In addition to water coming into the basement from the downspout, groundwater can flow down a hill toward the house, which then serves as a dam. You can place a drain field around the house using deco-drain piping in two tiers. Contact your local hardware store for more information. If a high water table is the problem, a sump pump is needed. Thoroseal, a dense cementlike material, can be applied to the outside block foundation as caulking to keep water out.

If the basement is still damp, a dehumidifier can help, but these work well only above a temperature of 50 to 60 degrees Fahrenheit. Chemicals such as baking soda are only temporary measures. The best way to remove the mold is to scrub the area with sulfur water. The basement can be hosed down and the water removed with an industrial vacuum.

THE KITCHEN

What's the most dangerous toxin in most kitchens? Gas. You should always have a vent in the kitchen; it has been shown that cerebral allergies are often directly attributable to the gas burnoff of pilot lights on stoves, which leak constantly. If you often have headaches and suspect that they are more common when you're spending time in the kitchen, try disconnecting your stove when you're not using it. If this makes a difference, you should consider replacing the gas stove with an electric one. Not only are gas ovens a health risk, microwave ovens can leak; a defective microwave creates a very unhealthy environment within about eight feet around it.

The freon in the condenser of the refrigerator is a highly volatile, dangerous chemical. It is a very good idea to replace refrigerators that are more than ten years old.

The refrigerator contributes to another seldom-considered form of pollution found especially in the kitchen: noise pollution. You should be able to tolerate background noise of about 30 to 35 decibels. Noise higher than 50 decibels becomes uncomfortable. Above 80 decibels, you become substantially irritated, and noise above 100 may cause ear damage or central nervous system overstimulation. The compressor in most refrigerators is up to 60 decibels. You don't appreciate this until you turn on a refrigerator when everything else is totally quiet. But think of a kitchen with a television or a radio on, things cooking, telephone conversations—you can't even hear the refrigerator, and the noise level may be up around 100 decibels. The kitchen is one of the most stressful places because of this level of background noise. Even if you are unable to replace appliances such as refrigerators and air conditioners with less noisy ones, you can cut down on the number of noisemakers you are using at the same time.

Street noise can be irritating in any room. Noise-buffering double-fold drapes can keep noise down as well as insulate.

Mold and mildew are common invisible toxins in a kitchen. When was the last time you changed the water tray in your refrigerator? Under the condenser coil is a tray to collect water, but it can also collect all kinds of mold. Mold spores are in the air all the time, and you're inhaling them. If you're sensitive and your immune system is low, you'll feel it: Your eyes will get puffy, your nose will clog, and your throat will get sore. Keeping this area clean and dry could make a big difference.

Look under your kitchen sink; you'll be amazed at the range of toxic chemicals you keep there, so close to your food. Cleansers, for instance, especially ammonia-based products, often vaporize easily. Ammonia is very toxic and will stay in your blood for hours after you've smelled it. When you wax the kitchen floor, the floor wax will evaporate and you will breathe it in. Try to install floors that will not need waxing, but if you don't want to tear up your current floors, you might want to settle for a matte finish rather than a high sheen if you have to constantly apply volatile chemicals to maintain that sheen. As with the weed killers and insecticides in your garage, there are alternatives to chemical cleaners in the kitchen. Apple cider vinegar and hydrogen peroxide mixed half and half in cold water do the same job as ammonia. This preparation will clean windows and glassware perfectly too.

Roach sprays are very stable. They can last for months and vaporize constantly. A dog or cat licking the floor can pick them up directly. A safer alternative is to use boric acid. You can mix it with sugar as a bait, but be sure pets and children can't reach it; line all the counters and fittings underneath with a strip of this no thicker than a pencil. This mixture is not volatile and is safe as long as it's put only in inaccessible places. Diatomaceous earth is safe and works well too. Or use the roach motels that use resin instead of poisons.

Aluminum-based cookware in which the aluminum can come into contact with food should not be used. Aluminum has been implicated in Alzheimer's disease. It is a heavy metal that lodges in the blood, brain tissue, and central nervous system, where it can cause motor problems. Aluminum foil is all right to store cooked food but should not be used in cooking, where it can oxidize in microscopic amounts. You can't see this, but it can get into your food and your body. Teflon and all other nonstick coatings should also be avoided. They easily scratch or flake off with age, getting into food as well as exposing it to the often inferior metal underneath.

Water from the kitchen tap may contain over a thousand chemicals, including those which the government puts in, such as fluoride; traces of herbicides and pesticides that have leached down into the water supply from fields; and traces of metal, rust, and molds from the inside of your pipes. Most water filtration systems can remove only a portion of these; the finer particles, including toxic chemicals such as pesticides, come through. If you live in a polluted area and your water supply is from underground streams, buy bottled water. I would buy plain distilled water. You get minerals from food; you don't need them from water. Since 72 to 74 percent of our bodies consist of water, we should be sure it is the purest water possible.

THE BATHROOM

One of the most common causes of allergy is what we put on our bodies: soaps, deodorants, and cosmetics. We use these things day in and day out, rarely thinking about their effect on us. For example, women who wear lipstick every day and lick their lips are absorbing chemicals never meant to be eaten. Perfumes vaporize and get breathed in. Read the ingredients of your antiperspirant; most likely it contains an aluminum-based compound that can be absorbed through the skin and carries the risks of aluminum outlined above. You can minimize these sources of toxins by using natural soaps and shampoos made out of vegetable ingredients, a nonfluoride toothpaste such as Dr. Bronner's or Tom's, and mouthwash you can make yourself with a little ascorbic acid in water.

It's important to air out the bathroom after a shower or bath and let it dry out. A window fan to evacuate the moist air is a good idea. Bathrooms are too often closed up most of the time and can be like little chambers that trap the perfume, deodorant, and cleaning-fluid fumes in a small space. Odor disguisers such as pine- or lemon-scented aerosol sprays are worse than useless; the odor is a molecule floating around in the air that can be removed only by letting the air escape. Products that claim to take away odors only cover them up with a chemical that probably smells worse and is certainly worse for you.

The "disinfectant" cleaners so popular for bathroom tiles and tubs are virtually useless. To disinfect something, you have to boil it for twenty minutes, but within one minute it will be covered with germs again. Those germs are not going to kill anyone despite the fear tactics used to market these cleaners. Their heavy aromatic odors are often more of a problem than the germs; pine, for example, is a resinous material that is quite troublesome to allergic or sensitive people.

Never store medications in the medicine chest; it's hot and humid in the bathroom, and this can cause them to go bad. Store medicine and vitamins in the refrigerator.

As in the kitchen, look around the bathroom and think about potential toxins: cleaners for the tiles and sink, toilet fresheners, and so on. Do you need all those things? Can you substitute natural, nontoxic products?

THE BEDROOM

We spend a third of our lives in the bedroom; if you live seventy-two years, that means twenty-four years in bed. An ecologically ideal, safe place to spend all this time should be as free of dust as possible. Many bedrooms have wall-to-wall carpeting, which is an ecological disaster. Carpeting is toxic in several ways. Whereas new synthetic-fiber carpeting contains chemicals, such as formaldehyde, which will vaporize for a year or more, old carpets collect dirt, yeast, fungus, and mold. Dust mites live in rugs. Through an electron microscope these mites look like tiny dinosaurs; their diet is chiefly composed of the shed human skin cells that are another large component of dust. House dust mites can be wafted into the air by currents and breathed into the lungs. People who are allergic to them react as they do to cat or dog dander. Like dander, they can get into your eyes and make them red and puffy.

Think about ripping up your old carpet and putting in nice hardwood floors. They're easy to maintain and nontoxic. The Japanese have never had polyvinyl fluoride or no-wax floors; they use natural resins on wood, and some of these floors are 500 years old. If you feel you must have carpets, buy wool or natural fiber rugs with natural dyes. Stay away from synthetic carpets. And learn to vacuum efficiently. Most people just zip the vacuum over the carpet; by the time the dust has had a chance to get up through the nap into the air, the vacuum has moved on and has only raised the dust. You've actually increased the pollution in the air. Run the vacuum very slowly over the carpet, giving the dust you raise time to get into the vacuum.

You may be sleeping on foam-filled synthetic pillows and using synthetic-fiber pillowcases and sheets. Replace them with down-filled pillows and comforters and pure cotton sheets. Be aware of what you're putting in your sheets when you wash them; bleaches and fabric softeners are potential irritants. Many manufacturers of bedding use chemicals to which many people are allergic in order to fireproof the material. The way to test for this is to sleep on bedding that is not treated to be fireproof and see if your symptoms disappear. Again, if you feel better when you are sleeping away from your house on vacation, it should alert you to the fact that something in the bedroom is causing trouble.

Sleeping on clean sheets that are changed frequently reduces possible reactions to dust and dust mites. When you wash bedding, it's best to avoid perfumed detergents, antistatics, and softeners and to use biodegradable brands. Bleach should be oxygen bleach, not chlorine, which leaves an irritating residue. Miracle White, made by Beatrice Food Company, works well. If you suspect that a pillowcase, for example, is bothering you, wash it with a simple unscented detergent, rinse it three or four times, and try it again to see if the problem goes away.

Even your closets can affect your health. Mothballs emit a dangerous gas. Try a mixture of rosemary, mint, thyme, ginseng, and cloves, which has the additional advantage of smelling good.

AIR QUALITY

If you ever see the sun slant into a room at a certain angle, you know how much dust and smoke are in what you thought was clear air. It's there all the time. An air purifier with a negative ionizer is the best way to eliminate airborne toxins: spores, dust, cigarette smoke, hydrocarbons and pollutants from the street, cat hairs, and positive ions. The ionizer bombards the room with negative ions that attach themselves to the positive ions of pollutants, which then drop to the ground and can be filtered out by the filtration system.

Humidifiers are fine for improving air quality as long as you use distilled water in them. Otherwise mineral deposits from the water will end up all over your carpet, floor, and furniture.

PLANTS

One efficient and natural air-quality *improver* is living greenery in your house. The more plants in your environment, the better. A large number and variety of houseplants will increase the oxygen level in the air. Green, nonflowering varieties are best, since they will not give off pollen. Plants are also a great natural air pollution filtration system. They help maintain humidity levels and a proper electricity balance in the air. They also create a living energy field that we can share and be invigorated and calmed by.

LIGHT

Your visual environment is more important than you might realize. If you feel tired, ill, or depressed inside in the winter, especially if you live at a high latitude where the days are very short, and if you spend most of your day indoors, you may be suffering from seasonal affective disorder. In this condition the hypothalamus of the brain is deprived of full-spectrum natural sunlight—most artificial lights use only a part of the spectrum. The best solution is to allow plenty of natural light into your house; use double-glazing rather than small windows or heavy drapes if insulation is a concern. Try to spend time outdoors or arrange your activities so that you're near a window.

If getting more daylight is beyond your control—the days are short, your house is dark, and you must stay indoors—the situation can be improved with full-spectrum light bulbs. Full-spectrum incandescent lighting works on a completely different principle from that of fluorescent lighting (discussed in the section on the workplace below) and is more natural for the eyes. These bulbs are available in health stores in all sizes; using them in your office as well as in your home can make a big difference in your energy level and mental state.

HEAT

In cold areas we shut down for the winter, closing and sealing the windows to avoid ventilation from the outside. These practices contribute to the toxic state of the air inside.

Oil heaters often burn inefficiently and release unburned oil fumes into the house. An afterburn catalyst that is available on the market can now recycle these fumes, creating a clean air burn. Electric stoves are not a problem. Gas or oil space heaters are one of the worst offenders. Dry radiated heat can dry up your nose and skin. Wood-burning stoves may seem rustic and natural but can be one of the worst sources of indoor pollution.

In forced-air combustion heating systems that use gas or oil, a little pinhole not infrequently develops between the heat exchanger, which is next to the combustion chamber, and the air going past it to be heated. As the air that you're going to breathe goes around that heated chamber, it sucks in the partially combusted gases. You may not even perceive this in the air, because it's at a very low level, but over a six-month period this air can produce severe illness. Therefore, you must have your forced-air system checked out electronically for these pinholes every year. The smell test is not satisfactory. If you don't do this, you're at risk.

THE WORKPLACE

The energy crisis of the 1970s led to a generation of very well insulated but poorly ventilated office buildings. People who work in these buildings often complain of fatigue, nasal congestion, dizziness, and a host of other mysterious symptoms, yet there has been clear-cut documentation of toxic levels of pollutants in very few cases. The levels of toxins in these buildings are rarely high enough to provoke official alarm, but they are high enough to cause fatigue and illness through long-term, chronic exposure. Even low levels of organic chemicals, pesticides, formaldehyde, carpet cleaners, and tobacco smoke can affect those exposed to them for a long enough period.

The individual pollutants can be located and reduced, but the single most important factor is ventilation. Monday is the worst day for headaches and stress, at least partly because the ventilation systems have often been shut down over the weekend; you're breathing old, stale air. The ducts of your office air-venting system probably haven't been cleaned in years. Dust and molds have built up inside them and are coming out into the air you breathe when the system is restarted. Ask the maintenance people to clean them; if they won't, get a heavy-duty charcoal filter and put it in the vent with a thick white insulation pad over it. These filters can be bought inexpensively at any hardware store. In one week the insulation pad will be covered with black particles large enough to see.

If it's noisy where you work, wear earplugs. You can also make your desk more pleasant with a small portable ionizer. The ionizer can actually fit in your pocket and is also useful in airplanes or on the dashboard of your car.

The fluorescent lighting often used in offices flashes on and off rapidly and constantly, placing great stress on your central nervous system. Although you are not consciously aware of this very rapid flickering, your eye and nervous system are overstimulated by it; two or three hours of work under fluorescent light can have the effect of three or four cups of coffee. At a certain level of overstimulation the central nervous system will shut down, and you will find yourself deeply fatigued. Replace the fluorescent lighting at your desk with a lamp that uses incandescent bulbs and use natural full-spectrum light bulbs. It's best to have an office with a window or skylight for true natural lighting; if you don't have one and can't arrange it, it's especially important to have natural—and sufficiently bright—lighting.

Stay away from the photocopier at the office as much as possible; it uses volatile chemicals. Don't leave typewriter ink or correction ribbons lying around open; put them in a sealed plastic bag when they are not in use. An exhaust fan on the ceiling will help draw away vaporizing fluids.

Research Update

An increasing body of evidence is showing the benefits of natural modalities to overall health and well-being. The following is a sample of recent peer-reviewed scientific studies in the area of environmental illness.

A 2015 report in *JAMA Psychiatry* concluded that that prenatal exposure to polycyclic aromatic hydrocarbon (PAH) air pollutants may affect the development of left hemisphere white matter and is associated with cognitive and behavioral problems in childhood, including slower processing speed, attention-deficit/hyperactivity disorder symptoms, and externalizing problems. A 2014 article in *Townsend Letter* reviewed the literature and determined that mycotoxins—toxic chemicals produced by both molds and yeasts—may disrupt endocrine, thyroid, and adrenal function. Mycotoxin exposure has been linked to many adverse conditions, including fibromyalgia, chronic fatigue syndrome, various cancers, diabetes, atherosclerosis, cardiovascular disease, hypertension, autism, rheumatoid arthritis, inflammatory bowel disease, lupus, Crohn's disease, multiple sclerosis, Alzheimer's disease, Raynaud's disease, kidney stones, and vasculitis.

Chapter 34

Fibromyalgia

Fibromyalgia is a chronic disorder marked by muscle pain, fatigue, and multiple tender points. Although often considered an arthritis-related condition, fibromyalgia is different because it does not cause inflammation of the joints, muscles or other tissues like arthritis does. For the three to six million Americans afflicted with the condition, as many as 90 percent of whom are women, it can be debilitating, and difficult to diagnose and treat.

Symptoms

"Fibromyalgia is also called fibrositis," says homeopath Dana Ullman. "For those who aren't familiar with it, it's a somewhat newly defined disease. At first, there was controversy as to whether it existed or not, but now there's basic acceptance that it is a condition. It's not officially arthritis, although it is thought to be a type of rheumatism where the person experiences pain and discomfort in the joints. They can also experience fatigue and even emotional and mental changes such as poor concentration, anxiety, and irritability. There might also be an irritable bowel, headaches, and cramps. The syndrome comes on in exacerbations. The person may be fine at one point and then all of a sudden have all these symptoms."

Other symptoms may include sleep problems, painful menstrual periods, restless legs syndrome, and temperature sensitivity.

Because the symptoms of fibromyalgia are similar to those associated with other conditions, patient often see a number of practitioners prior to diagnosis. There are no laboratory tests specific for fibromyalgia. Many patients are reportedly told that their pain may not be real or that there is nothing that can be done to relieve it.

Diagnosis of fibromyalgia is based on two criteria established by the American College of Rheumatology: widespread pain that affects all four quadrants of the body and lasts more than three months; and the presence of at least eleven out of eighteen standard tender points.

Causes

The cause of fibromyalgia is unknown. Among the theories are trauma, stress, repetitive injury, illness, or genetic predisposition. Research is being conducted to determine the role of female reproductive hormones, as well as chemical interactions between the nervous system and the endocrine system.

Clinical Experience

Mainstream doctors tend to focus first on medication. In 2007, the Food and Drug Administration approved Lyrica as the first drug to treat fibromyalgia. Other medications are used to treat the symptoms. They include analgesics (painkillers), nonsteroidal anti-inflammatory drugs (NSAIDs), antidepressants, sleep aids, muscle relaxants, and benzodiazepines.

Beyond medicine, there are a variety of lifestyle modifications that have proven beneficial. Adequate sleep is very important. Exercise may be difficult but has been shown to be one of the most effective methods of relief. This includes aerobic and flexibility exercise, as well as strength training.

Fibromyalgia patients should maintain a healthy diet high in fiber, low in animal fat, and emphasizing whole grains, fresh fruits and vegetables. In her *Fibromyalgia Cookbook* and *Fibromyalgia Nutrition Guide*, Mary Moeller recommends eliminating four substances entirely from the diet: chocolate, carbonated beverage, coffee, and alcohol. Other items that should be avoided include high fat dairy foods, white sugar and white flour, fried foods, preservatives, salt, and red meat.

Among the complementary and alternative therapies for fibromyalgia are massage; movement therapies such as yoga, Pilates and the Feldenkrais method; sound resonance therapy; chiropractic; and acupuncture. Herbs and dietary supplements also have been found to be helpful. Dr. Ray Sahelian offers the following recommendations, some of which are based on recently published research: fish oil capsules, acetyl L-carnitine, SAM-e, coenzyme Q10 (50 milligrams or less), ginkgo (40 or 60 milligrams), mucuna puriens (100 to 200 milligrams), ribose. The hormone supplement DHEA is unlikely to be helpful, and may cause adverse effects.

Dana Ullman, a homeopath who has done a lot of work with fibromyalgia, tells about some useful remedies. "A study was published in the *British Medical Journal* on fibromyalgia. The researchers admitted into the study only those patients who fit the most popular homeopathic remedy used to treat the acute stages of fibromyalgia. It's a remedy called Rhus tox [Rhus toxicodendron], which is poison ivy, believe it or not. [With] actual poison ivy, not only [does] an overdose cause skin eruptions, but if taken internally, and I don't recommend it, at least in a crude dose, it can and will have effects upon connective tissue that make the person feel extremely stiff, re-creating many of the symptoms that people experience when they have not only fibromyalgia but even many types of arthritis.

"They found that 42 percent of the people they interviewed fit this remedy. So they admitted these people into this study. In the first half of the study, half the people got a placebo and half the people got the real remedy. Then halfway through the study they switched, and the people who got the placebo now got the real remedy, and the people who began with the remedy got the placebo. The researchers found that when people began the real remedy, the homeopathic medicine, that's when relief began."

Ullman recommends some other homeopathic remedies. "Another remedy that comes to mind is Bryonia. Bryonia is an herb called wild hops. This is not the same hops that you drink in a beer. It's a different botanical substance entirely. This is for people with various types of musculoskeletal problems where any type of motion exacerbates the condition. By contrast, people who benefit from Rhus tox have this rusty-gate syndrome where they feel worse only on initial motion and then loosen up and limber up. People who need Bryonia, the more they move, the worse they are. Here is a really obvious difference. That's one of the unique and nice things about homeopathy. We can be quite precise in finding a remedy that fits each person because the bottom line is that we are all biologically individual. We don't have the same type of joint disease or headache or depression or fatigue. We all have our own unique constellation, our own pattern of symptoms, and homeopathy is an exclusively effective, individualized approach to using these substances from the plant, mineral, or animal kingdom to augment the body's own defenses."

Another remedy Ullman describes is honeybee venom (Apis mellifera). "For those of us who have ever been stung by a honeybee, or at least we know what it's like, it's a burning and stinging type of pain, somewhat sharp. If you've ever had a bee sting, you also know that if you put ice on the bee sting, it provides some relief. But if you get near heat or you apply heat to it, it worsens the pain. Likewise, people who will benefit from homeopathic doses of Apis will have joint pain with swelling, much like a bee might cause, because the bee not only causes that burning, stinging pain, but also causes that inflammatory redness and heat. Thus, there will be swelling that will be increased by cold applications and aggravated by heat."

Research Update

An increasing body of evidence is showing the benefits of natural modalities to overall health and well-being. Following is a sample of recent peer-reviewed scientific studies in the area of fibromyalgia.

Research published in *Rheumatology International* (2013) found that eight weeks of supplementation with magnesium citrate (300 milligrams/day) in combination with amitriptyline (10 milligrams/day) was effective in reducing fibromyalgia severity and significantly improved pain, tender points, depression and anxiety, sleep problems, and irritability. A 2012 study published in *Clinical Rheumatology* determined that fibromyalgia patients who practiced tai chi twice a week for twelve weeks had notable improvement in pain, physical function, and mobility. Scientists from Tufts University Medical Center published similar results in the *New England Journal of Medicine* in 2010: in a twelve-week study of 66 patients with fibromyalgia, those who participated in tai chi had an 18.4 percent greater reduction in severe symptoms when compared with participants in a wellness education/stretching program. In 2010, a *Pain Management Nursing* study found decreased pain, depression, and anxiety, and improved sleep following music therapy along with other relaxation techniques based on guided imagery. Research published in 2011 in the *Journal of Pain Research* found that an eight-week course of yoga intervention yielded improvements in pain, psychological functioning and mindfulness, as well as changes in cortisol levels in women with fibromyalgia.

Chapter 35

Food Allergies

It is a classic case of overreaction. Your body incorrectly senses that the food that has just been eaten is a foreign substance to be repelled. Cells begin to exhibit disease-like symptoms as they react and overreact to the food.

Allergists conservatively estimate that up to 15 percent of the population suffers from a minimum of one allergy, frequently one that is serious enough to warrant medical attention.

Symptoms can range from a mild tension headache or irritability to criminal actions and full-blown psychotic behavior. Most common are fatigue, headache, insomnia, rapid mood swings, confusion, depression, anxiety, hyperactivity, heart palpitations, muscle aches and joint pains, bedwetting, rhinitis (nasal inflammation), urticaria (hives), shortness of breath, diarrhea, and constipation. Reactions can be immediate following exposure to the allergen or delayed for many hours after contact.

Allergic symptoms are so diverse that the reactions can occur in virtually any organ of the body. Reactions in the brain or central nervous system may lead to behavioral changes and to paranoia or depression. A response in the gastrointestinal tract may translate into bloating, diarrhea, or constipation. Different food combinations can cause multiple reactions in the same person. If a person has an allergy to wheat that manifests itself in the brain, while their gastrointestinal tract is sensitive to milk, they may experience both fatigue and irritable bowel syndrome from a breakfast of whole wheat toast and milk.

All forms of a potentially offensive food can cause an allergic reaction, not just the whole form. Corn sugars and syrup, including dextrose and glucose, for example, will cause symptoms in many corn-sensitive patients. In many instances, researchers find, corn sugars will cause a more immediate reaction than will corn starch or corn as a vegetable.

Environmental medicine experts, also known as clinical ecologists, say that one reason people are developing sensitivities to certain foods is their widespread occurrence in our diets in both the natural and processed forms. Just because you only rarely treat yourself to corn on the cob, for example, doesn't mean you're not eating corn every day. On a typical day you might eat corn flakes, a corn muffin, and processed food products containing both cornstarch and corn syrup. Also, many of the daily vitamin C supplements are derived from corn.

Types of Food Allergies

The foods we eat most frequently are also the most common causes of allergies. These include milk, wheat, corn, eggs, beef, citrus fruits, potatoes, tomatoes, and coffee. Food allergies can be divided into several categories:

FIXED FOOD ALLERGY—Each time you consume a specific food, you react. For example, whenever you eat beef, a reaction occurs.

CYCLIC FOOD ALLERGY—This is the most prevalent type of allergy. It occurs when you've had an abundance of a particular food. If exposure to the food can be reduced to no more than once every four days, little or no reaction occurs. The food, in other words, can be infrequently tolerated in small amounts. So, in a cyclic allergy, a person can remain symptom-free as long as she eats the offending food infrequently.

Of course, other factors can influence the degree of this sensitivity. Infection, emotional stress, fatigue, and overeating can increase susceptibility. The condition of the food (raw or cooked, fresh or packaged) may also be an important factor. Pollution, the presence of other environmental allergens, or marked environmental temperature change can also help trigger or subdue a reaction. A food eaten by itself may be tolerated. But if it is combined with other foods at the same meal, an allergic response may develop. The length and severity of the symptoms will depend in part on how long the allergens remain in your body after ingestion.

ADDICTIVE ALLERGIC REACTION—Here the person craves the foods to which she is allergic. In essence, she becomes addicted to the foods. When made to go without the food, depression and other withdrawal-like effects may appear.

Moreover, eating the food may momentarily alleviate the symptoms, only to aggravate them later. Over time, the symptoms of the addictive allergy may grow increasingly complex.

This type of allergy often remains hidden or masked—even to the individual who is suffering from the problem. Because of its insidious nature, the person never suspects that the foods that seem to alleviate the symptoms might contain substances to which she is allergic.

But allergies do not always fit neatly into one of the three categories. A fixed allergy in infancy can develop into an addictive allergic reaction later in life. Milk is a good example of such a food. When first introduced to a baby, it may cause an acute reaction in the form of hives or spitting up. However, if the parents don't recognize this as an allergic reaction and continue to keep milk in the diet, the symptoms may take on a more generalized and less obvious form.

What is first experienced by the body as an acute reaction will—in the body's attempt to adapt by assimilating the new foreign substance—lead to more chronic symptoms such as arthritis, fatigue, depression, or headaches. For example, if you drink milk or eat milk products every day, symptoms of allergic reactions may blur with your natural personality traits and may become an accepted, even unnoticed part of your everyday life.

Eventually, you may develop a chronic condition, such as arthritis, migraines, or depression. Your daily dose of milk would never be suspect at this stage. Your body has upped its tolerance levels in trying to adapt. At the same time, milk's harmful effects have been subtly registered. You keep on with a daily dose of milk, your own substance for abuse, to keep withdrawal symptoms at bay. Acute reactions are gone—except when the milk is withdrawn completely. Chronic reactions have replaced them.

Hidden or masked food allergies, no different from allergies generally, tend to be to the very foods we eat most frequently. In the United States, dairy products, including milk and eggs, are high on the list. Corn, wheat, and potatoes are also common allergens, as is beef. Yeast, which occurs in many foods, is often a cause. Finally, many people have a hidden allergy to coffee.

Causes

IMPAIRED DIGESTION

Most food allergies can be traced to an impaired digestive system. Proper digestion requires that the body secretes sufficient hydrochloric acid and pancreatic enzymes into the stomach to process foods. These substances break down large protein molecules into small molecules so that they can be absorbed and utilized. When too few digestive juices or enzymes are secreted, the large protein molecules go directly into the bloodstream. The immune system reacts to these large molecules as if they were foreign invaders—the allergic response.

ENVIRONMENTAL AND EMOTIONAL STRESSES

In addition, other stresses can affect a person's "allergic threshold." These include environmental stresses such as air, water, and food pollution; inhalants such as perfume, aerosol hair spray, or room freshener; and emotional stress. The less healthful the physical and mental environment, the less likely are our chances for achieving and maintaining a state of well-being.

Environmental pollution poses a particular problem. Over the past two centuries the barrage of chemicals introduced into our environment has disrupted the balance of our ecosystem. Residues of many toxic chemicals such as pesticides, herbicides, and insecticides are ingested into our bodies along with food additives and preservatives that are added during commercial food processing.

In many cases, the contamination of food is an irreversible result. Foods such as oranges, sweet potatoes, and butter can be dyed. Other processed and packaged goods, such as Jell-O, ice cream, sherbet, cookies, candy, and soda can contain large amounts of food additives.

Most of our commercially raised meats and poultry are riddled with residues of antibiotics, tranquilizers, and hormones. It is even common practice to dip certain fish in an antibiotic solution to retard their spoilage. A person allergic to these antibiotics and drugs may be unknowingly ingesting them continuously, provoking either long-term or short-term reactions or illnesses, the source of which might remain unidentified. It is estimated that more than 10 percent of all Americans are sensitive to food additives. But remember, even when a person eats only organically grown foods, he or she may still be food allergic.

In most cases, the more severe a person's food sensitivity becomes, the more numerous the allergens that induce it. One clinical study reported that the average person suffering from hay fever was allergic to five foods as well. A total picture of a person's allergen exposure, environment, habits, and history are vital for effective treatment.

The end result of repeated or prolonged sensitization of the body by recurrent allergic reactions is termed "breakdown"—the point at which diseaselike symptoms appear. They may be erroneously diagnosed as the onset of an illness. But the biochemical breakdown, although it manifests itself suddenly, was actually initiated years before by prolonged exposure to allergens.

GENETIC MAKEUP

You can inherit allergic sensitivities. If both parents suffer from allergies, their children have at least a 75 percent chance of inheriting a predisposition to this hypersensitivity. When one parent is allergic, the chances of an inherited allergy remain as high as 50 percent. The child does not have to inherit the same allergic response. What is inherited is a genetic makeup that is more likely to have allergic reactions in general. For example, the mother may have chronic indigestion while the child's allergy manifests itself as acne. A mother may be sensitive to corn while her child is sensitive to yeast. Infants can develop allergies to the same foods as their mothers while still in the womb, through the placenta, or through breast milk after birth.

THE MECHANISMS OF FOOD ALLERGY

Conventional allergists believe that the mechanism of food allergy is triggered by direct contact of the food antigens—the substances the body produces to fight the "foreign food invader"—with immune system antibodies in the gastrointestinal tract. The usually swift reaction that results is called an immune system–mediated response. This is the only kind of allergic reaction conventional allergists recognize.

But there is a second mechanism recognized by clinical ecologists, through the absorption of the allergen from the gastrointestinal tract into the bloodstream. Circulating in the blood, allergens can react with elements other than antibodies. The resulting reaction can occur in the blood, in the nervous system, or in the musculoskeletal system. Sometimes referred to as a sensitivity or intolerance, to distinguish it from a classic allergic reaction, this second mechanism can be extremely complex. However, tests to uncover these more subtle intolerances are available.

Hypersensitivity to foods can come at any time of life and continue to any age, although the onset occurs most commonly in infancy and early childhood. This is largely because the gastrointestinal systems of the very young are less efficient than in the adult. One researcher refers to the progression of allergies from childhood to adulthood as the "allergic march." Symptoms can move from one organ system to another. A child may suffer from asthma as a result of drinking milk. During teen years the allergy may take the form of pimples. Unfortunately, many people erroneously believe that they have outgrown their allergy because they no longer suffer from the original symptom. They don't consider that their current problems may have the same underlying cause. Their allergic symptoms may continue to vary throughout their lives because of an underlying imbalance that remains constant. Hyperactivity as a child may be the result of ingested food additives. In later years, these same ingredients may cause migraines and fatigue.

Clinical Experience

TESTING FOR FOOD ALLERGIES

In some cases, a comprehensive medical history will provide significant clues about a person's allergic profile. A trained clinical ecologist may find the needed information from such a medical history alone.

The skin test performed by the traditional allergist has minimal use in identifying food allergies. In some cases, however, it may be helpful. A similar test takes another approach, putting extracts of food mixed with glycerin under the tongue, instead of into the skin by injection. A technique called applied kinesiology is based on the principle that there is a reflex response between a suspected allergen and the patient's body, in the patient's muscles. In this test, a doctor offers food to the patient and then measures or evaluates the energy or muscle function after the food is ingested. Here many foods can be tested in each session. However, the results may not be highly accurate depending on the nature and experience of both the person administering the test and the person being tested.

Newer tests are being developed. Some, such as the cytotoxic test, mix blood samples with food extracts and measure how many white blood cells burst. In allergy smears, samples of different body fluids or secretions are evaluated in the laboratory to look for a specific type of white blood cell. The various immune system cells may also be evaluated. In the Arest program, radioactive atoms are used to determine how antibodies respond to particular antigens.

There are also less technical tests, some of which can even be done at home. A fasting test, which should be done under medical supervision, begins by cleansing the system. Symptoms may subside, remain unchanged, or, if the allergy is an addiction of some sort, worsen by the second or third day of the fast. Then foods are reintroduced one at a time to check for symptoms.

Another test that can be performed at home is the Coca Pulse test. First find your normal pulse range by taking it every two hours. Then take it again at specific, regular intervals after eating the suspected allergen. If your pulse rises more than ten points, the food eaten last becomes suspect. The pulse is rising as a reaction to increased adrenaline in your system. The adrenaline may be released in reaction to an allergy.

Another home test involves keeping a food diary and recording everything you eat for a week. Record symptoms and when they occur as well. After the week, look for a relationship between symptoms and the food eaten.

Elimination testing is yet another approach. Eliminate the suspected allergen until symptoms clear up over a twelve-day period. Reintroduce the food on an empty stomach. Usually, if symptoms are to develop, they will do so within an hour of testing. A variation on that is the elimination of all common allergens—wheat, corn, dairy foods, citrus fruits, food colorings, sugar—and foods you may crave, over the course of a week. Then reintroduce the foods, one per day. If symptoms develop, the food may be an allergen. Don't eat it for five more days and then reintroduce it to double-check the result.

A final home test—perhaps among the most effective and sensible of all tests—also doubles as a treatment for food allergies. It is called the rotary diversified diet. Plan a diet in which you eat no individual food more often than once every four days. After five days, start a food and symptom diary. After reviewing correlations that may crop up through your recordkeeping, eat any suspected food the next time it comes up in the four-day rotation alone as one full meal. Note symptoms. Eliminate foods that stimulate adverse symptoms from your diet—permanently. The theory here is that food sensitivities become even more pronounced when a food is eliminated and then reintroduced into the diet. With this diet, your symptoms—and with them the responsible food—are clearly highlighted. This approach is also useful as a maintenance diet, enabling people who are prone to food allergies to prevent the emergence of new allergies, since they never eat any food too frequently. And even then, if a new food allergy does develop, it is spotted and quickly eliminated.

ALTERNATIVE TREATMENTS

ELIMINATION AND ROTATION DIETS

Elimination and rotation diets as described above can be used to treat food allergies.

NEUTRALIZING-DOSE THERAPY

Neutralizing-dose therapy is a treatment method that is especially useful in cases of multiple food allergies, and when avoidance of chemicals and medicinal inhalants is difficult, as during the pollen season. A neutralizing dose is determined for each allergen, and when it is injected or administered under the tongue, this dilution can bring about relief from the allergic symptoms.

These treatments are administered in a series during which the dose of the allergen is progressively increased, causing desensitization to this substance. (They work on the same theory as allergy shots or vaccines. The only differences are in the dilution of the substance and the wide variety of the substances that can be tested in this way.) Eventually, the person can tolerate contact or ingestion of the allergen with only a mild reaction or no reaction at all.

With the neutralizing-dose treatment, the allergist is first determining the amount of a particular allergen that causes an allergic reaction. The physician can work with many substances that the traditional allergist would be unable to treat, including foods, chemicals, perfumes, and cigarette smoke. The neutralizing-dose approach seems to be effective in eight out of ten patients.

Like the traditional allergy shot, the neutralizing dose can be administered by injection. However, it can also be given as drops under the tongue. Instead of taking approximately six months to find the optimal dose, the physician can usually determine the correct dosage in one or two sessions using this technique. Another advantage of the neutralizing dose is that the patient can be given the drops to take at home. It not only works as a preventive measure but can also block a reaction that has already started.

BOOSTING THE IMMUNE RESPONSE

Strengthening the immune system should improve resistance to current allergies and reduce susceptibility to new ones. There are several ways the immune system may be strengthened. Getting sufficient rest is essential, as is regular exercise. Keeping stress levels to a minimum will also help. You must also be receiving the right nutrients in the right amounts.

Many nutrients have been found to enhance the effectiveness of the immune system. These include vitamin C, beta-carotene, vitamin E, selenium, and glutathione. These are all antioxidants, which help to eliminate free radicals from the body.

Garlic has been found to be an immune stimulant, having both antifungal and antibacterial qualities. Garlic is most effective when eaten raw. It may be added to food or taken as a supplement in tablet or capsule form.

The essential fatty acids are also important to a proper immune response. Many researchers recognize the importance of omega-3 fatty acids, which are found in such oils as linseed and walnut, and in many fatty fishes, such as salmon.

It has been noted that 200 to 500 milligrams of pantothenic acid plus 50 milligrams of B complex vitamins can be useful in people with allergies. Vitamin C, in addition to its antioxidant properties, also has an antihistamine effect, which may benefit those with allergies by reducing the swelling of tissue and cell membranes. One study found that people with asthma who took 1,000 milligrams of vitamin C daily had 25 percent fewer asthmatic attacks than those receiving a placebo. Another study found that asthmatic children benefited from magnesium supplementation.

STRESS MANAGEMENT

A number of techniques are available to recondition the body to learn a new, more healthful way of responding to and dealing with stress, including that associated with food allergies. These include progressive relaxation, biofeedback, self-hypnosis, visualizations, meditation, yoga, and tai chi. Stress management techniques can improve the digestion of allergy sufferers.

THE LINK BETWEEN FOOD ALLERGIES AND CHRONIC DISEASE

If food and chemical sensitivities were routinely considered in each case of chronic disease, there would be a tremendous increase in well-being in this country.

An overly analytical medical system insists instead on classifying patients into narrowly defined disease states. Environmental aspects, including a patient's diet, are considered to be nonmedical. The person's whole experience—including diet, environment, lifestyle, emotional life, and work life—may also be considered to be outside the physician's domain, although few physicians would deny that the cause of almost any patient's illness will involve one or more of these factors to some degree.

FOOD ALLERGIES AND MENTAL HEALTH

It may be that up to 70 percent of symptoms diagnosed as psychosomatic are probably due to some undiagnosed reaction to foods, chemicals, or inhalants. Different allergic reactions occur. There are localized physical effects, such as gastrointestinal disorders, eczema, asthma, and rhinitis (nasal inflammation). There are acute systemic effects, such as fatigue, migraine headaches, neuralgia (nerve pain), muscle aches, joint pains, and other generalized symptoms. And there are acute mental effects, such as depression, rapid mood swings, hallucinations, delusions, and other behavioral abnormalities. It has been estimated that over 90 percent of schizophrenics have food and chemical intolerances.

Researchers now believe that food allergies may directly affect the body's nervous system by causing a noninflammatory swelling of the brain, which can trigger aggression. Despite studies at various correctional centers clearly showing the connection between diet and behavior, little is being done to change the dietary standards of correctional facilities throughout the nation. Routine screening programs for food allergies and nutritional deficiencies in chronic offenders do not exist.

While many other factors—not food alone—mitigate criminal, antisocial behavior, or mental illness, a case can be made for testing for and evaluating food sensitivities in any overall treatment, prevention, or rehabilitation program.

FOOD ALLERGIES AND HEADACHES

Migraines are an example of a condition in which recognition and elimination of food allergens can make a tremendous difference. The trick is to recognize the possibilities.

Right now, about 25 million people who consult their physicians each year complain of bad headaches. Although there are various types of headaches, about 50 percent of these people suffer from migraines. While conventional medicine has very little to offer the migraine sufferer, clinical ecologists see migraine as a disorder frequently resulting from food allergies. The nontraditional medicine offered by the clinical ecologist may offer a unique opportunity to relieve the suffering.

Headaches due to food or chemical sensitivities can often be treated simply by eliminating the allergy, once it has been identified, with an elimination or rotation diet. Yet, as a rule, food sensitivities are not investigated in the diagnosis and treatment of headaches.

While the pain may sometimes appear immediately after eating a particular food, it may also be delayed until hours afterward. For this reason it is not unusual for a person to fail to identify the correlation between what they're eating and the onset of their headache. A food may even seem to relieve migraine symptoms temporarily—a classic example of an addictive allergic reaction.

Of course, allergic headaches typically occur as the result of combinations of factors, rather than from food allergies alone. Emotional stress, for example, may play a large role in triggering an episode. Thus, even when a food allergy is at cause, the specific food source may not produce the same symptoms on every occasion, depending on the array of associated circumstantial factors. In some individuals stress may be compounded when the allergic reaction triggers further emotional symptoms. A vicious cycle is created. Sudden changes in temperature or light may also affect one's susceptibility, as well as the presence of any other health problems.

Environmental-medicine specialists have found that some of the foods that occur most frequently in the typical American diet are also the foods most commonly implicated in food allergy–related headaches. The list includes wheat, eggs, milk, chocolate, corn, pork, cinnamon, legumes (beans, peas, peanuts, and soybeans), and fish. Moreover, individuals with food allergies should avoid or limit their intake of fermented products, such as red wine, champagne, and aged cheese, because of the presence in these foods of a substance called tyramine. Tyramine has been associated with migraine occurrence in some cases.

Too often, conventional medical practitioners tend not to look toward nutritional solutions in cases involving allergies, including allergy-related migraines. In part, this is because the medical training they have received does not extend deeply into nutrition. And yet, a preponderance of evidence continues to point to the importance of nutritional solutions for an increasingly wide range of health problems.

FOOD ALLERGIES AND FATIGUE

Probably no allergic disorder is more puzzling and pervasive than tension fatigue syndrome. Indeed, for many of us, varying daily levels of tension and fatigue are the norm, tranquility and energy the rare exceptions. To compensate, we choose artificial solutions for moderating energy, from the first caffeinated gulps of coffee in the morning to the quick sugar, caffeine, or drug fix during the day, and the alcoholic "equalizer" in the evening. The result is that energy levels are either depressed or falsely elevated most of the time. In many cases, these quick pick-me-ups are responses to allergic disorders with their roots in food and nutrition.

Next to headaches, tension fatigue syndrome is the most common manifestation of cerebral and nervous system allergy. Yet, too often, this far-reaching malady is not even recognized by physicians or allergists. Its symptoms are usually assigned a psychiatric origin and treated with drug therapy or some other conventional modality when, in fact, a simple elimination and rotation diet is the best medicine.

There are several reasons for this all too common oversight. First, there are similarities between tension fatigue syndrome and psychiatric disorders. And second, there is the failure of standard scratch tests to identify many food and chemical reactions. The scratch tests simply have not been shown to be effective in the diagnosis of food and chemical sensitivities. And yet they continue to be used by allergists.

Of course, tension, extreme nervousness, irritability, depression, and emotional instability may be symptoms of psychological disorders in some cases. But too often this is the only possibility that is considered. The allergy may be due to any number of foods, and it is only through careful testing that a definitive diagnosis can be made. In all cases where such symptoms appear, food allergies should be ruled out first—before further traditional medical sleuthing occurs. This can save a lot of trouble and mistaken diagnoses.

Symptoms

The symptoms experienced in tension fatigue syndrome can include fatigue, weakness, lack of energy and ambition, drowsiness, mental sluggishness, inability to concentrate, bodily aches, poor memory, irritability, fever, chills and night sweats, nightmares, restlessness, insomnia, and emotional instability. Mental depression is another common symptom, ranging from mild to severe episodes of despondency and melancholia. Generalized muscle aches and pains, especially in the back of the neck or in the back and thigh muscles may also be present, as well as edema (fluid retention), particularly around the eye, and tachycardia (rapid heart beat). Gastrointestinal symptoms often associated with this syndrome are bloating, abdominal cramps or pain, constipation, diarrhea, and a coated tongue. Chills and perspiration are also frequently experienced in association with fatigue during food testing of symptomatic patients.

The disorder can begin at any age. It can last from several months to several decades. In some adults the extreme fatigue, bodily aches, depression, and mental aberrations that come from this continuing allergic state can be so severe that they interfere with work and domestic life.

As headaches or gastrointestinal upsets caused by allergy increase in frequency, the fatigue is more likely to remain even between episodes. Fatigue soon becomes the allergic individual's major complaint. The allergic origin of the fatigue and weakness commonly remains a mystery.

It's not unusual for allergic individuals to sleep up to fifteen or more hours for several successive nights to try to overcome their fatigue. Unfortunately, in most cases, these efforts prove futile. The fatigue experienced in allergic fatigue is quite different from the fatigue that naturally follows physical exertion. It cannot be relieved by normal or even excessive amounts of rest. It can be relieved only by eliminating its cause—the allergen.

DIFFERENTIAL DIAGNOSIS

Before the diagnosis of allergic fatigue can be defined, a complete medical workup should be done to exclude both organic and functional origins. This should include a comprehensive case history, complete physical examination, and diagnostic laboratory blood testing. Other causes for nervous fatigue include chronic infections and metabolic disorders, including diabetes, hypoglycemia, hypothyroidism, neurological disorders, heart disease, anemia, malignancy, and various nutrient deficiencies. Even if another disease is found, allergic fatigue may still be a causal factor. In some cases, fatigue is caused both by an allergic reaction and an underlying chronic disease state.

FOOD ALLERGIES AND OBESITY

Many obese women believe that they are overweight due to heredity, because they have a thyroid or metabolic problem, or because they simply eat too much. They may blame it on a lack of self-control, or become convinced that they have psychological problems. However, some experts believe that roughly two out of three obese individuals suffer from some form of allergy.

Of course, allergy may be only one of several factors affecting an obese person's weight. The presence of a thyroid condition or psychological problems can cause or aggravate a weight problem. Obesity is also related to many diseases including high blood pressure, heart disease, kidney problems, and diabetes. For obese individuals with allergies, the problems of each condition may adversely affect the other. Typically, someone who is obese will have allergic responses more often than a person who is not obese. The extra weight is a burden on the immune system, and the weaker the immune system, the greater the effects of allergies. People who are obese may also have difficulty breathing.

We store chemicals in the body in fat. Very often, allergies are triggered by a response to chemicals stored in this way. Because the obese person may naturally hold more chemicals in the body, she may tend to experience more frequent allergic responses. This may also explain why she feels worse, or has strong food cravings, at the beginning of a diet. Chemicals are stored in fat, and as the fat is burned, a large quantity of chemicals is passed into the bloodstream, often causing such cravings.

The mechanism by which an allergy can trigger obesity may be that of the hidden addictive allergy, whereby a person is addicted to the very foods to which she is allergic. Often, these are high-calorie foods, such as chocolate, cheese, or sugar. So the person may gain weight because she eats these high-calorie foods too frequently.

Hunger itself can be an allergic response, and compulsive eating and intense cravings for particular foods may also result from hidden allergies. In some cases, compulsive eating of the food one is allergic to may really be an attempt to stave off withdrawallike symptoms induced by going without the food for too long. Such withdrawal symptoms might include headaches, drowsiness, irritability, or depression.

Allergies can cause weight problems if they interfere with the body's natural ability to regulate itself. As noted by Dr. Arthur Kaslow, physician and author, both humans and animals naturally attempt to maintain their bodies in a state of bio-chemical equilibrium known as homeostasis. Unless there is a flaw in their reg-ulatory system, human beings will maintain their proper weight by eating the amounts and types of foods their bodies need to function properly. When the body needs food, it will send out a hunger signal. When it needs water, it sends out a thirst signal. If this mechanism breaks down, an individual may feel hungry when she does not really need food. It is possible that allergies can temporarily impair the cells responsible for sending out these signals.

FOOD ALLERGIES AND ARTHRITIS

Some clinical ecologists estimate that 80 to 90 percent of all cases of arthritis are either allergy induced or are allergylike reactions to some food the patient has eaten. The arthritis may also be related to an environmental factor to which the patient is sensitive, such as gas inhaled from constant proximity to a gas stove. Examining arthritics for both food and environmental allergies may help reduce current symptoms, prevent recurrences of symptoms, and minimize the damage that eventually results from joint inflammations.

Dr. Marshall Mandell successfully treated hundreds of arthritis patients by putting them on a five-day distilled-water fast and then allowing their usual foods, one at a time, back into their diet. If a food causes the arthritis symptoms, the symp-toms will return when it is reintroduced into the diet and should be permanently eliminated.

PATIENT STORY

I had an interesting case a few years ago where this woman had developed chronic intestinal problems seemingly out of the blue. We tested her for food allergies and I told her it has to be something you're eating all the time for it to be such an ongoing problem. For something you eat only twice a year well then you know it's not going to cause prob-lems like that. So we tested her and the only thing that came up was hazelnuts, and I thought well this can't possibly be what's causing these chronic issues. But sure enough when we went back through her diet she had started drinking hazelnut flavored coffee every day, and just that little bit of flavoring was enough to make her really sick. She had been to so many doctors, and you know so that's where the value of the testing sometimes comes in. But it brings up the point that it doesn't take much of a food if you're allergic to it to really cause pretty dramatic symptoms in your system, but you do need to be exposed to it on a regular basis.

—*Dr. Christine Doherty*

Chapter 36

Heart Disease

In nearly every year for which we have records, heart disease has been the number one cause of death in the United States. According to 2015 data from the Centers for Disease Control and Prevention (CDC), more than 600,000 Americans succumb to heart disease annually. It is a much greater threat to women than many people believe: one in every four women dies from heart disease, and two-thirds of women who have heart attacks never recover fully. Over the past three decades, more women than men have died of heart disease, and the survival gap continues to grow. Sadly, as Dr. Sherrill Sellman explains in this chapter, in their mad-dash attempt to prevent heart disease in women many doctors rushed into hormone replacement therapy (HRT) without knowing the alarming facts that later emerged—not only does HRT not protect the heart, it also increases the risk of stroke and cancer. Fortunately, there are many natural ways to maintain the integrity of the heart, not just in terms of physical health, but mental, emotional, and spiritual as well.

Causes

"Overall, there are 247 risk factors that can damage the heart," states Dr. David Steenblock, a complementary physician from California. "A risk factor is anything that injures the inner lining of the blood vessels that supply the heart with oxygen and nutrition. Any agent that injures this inner lining, such as tobacco, air pollution, food additives, high blood pressure, and gasoline fumes, can initiate atherosclerosis, the so-called hardening of the arteries. Then the accumulation of such things as cholesterol, calcium, scar tissue, and fat causes atherosclerotic lesions, which gradually go on to occlude, or block, the arteries to the brain and the heart. When the arteries to the brain [the carotid arteries] are blocked, you have a stroke, and when the arteries to the heart [the coronary arteries] are blocked, you have a heart attack."

High blood pressure (hypertension), which affects some 50 million Americans, increases the risk of heart attack and stroke. Dr. Michael Janson, former president of the American Preventive Medical Association and author of *The Vitamin Revolution in Health Care* says, "High blood pressure can be the result of dietary habits; lack of exercise; high stress; being overweight; having too much caffeine, sugar, alcohol, or, in particular, salt in the diet. In the past few years, some reports have said that salt does not make much of a difference for most people. The fact is, that's not true. Even a slight elevation in blood pressure is enough to increase the risk of heart disease."

Among the more recently identified potential risk factors for heart disease are high levels of the amino acid homocysteine, high fibrinogen (a blood-clotting protein), and certain viral and bacterial infections. An elevation in the level of C-reactive protein, a substance in the blood that indicates the presence of inflammation, is also thought to be involved.

Dr. Janson describes other common heart ailments, some of which are precipitated by atherosclerosis. In angina pectoris, he explains, "clogged arteries leave the heart muscle with inadequate oxygen. As everyone knows, muscles hurt when exercised beyond their oxygen capacity. When not enough blood flows from the coronary arteries to the heart muscle, people experience pain in the chest. Sometimes they feel pain in the jaw, the shoulder, or even the wrist. Often they do not realize that this is referred pain coming from the heart itself."

Congestive heart failure is another common heart problem. "Hardening of the coronary arteries can lead to a number of other problems," Dr. Janson explains. "When heart muscle tissue functions inefficiently, more blood comes in than is pumped out. In other words, with each beat the amount of blood being returned to the heart is more than the heart muscle can handle. Fluid backs up, and other tissues, such as the lungs and legs, can get congested. Congestive heart failure leads to shortness of breath, water in the lungs, and swelling of the ankles."

Symptoms

Heart disease is a gradual process that takes years to develop into a serious condition. At first there are no warning signs. There may be an increasing sense of tiredness and fatigue, as well as lack of stamina. If the coronary arteries become severely blocked, a woman may experience shortness of breath or chest pressure and pain (angina pectoris) that is relieved by rest. Other signs of an impending heart attack may include light-headedness, sweating, nausea, and pain spreading to the shoulders, neck, or arms. Unfortunately, many people are unaware of or overlook these signs: 50 percent of all people who have heart attacks wait two hours or longer before seeking treatment, and many die before reaching the hospital.

Diagnosis is an important first step. Before anyone begins a cardiovascular health program, a doctor should take the following factors into account: family history, blood pressure, cholesterol level, weight, and stress electrocardiogram (ECG) tests. After assessment of a woman's risk factors, the program can begin.

Clinical Experience

CONVENTIONAL TREATMENT

Conventional treatment of heart disease often involves the use of medication to address symptoms such as high blood pressure and high cholesterol. And every year, well over 1 million Americans undergo surgery such as coronary bypass and angioplasty (in which a balloon catheter is used to open clogged arteries) to restore their hearts.

Dr. Janson believes the general public is being misled into believing that medications for high blood pressure are safe and always necessary. "We all hear advertisements on the radio telling us to stay on these medications for life. They say that no symptoms tell you whether or not your blood pressure is high. Therefore, if you are taking medication for high blood pressure, you must stay on your medication and never, ever stop. That so-called public-service announcement is really a sales pitch from the drug companies that make the medications. We know that these medications actually cause more heart disease and that they create side effects in addition to the high blood pressure."

Dr. Cynthia Thaik, who has developed a national foundation that educates people and physicians on the prevention and treatment of cardiovascular disease, and wrote *Your Vibrant Heart: Restoring Health, Strength and Spirit from the Body's Core*, agrees. "We are so quick to diagnose diseases and so quick to use the quick fix in terms of pharmaceuticals. . . . I always tell my patients: when we use pharmaceuticals to lower your blood pressure, your cholesterol, or diabetes, those lower the numbers. They don't change anything regarding the metabolism, the inflammation, or the actual derangements that are occurring within your body."

Dr. David Steenblock warns, however, that patients who depend on medication to control high blood pressure should not self-discontinue. "Many people have this idea that since the doctor is not getting at the cause of their high blood pressure, it is somewhat illogical for them to take their blood pressure medicine. True, doctors often do not have the answer. Still, if you fail to take your medicine and your blood pressure gets out of control, you can develop heart disease and go on to have a stroke."

Statins such as Zocor and Lipitor are often prescribed to lower cholesterol levels, and thereby prevent heart attacks and stroke. Many women who have high cholesterol but no sign or history of heart disease are taking these drugs, and facing the risk of serious side effects without even attempting natural therapies. Dr. Sherill Sellman, a natural health practitioner and internationally respected lecturer and author on women's health, tells us more.

"The fact of the matter is there's only one population that really seems to benefit, if at all, from statins and that's men who've already had a heart attack. It has not shown to really be effective for women prophylactically. . . . The story about cholesterol is really a story of inflammation, the result of damage in the arteries from inflammatory response. We've got to reduce inflammation and part of that process, obviously, is getting the hormones balanced and reducing that estrogen excess pattern that can drive the very reasons that the arteries become damaged. It's not a statin drug that we need."

HORMONE REPLACEMENT THERAPY (HRT)

Nothing illustrates the problem with medication better than the debacle related to hormone replace therapy (HRT). In the 1990s, many doctors began prescribing HRT to help prevent heart disease in women. A Harvard study of about 46,000 female nurses had found that those who had taken HRT had a lower incidence of heart disease by up to 50 percent. However, when that study was more fully investigated, it turned out that the women with lower rates of heart disease were actually women who were healthier in general. Compared to the group who were supposed to have a greater incidence of heart disease, they were wealthier, more likely to exercise, and had better diets; fewer of them had diabetes, and they smoked less. The women who didn't take HRT were more likely to have diabetes, smoked, were poorer, and didn't visit their doctors. Also not reported in the study was the fact that the women who took HRT had a 50 percent increase in strokes. This, then, was a flawed, biased study.

"The rationale for giving HRT to postmenopausal women was that when you arrive at menopause, your risk of getting heart disease or stroke will skyrocket and, therefore, you need protection," says Dr. Sherrill Sellman, a naturopath, psychotherapist, and author the best-selling book *Hormone Heresy*. But, she says, studies from reputable researchers showed that this was a myth. There was no rapid increase of heart disease in postmenopausal women. There was simply a rise in heart disease as women move on in life in general. The doctors who pushed HRT as a preventive for women's heart disease seemed not to take into account the fact that men also have a higher incidence of heart disease as they age.

Studies began to come in challenging the theory that hormone replacement therapy was beneficial to the heart. A study published in 2001 found that postmenopausal women with heart problems who took hormone supplements for less than one year actually had a greater risk of another heart attack or death from heart disease than women who were not on HRT. An earlier study, sponsored by Ayerst, the company that manufactured the number-one replacement estrogen, Premarin, yielded similar results. Dr. Sellman explains, "They gave half the women hormone replacement therapy and the other half a placebo. After five years, they discovered that in the first year of treatment, the women taking the HRT had a 50 percent increase in heart attacks. Over the five years, the risk decreased. The conclusion was that women who already had heart conditions got no overall benefit from HRT. But this glossed over the horrible fact that HRT increased heart problems the first year. What was more, women taking it had three times as many blood clots in the legs than women taking the placebo. There was also an increase in gallbladder disease."

In 2001, the American Heart Association finally took heed of the growing scientific evidence and shifted its stance, advising against the use of hormone replacement therapy to prevent heart disease in women. And, in 2003, a major government trial, known as the Women's Health Initiative (WHI), definitively linked the long-term use of combined estrogen and progestin as menopausal hormone therapy to an increased risk of heart disease, as well as stroke and breast cancer. As described in a 2007 press release issued by the National Institutes of Health, "both the estrogen plus progestin and estrogen-alone trials of the WHI were stopped early because of increased health risks and the failure to prevent heart disease. Specifically, the estrogen plus progestin trial was stopped after 5.6 years because of an increased risk of breast cancer and because overall risks, including increased risks for heart attack, stroke, and blood clots, outnumbered benefits. The estrogen-alone study was stopped after 6.8 years because of an increased risk of stroke and no reduction in risk of CHD [coronary heart disease]. The estrogen-alone study also found an increased risk of blood clots." The findings suggested that risk due to hormones may differ depending on age or years since menopause.

THE COMPLEMENTARY APPROACH

The solution here is to work with a complementary medical physician until your heart health is restored. In some cases, medication may be needed long term, even for a lifetime, but no one can fail to benefit from improving lifestyle and diet. A number of full alternative therapy programs are available to combat heart disease, including those developed by Dean Ornish, Julian Whitaker, John McDougall, and Eric Braverman. To varying degrees, these and other programs incorporate the following approaches.

DIET

The typical American consumes an overload of calories, total fat, saturated fat, added sugar, sodium, and refined grains, and not enough omega-3 fats, fiber, and whole grains, fruits, vegetables and phytonutrients. The average daily intake for adult women is 51 grams of total fat, including 23 grams of saturated fat, 19 grams of monounsaturated fat, and 10 grams of polyunsaturated fat.

There is not much controversy about what is wrong with the standard American diet. But there is controversy over the proper foods for those with heart disease. There are tens of thousands of dietitians in the United States, and they have been a primary source of information on what a sick person should eat. After all, physicians graduate from medical school with only an hour or two of learning about nutrition. However, even though dietitians are well trained, there is a split in the field. Only a very small percentage believe the standard American diet plays a large role in causing the diseases we are beset with, including heart disease.

The American Heart Association recommends that we limit cholesterol intake to less than 300 milligrams daily, and less than 200 milligrams for those with high levels of "bad" LDL cholesterol. Sodium should be less than 2,300 milligrams per day (about 1 teaspoon). Fat should be 25 to 35 percent of total calories daily, with only 7 percent of this in the form of saturated fats (fats found particularly in land animals, palm and coconut oils, and hydrogenated vegetable oils). We have been told that margarine, made from "polyunsaturated fats," is good for the heart and will lower cholesterol. That is simply not true; margarine is loaded with the fatty acids that contribute to heart disease. Instead of margarine, use olive oil, canola oil, or flaxseed, almond, safflower, sunflower, or soy oil. Of these, olive oil would be at the top of my list. But don't have margarine.

Dr. Janson adds that people should avoid foods such as sugar, salt, white flour, white rice, and particularly any shortening or hydrogenated vegetable oils found in products like margarine and vegetable shortening: "Whenever you see vegetable shortening, hydrogenated vegetable oil, or partially hydrogenated vegetable oil on a label, avoid that product. These are not foods. In fact, I consider margarine an industrial waste product that is fashioned to resemble food."

While the dangers of saturated fats to heart health are well known, Dr. Ray Peat, a distinguished scientific researcher in Eugene, Oregon, says unsaturated fats can be just as damaging. "Many people have been soaking their bodies in unsaturated vegetable oil diets for years. As a result, every time they get hungry or face stress, their blood sugar falls, their adrenaline rises, and these unsaturated fats are drawn out of storage. Once released, they immediately start poisoning the lining of the blood vessels and all the cellular energy-producing systems. In 1960, this effect was demonstrated by a group in England, which saw that adrenaline, either natural or synthetic, caused damage to the circulatory system. It turns out that this occurs after unsaturated fats become mobilized. They hit the lining of the blood vessels, where they cause lipid peroxidative damage."

HEART-HEALTHY FOODS

The power of a vegetarian diet in a cardiovascular health program was recognized in a now-famous study by Dr. Dean Ornish. The Ornish study placed heart patients on a protocol of healthy vegetarian foods, as well as daily aerobic exercise and relaxation. At the end of a year, a significant number of patients showed improvement in their heart condition, and in some the disease was even reversed.

The late Dr. Paul Cutler, a complementary physician from Niagara Falls, New York, said, "Medicine in general owes Ornish a great deal of gratitude. He showed that a drastic reduction of fats was most important. I believe that the total dietary fats should be well below the typical average. Modern nutritionists are saying 30 percent. I try to get fat content down to 10 percent of the total calories. I see improvement in angina just by reducing the fats to that degree."

Dr. Janson continues, "The diet should be high in complex carbohydrates, including whole grains, beans, vegetables, and fruits. Remember, flavonoids, which are plant pigments, are present in fruits and vegetables and in some beans and grains. These are very protective, and most of them are not available as supplements.

"I think the diet should be largely vegetarian, although a number of studies show that fish also reduces levels of heart disease and cancer. Fish may or may not be the reason for this. It may be that eating more fish means eating less chicken and meat. Cutting those foods out of the diet helps cut down on heart disease.

Dr. Caldwell Esselstyn, a clinician and researcher at the Cleveland Clinic and author of *Prevent and Reverse Heart Disease*, explains that while certain foods are "lethal" to the delicate cells that line the arteries (the endothelium), others are extremely valuable. "The type of food that one wants to consume to restore these endothelial cells is largely plant based," he says. "That includes grains for your cereal, breads and pasta, but they should be whole grains. You should have all the different type of legumes. Then there are the green leafy vegetables: bok choy, Swiss chard, collard greens, beet greens, mustard greens, turnip greens, napa cabbage, brussels sprouts, broccoli, spinach and kale. We have seen striking reversal of symptoms often within two and three weeks in patients with angina or chest pain when they really eliminate all the foods that are going to injure their arteries and pour in all those wonderful foods."

Broccoli and other types of produce, seeds, legumes, and grains provide necessary vitamins, and they also contain important phytochemicals. The phytochemicals include beta-carotene, alpha-carotene, ascorbic acid, ash, boron, caffeic acid, calcium, chlorophyll, chromium, citric acid, copper, glycine, iron, linoleic acid, lysine, magnesium, niacin, oleic acid, phosphorus, potassium, riboflavin, selenium, thiamin, tryptophan, and zinc, among others. These chemicals have all kinds of healing properties. Chlorophyll, for instance, helps purify the blood and acts as a detoxifier.

You should have at least nine servings of vegetables and five of fruits each day, raw, steamed, or juiced. Once you start, you will notice a world of difference in your overall vitality. Other valuable heart foods are rice and beans, which are complete proteins rich in fiber and B-complex vitamins.

Many people grow up with the pernicious myth that if it is not an animal protein, it is not a complete protein, and so is not really nutritious. I did studies at the Institute of Applied Biology that proved conclusively that beans, legumes, and all grains contain complete proteins just like animal proteins, without the saturated fats. They are not high in calories and are rich in vitamins, minerals, and essential oils.

Nuts, despite their high fat content, are being found to have some important benefits as well. Not only do they provide protein, they also contain nutrients that can protect against heart disease, high blood pressure, and stroke. The protein in peanuts, hazelnuts, and walnuts, for example, is a good source of arginine. This amino acid is noted for its ability to produce nitric oxide, which helps blood vessels to widen and may stop or even reverse plaque buildup. These nuts also contain folate, which has been found to lower blood levels of homocysteine. High levels of homocysteine are associated with increased blockage in the arteries.

A Harvard study of 86,000 nurses found that those who ate more than 5 ounces of nuts a week were 35 percent less likely to develop heart disease than those who rarely ate nuts. Other studies have reported similar findings.

EXERCISE

"Aerobic exercise and an improved diet should go hand in hand," noted Dr. Cutler. "Aerobics help the good cholesterol go up significantly, which in turn helps remove cholesterol from arterial walls after the cells are through with it, so it is less likely to form plaque." Exercising aerobically means getting the heart rate up three or four times a week. A doctor can help determine how much exercise is needed.

Dr. Janson adds that people should stretch before and after an aerobic workout. "The stretching has another benefit in that it relaxes the body and keeps people limber and more flexible. That makes it easier to continue an aerobic exercise program."

Exercise is not a panacea, however. Some people mistakenly assume that cholesterol can be burned off by exercise and activity and that as a result, people who engage in athletics and body building can eat more meat and eggs without suffering ill effects. There is no scientific basis for this notion. To the contrary, studies have shown that good conditioning and muscle tone do not necessarily put a person in good cardiovascular condition.

Dr. Julian Whitaker refers to studies done on marathon runners in South

Africa, in which five died of heart attacks. "These were conditioned long-distance runners. They all had cholesterol levels of 270, 290, et cetera. They were very fit but not very well."

SUPPLEMENTS

Supplements provide wonderful support for the heart and sometimes help eliminate or reduce dosages of medication. Antioxidants help protect the heart from free radical damage, also known as oxidation. Antioxidant nutrients include vitamin E, vitamin D3, and vitamin C (see below), beta-carotene, and selenium. Free radicals damage the tissues lining the arteries, which leads to atherosclerosis and plaque deposits. Antioxidants, particularly vitamin C, can prevent this from happening by protecting the lining of the arteries. The following are nutrients you should know about.

L-ARGININE—L-arginine is an amino acid that has been receiving well-deserved attention in the medical literature for its ability to produce nitric oxide. Nitric oxide benefits the arterial walls in several ways. It helps the smooth muscles in the arterial walls relax, promoting an antianginal, antihypertensive, and antistress effect. Additionally, research shows that L-arginine reduces the activation of platelets, the small bodies that can initiate arterial spasm and plaque development. Other studies show that L-arginine slows plaque development and even reverses small amounts of plaque buildup. "I've seen it work," said Dr. Cutler. "Taking 2 to 3 grams of L-arginine per day has quite a marked antianginal effect. L-arginine is now a must in my protocol for nutrients. Usually I start with about 1,000 milligrams per day, and raise the levels if that amount isn't helping."

L-CARNITINE—The heart muscle needs to burn fat for energy, and L-carnitine allows this to happen. Dr. Janson explains: "L-carnitine gets fat into the little engines inside the cells called mitochondria. These little mitochondrial engines are where fat is burned for energy. Your heart muscle needs to burn fat for energy, and the only way it can get the fat into that little engine is with the amino acid L-carnitine. At the same time, that inner mitochondrial membrane requires another nutrient to burn the fat: coenzyme Q10." Dr. Janson recommends that people take 500 milligrams L-carnitine two to three times a day. You should take L-carnitine along with vitamin E, because they work together synergistically.

CHROMIUM PICOLINATE—Chromium picolinate has been shown to be beneficial both for the heart and for blood sugar levels.

COENZYME Q10—Coenzyme Q10 is a nutrient that should be taken by anyone who has heart problems or who wants to avoid getting them. Along with L-carnitine, it helps prevent angina and protects the heart muscle by letting it burn fat for energy more easily. It also improves heart health by reducing blood pressure and arrhythmias. As an antioxidant, it prevents the damage to blood vessels that leads to hardening of the arteries. Therapeutic levels are between 50 and 200 milligrams for mild heart disease. More severe heart disease may respond to 200 to 300 milligrams.

LECITHIN—Lecithin is made from soy. Not only does it keep the arteries strong and healthy, but it also helps emulsify fats, helps the brain, and is good for memory.

MAGNESIUM—Magnesium increases blood flow by allowing muscles in the arterial wall to relax. Usually 1,000 milligrams are needed.

MAXEPA—MaxEPA, a combination of EPA (eicosapentaenoic acid) and DHA (docosohexaenoic acid), also known as fish oil, is part of the omega-3 and omega-6 fatty acids found in salmon, sardines, and mackerel. Since many people do not eat these fish, they should be getting these fatty acids in fish oil. The recommended daily dose is 500 to 1,000 milligrams. Clinical and epidemiological experience as well as scientific studies have found that people who eat a lot of fish have less heart disease than people who do not.

NIACIN (VITAMIN B3)—A fifteen-year study on the effects of niacin published by the American Heart Association in the mid-1980s connected the use of niacin to a significant reduction in heart attacks and death from heart disease. Long-term niacin use has also been associated with decreased rates of cancer. Niacin should be taken under medical supervision, since it can affect liver function.

TAURINE—Taurine, an amino acid, is another important antioxidant that helps prevent atherosclerosis. Additionally, it can avert heart failure by improving the strength of the heart's contraction. That increases the outflow of blood from the heart and reduces congestive heart failure. Generally, 500 milligrams are taken twice a day.

THYROID SUPPLEMENTS—Thyroid supplementation may normalize high cholesterol. According to Dr. Ray Peat, "High cholesterol indicates a thyroid hormone deficiency. A clear demonstration of this was seen in patients whose thyroid glands were surgically removed. After the operation, cholesterol levels became abnormally high, but they returned to normal with thyroid supplementation." He adds that thyroid extract is linked to fewer heart attacks. "One of the foremost American researchers in the field, Broda Barnes, wrote *Solved: The Riddle of Heart Attacks* after finding that patients in one group had far fewer heart attacks than did patients in another group. All the low-heart-attack group did differently was take thyroid when they needed it."

B VITAMINS—Vitamin B_1 (thiamine) is the most important B vitamin for the heart: 25 to 50 milligrams daily are recommended. Dr. Janson says that other B vitamins, such as folic acid and B_{12}, can help lower blood levels of homocysteine.

VITAMIN C—If there is one vitamin everyone needs to take every day, it is vitamin C. Get over that old-fashioned idea that all you need is one glass of orange juice to get the necessary vitamin C. Now we have thousands of studies of the valuable properties of vitamin C, which can help with everything from cancer to heart disease and diabetes. I would take 500 to 1,000 milligrams, five times a day. Vitamin C washes out of the system, so you need to take it throughout the day. Two well-known specialists in coronary heart disease recommend that their patients take vitamin C before going to bed at night because they find it helps prevent heart attacks during sleep and in the morning, which is when the majority of heart attacks occur.

VITAMIN E—Vitamin E has several functions. Aside from being a protective antioxidant, it reduces the stickiness of the platelets, little blood fragments that initiate blood clots. This effect is helped by the addition of essential fatty acids and garlic to the diet. Minimizing free radical damage and keeping platelets from clogging the arteries give arteries a chance to heal and recover. There is more room for oxygen to flow through the arteries to reach tissues. It is estimated that between 400 and 800 international units (IU) are useful in preventing stroke. You may go higher, up to 1,200 or 1,600 units, unless other medical conditions preclude a higher level. I believe we would cut the incidence of stroke by 20 percent, saving 50,000 to 100,000 people a year, just by having everyone take this little, inexpensive supplement.

OTHER—In addition, other beneficial supplements are chondroitin sulfate A, evening primrose oil (1,500 mg/day), Rejuna (300 mg), Oligomeric Proanthocyanidins (30 mg), Omega3 Fatty Acids (3000 mg), Olive extract (500 mg), PQQ (20 mg), curcuminoids (700 mg), decaf green tea (1000 mg), and Cytokine Supress with EGCG (300mg).

HERBS

In addition to the herbs listed below, consider taking barberry, black cohosh, and butcher's broom.

BUGLEWEED—Bugleweed is a remedy for heart palpitations and elevated blood pressure. It may also alleviate anxiety, since elevated blood pressure is frequently associated with a rapid pulse rate, anxiety, and agitation.

CAYENNE—Capsaicin, the active ingredient in cayenne, helps the heart in many ways. It stimulates circulatory function, lowers cholesterol, reduces blood pressure, and lessens the chance of heart attacks and strokes. By decreasing blood levels of fibrin, it also reduces the risk of forming blood clots that cause heart attacks and strokes.

GARLIC—Among its many benefits, garlic helps lower blood pressure and decrease cholesterol. When combined with vitamin E, it lessens the frequency of blood clots in arterial walls, which in turn helps prevent heart attacks and strokes. The recommended amount is 2,000 milligrams per day.

GINKGO BILOBA—Ginkgo biloba helps improve small blood vessel circulation.

HAWTHORN BERRY—Hawthorn is an overall heart tonic that works against arrhythmia (irregular heartbeat), angina, high blood pressure, and hardening of the arteries. It aids circulation and ameliorates valvular insufficiency and an irregular pulse. Hawthorn berry can also correct acid conditions of the blood. It can be safely taken every day.

MISTLETOE—Mistletoe is a cardiac tonic that stimulates circulation. Fifteen drops of tincture taken three times a day or three cups of tea daily can help lower blood pressure and alleviate heart strain. Mistletoe should not be overused, nor should the berries be eaten.

MOTHERWORT—Motherwort helps stabilize the electrical rhythm of the heart. The amount taken should be monitored by a doctor.

WILD YAM—Wild yam stimulates production of DHEA. Low levels of this hormone have been related to higher incidences of heart disease.

CHINESE HERBAL THERAPY

Letha Hadady, one of the leading herbalists in the United States, says most Americans do not go to the doctor when they are a little sick; they wait until they are really suffering. They may have chest pains or difficulty breathing, but they generally don't go to the doctor or, of course, to the herbalist. They say, "I'm tired; I'm under stress," and ignore it. That is a problematic approach because some of the associated conditions of heart disease are the ones they are complaining of: fatigue, stress, and poor digestion. Poor digestion and fatigue lead to cholesterol buildup, which leads to pain and heart congestion. People try to breathe more deeply and reduce stress when they experience these early symptoms, but that does not help. However, changing your diet, taking herbs and foods that reduce cholesterol will definitely help.

Hadady's clients often have conditions that they believe are unrelated to heart disease, but her special training as an herbalist enables her to see a connection to the heart. Mind, body, and spirit are interconnected, and the heart is affected by all of these. Depression, for example, is related to a weak heart. Insomnia, poor concentration, and palpitations are all signs that poor circulation could be affecting the heart.

Many Western doctors will say that herbs have not been tested. But when you go to a public library or consult an online medical search and reference service such as Medline, which is available free to any interested person, you find 3,500 studies on Chinese herbs alone. The majority of the research is done in Asia.

Quite a number of these remedies are available in health food stores, by mail order, or in your local Chinatown. The ingredients are always in English or Latin on the back.

Hadady points out that one of the major underlying problems associated with heart disease is fatigue. Chinese doctors link the heart's health to the strength of the adrenal glands—not an obvious connection. Hadady states, "If I had a patient complaining of fatigue and being overweight, I would suspect heart problems— if not then, somewhere down the line, so I would work on the adrenals. To strengthen the adrenals, you can get the herbal preparation from Chinatown called Goldenbook. It adds to immune energy and will help with kidney and heart problems. We strengthen what is weak so that the heart will not falter."

Hadady explains that clove is a strong stimulant. A pinch in the late afternoon will act like coffee. Coffee is a major problem because it increases painful, sluggish circulation in the gastrointestinal tract that affects the whole circulation, meaning that the heart will not run smoothly. A pinch of clove will replace coffee better than anything else can.

Siberian ginseng, a blend of various ginsengs, is beneficial. The ginsengs are adaptogens; that is, they help us maintain energy as well as aid us in living under a high level of stress. They support the nervous system. Raw Tienchi ginseng, one that Americans are less familiar with, comes in powdered form. A half teaspoon in cool water, taken every day, will reduce cholesterol and pain around the heart.

One Chinese remedy that is especially valuable in relation to heart pain and blood vessel congestion is dan shen wan, which combines salvia and camphor. The camphor dilates the blood vessels while the salvia increases the heart's action. Another valuable remedy is guan xin su he wan, which contains frankincense. Both frankincense and myrrh improve circulation. Frankincense increases blood flow around the heart. You can take it once a day to prevent heart attack. It can be chewed and swallowed. Hadady recommends it even if you have no heart symptoms. It has healthy ingredients such as liquid amber and sandalwood, which keep the esophagus and chest cool.

Yang shen jia jiao wan is a combination of ginseng and other herbs that free the circulation of the blood in the brain. This is not just for victims of heart attack but also for those with stroke and hemiplegia (paralysis of one side of the body).

People with high cholesterol and those at high risk of heart trouble can take one dose a day as a preventive measure.

Baoxin wan is a remedy for heart attacks. If you feel faint and experience pain and weakness, you sniff it like a smelling salt. If the pain is great and you feel the onset of an attack, take it orally. It includes ginseng and liquid amber. It treats the congestion of the blood vessels around the heart and opens them up.

Some of the underlying problems leading to a heart attack, such as excess weight and cholesterol, are well countered by herbal remedies. One preparation whose name is self-explanatory is Keep Fit, Reduce Fat. The ingredients are ginseng, hawthorn, and other herbs that are good for the heart. Hawthorn, a slightly bitter, slightly sour berry, works as a digestive. You can take a capsule of Keep Fit after meals. Cholesterol is reduced, and the muscle of the heart is made stronger.

Evening primrose oil is another useful herb for reducing cholesterol. Chinatown is an excellent place to purchase this remedy since the prices are apt to be considerably lower than those for comparable items in health food stores.

Another popular remedy in Asia is green tea, which has been reported in the popular press as being very good for reducing cholesterol. "This is a good alternative to other caffeine teas," Hadady notes, "because the caffeine in it is very low. It gives the satisfaction of a bitter tea while reducing cholesterol."

Bojemni slimming tea protects the heart. It includes hawthorn. Xiao yao wan, a digestive remedy that boosts circulation and combats depression, contains ginger, mint, and other herbs; it eases the flow of bile, eases the digestive process, and reduces chest congestion.

Digestive Harmony is an American-made product that contains Chinese herbs, one of many such products that are now on the market and sold door to door or through mail order. "This is part of a trend now," Hadady explains, "a very important trend in herbalism, of using Asian herbs manufactured with American standards. Digestive Harmony can be ordered from Oakland, California. It will ease the underlying troubles related to heart disease.

"Remember that depression is in part a heart problem," Hadady goes on. "The heart is not just a circulatory center, but is related to our emotions. Depression is rightly associated with heart disease since it affects the heartbeat. When we are not happy and our emotions are not smooth, we feel it in the heart.

"Some remedies that combat depression come to us from China. Schizandra strengthens the energy level and keeps us from losing the energy we have. It is good for both the adrenals and the heart. It fights against poor memory, poor concentration, and depression. Also try anshen bu nao pien, available in all the Chinatowns in the United States. It is for depression, blood deficiencies, and heart-related problems such as panic and anxiety.

"Also useful is mao dong qing, which is the Chinese name for holly, and it comes in capsule form. It is for chest pain and prevention of heart trouble. You can take several of these capsules each day as a preventive. If you already have heart problems, it reduces cholesterol, congestion, and pains.

"In general," Hadady concludes, "Chinese remedies for the heart treat not just pain but also emotional problems: sadness, anxieties, and other mental suffering."

CHELATION THERAPY

Chelation therapy, which is being administered to hundreds of thousands of heart disease patients, is proving quite successful, and is considerably safer and substantially less expensive than bypass surgery. It is not new, having been in use since the 1950s. In 2013, the skeptical mainstream medical community was surprised when the procedure received a stamp of approval from the US government: a $30 million, multicenter study of chelation therapy for coronary artery disease conducted by the National Institutes of Health showed a "modest but statistically significant" reduction in cardiovascular events, with the greatest benefit seen in people with diabetes when high-dose vitamins and minerals were also used.

Chelation involves the infusion into the bloodstream of the amino acid EDTA. The EDTA bonds with toxic metals and calcium and carries them out of the bloodstream through the kidneys, slowing or reversing some plaque formation in the arteries and thus retarding the degenerative process. EDTA enhances blood flow, permitting more essential oxygen and nutrients to circulate and be absorbed by the body. As chelation therapy is more commonly used, chelation specialists feel that it will become the most important heart disease therapy offered in the future.

As Dr. Steenblock describes, "EDTA binds with calcium that has deposited in artery walls and is excreted from the body through the kidneys. In addition, it breaks down scar tissue and allows the arteries to become softer. In other words, it takes the *hard* out of *hardening of the arteries*."

When deciding whether or not to administer chelation therapy, Dr. Cutler tests patients for heavy metal buildup. "I look for elevated iron and copper levels in the blood. I also measure something called the serum ferritin, which reflects artery tissue levels of iron. If I start chelation, as the iron levels come down in the blood, there are also clinical improvements in angina and exercise tests. And there are angiogram and treadmill test improvements as well.

"If I do not find any abnormality in these metals, I do what is called a challenge, which means I give one chelation treatment, collect urine for twenty-four hours afterward, and observe the metals that come out. Based on these results, I make the decision as to whether I want to chelate the person."

Dr. Steenblock, who has administered chelation therapy for more than twenty-five years, uses the treatment more extensively. He explains why it is so valuable for most individuals. "In their forties most people develop some degree of atherosclerosis due to cholesterol, scar tissue, fat, and calcium, which accumulate in the artery walls.

"You have to try to prevent all these risk factors by keeping your diet low in fat and cholesterol and by exercising, thinking properly, avoiding chemicals, and taking antioxidants to protect the inner lining of the blood vessels. In addition, you can break down scar tissue and remove calcium with chelation.

"Studies show that if you start chelating in your forties, you can actually reverse all the atherosclerosis as soon as it starts to develop. If you have done things that have not been perfect in your life—you haven't eaten right, you have been under too much stress, you have smoked—by the time you are forty, you will have some degree of atherosclerosis. Chelation can reverse this process and keep those arteries more pristine.

"By the time you are sixty, the amount of calcium that has been deposited in your arteries is ten times what you had in your arteries at ten years of age. Al Fleckenstein, a leading cardiovascular drug researcher, says in one of his books that the amount of calcium present in the walls of the arteries is the single most important risk factor in the development of atherosclerosis. In other words, as calcium accumulates in the arterial walls, it promotes the development of atherosclerosis; atherosclerosis develops because you are gradually accumulating this calcium. If you can remove the calcium somewhere between the ages of 40 and 60, you can change that ratio, reverse the whole process, and put off the development of atherosclerosis for a number of years. That's for prevention.

"Of course, if you have outright disease, you can be helped as well. I have been doing chelation since 1977, so I have treated thousands of patients, and most do not come for prevention. They come for treatment of disease. They come in with angina or claudication [lameness due to leg pain]. With chelation, most of the time these symptoms disappear. If they do not, it is usually because the person has advanced disease and needs more than the standard thirty treatments. When people who are seventy-five or eighty years old come in with advanced disease, I tell them that they need to start out with thirty treatments—that's one treatment twice or three times a week. They wait a month or two, and then come back and do another thirty. This process continues until we clean out these arteries, because it takes time to reverse all of the terribly occluded blocked arteries that develop over many, many years of bad living."

STRESS MANAGEMENT

Virtually all the authorities agree that if you want to get a handle on heart disease, you have to deal with stress. Stress or distress is a major problem for the American psyche.

For a long while we have known that stress is a contributor to heart disease, but only recently have we begun to understand the physiological basis of the connection.

Dr. Richard Friedman of Harvard Medical School remarks that when confronted with stressful situations, most people try to oversolve the problem. We constantly try to fit square pegs into round holes, and when we find that is not going to work, we turn inward, brood, and look for ways to dissipate stress, frequently by acting inappropriately, such as overeating, drinking, or taking inappropriate drugs or medications. This contributes to the disease process.

Dr. Friedman says there is a link between stress and cardiovascular disease. When we are stressed by a fear of physical or psychological danger, the body exhibits a fight-or-flight response as it prepares to deal with an enemy. Recent research indicates that the body readies itself not to bleed if it is cut or injured, which makes a lot of sense from a biological and evolutionary perspective. However, if the threats are psychological and you have a bad diet, you may be going through stressful incidents twenty or thirty times a day, triggering the fight-or-flight response. Each time this happens, the body prepares not to bleed by making the blood platelets stickier. This internal clotting takes place every time you get angry, whether on a supermarket line or in a traffic jam. Over time this continual clotting can contribute to plaque buildup in the arteries.

Stress also contributes to heart disease by increasing free radical damage to tissues and increasing spasms in the arterial walls.

When you are exposed to a biochemical or psychological stress, a host of changes take place in addition to platelet stickiness. The body's ability to fight off viral and bacterial infection is lessened by the weaknesses induced by stress. Stress compromises the immune system's ability to fight off opportunistic diseases.

There is some good news, though, about our ability to fight off the debilitating conditions that lead to a heart attack. Dr. Friedman notes that just as continued stress leads to a weakening of the system, there is an opposite effect, one that has been labeled by his colleague at Harvard, Dr. Herbert Benson, the "relaxation response." Eliciting this calming response on a daily basis makes it less likely that you will have high blood pressure, arteriosclerotic plaque buildup, or a heart attack down the road.

The relaxation response should be combined with other behavior modifications to create a healthier response to stress, and all these techniques should be combined with the best medical care. That is the way to optimize your health.

Dr. Friedman tells us how the relaxation response is induced: use whatever strategy you have available to let go of any muscle tension you may be experiencing. Make sure your muscles are loose and your jaw lets go. After you feel a bit more comfortable, focus your attention on your breathing. If you find yourself having any distracting thoughts, do not let them bother you or take you away from the process. As soon as you have a distracting thought, simply say to yourself, "Oh well," and return to a concentration on your breathing and to a thought or image that allows you to stay calm, peaceful, and relaxed. Become aware of the cool air coming into your nostrils and the warm air going out. Keep this up till you are deeply relaxed.

HeartMath is a program that uses specific techniques and exercises to improve physical, emotional, spiritual health by making a deeper connection with the heart. It uses biofeedback and positive emotional balancing. "In terms of really changing our being, HeartMath is doing a lot of work in looking at the heart as having more neuroconnectivity," says Dr. Thaik. "The emotions that we resonate with in our heart then turn around and have impact on our brain biochemistry. It has affects within our GI tract and our immune system in terms of allowing us to protect ourselves."

Other ways to overcome stress are exercise, deep breathing, visualization, tai chi, yoga, meditation, qi gong, mantras, massage, Reiki, biofeedback, and aromatherapy. An essential oil blend of ylang ylang, lavender or peppermint, and marjoram added to oil and applied during massage helps calm the system and may even lower blood pressure.

TREATMENT OF HELICOBACTER PYLORI

Dr. Paul Cutler said that research links the Helicobacter pylori bacterium to high incidences of heart attacks and strokes. "Helicobacter pylori causes ulcers and chronic gastritis. Most practitioners are well aware of the higher incidence of stomach complaints in patients with heart disease. Apparently, this little bacterium, which comes from contaminated foods, burrows its way into the stomach wall. In its attempt to fight off the body's defenses, it produces toxins that initiate plaque development and thickening of the blood. This points to a strong correlation between stomach ulcer disease and coronary artery disease."

Fortunately, this problem is simple to cure, said Dr. Cutler: "You can use one particular type of honey that is high in hydrogen peroxide or cider vinegar, bismuth, and extracts of licorice. Or you can take a one-week course of three antibiotics to kill this bacteria, probably 97 percent of the time. It is very gratifying as a physician to see not only stomach symptoms but angina improve, sometimes dramatically, with the treatment of this common bacterial parasite."

HOMEOPATHY

The late Dr. Ken Korins explained how his specialty, homeopathy, seems to get results with heart disease. "Homeopathy works by giving very small doses that are extremely individualized to the person's symptoms and physical state. These doses work by means of a type of vibration or energy that stimulates the body much as acupuncture does."

Many traditional practitioners dismiss homeopathy. These physicians say this therapy has never been proven by randomized, double-blind studies in the way more scientific procedures have been. Dr. Korins argued that is absolutely incorrect. He told us that nearly twenty years ago the *British Medical Journal* reviewed 107 clinical studies of homeopathy. About 80 percent found that homeopathy had positive effects. Many of these were extremely rigorous studies. A double-blind study in the *Journal of Pediatrics*, for example, showed extraordinary results from homeopathy.

What kinds of heart problems improve with homeopathy? Hypertension is one. Homeopathy can also help people recovering from congestive heart failure, cerebrovascular accidents, arteriosclerotic heart disease, and a wide range of other conditions.

In classical homeopathy, the specialist selects a single remedy. Korins elaborated: "We don't rely on a lot of tests and the high technology that goes with them. We prefer to look at what symptoms a person has and how they present themselves. For example, if a person is having angina, tightness, a squeezing sensation, a remedy such as hawthorn cactus, which is extremely effective in treating angina, is called for."

QI (CHI) MANIPULATION

An Asian treatment that has some success with heart patients is the manipulation of qi (chi) energy. This term refers to all the nonliquid, biological energy that circulates through the body. Dr. Jeie Atacama uses qi to accomplish healing. He estimates that he has helped some 5,000 people. Rebalancing qi energy can help greatly with heart disease by rebuilding the body's health and restoring its self-healing powers.

This practice works exactly like acupuncture. It does not use needles, but it shares with acupuncture a focus on the meridians of the body. In a technique he learned from his father, Dr. Atacama uses his fingers directly on the patient's skin. Points are found on either side near the base of the spine. The treatment session should be done three times a week for as many weeks as are called for by the condition. If the problem is cramps in the leg due to poor circulation, ten sessions will get rid of the problem.

Healing practices such as tai chi and qi gong depend on channeling internal qi energies to rebalance the body.

PSYCHOLOGICAL, SOCIAL, AND SPIRITUAL FACTORS

Most healing programs focus on physical modalities. We look at diet, exercise, supplements, and substances to avoid, but people are beginning to understand that more subtle factors have a powerful influence as well. Dr. Ron Scolastico, a spiritual counselor and author of *Healing the Heart, Healing the Body*, believes that the process of remaining healthy involves four important elements: "The first element is our physical life, which most people know a great deal about. The second element looks at our mental life. It is becoming clearer and clearer that our thoughts promote or hinder health and in some cases actually cause disease. The third element addresses our emotional lives. Feelings, particularly love, have a profound effect. The fourth element addresses spiritual factors. I believe those energies come from the soul, which is an incredible source of power, love, and wisdom inside each of us."

Dr. Scolastico says we must draw on each of these factors as needed. Sometimes we must take physical steps such as seeing a doctor and taking medications or herbs, but sometimes that is not enough. "For example, one of my clients developed congestive heart failure after a painful divorce, along with pericarditis, which is an inflammation of the membrane surrounding the heart. She failed to respond to medical treatment, and her condition began to worsen. As I worked with her, she realized that she had lost touch with her soul. The divorce had wreaked such havoc in her emotional life that she could no longer feel love.

"Every day for six months she took an hour to connect with her soul. By doing this, she was able to regain a feeling of deep love for her body and herself. Today she is symptom-free and believes that without inner work she might be dead. So, many times, we need not only physical treatment but mental, emotional, or spiritual work to augment that process."

To promote health at every level, Dr. Scolastico advises the following:

- Connect with your spiritual nature. Religious or not, we need to accept the existence of some benevolent, healing force larger than our personality and physical being. Once we realize we are never alone or abandoned, amazing changes can happen.
- Be mindful of your thoughts. We all have negative thoughts, but this alone does not cause illness. Swallowing them and actualizing them does. We must learn to release negative ideas. This work takes time, and we should not be hard on ourselves when our thoughts are less than perfect.
- Follow the physical principles of health. Living in a healthy way includes eating the right foods, exercising, and getting enough rest, play, and social activity. Giving to others has a beneficial impact on health.
- Create love in your life every day. This is perhaps the most important principle of all. Research shows that love affects

every aspect of our beings, including the physical. When we feel love, all body systems work better. The endocrine system produces beneficial hormones. Muscles relax, so that the flow of oxygen to the cells increases. Immune system function is enhanced. When we are filled with self-love, our health is strongest and our lives improve all around. Recent studies show that self-esteem improves academic performance and promotes emotional stability and greater health.

"A powerful way to enhance self-love," advises Dr. Scolastico, "is to notice when you are creating negative thoughts and feelings about yourself. Then consciously create an experience of love for yourself right at that moment, using the power of the word to augment the process. You can say, 'I just noticed I'm creating these negative thoughts and feelings about myself. I now choose to use my imagination, my creativity, and my will to create an inner experience of love for myself right now, in this minute.'"

Another way to build love into our lives is to set aside time each day for cultivating loving energy. Dr. Scolastico says, "For at least five minutes, use your mind, open your heart, and create love in your feelings. You can do that by imagining a person you love. Let your feelings for that person fill you as you bring that loved one fully into your thoughts and feelings. Let the corners of your mouth lift up in a smile. Just let your heart swell with love. You won't need a scientific test to prove the benefits."

Equal in importance to self-love is the love we share with others. Connecting with family, friends, and community gives us a sense of belonging that is invaluable to our well-being. A link between social bonds and heart health was reported in *Natural Health*. The magazine summarized 30 years of research on the town of Rosetto, Pennsylvania, and concluded that the most important risk factor for heart disease is a lack of community and intimate relationships. In this town, people lived in three-generation households with grandparents, parents, and children. There was a lot of interaction among families and much participation in community organizations. The incidence of heart disease was virtually nil even though residents ate high-fat diets and did not go out of their way to exercise. In fact, there was less coronary heart disease in Rosetto than in any other population in the United States.

Dr. Thaik adds that it's really about learning how to handle the stresses in life and leaning toward the positive vibration and vibrational energy. It's about having love and gratitude, and looking at the things that bring us joy and happiness. "I tend to tell people that every thought, every motion, leads to instantaneous cascades of hundreds and thousands of neurotransmitters, inflammatory markers, cytokines that we haven't even begun to touch the surface of. The things such as cortisol and epinephrine. The buildup of hormones then turns around and has actual effects within the body in terms of blood sugar, blood pressure, and heart rate."

Research Update

An increasing body of evidence is showing the benefits of natural modalities to overall health and well-being. Following is a sample of recent peer-reviewed scientific studies in the area of heart disease.

According to a 2013 study in the *International Journal of Cardiology*, aged garlic extract (250 milligrams) with a supplement of vitamin-B_{12}, folic-acid, vitamin B_6 and l-arginine was found to reduce the progression of coronary atherosclerosis. A 2015 report in *PLoS One* described Whole Body Periodic Acceleration (pGz), a noninvasive technology that improves cardiac function after myocardial infarction by increasing pulsatile shear stress to the endothelium. A 2011 article in the *Townsend Letter* provided abstracts of research confirming that magnesium may reduce risk of sudden heart failure, multivitamins may decrease risks of heart attack, and healthy proteins lower heart disease risk. Using data from nearly 90,000 women in the long term Nurses' Health Study, scientists at Harvard Medical School reported in the *American Journal of Clinical Nutrition* in 2010 that women with the highest dietary intakes of magnesium had a 37 percent reduction in risk of sudden cardiac death. A 2010 report in *Circulation* also cited data from the Nurses' Health Study indicating that women aged thirty to fifty-five who substituted other protein-rich foods for one serving of red meat per day had the following reductions in risk of coronary heart disease: 30 percent with one serving of nuts, 24 percent with one serving of fish, 19 percent with one serving of poultry, and 13 percent with one serving of low-fat dairy. Swedish researchers reported in *American Journal of Clinical Nutrition* in 2010 that daily multivitamin intake was linked with a 27 percent lower risk of myocardial infarction among the women in a target group of 30,000 aged forty-nine to eighty-three years without a history of cardiovascular disease.

Chapter 37

Herpes

Some viral infections, such as a cold or the flu, are like bad party guests you can't persuade to go home. They seem to hang around forever, although you know they will eventually leave. After a few weeks of misery, the cold and flu depart. But there are other viruses, notably herpes, which come to the party with a bedroll and tablecloth, planning to take up permanent residence.

There are a number of types of herpes. One is the common cold sore, which usually occurs before another, more aggressive virus, such as a cold, is going to take hold in the body. Cold sores on the lips are usually referred to as fever blisters. A cold sore is typically classified as herpes simplex virus 1 (HSV-1). A more serious kind of herpes is genital, sexually transmitted herpes, called herpes simplex virus 2 (HSV-2). Herpes zoster (shingles) is a painful skin rash caused by the varicella zoster virus (chicken pox). Herpes also can cause mononucleosis and meningitis, infect the eye, and increase the risk of HIV infection. For the numerous people who already have a diminished or compromised immune system, recurrent outbreaks of herpes can put a further strain on their immune reserves.

According to a 2014 fact sheet from the Centers for Disease Control and Prevention (CDC), one of every six people aged 14 to 49 years, is infected with genital herpes. Women are affected twice as often as men are. It is estimated that as much as 90 percent of the population has been exposed to HSV-1. Over the past decade, the percent of Americans with herpes infection appears to have decreased.

Controversy and Risks

Michele Picozzi, a health writer who specializes in natural medicine and the author of *Controlling Herpes Naturally*, points out that there is some controversy about the relationship between the two HSVs. There is no agreement on the status of "herpes simplex 1, which occurs, technically, above the waist, most often on the face or the lips, and simplex 2, which occurs below the waist. There is a body of evidence that they are actually different viruses, and they are classified as such. However, some researchers think they are both the same virus, which acts differently in different parts of the body. This would indicate that there is merely a herpes simplex 1 that is appearing at different sites."

Herpes can be pervasive, persistent, painful, and embarrassing. It also represents a fairly serious health risk both to the individual and to the community because many people who have herpes, particularly genital herpes—that is, anywhere from 20 to 25 percent—don't know they have the disease, since they don't experience symptoms. Even without symptoms, they can transmit the disease. Herpes is very contagious, and it has no cure.

As Picozzi notes, "Herpes has remarkable staying power. Once you contract it, you have it for life. It never leaves the body. It lies dormant in the nerve endings at the base of the spine. Thus the possibility of infecting people over a lifetime is considerable if there are recurrent outbreaks."

Causes

Some factors involving both food and emotional and physical states can cause herpes to recur, although the exact mechanism by which this happens remains a medical mystery.

According to Picozzi, "Stress is considered to be the number-one precursor to a herpes outbreak, and this applies to all types of stress: emotional, mental, or physical. Physical stress would include such things as overexertion, exercising too long, exercising in the sun, and doing a type of exercise for which your body is not ready. For example, you may be lifting weights and trying to increase your weight load. That may put a strain on the body. Stress inhibits the production of interferon, the body's antiviral agent. That's important, because herpes is a virus. Stress also inhibits the body from creating antibodies to fight off infection."

Certain foods have been found to cause herpes recurrences. These are primarily foods high in the amino acid arginine, including chocolate, peanuts, sunflower seeds, soy, and coconut. There are also some foods that raise the acidity of the blood. A high blood acidity level can irritate soft tissues, which is usually where herpes appears. These foods are sugar—that is, processed sugar—white flour, and red meats.

Exposure to strong sunlight—ultraviolet B (UVB)—has been shown to be a major factor in causing facial herpes, that which occurs on the lips, around the nose, or on other parts of the face.

Some people have a recurrence of facial herpes because there has been a trauma to the skin, for example, when they have dental work. Some people have a sensitive mouth, so just the friction of the dentist working in that area can cause the virus to recur.

Also implicated are seasonal changes, particularly the transitions from winter to spring and summer to fall, when the body goes through certain adjustments and detoxifying periods. This can also cause herpes to recur, depending on how well you are taking care of yourself at that particular time.

Genital herpes can be sexually transmitted, and pregnant women can transmit the virus to their unborn children. Moreover, prescription drugs that lower immunity, such as antibiotics, steroids, and antidepressants, can set off an attack.

Symptoms

About 50 percent of people who have recurrent infections of herpes virus experience warning signs. Medically, these signs are known as a prodrome. These sensations are usually experienced in the area where a previous infection has occurred.

Picozzi explains, "The most common of these is a tingling or an itching, twitching sensation. Some people feel heat or a crawling beneath the skin, or 'pins and needles.' Some feel as if they are coming down with the flu. They feel fatigued. Their lymph glands are swollen, and they have other muscular aches and pains throughout the body. These signals from the brain can last anywhere from a few seconds to a few days."

She describes some recent work on the emotional triggers of an outbreak: "The most interesting thing I have found in researching herpes is the mind-body connection. Most people with genital herpes will tell you that for them, stress is the biggest precursor for an outbreak. I have found that this connection goes even deeper. I call it the overlooked psychological connection.

Genital herpes causes surface sores on the skin and the lining of the genital area. In women, sores can appear on the cervix, vagina, or perineum and may be accompanied by a discharge or vaginal blisters. There is often a burning sensation, especially at the onset of an outbreak. Other symptoms may include urinary problems, fever, and lymphatic swelling. Intercourse is painful and should be avoided during an outbreak to prevent transmission. HSV-2 occurs intermittently and usually lasts five to seven days.

As the name implies, facial or oral herpes tends to attack the skin and mucous membranes on the face, particularly around the mouth and nose. These cold sores tend to appear as pearllike blisters. Although they don't last very long, they can be irritating and painful. Herpes zoster, the result of the varicella zoster virus, causes agonizing blisters on one side of the body, usually on the chest or abdomen. Pain is usually felt before effects are seen, the result of overly sensitive skin covering the affected nerve. The symptoms may last from a few days to several weeks.

Clinical Experience

CONVENTIONAL TREATMENT

There is no conventional medical cure for herpes, although drugs are commonly given to lessen symptoms. Acyclovir, valacyclovir, and famciclovir may be used to decrease the frequency, duration, and severity of genital herpes outbreaks. Herpes medications have many potential side effects, including dizziness, headaches, diarrhea, nausea, vomiting, general weakness, fatigue, ill health, sore throat, fever, insomnia, swelling, tenderness, and bleeding of the gums. In 2000, the FDA approved Abreva (docosanol 10 percent cream) as the first over-the-counter treatment for cold sores.

NATURAL REMEDIES

Herpes sufferers will be glad to learn that natural remedies are often highly effective in shortening the length of outbreaks and diminishing their frequency. Here are some of the important ones to know about.

NUTRITION AND LIFESTYLE CHANGES

When herpes strikes, it is always a good idea to rest and eat lightly. Short fruit fasts, with plenty of pure water and cleansing herbal teas, can be very helpful. Good herbs to include are sage, rosemary, cayenne, echinacea, goldenseal, red clover, astragalus, and burdock root. Beneficial bacteria, such as those found in nondairy yogurt and in supplements containing lactobacillus and acidophilus, support the digestive processes necessary for the maintenance of the immune system. Other nutrients that directly enhance the immune system include garlic, quercetin, zinc gluconate, buffered vitamin C, and beta-carotene. Bee propolis is anti-inflammatory, while B vitamins combat stress. Also good are bee pollen, blue-green algae, and pycnogenol.

Dr. Steven Whiting, author of *The Complete Guide to Optimal Wellness*, has spent a great deal of time looking at the value of lysine. "Lysine is an isolated form of an amino acid. Herpes, like so many viruses, requires complete protein in which to replicate. The lysine molecule mimics the virus's favorite protein structure, yet it is missing several bonds that are vitally important to the virus's lifestyle. When you increase lysine in the blood, the herpes virus attaches itself quite quickly to the molecule, and then it is too late. It is unable to replicate. You can shorten the outbreak of herpes down to a matter of a few hours with this treatment. In fact, if you catch it soon enough, you can keep the outbreak from occurring."

Dr. Whiting recommends a full-spectrum program for the management of herpes. "First take vitamin C, which is a powerful antioxidant and should be used in the presence of all viral infections. Take 2,000 milligrams as a minimum per day. Vitamin E used topically, for example, on the lips, will relieve pressure and irritation quite rapidly. It is also a powerful antioxidant and helps prevent cross-linkage at the outbreak. Take zinc, 100 milligrams per day, and copper, 2 milligrams per day. Acidophilus is certainly very important in any viral condition because of the die-off of the viral material, which eventually has to be processed in the colon. Take four to six capsules once or twice a day. Finally, and most important, is L-lysine, which can be purchased at your health food store in isolated form. In order to achieve saturation at the cellular level, you'll need 1 to 3 grams a day, but take that only for an actual outbreak."

However, as Picozzi notes, lysine is not useful for everyone. "Some people don't do as well as others using lysine alone to control herpes. Some dietary supplement manufacturers have come out with formulas containing lysine with some supporting herbs and vitamins that some people may find more effective."

Nervous system stressors, such as caffeine, alcohol, and hard-to-digest foods such as meat, should be avoided, especially at the onset of an attack. Foods high in the amino acid arginine, such as chocolate, peanut butter, nuts, and onions, are also associated with higher incidences of outbreaks.

Since stress promotes outbreaks, it is important to make time for activities that alleviate tension. Among the many possibilities are biofeedback, yoga, meditation, deep breathing, and exercise.

Toothbrushes should be changed frequently and completely dried before reuse to prevent reinfection. Soaking them in baking soda also fights germs.

HERBS

Picozzi also sees herbs as an important part of the treatment. "Some herbs are very good for building and maintaining immunity. They include echinacea and licorice root, both of which have been shown to have interferon-like properties. Echinacea also has some antiseptic qualities. It helps the body regulate the glandular system."

Also recommended is goldenseal, which is very important because it regulates liver function and in addition is reported to cleanse and dry the mucous membranes, the site where herpes often appears.

Siberian and American ginseng are invaluable in helping the body boost its resistance to stress and infection because they support the adrenal glands and the nervous system.

Tarragon is good because it contains caffeic acid, which has been found to prevent herpes. Tarragon has been shown to be beneficial for fatigue, particularly when taken in combination with lemon balm. Lemon balm has become very popular for both internal and topical use. It's best taken as a tea, two to four cups a day.

Herbs should only be taken for short periods, say one or two weeks, and under the supervision of a health care practitioner.

HOMEOPATHY

According to Dr. Erika Price, a practitioner of classical homeopathy and holistic healing, the following remedies may prove extremely helpful for cold sores:

NATRUM MURIATICUM—When sores are on the lips, especially in the middle of the lips, the 30c potency of this remedy should be taken twice a day.

PHOSPHORUS—Cold sores that manifest above the lips, accompanied by itching, cutting, and sharp pain, should be treated with the 30c potency of phosphorus twice a day.

PETROLEUM—For cold sores that erupt in patches and become crusty and loose around the lips and mouth, Petroleum is indicated. A 9c potency is needed three times a day.

APIS—Apis helps cold sores around the mouth and lips that are accompanied by stinging; it also helps painful blisters that itch and burn. A 6c potency is needed three to four times daily.

The following remedies may be helpful for female genital herpes:

NATRUM MURIATICUM—This remedy is indicated when the herpetic lesions are pearllike blisters and the genital area feels puffy, hot, and very dry. A 6c potency, four times a day, may be beneficial.

DULCAMARA (BITTERSWEET)—Women who tend to get a herpes outbreak in clusters on the vulva or the hair follicles around the labia and vulva every time they catch a cold or get their period probably need Dulcamara in a 12c potency two to three times a day.

PETROLEUM—Petroleum may be beneficial if herpes eruptions form in patches and the sores become deep red and feel tender and moist. Outbreaks usually occur during menstrual periods, and most often affect the perineum, anus, labia, or vulva. A 9c potency should be taken three times a day.

The following remedies may be helpful for shingles:

ARSENICUM ALBUM—This remedy benefits most cases of shingles, especially when the individual feels worse in the cold, worse after midnight, and better with warmth. If taken at the onset of an attack, it is best in a 30c potency twice a day for two to three days. After the first three days, it is indicated if there is a burning sensation in the areas that were affected by the zoster eruptions (typically the chest and abdomen). At this point 12c, taken two to three times a day, is best. This remedy is excellent for getting rid of the burning sensation that is often present.

HYPERICUM PERFORATUM (ST. JOHN'S WORT)—This is a wonderful remedy for any kind of nerve pain. It is indicated whenever there is intense neuritis and neuralgia with burning, tingling, and numbness along the course of the affected nerves. Take this remedy in a 30c potency, two to three times a day, as needed.

AROMATHERAPY

The use of essential oils has recently gained popularity in the United States, where they are used widely in skin and body care products. However, the medicinal value of certain oils has long been accepted in other countries, particularly France, where in many instances, their antimicrobial properties make them an acceptable replacement for drug therapy.

Aromatherapist Valerie Cooksley, author of *Aromatherapy: A Lifetime Guide to Healing with Essential Oils*, says that pure essential oils, properly used, can heal cold and canker sores. One mouthwash she recommends combines 5 drops each of peppermint, bergamot, and tea tree oil with raw honey, which is used as a carrier. This is important, as oils do not mix with water. The mixture is then added to a strong sage or rosemary tea. Rinsing with the formula several times a day balances the pH of the mouth and helps heal infections. Using this daily may even prevent outbreaks.

Additional spot treatments alleviate pain and restore health. One that Cooksley recommends involves dabbing a cotton swab with myrrh oil and applying it directly onto cold and canker sores. Another aromatherapist, Sharon Olson, dabs a cotton swab with diluted tea tree oil and places it on the cold sore to kill the virus. She follows this up later with lavender, which soothes the sore and stimulates the growth of new skin. The addition of fresh aloe vera gel further promotes healing. A side benefit of the therapy is its ability to lift the spirits. "When I get a cold sore, I get depressed," reveals Olson, "so I usually inhale some rosemary or basil to lift my spirits and clear my mind."

Research Update

An increasing body of evidence is showing the benefits of natural modalities to overall health and well-being. Following is a sample of recent peer-reviewed scientific studies on herpes.

An article published on the *Life Extension* website noted that although more research needs to be done, bioidentical progesterone may offer some protection against vaginal HSV-2 infection. In *Antiviral Research*, a 2012 study found that zinc oxide prevented HSV-2 from entering cells, and a 2011 report indicated that the natural cardenolide, glucoevatromonoside, isolated from a Brazilian cultivar of *Digitalis lanata*, inhibited HSV-1 and HSV-2 replication at very low concentrations. Bee propolis was shown in 2010 research in *Phytomedicine* to have antiviral activity against HSV-2.

Chapter 38

HIV/AIDS

According to 2014 data, an estimated 35 million people worldwide are now living with HIV infection, about half of whom are women and girls. Approximately 1.1 million people in the US have HIV, with 50,000 new infections occurring each year. Women account for one in five new infections and deaths caused by AIDS. The proportion of AIDS diagnoses reported among women has more than tripled since 1985, with African-American and Hispanic women disproportionately affected.

In 1984 at a conference in Maryland, Dr. Robert Gallo claimed to have isolated the HIV retrovirus, which he conjectured was the active agent causing AIDS. The press front-paged the story, not only lauding Dr. Gallo and his fellow researchers but also predicting a cure was just a short distance down the road.

Well, more than thirty years have passed and we find that in relation to AIDS, we are not on the high road of hope but slogging through a quagmire of failed studies that provide little sense or information about how the disease progresses; confusing and expensive treatments; and toxic drugs that often do more harm than good. That's the bad news coming from the medical establishment. The good news is where the establishment failed, that is, in the accuracy of their doomsday predictions about the inevitable, plague-like spread of AIDS. AIDS has not spread with either the speed or decimating broadness that was foreseen. On the other hand, if there is to be any good news on the treatment front, it will have to come from the alternative doctors who concentrate on such healing remedies as the use of nutritional and lifestyle changes as well as oxygen and ozone therapies.

Current Outlook

On December 2, 2013, President Obama marked the 25th Anniversary of World AIDS Day by pledging $100 million to research on finding a cure for HIV. Discussing his new push for funding, Obama remarked that, "The United States should be at the forefront of new discoveries into how to put HIV into long-term remission without requiring lifelong therapies, or better yet, eliminate it completely." However laudable this commitment to ending the war on HIV/AIDS is, we must question how it is that billions of dollars spent for decades on a pharmaceutical-based treatment has not yielded better results.

For our answers let's go back to December 9, 1993, when more than 100 persons assembled with their physicians and their medical records in New York City at a major press conference. They had been selected over a twelve month period if they could prove with medical verification, including blood work up, viral load, CD4 and CD8 count, that they had made major improvements without relapse with their AIDS diagnosis. These individuals followed more than 20 different alternative treatment programs. An independent panel of medical and scientific experts brought to the press conference more than 25,000 scientific references from the peer-reviewed literature to verify the medical veracity, efficacy, and safety of any given protocol used by the patients. Herbs, botanicals, homeopathic and naturopathic remedies, intravenous vitamin drips, ozone therapy, meditation, detoxification, stress reduction, a plant-based diet, and antioxidant therapy were all examined for their antiviral, antibacterial, and anti-yeast and/or immune-modulating impacts. Therefore, if one of the patients were to suggest that they were following the Louise Hay, Gerson, or Ann Wigmore protocols, it would not have been difficult to understand how these protocols were helping these individuals' bodies.

All of this was precipitated more than a year and a half earlier by a group of AIDS patients who came each day to a medical facility in the Upper West Side of Manhattan to be attended by a group of physicians, nurse practitioners, and other therapists helping them to restore their immune systems and adopt a more positive, optimistic state of mind. The theoretical framework behind our program was simple: instead of trying to kill the virus with antiretroviral pharmaceuticals designed to stop viral replication before it kills patients, we focused on what benefits could be gained by building up the patients' natural immunity and restoring biochemical integrity so the body could fight for itself.

As they began to make major improvements, one of the patients spoke up one evening. He explained that in addition to his own progress in combating AIDS naturally, he knew of other individuals who were using more natural and holistic modalities all across the country and that the world didn't know of this. The world only knew of the official AIDS treatment: AZT. He and the other people being treated at the facility all feared the mainstream treatment because they had seen how many of their friends and partners as well as other AIDS patients had died or become extremely sick using these aggressive drugs and yet the natural modalities had been virtually ignored in any public discussion on AIDS. So it was at their urging that the press conference evolved.

That day in December could have been historic if only members of the press, scientific community, government agencies, activist organizations, and foundations had chosen to attend and been open to a different medical paradigm. Despite the fact that more than 7,000 individuals from the media and these other groups had been invited on three separate occasions in the months leading up to the press conference, not one showed up. Clearly this was an intentional boycott. As a result, the patients spent the entire afternoon giving their own testimonials, showing their records and having their physicians speak about the remarkable improvements they saw, but the findings presented largely remained a secret from the rest of the world.

Tony Brown, of PBS, learned of the press conference and began to look carefully and meticulously at the AIDS patients who had made remarkable recoveries, inviting more than eight to appear on his national television program. I was also invited to appear on Tony Brown's program since these were my protocols and I had been working every day with these specific individuals for more than sixteen months. The program profiled one man named Louie, who submitted medical records showing that he experienced a life-affirming reversal of AIDS and all of its conditions.

Up to that point, I had spent every day for years working with people with AIDS-defining conditions, written twenty-two articles on living with AIDS naturally and a 750 page reference book with nearly 100 pages of it covering how to treat AIDS naturally. Further, I had produced a documentary, *Living with AIDS Naturally: The Real Heroes*, chronicling the story of AIDS patients in the nineties that did not respond well to orthodox therapy but improved after incorporating natural holistic protocols to their treatment programs.

After all this, one would have thought that this information would have permeated into the mainstream AIDS dialogue. In fact, just the opposite occurred. Because I challenged the safety and efficacy of AZT and called into question the science behind conventional AIDS treatment, I was personally attacked as an AIDS denialist, which I categorically deny. There is no debate that HIV exists and that it attacks the immune system. What is still up for debate is whether pharmaceutical drugs are the complete answer. Back then and still today, there is no opportunity for questioning, you are either on board or thrown overboard and then attacked.

Despite the array of devastating side effects that AZT is known to produce, it is still used today in combination with other medications, albeit at much lower doses. Today, if any physician were to prescribe AZT in the same amount that was typical in the 1980s and early 1990s, they would more likely than not be brought up for medical malpractice. While survival rates have increased with the introduction of new anti-retroviral treatments, the mainstream treatments continue to focus on pharmaceutical drugs to the exclusion of holistic lifestyle therapies. This is especially alarming given the extensive body of independent scientific research spanning decades that indicates that we were right all along about the critical importance of treating AIDS patients by incorporating a comprehensive, immunity-enhancing behavior and lifestyle modification approach that incorporates diet and nutritional therapies, detoxification, exercise, meditation, and stress reduction.

As public awareness about the therapeutic value of alternative approaches to health and wellness increases, a growing number of individuals and groups within the scientific community are calling attention to the benefits of an integrative approach to AIDS. Given President Obama's recent pledge of $100 million towards a cure for HIV/AIDS, it is clear that drugs alone are not the answer. By shifting the paradigm to one that embraces and incorporates proven natural methods, we have the potential to revolutionize modern HIV/AIDS treatments and empower individuals to achieve greater health and longevity.

Conventional Treatments

Among the difficulties I have with conventional programs is that they are restricted in purview almost exclusively to drugs. Various drugs are used to treat the opportunistic infections and illnesses, and to prevent HIV from reproducing and attacking the body's immune system. Since 1995, the number of medications used to treat AIDS has more than tripled. Among the types of HIV drugs available are reverse transcriptase inhibitors, protease inhibitors, fusion inhibitors, entry inhibitors, and integrase inhibitors. Many people take several of these drugs in antiretroviral combinations, or "cocktails."

If one brings up measures to help the AIDS patient that go beyond ingesting pharmaceuticals, says Dr. Dean Black, "this opens up the door to all the lifestyle measures that medicine has so long discounted, the idea that it could be in the behavior of the AIDS victim, in the diet, in the lifestyle in some fashion."

Researcher Bill McCreary points to the absurdity of doctors ignoring their own intuitions about the people they are treating in order to await orders from on high: "Doctors say it's not approved by the FDA so we can't touch it. . . . Doctors usually do a better job because they're there, they know the patient. . . . Today, the doctor works from a cookbook that is issued out of the federal government. They have to abide by that cookbook or they may be found guilty of malpractice."

AZT was developed as a chemotherapy agent in the late 1960s for the treatment of leukemia, but was never patented by its creator, Dr. Richard Beltz, after he established that his chemotherapy compound was "too toxic for even short-term use" and "caused cancer at any dose." Because of this, AZT was never used for its intended purpose as a cancer chemotherapy. Laboratory studies revealed some of its side effects to be hair loss, weight loss, muscle loss, anemia, and the very same pneumonia associated with AIDS. The drug was then shelved.

The drug's antileukemic mechanism of action is to kill growing lymphocytes by termination of DNA synthesis. The rationale of AZT therapy is simple, if not naive: the retrovirus HIV depends on DNA synthesis for multiplication, and AZT terminates DNA synthesis. Thus AZT should stop AIDS.

It should—but there's one catch. As Huw Christie explains, "Cancer cells, which AZT was designed to kill, grow faster than normal tissue cells, the idea therefore being that, when incorporating AZT, they die more quickly than normally replicating cells too. When the treatment is finished and the chemotherapy stopped, the normal tissue cells can set about making up for their own lower rate of loss." Studies show, on the other hand, that no more than one in a thousand lymphocytes are ever infected by HIV—even in people dying from AIDS. Since AZT cannot distinguish between an infected and an uninfected cell, 999 uninfected cells must be killed in order to kill just one HIV-infected cell.

In 1984, the US Department of Health granted a contract for AZT to Burroughs-Wellcome, which remarketed AZT to AIDS doctors as an "antiviral." AZT was first given to human beings in the initial AIDS treatment trials.

A campaign was then waged to get every HIV-positive person on AZT. Researcher John Lauritsen explains: HIV-positive patients "were told that they should go for what was called early medical intervention. There were slogans put out, 'Put time on your side.' The early intervention meant purely and simply AZT. And rather than putting time on the side of these people, what the drug did and is doing is to terminate their lives."

Here's another difference from cancer treatment. In cancer, you begin to take chemotherapy after you contract the disease. AZT, which, as we saw, was originally developed for chemotherapy, has become the first "chemotherapy" prescribed as a preventative before a person shows any symptoms.

Activist G. Hazlehurst put it like this: AIDS "is the only disease I know of where treatment with powerful drugs is begun several to many years prior to the actual onset of any illness, when there is still the possibility it may not even develop."

Drugs like AZT, as Dr. Martin Feldman points out, "tend to severely weaken the immune system and make the body have to work harder to have immune strength. The body uses up its basic nutrients in the process. Really, the body is fighting against the AZT."

Natural Therapies

Advocates of alternative treatment tell us that we need to change the focus of treatment toward "stimulating, activating, and increasing" the body's antibody system. The best direction of treatment, according to this perspective, would be to help the body to use the immune system it already has instead of forcing it to tolerate an artificial one.

A number of alternative treatments are having some success with AIDS. In this chapter we will highlight three approaches: supporting the body's own methods of healing and defense by bringing nutrient levels up to optimal levels and making lifestyles changes; working on improving the body's metabolism using a special fatty acid preparation; and elevating the level of oxygen in the blood to boost the immune system and cell activity. We also include my sample protocol. It is important to discuss with a medical professional any alternative therapies you are considering or already using.

Theories and methods that seem very different can have broadly similar results. All of the treatment approaches mentioned below, at the very least, have reversed some of the symptoms of HIV infection in some patients and have improved the quality of life, according to the patients themselves, in many cases.

The approaches are not mutually exclusive. Is there any reason why they should not be used together, complementing each other? For example, it is noteworthy that some of the reported actions of the vitamin C infusions were very similar to those of the ozone infusions used by Dr. Pittman. Both were found to be highly effective in inactivating many viruses, and HIV in particular; and both seemed to augment the effectiveness of the immune system. Perhaps if they were used together, the effects of each would potentiate the other, with results better than either alone.

One of the very important advantages of many of these "nonconventional" methods is that, whether or not they are effective (and there is evidence that some are), they are generally safe. Most nutritional and herbal methods cause far fewer side effects than the pharmaceutical and surgical methods now in favor. This is a major argument for permitting them to be used at the discretion of the individual.

That is a reason for not bringing these modalities under the regulatory authority of the state or organized medicine. It is a matter of constitutional freedoms. But there are also strong economic arguments. The costs of these alternative techniques are almost always far lower than the treatments now approved by organized medicine for the same disorders. Thus, encouraging the use of these other approaches can save the American public, both as taxpayer and as health care consumer, vast amounts of money.

Yes, the physicians whose work with HIV infection we have examined approach health and illness from different perspectives. But they do share a basic worldview that separates them from the practitioners of conventional medicine.

According to the conventional view, my body consists of congeries of mechanisms, with subsystems that can be adequately understood separately, with little regard to the status of the myriad other subsystems. The view of the body found in alternative health care is one that sees its level of interconnectedness as far higher. In a healthy organism all the subsystems are supporting each other in myriad ways, most of which are not yet observable or understood. In the first (allopathic) worldview, most disease originates through the breakdown of some one mechanism, or a few discrete mechanisms; disease, then, is to be treated by fixing or bypassing the defective mechanism. In the second (holistic) worldview, however, disease has to do not only with individual mechanisms but also with weakening of many kinds of couplings between mechanisms, and with over-stressing supporting systems through excessive demands for support.

OPTIMIZING NUTRIENT LEVELS AND MAKING LIFESTYLE CHANGES

Evaluations of the health conditions of HIV-infected persons before they show any disease symptoms indicate that many have poor nutrition, including decreased body mass, fat, and protein, resulting from malabsorption. Malabsorption can lead to immunosuppression, infection, and mucosal damage. Dr. Christopher Calapai sees the body's inability to profit from food nutrients as stemming not only from absorption problems but also from anorexia and high resting energy expenditure (REE). REE means that the body is overstimulated. While it should have slowed during rest, the metabolism is still using up nutrients at an accelerated pace. In any case, the HIV-infected person is either not getting or using too quickly the nutrients he or she needs to support bodily functions.

There is no question that certain vitamins are needed to maintain immune response. These include E, B_6, C, and beta-carotene. In fact, there is evidence that certain vitamins as well as herbs can counter the progress of AIDS as they bolster the immune system. The Institute for Traditional Medicine in Portland, Oregon, has done some vital work in looking at how Chinese herbs can be used in treating AIDS. The founder of the institute has developed a specific herbal combination that combines strong tonic herbs with those that fight inflammation and infection. Of 150 patients who have undergone therapy with this herbal formula over three months, 76 percent experienced an increase of energy, and 62 percent of the patients who suffered from diarrhea saw a cessation of the problem. Other symptoms were similarly improved.

Dr. Chang of the Sun Yat Sen Medical Center also found a mix of Chinese herbs to work strenuously against AIDS. He found that extracts from eleven different herbs inhibit the activity of HIV. Dr. Quingcai Zhang notes these Chinese herb treatments are effective because they work with the body to fight infection, rather than by trying to override the body's own creative functioning, the way drugs such as AZT do.

Some of the vitamins and herbs that have been used for treating people with AIDS with positive results are listed below.

VITAMINS

GLUTATHIONE—Glutathione is an antioxidant that protects against cellular damage. It stimulates lymphocytes that help defend the body against viral illnesses, such as AIDS. When N-acetyl-cysteine (NAC) is given to a patient, the body will convert it to glutathione.

A study in *Nutrition Review* indicates that HIV-positive individuals are deficient in glutathione. On the other hand, results have been reported from a number of studies that indicate HIV activity is reduced by glutathione's presence.

Dr. Joan Priestley gives her HIV-infected and AIDS patients intravenous glutathione, because, she says, "Glutathione specifically attacks the AIDS virus in about four different steps."

At an AIDS symposium, Dr. Calapai stated, "When we add glutathione intravenously with vitamin C, we see a significant turnaround in the patient's comfort, attitude, and well being. . . . NAC taken intravenously can inhibit reverse transcriptase [HIV replication] activity better than 90 percent. There is no drug available for any treatment or disease that can do better than 90 percent with minimal or no side effects."

BETA-CAROTENE—Beta-carotene is a safe form of vitamin A, which stops damage from bodily pollution, bolsters the immune system, inhibits viruses, and prevents premature aging.

A study done by Dr. Semba of Johns Hopkins showed that a vitamin A deficiency found in HIV-positive and AIDS patients was a serious risk factor for the disease. In a different study, Dr. Semba's team found that a lack of vitamin A was positively correlated with death from AIDS.

On the other hand, a number of studies chart improvements when beta-carotene is administered. In one, eleven HIV-positive patients received 60 milligrams of the vitamin per day for four months. They recorded an increase in natural killer cells and other vital parts of the immune system, which HIV infection tends to diminish. Another study was done on ten patients who had just gotten off AZT and began taking 120 milligrams a day of beta-carotene. Although one died a few months into the treatment, the other nine experienced an HIV-burden diminution, clinically measured improvements in health, and evaluated themselves as having a better quality of life.

VITAMIN C—Vitamin C is one of the stars among the vitamins in treating AIDS. Basing his opinion on numerous clinical studies, the late Dr. Robert Cathcart confidently stated, "Vitamin C can double the life expectancy of AIDS patients." He said that his treatment, which involves using massive doses of buffered ascorbate of 50 to 200 grams every twenty-four hours (in combination with other treatments for secondary infections), will produce a clinical remission of the disease that shows every evidence of being prolonged if the treatment goes on.

Other doctors report similar results. Dr. Raxit Jariwalla, a virologist from the Linus Pauling Institute, says, "In laboratory cultures of HIV-infected cells . . . vitamin C can significantly suppress both the activity and the replication of the AIDS virus."

Joy DeVincenzo, who is HIV positive and has used massive doses of vitamin C, explains, "A lot of doctors . . . do not believe in giving me vitamin C . . . [but] without it, I know I wouldn't have stayed stable for so long."

These statements are supported by a host of studies, such as the one that appeared in the volume *Nutrition and AIDS*, which summarized the results of various examinations of C's value. The authors point out, "A striking property of ascorbic acid is its ability to inactivate viruses and inhibit viral growth in their host cells." Experimental studies reported in the same volume show that vitamin C will directly interfere with HIV replication, carrying the assault on the disease into the enemy's camp.

VITAMIN E—Vitamin E is an antioxidant that seems to prevent many diseases caused by environmental stressors. It is found in fish and vegetable oil, nuts, and whole grains. However, most Americans do not get enough of this vitamin in their foods and need supplementation.

Studies are piling up showing that vitamin E is a warrior against AIDS. One study showed that the administration of 50 milligrams per kilogram per day over five days already began to inhibit the replication of HIV. Another study showed that if the dosage of E was increased fifteen-fold (to 160 IU/liter), immune system functions that had been suppressed by HIV presence were restored.

HERBS

ASTRAGALUS—Astragalus root has been used for centuries in China because it was thought to strengthen the immune system. Current research shows the truth of this belief, since astragalus is now known to correct T-cell (part of the immune system) deficiency and to promote antiviral action.

A study at the University of Texas showed that taking astragalus extract stimulates T-cell production in healthy animals and restores it in cancer patients who have seen their T-cell production impaired. In another study involving nineteen cancer patients with weakened immune systems, an extract of astragalus induced such a complete recovery that it was noted, "People whose immune systems were devastated by cancer experienced full restoration of immune function."

Of course, studies need to be conducted on AIDS sufferers, but astragalus's aid to the immune system is evident.

GARLIC—Garlic has a number of antitumor and antiviral mechanisms. It stimulates the immune system's production of phagocytosis, which eliminates abnormal cells from the body. It is toxic to some abnormal cells and inhibits the implantation of others. It has even proven effective against some bacteria that do not respond to antibiotics.

In fighting AIDS, it is especially good in eliminating the opportunistic infections that set in once immune systems have been weakened. A German study of seven AIDS patients who were given 5 grams of garlic daily found that five of them showed significant improvements in their T cells, along with other improvements in health and fewer outbreaks of opportunistic infections.

GINSENG—Numerous studies of ginseng's benefits were conducted in Russia in the 1960s and 1970s. Norman Farnsworth collected and translated many of these studies, which indicated that various types of ginseng acted to normalize body temperature, enhance the body's ability to resist infection, improve cells' ability to dispose of the by-products of metabolism, and counter the effects of environmental pollution.

Its effects in treating AIDS patients have also been shown. In a study by Y. K. Cho and others, Korean red ginseng improved weakened immune response in subjects infected with HIV.

LICORICE ROOT—Licorice root has also been effective in stopping the HIV virus from replicating. A study, done at the World Life Research Institute, recorded no toxicity to normal cells.

The plant is known to strengthen the immune system by increasing macrophage activity and that of interferon-gamma, both vital actors in combating infections and viruses. Licorice is a detoxifying agent and has anti-inflammatory, antiallergic, and antispasmodic properties.

ST. JOHN'S WORT—Studies at New York University have shown that St. John's wort contains two potent chemicals that are highly effective in preventing the spread of retroviruses, such as HIV, both in laboratory samples and in patients.

One of the researchers found that one of these chemicals would stop the spread of AIDS, even crossing the barrier into the brain, which serves as a reservoir of HIV cells, to combat the disease there. This researcher comments that St. John's wort's "antiviral activity is remarkable both in its mechanism . . . and in the potency of one administration of a relatively small dose of the compounds."

PHYTOCHEMICALS

Phytochemicals are disease-preventing or healing substances found in edible plants, such as those found in licorice root, which are believed to account for the plant's valuable immune-system strengthening qualities. These chemicals are found in frequently consumed foods such as fruits, vegetables, grains, legumes, and seeds as well as in less common foods such as soy and green tea. They have already been associated with the prevention and treatment of four of the leading causes of death in this country: cancer, diabetes, cardiovascular disease, and hypertension. Although not enough studies have been done on these substances, those that have been done hint that quite large benefits are to be expected.

Research on limonene, found in citrus fruits, shows that it increases the body's production of enzymes that help it dispose of potentially carcinogenic substances. It is well known that people whose diets are heavy in fruits have lower rates of most cancers than do those who don't have such diets. Many are attributing this low cancer rate to the effect of the phytochemicals.

LIFESTYLE CHANGES

Research supports the long-term efficacy of dietary counseling and use of nutritional supplementation for people with AIDS to increase or maintain weight, restore lean tissues, and lessen the effects of the disease. Patrick Donnelly, program coordinator for the Whole Foods Project, says AIDS patients must be made aware of the need to eat nutritious foods. He advises working with "the new four food groups, which are grains, legumes, fruits, and vegetables." These foods are high in antioxidants and have nutrients like beta-carotene, vitamin C, zinc, and selenium. Such nutrients are not found in the high-fat, high-protein standard American diet. Donnelly says, "We're trying to get people to look at a new way of eating that is not about providing calories so much as supporting the immune system."

Another member of the project staff, Richard Pierce, comments, "You only have to look at this food [we provide] to see that it's full of life. . . . The vitality of the food is what nurtures us."

Along with eating healthy foods, one must learn to avoid the foods that contribute to the growth or virulence of disease, counterproductive foods, particularly yeast and sugar. Yeast is a natural part of our makeup, but it can wreak havoc on the body when it gets out of control. Sugar is an immune suppressant. If one takes 100 grams of sugar, it will cut antibody production by 50 percent for twenty-four hours.

Studies have shown that regular exercise has long-term benefits on the biological condition of HIV and AIDS patients as well as on the course of the illness. Researchers have found that exercise will improve a patient's health at all stages of the disease. Moreover, it seems that complications of the disease will be delayed by exercise.

ACUPUNCTURE

Acupuncture has proven to be one of the most popular treatments for people with HIV. One study found that people with HIV who use the treatment have extended survival rates. In addition, they regularly report a substantial reduction in symptoms and side effects from HIV-related drugs. Acupuncture frequently provides relief from AIDS-related diseases, and most patients report a reduction in fatigue, abnormal sweating, diarrhea, and acute skin reactions after four to five treatments. Some patients have a fifteen- to twenty-pound weight gain and return to long hours of work.

Abigail Rist-Podrecca, a registered nurse, notes that acupuncture works by "dilating the blood vessels, so that the vessels can open. You get more circulation, more of the nutrients, more oxygen flowing through those meridians [the places where the acupuncture needles are stuck]."

She believes one of the reasons people with AIDS weaken is that they lose the ability to take up nutrition through the intestines. Acupuncture acts to reverse this digestive problem as well as working on the lungs and other bodily centers.

Studies conducted at the Lincoln Hospital Acupuncture Clinic in New York, the AIDS Alternative Health Project in Chicago, and the Quan Yin Herbal Support Program in San Francisco have reported symptomatic relief and overall physical improvement following acupuncture.

REFLEXOLOGY AND AROMATHERAPY

Reflexology is a form of relaxation treatment. It was used in an AIDS program in Uganda. Four months after the program began, 85 percent of those treated noted pain relief, better relaxation, and better sleep following the reflexology sessions.

Aromatherapy is the use of plant essences in healing. Pure oils are used, some of which have already proven to have antifungal and antiviral effects. One study looked at the effect of aromatherapy when used in conjunction with other therapies to see if it would lessen the need for toxic drugs. Using eighty randomly selected AIDS patients, the study concluded that the group that utilized aromatherapy, in contrast to the control group, reported fewer aches and pains, faster healing of wounds, greater physical strength, and a better ability to cope.

IMPROVING METABOLISM

The late Dr. Emmanuel Revici also believed that AIDS must be managed by addressing nutritional deficiencies. His approach, though not based on Chinese medicine, did resemble the Asian system in viewing the body as driven by two cross-currents, *yin* and *yang*, that create the body's vitality. The body's health depends on their balance. Dr. Revici's program saw two basic processes in the body: the anabolic, which builds up, and the catabolic, which breaks down. When an organism is working normally, it maintains its characteristic rhythms and intensities by means of this oscillation. However, when there is a breakdown, it will be because the alternations are lopsided, and either catabolic or anabolic influences are unduly dominating. It is as if a pendulum's swing were being artificially pulled to one side.

In the case of AIDS, there is a deficiency in certain of the body's phospholipids (a type of fat), which normally play a role in disease prevention. The course of the disease is as follows: A primary viral infection occurs, which brings about the weakening of the body's line of lipidic defense. This is followed by secondary, opportunistic infections that are allowed to run wild due to the body's lowered defense threshold. Then comes an exaggerated catabolic imbalance whereby the body's breakdown of substances is outrunning its construction of others.

The treatment called for in such a case is a four-pronged one. To deal with the viral infections, antiviral agents should be introduced into the system. To deal with the lipid deficiency, these lipids have to be reintroduced by injection. For the secondary opportunistic infections, proper antibiotics are applied. And for the catabolic imbalance, balancing agents are prescribed.

I examined ten of Dr. Revici's cases and I can make these generalizations about them: Of these patients, only three seem not to have improved during therapy. Yet, of these three, one, though worsening in immunologic markers, nevertheless felt "well" at the end of ten years of treatment. Another, though his T4 count also declined considerably over four years of treatment, was still "feeling fine" at the end of that period. Thus, of the ten patients, eight currently (or recently) report feeling well after an average period of 5.2 years of therapy. Five of the eight also report no remaining symptomatic complaints, and two of those have had a marked improvement in immune markers. All are currently continuing in therapy.

OXYGEN AND OZONE

Dr. John Pittman of the Carolina Center for Integrative Medicine has developed a treatment based on the use of ozone and oxygen. Oxygen is an essential nutrient. It is, in fact, the most essential, as it is the only one that must be continuously available, at pain of quick death. As we all know, life ceases if the supply of oxygen is cut off for more than a few minutes. A number of studies indicate that ozone inactivates HIV at low and safe concentrations. It has been conjectured that ozone kills HIV cells. Ozone is also able to strengthen immune responses.

Dr. Pittman believes that ozone can arrest the progression of AIDS diseases and turn the syndrome into a manageable condition. He values ozone's ability to help alleviate chronic problems that plague patients, including dermatological conditions and low-level infections. He also notes a relationship between ozone and improved T-cell and CD4 counts. Best results occur when an intensive series of treatments is taken every four to six months.

Dr. Pittman uses ozone as an integral part of a wider treatment protocol. He explains, "The first ten days of their program entails a modified juice fast. Everyone drinks fresh-pressed vegetable juices and eats no solid food." Patients are then put on an intensive detoxification program. Nutritional supplements are given. The patient begins autohemotherapy. This involves the removal of blood from the body so that it can be filled with ozone and then reinfused.

After five days of autohemotherapy, Dr. Pittman says, "if the patient has tolerated that . . . we begin with the direct intravenous infusion of ozone gas . . . on a daily basis, gradually increasing concentrations and volume until we observe a healing crisis in the patient." The patient will experience fevers, chills, and sometimes flu symptoms. When the healing crisis passes, the doctor tapers off dosage and concentration, and goes into lower doses, "which have a more immune-stimulating effect."

Concurrent with ozone therapy are other intravenous therapies, which include intravenous vitamin C and mineral infusions as well as EDTA chelation therapy. The doctor also employs acupuncture and other dietary therapies throughout the program.

Although I was not able to obtain the same detailed case histories from Dr. Pittman that I had from the other practitioners mentioned here, I did gather very positive anecdotal evidence, including the story of a man who came to the clinic with a CD4 count of 42. In two weeks of intensive therapy, his count soared to 285.

As you can see, Dr. Pittman believes in a nontoxic multifactorial approach in the treatment of AIDS. He says, "I think the approach for AIDS has got to be one from a multimodality standpoint. There is no one single approach. It is only through the combination of appropriate antiviral therapy, immune-stimulating therapy, diet, and detoxification programs that a patient is really going to be maintained and have any hope of improvement."

Gary Null's Protocol for HIV/AIDS

Here is a sample AIDS protocol outlining the program I have used for decades to help countless individuals deal with their HIV/AIDS naturally. As with other protocols in this book, it is not in any way to be construed as a prescription to cure the condition, but as nutritional, lifestyle, and behavior modification suggestions only. Always consult with a physician for guidance on specific health issues and before following this or any other protocol. A patient's diagnosis, treatment, and medications must be considered in determining if any of the suggested vitamins, minerals, foods, and herbs are contraindicated. Special consideration should be given to pregnant and nursing mothers. Many supplements do not have a suggested dosage. Individual clinicians must make individual recommendations based on the patient. Finally, the protocol below must be implemented in gradual steps. It is suggested to begin with low doses of one or two items to determine the patient's acceptance and tolerance. Once it is determined that the patient has adapted, the dosage should be increased in gradual steps.

DIET

The diet is an immunosupportive DNA-reparative, cleansing, and pH-rebalancing program. It is recommended to begin the day with a large smoothie containing a tablespoon of one of the following healthy oils: black cumin seed oil, coconut oil, or flaxseed oil. Add a handful of either walnuts, almonds, cashews, pistachios, sunflower seeds, pumpkin seeds, or chia seeds; concentrates from blueberry, pomegranate, tart cherry, noni, or papaya; a teaspoon of probiotic powder containing at least 5–10 billion CFU, as well as 30–40 grams of a high-quality, non-GMO protein, either from rice, pea, hemp, or soy.

Include smaller meals throughout the day with a full spectrum of sea vegetables, fermented foods, starchy vegetables, legumes, whole grains, and liberal amounts of garlic and onion, and wild fish (preferably sardines and salmon).

Drink either wheatgrass juice, bitter melon juice with raw honey and bee propolis, or combinations of vegetable and fruit juices throughout the day, ideally 16 ounces each.

SUPPLEMENTS

L-Carnosine/Acetyl L-carnitine
Whey protein: 30–60 g/day
SAMe: 400–800 mg/day
Magnesium: 400–500 elemental mg
Calcium: 400–500 mg
Vitamin B_6 (pyridoxine)
Vitamin B_{12}
Folic acid
SOD
DMG
Pancreatic and proteolytic enzymes

Multimineral supplement

EFAs: borage, omegas 3 &6, GLA, EPA

Lecithin

CoQ10: 1,000 mg

Curcumin

DHEA

Citrus bioflavanoids

Ginseng

Milk thistle

Green tea extract

Monolaurin

Melatonin

NAC: 1000–1,800 mg three times a day

Grape seed extract: 400 mg

Alpha lipoic acid: 300 mg twice a day

Vitamin B2 (riboflavin)

Beta-carotene/vitamin A

Vitamin B1 (thiamin)

Vitamin B3 (niacinamide)

Vitamin B5 (pantothenic acid)

Evening primrose oil

Vitamin C: 2,000–10,000 mg/day

Quercetin: 3,000 mg

St. John's wort: 300 mg

Vitamin E—mixed tocopherols

Vitamin K

Zinc

Vanadium

Garlic/cayenne

MSM

Selenium: 200 mcg twice a day

Chromium picolinate

Activated lipids (AL 7/21)

Germanium

Astragalus

Silymarin

Eurocel
Lactoferrin
Probiotics

OTHER MEDICALLY SUPERVISED THERAPIES
Ozonated colonics/coffee enemas
HBOT—hyperbaric oxygen therapy
IV Vitamin C drips and bio-oxidative therapies require MD orders
IV DMSO
Chinese herbs/AMMA/Acupuncture
Bach flower remedies
Hyperthermia
Homeopathic remedies
Positive visualization
Guided imagery
Stress management therapy
Hydrazine sulfate if wasting syndrome occurs
Check cortisol levels regularly

TOPICAL TREATMENTS
Virgin castor oil
Calendula
Aloe/avocado oil baths
Colloidal copper spray

SAMPLE DETOXIFICATION LIFESTYLE PROTOCOL
Take the following daily as directed:

The First Four Weeks:
Two (2) – 16 oz. glasses of green juice per day:
Juice 4 oz. dark & light green vegetables. Add 12 oz. water
or
1 tbsp. of powdered dry green concentrate. Add 12 oz. water.
In the above juices, add 1 oz. of aloe concentrate and 1 tsp. of red fruit dried concentrate.

At Night:

Antioxidant complex: Follow the instructions on the label

Garlic with cayenne powder: Follow the instructions on the label

Psyllium bifidis fiber: Follow the instructions on the label

Vitamin C: 500–2,500 mg

After 4 weeks add:

Quercetin: 550 mg 3X/day

Pycnogenol: 50 mg 3X/day

L-Carnitine: 250 mg 2X/day

After 4 more weeks add:

Brain complex, 3 capsules per day or

Ginkgo biloba: 100 mg (consult your doctor if on blood thinners)

L-Phenylalanine: 5 mg

L-Glutathione

L-Taurine

Choline bitartrate complex

Inositol

L-Glutamine

L-Tyrosine

Phosphatidyl Serine Naturleaf (enzyme enhanced)

Plant-Sprout sterols/sitosterolins: 500 mg 4x/day

MGN 3: 500 mg 3x/day

Increase antioxidant complex to 5 times per day

B-Complex: 50 mg

DIETARY GUIDELINES

1. No meat: Includes beef, poultry, and shellfish.

Replace with: cold water fish (wild salmon, sardines) 4 times/week; nuts, nut butters, seeds, soybeans and soy products, organic eggs, quinoa. Mix grains with beans.

2. No dairy: Includes milk, yogurt, cheese, butter, ice cream, cream sauces.

Replace with: rice milk, soy milk, almond milk, Amazake, Silken tofu, oat milk. Nothing with "casein" in the ingredients.

3. No caffeine or alcohol: Includes chocolate, coffee, tea, wines, hard liquor, etc.

Replace with: herb teas, grain beverages (postum, cafix, Rajs's cup), lemon water, and green tea.

4. No sugar/artificial sweeteners.

Replace with: stevia root, raw manuka honey, molasses, brown rice syrup, and pure maple syrup. May use chromium picolinate (200 mcg) for sugar cravings.

5. No carbonated drinks: Includes sodas, seltzer.

Replace with: spring water, distilled water, filtered water, or fresh-squeezed organic fruit juice.

6. No bread or wheat.

Replace with: spelt bread, sprouted whole grain bread, rice bread, Essene bread. Read the labels.

7. No non-organic produce.

Replace with: organic produce, include potatoes (NOT Idaho), squash, sweet potatoes, yams, grains, beans, fruits, vegetables.

8. No fried/processed foods.

Replace with: steamed, sautéed, stirfried, grilled, broiled meals. Oils for cooking: coconut, macadamia, safflower. For baking: hazelnut, macadamia nut. For salads: Walnut, flax seed. Extra virgin cold pressed olive oil is okay to add to cooked foods; avoid cooking with the olive oil.

9. No food additives, preservatives, coloring agents, flavorings, MSG, or miso.

Eat primarily during the day; have your large meal between 1 p.m. and 3 p.m., a very light breakfast and a light dinner (grains and any salad with dressing, sea vegetable and/or soup).

ORGANIC MEAL PROGRAM

Quality protein and amino acids: 9/10th gr/kg of body weight/day

Approximately 40–60 g/day for women and 50–80 g/day for males

(Suggestion: Begin by getting your protein from grains, legumes, and seeds. If needed, protein powder supplements are useful in guaranteeing sufficient amounts. The diet should provide you with 40–50 g of fiber per day.)

Tofu and tempeh

Grains and sprouts: millet, buckwheat, brown rice, spelt, rye, quinoa

Organic raw vegetables and fruits—all types

Fatty deep water fish: salmon or sardines, 6–8 oz.

Raw seeds and nuts

Tubers: yams, potatoes, or sweet potatoes

3–4 servings of cruciferous vegetables daily: broccoli, cabbage, cauliflower, and onions.

Sea vegetables.

Drink a minimum of 1 gallon of liquids which include purified water and juice.

1–2 cups green tea daily.

Lemon juices daily—to alkalize the body.

Digestive enzymes for fatigue.

If candida is present: use grapefruit seed extract, 5–10 drops in water 3x/day

Oil of oregano—as directed

Olive leaf extract—as directed

EXERCISE

Build up gradually to 1 hour/day of aerobic activity. Take your pulse throughout your aerobic workout to make sure you are neither under- nor over-exerting yourself. Generally, your target rate is determined by taking 220 and subtracting your age and then multiplying the result by 70 percent. So a thirty-one-year-old person would have a rate of 220 minus 31 times 70 percent or 132. In addition to aerobic exercise you must do weight training three times per week.

Research Update

An increasing body of evidence is showing the benefits of natural modalities to overall health and well-being. Following is a sample of recent peer-reviewed scientific studies in the area of HIV/AIDS.

Publishing in *PLoS One* in 2014, German researchers found that extracts of the geranium plant *Pelargonium sidoides* inactivate HIV-1 and stop the virus from attacking human cells. Scientists at the University of Missouri reported that EFdA, a nucleoside analog related to a component used in soy sauce as a flavor enhancer, was significantly more effective than the first-line HIV drug Tenofovir, and less likely to cause resistance and lose effectiveness over time. Their research was published in 2014 in the journals *Retrovirology*, *Antimicrobial Agents and Chemotherapy*, and the *International Journal of Pharmaceutics*.

An article on the *Life Extension* website details numerous other recent scientific studies confirming the effectiveness of natural compounds and treatments. For example, in 2011, researchers at the 29th Annual Scientific Meeting of the Obesity Society reported that green coffee extract produced high levels of chlorogenic acid and other polyphenols that promote healthy blood sugar control and reduce the risk of disease in HIV-infected patients. This is important because long-term antiretroviral drug therapy can cause metabolic problems, including insulin resistance and diabetes. Subjects who took 200-milligram supplements experienced a 14 percent decrease in blood sugar, and those who took 400 milligrams had double the effect at 28 percent. Another 2011 study, published in *Clinical Therapeutics*, added to the evidence showing the benefits of omega-3 fatty acids: 48 HIV-infected patients given 4 grams per day for twelve weeks had significant reductions in triglyceride levels when compared with placebo.

Additional 2010 reports, in the *Scandinavian Journal of Medicine & Science in Sports* and *AIDS Research and Human Retroviruses*, found that physical activity supports immune function and reduces the risk of metabolic abnormalities in HIV-infected patients.

Chapter 39

Hormonal Imbalance and Hormone Replacement Therapy

Disturbance of a woman's hormonal cycle can play a major role in the development of various medical conditions. Women are affected both by their monthly hormonal cycle and by the hormonal phases associated with the life cycle of adolescence, maturity, pregnancy and childbirth, and menopause. Knowledge of these natural events is invaluable in understanding and treating a multitude of symptoms.

"A wide variety of symptoms and seemingly separate diseases can result from hormonal imbalance," says Dr. Michael Wald. "This is where medicine gets confused because they think of hormones only in the narrow range of reproduction. Finally, we are hearing about cardiovascular connections. But there are many other subtle concerns. A loss of estrogen usage in the brain has been associated with dementia and even Alzheimer's. A loss of progesterone usage in the gut is associated with various gastrointestinal symptoms. Chronic inflammation of tissues is a result of hormone imbalance in general. These look like different concerns. Fundamentally, there is hormone disruption."

Among the common problems associated with hormonal imbalance are premenstrual syndrome (PMS), infertility, breast cancer, osteoporosis, heart disease, fibroids, endometriosis, memory loss, mood disorders, and hot flashes.

For more than 40 years, women have been led to believe that the best approach to hormonal imbalance, re-mineralization of the bones, and turning off hot flashes is synthetic estrogen replacement therapy. At any given time, ten million

American women are using it. Now, according to the best scientific literature we have, about 14 percent have adverse effects. Those adverse effects include heart attacks, strokes, breast cancer, ovarian cancer, colorectal cancer, and dementia.

When you consider that we have no monitoring system whatsoever in the United States to determine if a person's heart attack or stroke came from synthetic hormone replacement therapy, then we're talking about numbers that could be in the multiple millions, and yet we don't know. All we know is that a person is more likely to have an effect. The extent of that effect, again, has never been quantified.

Despite known risks, mainstream medicine continues to claim that synthetic hormones remain the most effective solution for the symptoms of menopause, while denigrating any form of natural hormone replacement therapy or rebalancing as nonsense, anecdotal, and quackery. Natural, or bioidentical, hormones are very similar to the ones that are made by the body, and therefore do not carry many of the risks associated with synthetics. However, their use is still a matter of debate, among conventional practitioners as well as in the alternative medicine community. (See chapter 43 for more discussion on the debate over bioidentical hormones).

As you will see in the sections below, hormones of any type are just one part of the solution for hormonal imbalance and not necessary for many women, as lifestyle changes, exercise, herbs, and supplements can often provide relief and restoration of health on their own.

Causes

Dr. Sherrill Sellman, a naturopath, psychotherapist, and author of the best-selling book *Hormone Heresy*, tells us that for the body to function properly, estrogen and progesterone have to be in balance. These hormones stimulate and help balance each other. One function of estrogen is to stimulate estrogen-sensitive tissues, which include cells in the breast, ovaries, and uterus. Estrogen helps develop the curviness of women. It produces their secondary sex characteristics. It is a very powerful stimulant of these tissues. Progesterone, on the other hand, helps slow down the growth of cells and stabilizes mature cells so that their growth doesn't get out of hand. The proper relationship, as Nature designed it, is one of checks and balances.

"We are seeing a predominance of estrogen in relation to just a little progesterone," Dr. Sellman says. "That's caused by the drugs and food we eat and the disharmony in our own bodies. It's been noted that 50 percent of women over the age of thirty-five are not ovulating each month. Now, only if women are ovulating, releasing an egg, can a little endocrine gland called the corpus luteum, which is the primary source of progesterone, be formed on the surface of the ovary. If a woman doesn't ovulate due to stress or bad diet, she can go a whole month without producing the progesterone to balance the estrogen. As a result, women are progesterone-deficient."

DIET AND LIFESTYLE FACTORS
Dolores Perri, a nutritionist from New York City, lists factors that can interfere with normal hormonal production and balance:

ALCOHOL—Alcohol blocks the body's gamma linolenic acid (GLA) production, preventing the manufacture of natural hormones. This quickens the aging process. Alcohol creates deficiencies in B vitamins, magnesium, and calcium, which upset hormone balance. Further, alcohol damages the liver, which in turn interferes with hormone metabolism.

ANIMAL PROTEINS—Animal proteins are loaded with hormones and synthetic antibiotics that throw our own hormone levels out of balance.

BIRTH CONTROL PILLS—Birth control pills deplete the body's B vitamins, which are needed for natural hormone production; increase susceptibility to allergies; and may cause liver damage, which can affect hormonal balance.

CAFFEINE—Caffeine is found in coffee, tea, chocolate, soft drinks, and certain medications. Like alcohol, it blocks GLA production. Chocolate inhibits the liver's breakdown of hormones. Tea interferes with the absorption of iron and zinc, particularly if drunk with meals. Caffeine also raises adrenaline levels and increases stress.

EXERCISE—Professional athletes and women who train vigorously may use up so many vitamins and minerals that the body has insufficient means to maintain normal hormonal production. This can lead to an abnormal menstrual cycle and even the absence of menstruation altogether.

PHOSPHATES AND POLYPHOSPHATES—The phosphates and polyphosphates found in many food products—such as soft drinks, processed meats, and cheese—can interfere with the absorption of nutrients.

SMOKING—Cigarettes contribute to hormonal problems by increasing the need for vitamins and minerals to detoxify the poisons in tobacco smoke. This reduces the amount of nutrients available for hormone production.

STRESS—Stress is a major contributor to hormonal imbalance. Any type of adverse stimulus that requires the body to change and adapt, such as day-to-day hassles, psychological trauma, financial problems, and environmental pollution, can cause stress. External stress can cause hormones to decline, which puts stress on internal body systems. This further diminishes hormonal production and can interfere with immune function, which can lead to the development of allergies and autoimmune illnesses such as thyroiditis and lupus. Conversely, stress can create problems by causing the body to secrete too many hormones.

SUGAR—Sugar interferes with nutrient absorption, particularly of B vitamins. It also interferes with the circulation of hormones throughout the body.

WEIGHT PROBLEMS—Excess weight adversely affects hormonal balance. The ratio of fat-to-lean body mass is critical in the initiation and continuation of the ovarian cycle. Being too thin is equally undesirable. If you fall below a certain weight, the pituitary hormone stops sending messages to the ovaries, and ovulation and menstruation stop.

OTHER FACTORS—Other conditions that contribute to hormonal imbalance include food sensitivity, allergy, chronic illness, candidiasis, menstrual and gynecological problems, drugs taken over long periods of time, and low levels of thyroid hormone.

Symptoms

Dr. Elizabeth Vliet is founder of the Women's Center for Health Enhancement and Renewal at All Saints' Hospital in Fort Worth, Texas, and author of *Screaming to Be Heard: Hormonal Connections Women Suspect and Doctors Ignore.* She describes some of the conditions that hormonal imbalance can trigger and tells when they are likely to occur. "Women's bodies are cyclic in their response to hormones. They have a monthly rhythm of hormonal changes from puberty to menopause, which have a critical bearing on many dimensions of health. Men's bodies, on the other hand, have a tonic pattern of secretion, which means that the same amounts of key hormones are produced every day. They vary within twenty-four hours in terms of their hormone production. But basically each day is similar to the day before and the day after.

"For women, the first half of the menstrual cycle is dominated by a rise in ovarian estradiol. This is the primary estrogen that is active at receptor sites on all the cells in the brain and body, from puberty to menopause. This rise in estrogen allows the ovary to prepare the follicle that will become the egg released at ovulation.

"At ovulation, when the egg is released, the estradiol level drops briefly. The egg then takes over and produces progesterone for the second half of the cycle. Progesterone levels rise, and estrogen levels rise again, though not as high as in the first half of the menstrual cycle. Progesterone and estrogen drop prior to bleeding, when the egg is not fertilized. The body sheds the lining of the uterus and starts over."

At this time there is also a decrease in certain critical brain neurotransmitters. "This is associated with mood changes women describe—feelings of irritability, insomnia, depression, or anxiety," Dr. Vliet says. "This may be a time in the cycle when women get migraines. The drop in estrogen that triggers changes in serotonin, norepinephrine, and endorphins sets off a cascade of blood vessel spasms that are involved in migraine headaches. That also affects chemical messengers involved in regulating the immune system, the gastrointestinal tract, the heart, heart rate, blood vessels, and as many as 400 other functions.

"We also see hormonal connections in women who have the diffuse muscle aches of fibromyalgia. These women often develop aches, pains, and tender points after some type of hormonal change, such as postpartum or post–tubal ligation, or following a hysterectomy, even if the ovaries are left in place. We see this in menopause too. If we look at the patterns of this type of pain in women, we see that 80 percent of fibromyalgia patients are female, and that the average age when fibromyalgia appears is about forty-four or forty-five."

Dr. Sherrill Sellman notes that infertility and miscarriage are both directly related to hormonal imbalance: an excess of estrogen and a deficiency of progesterone.

IN BALANCE OR OUT: HOW DO WE KNOW?

How does a woman know that she has a hormonal imbalance that requires some form of professional intervention? Dr. Sangeeta Pati, president and medical director of the Sajune Institute for Restorative and Regenerative Medicine in Orlando, Florida, who has been practicing both conventional and alternative medicine for over 20 years in the United States and abroad, helps us understand.

Hormonal fluctuations actually start early in life, she says. "Cortisol fluctuations start in our very early teens. When we have stressors, cortisol goes up. When the stressors go away, cortisol goes down. When we are in our teens, our reserve is high. If we're in good shape, we recover well after the stressors are gone. What happens as we get into our late twenties and early thirties is that this reserve starts to dwindle."

The first hormone that drops in young women is progesterone. "The main reason is because progesterone can feed the cortisol pathway," Dr. Pati says. "When our adrenal gland becomes more deficient in making cortisol, we're able to make up for it with progesterone. As the ovaries start to decline in production of progesterone, we start to feel the symptoms. The more stressors we have, the more nutritional depletion we have, the earlier we start to feel these symptoms."

Among the symptoms of low progesterone are anxiety, irritability, mood swings, and the feeling of being overwhelmed. In addition, there may be sleep disturbances, mid-abdominal weight gain, and decreased sex drive. "Because progesterone is the hormone that stops proliferation of breast, uterine, and ovarian cells, we start to see all those cells proliferating and dividing," Dr. Pati says. "There is more bleeding, breast cysts, and fibroids. As women continue with these symptoms, we see an increase in hysterectomies because of the bleeding, breast cancers, and bone loss."

The next hormone that declines is thyroid. "With nutrient deficiencies and toxicities, stress, and the inordinate amount of electromagnetic radiation that we're being exposed to, we find thyroid dysfunction starts a lot earlier," Dr. Pati says. Among the symptoms are low energy; less mental clarity; difficulty with memory, focus, and concentration; and depression. About 30 percent of people have weight gain. This number is important because many people assume that if they are not gaining weight, they must not have a thyroid issue. But only a third of people who have low thyroid will have the weight gain. Other symptoms include dry hair and skin, cold hands and feet, hair loss, constipation, and loss of motivation and joy in life.

After thyroid, testosterone starts to dip. This can cause changes in sexual function and sex drive, body composition, muscle to fat ratio, bone building, and blood flow to the frontal lobes of the brain. Cognition, memory, and mental clarity also decrease.

By the early fifties, women feel the decline of estrogen. Estrogen levels have actually been dropping since the age of twenty-five. "At some point, when you stop having the periods for a year because it's low enough, we call it menopause," Dr. Pati says, "but usually what women experience in the late forties and early fifties is a wild fluctuation of estrogen. It swings way up high and way down low, and way up high and way down low until, finally, we get to the point where the estradiol production stops all together. This is the point in time when one could consider using a bioidentical estradiol to support brain, bone, and heart."

The final hormone to discuss in more depth is cortisol. "Cortisol is considered to be the life hormone," Dr. Pati says. "It responds by increasing your blood pressure, when you are under stress. It mobilizes the body for the flight or fight response, and the body will, basically, shunt everything towards the cortisol system when there is an emergency. . . . Because all other hormones can make cortisol, when we are exposed to an inordinate amount of stress and the adrenal gland is not able to recover, we draw and shunt all the other hormones there. This is one of the reasons that we're starting to see so many young women with premature ovarian failure. Partly because of nutrient deficiencies and partly because of toxicities but very much, also, because of the amount of stress that their bodies are undergoing, and the fact that all of the ovarian hormones shunt to the cortisol system."

Symptoms include extreme fatigue, anxiety, hypervigilance, and being overwhelmed. Eventually there will be inflammatory diseases such as cancers, arthritis, diabetes, and heart disease. Because cortisol is responsible for keeping the body in an anti-inflamed state, there may be more allergies, psoriasis, eczema, gastric issues, salt cravings, and hypotension.

Clinical Experience

CONVENTIONAL MEDICINE

As mentioned above, synthetic hormone replacement therapy (HRT) was touted for decades as the number one conventional treatment for menopausal women with hormone imbalance. The situation changed in 2002, however, when the Women's Health Initiative reported that Prempro, one of the main drugs being used, was linked to an increased risk of breast cancer, heart attacks, and stroke. Still, HRT using Premarin, Provera, or Prempro is often recommended.

Dr. Ericka Schwartz is among many practitioners who have been sounding the alarm on synthetic hormones for years. "I think we need to understand first of all what these synthetic hormones are about because once we understand them, common-sense tells us that there is no use to taking them because it's just hurting ourselves.

"Conjugated estrogen, which is Premarin, is a toxic waste product of what the pregnant mare eliminates after she has used the hormones that she needs to sustain the fetus. It comes out of pregnant mare's urine, hence the name Premarin. It contains 200 molecules of estrogen, of which only two or three are similar to the molecule of estrogen that our body makes when we're young and healthy. The rest of them are foreign molecules that belong to the horse. What they will do is create reactions from the body because they're foreign to the body. So you will have immune response reaction. You will have abscess formation. You will have cancer growth. You will have increased thickness of the blood, creating increased incidence of strokes, thrombophlebitis, and blood clots. You will create all these horrible side effects because they're synthetic and they're not recognized by the body as their own. So that's what Premarin is about.

"A balance of Premarin is called Provera or Progestin, which has been created specifically to eliminate or negate the negative effects of Premarin on the uterus, which is increased uterine cancer. Progestin is supposed to be a kind of progesterone, but when you look at more of the formula it doesn't look anything like natural progesterone, and it is purely a synthetic medication made to basically countermand the negative effects of another medication. So that's the problem with synthetics. Why would anybody in their right mind prescribe them or take them?"

NATURAL APPROACHES

Alternative medicine practitioners use a variety of therapies to bring a woman's body back into balance. Dr. Beth McDougall explains her approach. "I try to work with vitamins, minerals, essential fatty acids, amino acids, or bioidentical hormones that are native to the human body and to remove things that are foreign to the body, because all of the toxins that we're exposed to in the environment or that come in the form of synthetic hormones or pharmaceutical medications tend to interrupt biochemical pathways and throw a woman's body off balance."

Dr. Vliet says women need to be aware of the relationship between hormonal cycles and medical conditions. "One of the ways to do that is to track patterns relative to cycles, and to test the blood for various hormones that women's bodies produce. I've developed an approach to doing that by measuring the hormonal levels at the right time of the menstrual cycle. This helps women know what is happening to their hormone levels at the time that they are having symptoms. I become frustrated when doctors tell me that we don't need to measure the female hormones because they vary. I respond that that's the whole point. They do vary, and how they vary, relative to women experiencing problems, is what we must find out in order to offer them the most constructive options."

Among the methods used by Dr. Michael Wald to measure hormone levels are blood tests, saliva tests, and urine tests. "When you put these three tests together in the context of the symptoms and the context of family history, you might really have something to go by," he says.

It is also important to check thyroid function. Thyroid hormone controls progesterone, cholesterol, and the ovaries. It acts as a cascading system. When not functioning properly, other hormones get out of balance.

Dr. Sara Gottfried, a Harvard-trained medical doctor and gynecologist, and author of *The Hormone Cure: Reclaim Balance, Sleep, Sex Drive and Vitality Naturally*, designed a three-step protocol after her own battle with hormone imbalance in her mid-thirties. Step one is to address the nutritional gap that occurs, and to make relevant lifestyle changes. "In my situation I had high cortisol, and I learned my top five strategies for how to hit the pause button when it comes to stress, and how to create that gap between stimulus and response," Dr. Gottfried says. Dietary changes included more green vegetables, green smoothies, low glycemic index fruits, and dark chocolate. She took supplements of phosphatidylserine and omega 3. Lifestyle changes included yoga.

Step two is to use proven botanical therapies. These have been used for thousands of years and have been shown to be effective in recent randomized trials.

"In my case involving cortisol, the key botanical therapies that were effective included rhodiola, ashwagandha, and ginseng," Dr. Gottfried says.

Step three is bioidentical hormones, but at the lowest doses and for the shortest duration. "It's amazing to me how much power foods can actually balance your hormones, and I think a lot of people don't realize that," Dr. Gottfied says. "They think that they need a prescription for the latest bioidentical hormone, and it turns out that much of your hormone balance, actually, comes with your fork.

"I don't think it's a good idea to just go on a dose of bioidentical hormones and stay on that dose forever. I don't think that's the best thing for the body. What we know is that just like with insulin resistance when your cells become numb to insulin, you can also develop thyroid resistance. You can develop cortisol resistance or glucocorticoid resistance. You can develop estrogen resistance or progesterone resistance. I would rather that people be working more in the step one and the step two, with the lifestyle changes and the food choices and the way you eat, move, think and supplement."

Lorna Vanderhaeghe, a medical journalist who has been researching nutrition for twenty-five years, agrees that not all women need hormones to adapt to change or imbalance. Lifestyle changes, rest, exercise, and supplements may be enough. If testing reveals that there is a need, she recommends estriol, a safe form of bioidentical estrogen, for women with thinning of the vaginal walls, vaginal dryness, recurring urinary tract infections, and painful intercourse. Progesterone along with melatonin and valerian is suggested for hormonal migraines and sleeplessness. Other useful substances include black cohosh, vitex, gamma oryzanol (from rice bran oil), and hesperdin (a flavonoid derived from citrus fruits).

NUTRITION

The typical American diet is high in fat, protein, caffeine, simple sugars, and salt, ingredients that interfere with optimal hormonal balance. These foods create a vicious cycle. They fuel premenstrual cravings for sweets and chocolate, and giving in to them worsens the cravings.

"I like to see a woman doing a strictly whole foods diet and really trying to avoid manufactured food products," says Dr. McDougall. "So you kind of shop around the perimeter of the grocery store. You're spending most of your time in the produce section and then if you choose to eat animal products then you're looking for free range, grass feed beef, organic poultry, and organic eggs. Ideally you should be getting those things from your local farmer. I really encourage women to add as many raw vegetables to the diet as possible. Not only do they have much greater nutritional value because a lot of vitamins are destroyed in the cooking process, they also have enzymes that are intact. Most foods contain myriads of enzymes that are destroyed in the cooking process, and these enzymes help you digest the food so that you can assimilate the nutrients better."

Perri advises us not to reach for a prescription drug for hormonal problems. It is better to eat high-quality organic foods and avoid foods that throw the system off balance. Beans and legumes are better sources of protein than meats, which are loaded with hormones. In addition, Perri recommends cold-processed oils, nuts, seeds, fatty fish, and beans. "These foods are all very high in GLAs," she notes. "The GLAs help us make natural estrogen in our own bodies."

Nutrition should be individualized to meet each woman's unique needs. According to Dr. Wald, nutrients are known as response modifiers. "Nutrients won't sharply raise hormone levels. They won't sharply diminish them. They help the body work better so hormone balance can be achieved as opposed to taking a synthetic/unnatural hormone, which will force it in one direction, which is almost never good."

SUPPLEMENTS

Dr. Schwartz has treated thousands of patients using natural hormones. "The natural, bioidentical hormones that I work with—which are FDA approved, prescription medications, with a molecular structure that's exactly like the structure of the hormones that we make—are the ones that we need to keep us from getting old, to keep us from getting sick, and to prevent and eliminate symptoms of hormone imbalance: hot flashes, night sweats, PMS, insomnia, weight gain, sexual dysfunction."

Wild yam and DHEA promote production of natural estrogens in the body, if the body needs them. If estrogen is not needed, these supplements are eliminated by the body, making them completely safe to use.

Dr. Wald recommends indole-3-carbinol (I3C). "You can eat indole-3-carbinol in cruciferous vegetables like broccoli, cauliflower, brussels sprouts, and cabbage, but if you're trying to deal with a hormone condition or really trying to prevent one, many of the studies I've read suggest that you need at least 150 milligrams of indole-3-carbinol daily. That's equivalent to about two plates of cruciferous vegetables a day. Whether you do that consistently or not I think it's a good idea to have some extra supplemental form of I3C. It has been proven to break down harmful estrogens."

Melatonin has also been shown to restore hormonal function. Other beneficial nutrients are licorice or glycyrrhizin, which inhibits the binding of the "bad" estrogens to cells and does not interfere with "good" estrogens, and lignans, which are from flaxseeds. "Two to three teaspoons of ground flaxseed meal daily can really help balance the hormone levels," Dr. Wald says.

In terms of vitamins, Dr. Wald suggests the following: vitamin C, vitamin E, and B vitamins. Magnesium and calcium may also be beneficial, since most women do not get enough of these nutrients.

HERBS

Chasteberry, blue cohosh, black cohosh, and yarrow help balance hormone production. Other balance-promoting herbs include raspberry leaf, dong quai, wild yam, passion flower, and red clover.

Janet Zand, a naturopath, doctor of Oriental medicine, and acupuncturist, uses programs that rotate the herbs being used in accordance with the four weeks of the menstrual cycle. Herbs used during the first two weeks nourish blood and balance hormones; those used during the second two weeks clear the liver, which tends to become congested during these last two weeks.

In an article on the HealthWorld Online website (www.healthy.net), Zand recommends the following general herbal program for balancing the hormonal system and building general resistance.

FIRST TWO WEEKS—Combination of red raspberry leaf and dong quai, as a tablet, capsule, tea, or tincture, three times a day.

THIRD WEEK—Astragalus, American ginseng, or Chinese ginseng. These adaptogenic herbs tone the deep immune system. Take as a tablet, capsule, tea, or tincture, three times a day.

FOURTH WEEK—Combination of goldenseal and echinacea. These herbs have antiviral, antibacterial, and anti-inflammatory properties. Take as a tablet, capsule, tincture, or tea, three times a day.

Dr. Sherrill Sellman would add a Peruvian herb called maca. "It is wonderfully supportive of adrenal function, thyroid function, and ovarian function," she says. "It helps with bones, and with a variety of health deficiencies."

Chapter 40

Infertility

About 6 percent of married women aged 15 to 44 in the US meet the criteria for infertility, being unable to get pregnant after one year of unprotected sex, according to 2015 data from the Centers for Disease Control and Prevention (CDC). The question of what can and should be done to conquer infertility is not only a complex medical issue, but also a potentially thorny ethical dilemma as well, with high emotional stakes.

After ten years of fertility tests and treatments, Carla Harkness, frustrated by the lack of consumer-oriented literature on the subject, consulted over one hundred medical specialists and put together *The Fertility Book*. Harkness sees infertility as an emotional life crisis that is largely unacknowledged by society. "Reactions include grief and mourning, loss of self-esteem, and impaired self-image. Couples often have difficulties communicating with each other. Their sexual relationship is tested and damaged. All in all, it is a traumatic experience."

She adds that an early end to pregnancy, due to miscarriage, produces the same frustrations. "The failure of a fertilized egg to implant is amazingly common. Often up to 50 percent of fertilized eggs do not make it past the initial two-week period to implantation. Up to 20 percent of confirmed pregnancies are miscarried in the first trimester in women under thirty-five years old. As a woman approaches forty, that number can exceed 25 percent, and by the age of forty-five, the miscarriage rate is almost 50 percent. The emotional impact of miscarriage is similar to the emotional impact of infertility. There is often grief and mourning that are not accepted as genuine mourning in our society. Couples often hear things like, 'I guess it was meant to be,' 'Something was wrong,' or 'You'll have another.' That is often of little solace to someone feeling this kind of loss."

Causes

Potential causes for infertility in women include endometriosis, a condition in which the glands and tissues that line the inside of the uterus grow outside the uterus; poor diet; deficiencies in folic acid, vitamin B_6, vitamin B_{12}, and iron; heavy metal toxicity; obesity; immature sex organs; abnormalities of the reproductive system; hormonal imbalances; and genetic damage from electromagnetic radiation. Among the toxicants linked to infertility are cigarette smoke, chlorinated hydrocarbons, polychlorinated biphenols (PCBs), bisphenol A (BPA), and phthalates.

The birth control pill and other sources of estrogen can add to the problem. The late Barbara Seaman, advocate for women's health issues, author of *The Doctors' Case Against the Pill* and coauthor with me of *For Women Only!*, concluded that the chemicals in the Pill may increase infertility in three ways: by suppressing the natural productions of hormones; by increasing the risk of sexually transmitted diseases (STDs), especially chlamydia; and by upsetting the assimilation of nutrients.

As Seaman reported, "Fertility experts confirm that many women who have been on the Pill for a long time have problems reestablishing their monthly cycles." Robin Wald, a nutritionist and health care writer who specializes in infertility, explains further how birth control pills can cause hormonal imbalances that affect fertility.

"The hypothalamus is the gland that produces gonadotropin-releasing hormone, the hormone that triggers the pituitary gland to secrete other hormones that are important for fertility. These hormones, follicle-stimulating hormone, which tells the ovaries to start producing and maturing an egg each month, and luteinizing hormone, which ripens the egg and allows it to be released, signal the ovaries to produce estrogen and progesterone so that you can have a normal menstrual cycle. It's a very complicated and complex system and must be in a very particular balance to function properly; for the egg to ripen and mature; for the egg to be released and travel through the fallopian tubes; and for progesterone to be there to build up the endometrial lining to nourish an egg, so that if it's fertilized it can be implanted and nourished and grow so that it doesn't miscarry. When you have too much estrogen that suppresses pituitary gland function, you disrupt the normal hormone balance."

The Pill can also promote the growth of chlamydia. "This condition has reached epidemic proportions in the United States," Seaman said. "Chlamydia causes pelvic inflammatory disease, which can then cause sterility. Usually, the first time it strikes, chlamydia does not render a woman sterile. Women who get the condition once should give up the Pill right away."

Another problem with the Pill is that it can cause nutritional imbalance. "If a woman has been on the Pill for a long time, she may be very low in folic acid; vitamins B_1, B_2, B_6, B_{12}, C, and E; and trace minerals zinc and magnesium; all essential to normal fertility," Seaman said. "Sometimes just getting on a really good diet with really good supplements can get her back into a fertile cycle without needing heavy-duty drugs. It should be noted, however, that any dietary supplements used should be low in vitamin A, niacin, copper, and iron, which tend to be elevated in Pill users."

Clinical Experience

ASSISTED REPRODUCTION

The laboratory options for infertile couples have exploded over the past four decades. "In 1978, the first 'test tube' baby was born in England through a process called in vitro fertilization," Carla Harkness says. "Since then, the process has been instituted [and expanded] worldwide."

Today there are three main methods of assisted reproduction: in vitro fertilization, fertility-enhancing drugs, and artificial insemination. According to the Centers for Disease Control and Prevention (CDC), in 2013, there were nearly 200,000 ART cycles performed at reporting clinics in the US, resulting in 68,000 live born infants. (The CDC definition of ART only includes fertility treatments in which both eggs and sperm are handled.)

"Now the boundaries have even exceeded menopause. Before, you had the practice of donor sperm for artificial insemination. Now there is the ability to fertilize donor eggs from younger women with the husband's sperm and to implant those eggs in an infertile woman who is over forty-five or fifty. She is able to carry a child to term that is not genetically related to her. These kinds of options have all become available, and they offer a great deal of hope to many couples."

ETHICAL ISSUES

While modern advances in fertility treatments offer a wealth of new possibilities, they also engender new ethical concerns. "A number of religious groups have raised questions about the intervention of technology in the natural process of reproduction," Harkness explains. "There is also a theme of pronatalism at any cost here, emphasizing that to be complete as couples or as women, people absolutely must birth a biological child."

Another issue revolves around extending maternal age past nature's deadline of menopause. Before, women in their mid-forties probably weren't able to get pregnant because their bodies would stop that function. Now it is possible for women in their fifties and even sixties to become pregnant. This raises a number of questions: Is that putting too much demand on their bodies? What about the age difference between them and their children? What about obligations to aging parents while having little ones in your midlife? Additionally, there is a legal and moral question revolving around the status of unused, frozen embryos in the event of death and divorce.

"There are further questions surrounding the availability of this expensive technology to those without the means or the medical insurance," Harkness says. "Unfortunately, these treatments are quite expensive. From the moment you walk into a specialist's office asking for an evaluation, you start incurring costs in the hundreds of dollars for examinations and tests, all the way to thousands of dollars for the in vitro techniques."

Many women distrust scientific intervention in general. Problems with intrauterine devices (IUDs) have caused pelvic inflammatory disease resulting in infertility. Diethylstilbestrol (DES), an estrogen replacement used as a "morning after" pill in the United States even after it was linked to cancer and anomalies of the vagina and cervix, has been another big problem, as has thalidomide. Now there are concerns about using female hormones to stimulate ovulation. With most infertility treatments, whether the problem stems from the man or the woman, it is mainly the women who undergo the drug treatments, the surgeries, and so forth. What are the long-term effects of exposing women to these drugs?

NATURAL OPTIONS

Dr. Marjorie Ordene, a gynecologist from Brooklyn, New York, believes that while there is a place for technology in fertility, women are too quick to seek out these methods. She suggests trying various natural options first.

PINPOINTING TIME OF OVULATION

Women should learn to recognize their time of ovulation by taking their temperature first thing in the morning, before getting out of bed. "Usually, temperature rises in the second half of the cycle, two weeks before menstruation." says Dr. Ordene. "The mucus that is produced around the time of ovulation has a clear, slippery quality. This is the kind of mucus that is needed for the sperm to penetrate the cervix."

WHAT TO AVOID

Robin Wald cautions that women trying to conceive should avoid exposure to toxic substances that not only may interfere with conception but have also been linked to miscarriage and birth defects.

"The first thing I tell people to avoid is tobacco smoke. If you're a cigarette smoker and you plan on getting pregnant, quit smoking. Tobacco is very high in chemicals, including cadmium, which is a toxic heavy metal that accumulates in the reproductive organs of both men and women. It interferes with sperm production in men and hormone production in women. Secondhand smoke can cause similar problems.

"I also encourage people to stop drinking, even if they only drink moderately. Alcohol interferes with fertility by causing liver toxicity. The liver is the primary organ for building up cholesterol to form the steroid hormones that are important to reproductive health. Marijuana and other drugs can also cause liver toxicity and should be avoided.

"In addition, I suggest that people eliminate caffeine, both in coffee and in sodas; switch to decaf coffee or herbal teas; and increase water intake. Although the subject of caffeine and fertility is controversial, studies have shown that as few as two cups of coffee a day or two cans of caffeinated soda can increase your chance of a miscarriage by four times and your infertility by 50 percent."

Wald further cautions women to avoid taking some over-the-counter medications. "A lot of women who experience menstrual discomfort think nothing of taking an aspirin or ibuprofen. But nonsteroidal anti-inflammatory drugs are also harmful to the reproductive system.

"One thing to avoid that cannot be overemphasized is pesticide—both pesticides that have been sprayed in your garden and pesticide residue from food that you buy. Pesticides are very toxic to the reproductive system. This is because pesticides are in a class of chemicals called xenoestrogens, synthetic chemicals that act like estrogen on the body. Overexposure to xenoestrogens can result in a condition called estrogen dominance. In estrogen dominance there is too much estrogen circulating in the body, which throws off the balance and production of other hormones that are essential for fertility."

Other sources of xenoestrogens are food additives, preservatives, and meat from animals that have been fed hormones. Dairy products also contain xenoestrogens, both from the cows' own hormones and from hormones given to them to promote milk production.

DIET AND LIFESTYLE

Women should maintain a healthy diet and follow a basic exercise program. Fertility specialists Dr. Talha Sawaf, Dr. Yehudi Gordon, and Marilyn Glenville, writing in *Positive Health* magazine, recommend eating organic foods as much as possible and avoiding food additives, coffee, and tea. They advise eliminating nonessential medications and avoiding exposure to radiation, hazardous substances in the workplace, pesticides, and pollutants such as toxic metals. They point out that becoming as healthy as possible before conception improves the quality of the egg and sperm, thereby maximizing fertility and reducing the risk of miscarriage. Conversely, fertility is decreased by poor nutrition, vitamin or mineral deficiencies, and too much alcohol, cigarettes, and stimulants.

After checking the nutritional status of a woman, Dr. Uzzi Reiss, a leading expert in obstetrical-gynecological practice and anti-aging medicine, recommends specific antioxidants according to individual need. "There is a report now, for example, indicating that if you add alpha lipoic acid, taurine, NAC [n-acetylcysteine], and high doses of vitamin C, you see changes in the ability of a woman to procreate. So that's one thing that I do."

Robin Wald, who suggests that the very first step in optimizing fertility is to examine your diet, says that the standard American diet does not promote either health or fertility. She recommends an organic, whole, live-foods diet. "The advantage of eating live food is that the nutritional value and the quality are that much higher. Good nutrition is vital when you're trying to get pregnant. Vitamins, minerals, fats, amino acids, and other nutritional components from our foods are essential for keeping the reproductive system healthy. Eat fresh fruit and vegetables, especially leafy green vegetables like collard greens, kale, Swiss chard, red chard, and beet greens, which are very high in folic acids and loaded with calcium. Folic acid is essential for preventing birth defects such as spina bifida, and calcium will aid in building your baby's skeleton as well as keeping your own bones healthy."

She suggests minimizing your intake of processed flour, bread, baked goods, and pasta, and incorporating more whole grains into your diet. She recommends brown rice, millet, quinoa, oats, and buckwheat. "Whole grains are loaded with fiber and have very high nutritional quality. Raw nuts and seeds are also good, as are chickpeas, lentils, black beans, and pinto beans, which are both high in fiber and a good source of nonanimal protein.

"Fiber is important in promoting the excretion of toxins and bound-up estrogens from the gut. If you have insufficient fiber to move things through your intestines in a timely way, these estrogens sit in the gut and get reabsorbed into the body. So instead of having environmental estrogens or estrogens your body has created circulating through your body once, they're now going through a second, third, or fourth time, which contributes to estrogen dominance."

Wald advises eating soy products, such as tempeh and miso. "Soy is a good source of phytoestrogens, which have a chemical structure similar to estrogen. Phytoestrogen tricks your body into thinking that it's getting estrogen, but the advantage of phytoestrogens is that they tell your body to lower its own estrogen production, which helps balance your estrogen levels. As well, phytoestrogens block the absorption of xenoestrogens."

EMOTIONAL AND SPIRITUAL ISSUES

The very first thing a woman (and her partner) should do prior to becoming pregnant is to go through a period of spiritual and emotional rebalancing. Often, a woman has apprehensions that need to be addressed about becoming pregnant. It may be reassuring to talk to the inner child and let her know that even though there will be another child, the little girl in her will still get the attention she needs. This kind of spiritual work is often important in achieving pregnancy.

Feelings of blame, guilt, anger, and frustration that infertile couples often experience will have a negative effect on their fertility. Discussing such issues, perhaps with a counselor, can resolve these negative feelings and improve the chances of conception.

Infertility is a very stressful, major life event, and stress can itself adversely affect fertility. Robin Wald describes how stress affects reproductive function. "Every time there is a stress response in your body, the adrenal glands secrete a group of hormones that have an inhibitory effect on the hypothalamus, which is the master gland that signals the production of the hormones needed for reproduction. When you have excessive stress, the hypothalamus does not function properly.

"Stress can also cause a condition called hypoprolactin anemia. Prolactin is another hormone that prepares the breasts for milk production. If a nonpregnant woman has high levels of prolactin, it will make conception difficult because it can shut down ovulation.

"If you're under a lot of stress, do whatever you can to reduce it," Wald suggests. She recommends yoga, meditation, breathing exercises, spiritual work and prayer, visualization and imagery, bodywork, and massage as ways to lower stress levels.

Nutritional supplements can also help. Wald recommends vitamins C and E, beta-carotene, alpha-carotene, coenzyme Q10, and antioxidants to protect against stress-induced free radical damage.

ASIAN NATUROPATHIC APPROACH

The traditional Eastern approach to fertility depends less on modern technology and more on time-tested knowledge. The late Dr. Roger Hirsch, a naturopathic physician from California, explained Chinese philosophy and infertility treatments based on this point of view: "We look at making the abdomen happy. This is an aphorism for correcting the digestion, menstruation, and hormones, so that women can conceive. Of course, raising the man's sperm count and sperm motility is important as well, because it is not just the woman who is infertile in an infertility situation. A key to this is the way the blood flows in the pelvic cavity."

Chinese medicine uses acupuncture, massage, heat, or crystals applied at points along the energy pathways, or meridians, to balance the flow of energy in the body. Changing the diet, decreasing emotional tension, and balancing heat and cold will increase the effectiveness of the basic treatment. Thus, acupuncture is more effective when used together with herbs to regulate the menstrual cycle, promote ovulation, and increase general vitality, all of which enhance fertility. Chinese medicine can be combined with assisted reproductive technology to minimize stress and help women tolerate drugs and surgery.

In Chinese medicine, every manifestation has a causative factor in the way someone is living her life, says Dr. Randine Lewis, a licensed acupuncturist and herbalist, who is the author of *The Infertility Cure* and *The Way of the Fertile Soul: Ancient Chinese Secrets to Tap into a Woman's Creative Potential.* "It may be on the physical level. How they are eating or how they are exercising. They might be exercising way too much, and a lot of people who are suffering from infertility have been put on certain exercise regimens, which aren't right for them that will say you must get down to this weight or you must no longer run. But individually I think as a whole we exercise and women especially exercise like men. They go to the gym and they exercise only their muscular skeletal system. What that does is it de-routes the body's energies away from the hypothalamic pituitary ovarian access and shunts the blood flow to the muscles. So most of our lives are spent really telling our bodies not to feed the reproductive system.

"I put people on an exercise regimen where in addition to whatever they're doing to increase the cardiac output and lose weight, they also work to bring the energy back to the pelvis, to the reproductive organs, to the hypothalamic pituitary ovarian access. That's often done with a mind body approach that reduces the response to stress in our lives. Some people are so overly concerned with, 'I've got to do this. I've got to do this. I've got to eat this way. I've got to take these herbs. I've got to take these supplements.' They are putting more stress in their bodies or in their lives than before they considered themselves to be infertile."

When people are in this state, overcoming infertility becomes extremely difficult.

Dr. Lewis explains, "There is no way that their bodies can even respond to their own reproductive hormones because we have been so programmed in our society to get whatever we want through struggle, through effort, through fighting, through trying, through competing, through being a little better, and through studying a little harder. Generally we get our goal from that approach. We can lose weight through that approach. We can get a degree through that approach. We can get a spouse. We can buy a house. We can get a job. We can get a profession. But something happens physiologically when we apply that same method to trying to get a baby. It works against us because it shunts our bodies' energies away from receptivity and into the fight-flight response and into what we have been conditioned our whole lives to do, which is fight for whatever we want.

"That's where most people come to me: in that state of fight. Whatever you tell me to do, I'm going to do it. I try to back them off a little bit from the frenzy.

This is not a program about following the rules. There are certain guidelines that you follow, but it's more of a process of learning to be receptive. Learning to shut down that fight. Learning to open up to life, which is what we're doing. We're not trying to force a certain chemical to appear through manipulating the outside. We're bringing the body into a state of relaxation and into a state of balance and into a state of harmony, so it can exert the appropriate chemicals and hormones at the right time and respond to them."

HERBS

"In Chinese medicine," said Dr. Hirsch, "herbs are used to tone renal/adrenal function because reproductive function is related to the kidney and to functions related to the kidney. The actual viability of the eggs for a woman over forty is related to kidney yang function."

HERBA EPIMETI—One herb that is very good for kidney yang is an aphrodisiac called herba epimeti, which translates as "horny goat weed." The Chinese noticed that goats become sexually active after eating this particular plant. They put the plant into the herbal formula for women who are kidney yang–deficient, and they noted that it increased sexual desire.

LUTAIGOU—Lutaigou, the gelatin that comes from boiling the antlers of deer, is used by the Chinese to help women over forty who are trying to extend their egg-producing years. It helps slow down the biological clock.

WORMWOOD—In the European system, we have wormwood, which creates more circulation in the pelvic cavity. The Chinese use this along with daughter seed and fructose litchi, a little red berry.

DONG QUAI AND CORTEX CINNAMOMI—Both of these help the circulation in the pelvic cavity. Cortex cinnamomi is not the cinnamon you put in your mulled cider, but a cinnamon with a very thick bark.

ACUPUNCTURE

In China, acupuncture has been used in the treatment of infertility for centuries. The Chinese look at five principal organ systems—the liver/gallbladder, spleen/stomach, heart/small intestine, lung/large intestine, and kidney/bladder—

and use acupuncture to release blockages from these systems so that energy, or chi, can move freely. This helps the body return to good health. Promoting fertility is one benefit that can be obtained.

Acupuncture to kidney points releases psychological blocks that interfere with reproduction. Dr. Hirsch used the treatment to help patients overcome deep-rooted fears connected to sexual abuse and low self-esteem. "In treating self-esteem issues, I work on the heart and kidney points. The acupuncture points that seem extremely valuable for this are Pericardium 5 and 6. If a practitioner is having a problem with understanding whether or not a psychological issue is involved in the infertility, and the patient does not know what the issue is, Pericardium 5 can be needled. If something is holding the person back, that will bring an event or dream to memory, and the patient will understand why she is stuck. In treating self-esteem issues, we may also release stress by needling the Heart 7 point, Heart 9, and sometimes Heart 7 to Heart 5.

"We also address Conception Vessel 17, which is between the breasts. This is a very important place for women because it opens their energy. It also helps relieve liver chi congestion. Remember, the liver and the liver hormones, both in Chinese and in Western medicine, govern the flow of blood in the pelvic cavity."

WESTERN NATUROPATHIC APPROACH

Dr. Joseph Pizzorno says that as a naturopath and midwife he saw numerous infertile couples and discovered two causes of the condition that were not generally recognized by the orthodox medical profession: pituitary insufficiency and pelvic inflammatory disease.

"The pituitary gland was not secreting enough of the hormones needed to stimulate the ovaries to mature, ripen, and produce a viable ovum," he says. "Most of these women had been on birth control pills for long periods of time. Even though they had been off the pills for several years, their pituitary never functioned fully again."

To address pituitary insufficiency, Dr. Pizzorno administered an herbal concoction using herbs that are commonly used for women's health problems, as well as raw pituitary gland from an animal. "There were surprisingly good results with this treatment," he says. "A urine test beforehand measured the level of hormones from the pituitary. If a patient had low hormone levels, I would then use this protocol with them. A surprising number became pregnant once their urinary hormone levels returned to normal."

In the case of pelvic inflammatory disease, Dr. Pizzorno detected infections in the fallopian tubes, which extend from the uterus to the ovaries. "Infections leave scars," he explains. "Then the ovum cannot penetrate the tube and get into the uterus for fertilization."

A simple method is available to combat this problem. Dr. Pizzorno describes the procedure: "A woman gets two big pots of water. One tub gets filled with hot water (as hot as she can stand it). When a woman sits in it with her arms and legs out of the tub, the water level reaches her umbilicus. The other tub gets filled with ice-cold water. That tub is filled to the point just below the umbilicus. In other words, there is more hot water than cold water. The woman sits in the hot water for five minutes, and then in the cold water for one minute. She alternates back and forth three times.

"The first time a woman does this, she will find it startling. But after a while she will actually start to like it. She does this every day. After a few treatments, she starts getting a discharge. As near as we can make out, this discharge is the body throwing off scar tissue and toxic material in the ovaries. This is a particularly dangerous time for a woman to have intercourse. The ovaries are starting to open up, and there is a high probability of an ectopic pregnancy. The egg will only be able to go partway down the tube since the tube is not yet open enough for it to get all the way into the uterus. We therefore tell women to have no unprotected intercourse for at least three months while doing these treatments every day. Again, a surprising number of them become pregnant."

RESTORING THYROID BALANCE

Even as far back as the 1930s, alleviating low thyroid conditions was found effective against infertility. Dr. Ray Peat says, "To keep thyroid levels up, women should snack frequently and eliminate unsaturated fats." Although unsaturated fats are often touted as beneficial, recent studies show them to inhibit thyroid secretion. More high-quality protein may be needed, especially by women following a weight-loss program or a vegetarian diet. "A daily minimum of 40 grams is recommended." Taking a thyroid supplement for a short period of time can greatly help. "People whose thyroid function is suppressed can benefit from a week or two of thyroid supplementation," Dr. Peat advises. "They don't need to take this indefinitely."

NATURAL HYGIENE

The late Dr. Anthony John Penepent followed the principles of natural hygiene when treating any medical condition. "Over the years, I have seen many wonderful things happen with natural hygiene that would not have been possible with allopathic medicine." Explaining infertility, Dr. Penepent said there are many causes, but that all of them can be treated similarly. "There are many mechanisms that can come into play. You can have basic amenorrhea or failure to ovulate. You can have any variety of hormonal imbalances or fallopian tube obstruction. In 40 percent of the cases it is not the woman's fault, although she may take the blame to save her husband's ego. The man may have a low sperm count, depressed sperm motility, or abnormal sperm morphology. These are all possibilities. Then again, conception may occur, but the egg or ovum may not have sufficient nutrients for the embryo to develop. What happens then is you have unrecognized spontaneous abortions that make it appear as if the woman is infertile, when in actuality she just has a nutritional deficiency.

"In many cases, an infertile woman can conceive and go on to have a successful pregnancy with a minor amount of dietary change. In the case of the fallopian tube obstruction, it may be necessary for her to fast for several days. I remember one patient, a rabbi's wife, who was childless. Because of their religious beliefs, it was absolutely essential for her to bear children. In her particular case, I put her on a fast for several days and followed that up with a nutritional regimen. She was able to conceive within six months."

CONSUMER ADVOCACY GROUPS

Carla Harkness recommends becoming part of a consumer advocacy group that can provide individuals and couples with support and information. One group, called Resolve, has a string of chapters across the country. "Resolve is a great ally that provides literature, referrals, and legal advocacy to the infertile. Chances are, wherever you live, there's a chapter by you."

Research Update

An increasing body of evidence is showing the benefits of natural modalities to overall health and well-being. Following is a sample of recent peer-reviewed scientific studies in the area of infertility.

In 2015, researchers reported in *Alternative Therapies in Health and Medicine* the results of a ten-year study of manual physical therapy on nearly 4,000 women with infertility. Whole-body, patient-centered treatments focused on restoring mobility and motility to structures affecting reproductive function. Results included a 61 percent rate of cleared fallopian tubes, with a 57 percent rate of pregnancy in those patients; a 43 percent pregnancy rate in participants with endometriosis; a 50 percent lowering of elevated levels of follicle stimulating hormone (FSH), with a 40 percent pregnancy rate in that group; and a 54 percent pregnancy rate in women with polycystic ovarian syndrome (PCOS). A 2008 study published in *Fertility and Sterility* followed 438 women over eight years, and found that regular use of multivitamin supplements, at least three times per week, may decrease the risk of ovulatory infertility.

In a 2013 article published on greenmedinfo.com, Dr. Kelly Brogan tells about recent research on the gluten-infertility link. A US study of 188 infertile women found that nearly 6 percent with unexplained causes were determined to have celiac disease, and all proceeded to get pregnant within a year after changing their diets. Several studies in Europe have shown that conception was achieved in women who switched to a gluten-free diet after blood tests showing antibodies to gliadin and/or tissue transglutaminase.

Chapter 41

Lupus

Lupus is an autoimmune disorder of the connective tissues that affects 1.5 million Americans, 90 percent of whom are women. *Lupus* is the Latin word for "wolf," and *erythema* means "redness." The typical red skin sores caused by the disorder are said to resemble a wolf's bite. The severity of lupus can range from mild to life-threatening. African American, Hispanic, and Asian women are disproportionately affected.

Causes

Lupus occurs when antigen-antibody cell complexes circulating through the body are deposited in various body tissues such as the kidney and skin, causing inflammation. Symptoms may be exacerbated by infections, extreme stress, antibiotics, and certain other drugs. Although the exact cause of this disease is unknown, hormones are believed to aggravate it, particularly estrogen, which is why so many women are affected. According to an article by Anthony di Fabio of the Arthritis Trust of America, lupus seems to be related to the use of estrogen therapy, indicating that it may be to some extent hormone-dependent.

Symptoms

Initial signs include arthritis, a red "butterfly" rash across the bridge of the nose and on the cheeks, weakness, prolonged and extreme fatigue, and weight loss. There may also be fever over 100 degrees, light sensitivity, skin sores on the neck, hair loss, chest pain, Raynaud's disease (a constriction of circulation in the extremities that causes fingers to turn white or blue in the cold), joint pain, muscle inflammation, anger, depression, and anemia. If the central nervous system is involved, seizures may occur.

Additional symptoms include mouth or nose ulcers and a nail fungus, which is an outgrowth of infection by Candida albicans. Often lupus sufferers have headaches. The characteristic skin sores are raised reddish patches that become scaly and crusted. When they fall off, they leave white scars. If these sores spread to other tissues in the body, tissue wasting may occur.

Lupus may begin abruptly with a fever, or slowly, with infrequent flare-ups. Those whose symptoms appear only in the skin have a better prognosis, while those whose kidneys and brains are affected have a poorer prognosis. In some patients, many different organs—lungs, heart, kidneys—are affected.

Clinical Experience

TRADITIONAL TREATMENT

Mild cases of lupus are treated with nonsteroidal anti-inflammatory and analgesic drugs such as aspirin, ibuprofen, indomethacin, and sometimes phenylbutazone. Prednisone, a form of cortisone, may be given for arthritis and muscle aches. In severe cases of lupus, steroidal drugs are prescribed for internal and external use. However, long-term use of these medications can damage the liver and weaken the bones. Steroids depress the immune system, leaving the body vulnerable to infection.

For both mild and severe forms of lupus, says Anthony di Fabio, traditional treatments only relieve symptoms; they do not get at its causes.

NATURAL THERAPIES

Alternative practitioners have successfully treated lupus with a variety of therapies, generally based on changes in diet and appropriate supplementation.

HERBS AND SUPPLEMENTS

To lessen inflammation, many people use pycnogenol, cat's claw, black walnut, omega-3 fatty acids, and flaxseed oil. Pau d'arco and aloe vera juice act as blood cleansers. A good nervous system tonic is gotu kola. Colloidal silver is antibacterial, antifungal, and antiarthritic.

According to Dr. Jonathan Wright, a physician and nutritionist from Washington, writing in *Nutrition and Healing*, vitamin B$_6$, up to 500 milligrams three times a day, will help relieve symptoms. People with lupus also need supplementation with hydrochloric acid. He adds, "All lupus patients have food allergies, and will improve when this condition is handled." In addition, over half of women have low levels of DHEA and testosterone and need to take these hormones as supplements.

INTRAVENOUS THERAPIES

According to di Fabio, Dr. Ronald M. Davis of Texas reports success treating lupus patients using EDTA (ethylenediamine tetracetic acid) chelation therapy with the antioxidant DMSO (dimethyl sulfoxide), and intravenous hydrogen peroxide. Dr. Davis initiates treatment of lupus and other autoimmune diseases by giving antifungal drugs such as metronidazole, since it appears that some antibodies related to autoimmune disease are produced in response to fungal microorganisms found to be present in such diseases.

ACUPUNCTURE

Acupuncturist and massage therapist Gina Michaels of New York City explains that she individualizes her acupuncture treatments according to each patient's unique profile. "Each decision an acupuncturist makes looks at the large picture. For example, if the person has a headache, along which meridian is that headache located? Is it the gallbladder channel? The stomach channel? Are they having other symptoms, such as fever or sweat? Is the central nervous system affected? All of this is very, very important in deciding what treatment protocol to choose.

"There are eight meridians formed during conception that go to a very deep constitutional level. Treating these is very useful for illnesses that are systemic or of a much deeper nature."

DIET

The Arthritis Trust of America recommends that women with lupus avoid overeating; minimize intake of cow's milk and beef; eat more green, yellow, and orange vegetables; eat nonfarmed cold-water fish several times a week; avoid alfalfa sprouts and tablets containing L-canavanine sulfate, a substance that can worsen lupus; and avoid taking L-tryptophan, which can exacerbate the autoimmune reaction.

The diet should be high in vegetables and low in grains. Wheatgrass is excellent for reducing inflammation. Foods detrimental to healing include peanuts, bread, corn, soybeans, and other foods that can produce fungi and molds. In addition, alcohol, spinach, and carrots may aggravate the condition. Acid-producing foods, such as orange juice, meat, and dairy products, can also be harmful.

FASTING

Di Fabio quotes Dr. Joel Fuhrman, who says, "Having fasted over a thousand patients with various diseases, I can say without hesitation that fasting is very often the only avenue that a patient can use to establish a complete remission.

"This is especially true with autoimmune illnesses such as lupus, where it is almost impossible to shut off the hyperactive immune system with nutritional modifications alone, without total fasting." Fasting, he explains, is not merely a method of detoxifying. "The body clearly has the mechanism to adequately handle the removal of endogenous wastes generated in the fasting state. In fact, fasting has been shown to improve or normalize abnormal liver function." No drugs of any sort should be taken while fasting.

OTHER METHODS

Regular exercise is important, because it helps to keep the joints moving. Lupus can flare up during times of extreme stress. Working at a job one dislikes can be a contributing factor, for example. It is important for people to examine their lives and to create circumstances that promote health and happiness. Aromatherapy may also be beneficial. Essential oils can help calm the emotions and eliminate flare-ups. Rubbing tree oils such as pine and cedar directly onto the joints can diminish swelling. A drop of chamomile, lavender, lilac, or neroli can be placed on the palms and breathed in for relaxation. When there is chest congestion, eucalyptus is excellent for clearing the nasal passages and lungs.

Research Update

An increasing body of evidence is showing the benefits of natural modalities to overall health and well-being. Following is a sample of recent peer-reviewed scientific studies relating to lupus.

An article on the *Life Extension* website describes recent advances that move away from mainstream medicine's reliance on immune suppression in treating lupus. These include the use of monoclonal antibodies, which are directed against immune system cells that cause lupus autoimmunity; stem cell therapy, in which healthy immune cells replace problematic ones; and vitamin D, which has been found to be deficient in people with lupus and to act as a modulator of immune cell activity. In 2015, a two-year prospective study of 34 patients with systemic lupus erythematosus (SLE), published in *Lupus*, found that vitamin D exerted important actions on T-cells. Research in the *International Journal of Clinical and Experimental Medicine*, also in 2015, found that a vitamin D analog (EB1089) could repair the defective bone marrow-derived mesenchymal stromal cells in these patients. Other natural therapies include lifestyle changes (exercise, avoiding sun, reducing stress), as well as supplementing the diet with fish oil, vitamin E, vitamin A, curcumin, ginkgo, pine bark extract, astragalus, and DHEA.

Chapter 42

Memory Loss

One of the most disturbing symptoms of aging is diminished brain function, which can cause everything from forgetfulness and loss of concentration to Alzheimer's and other serious diseases. Fortunately, modern research reveals that much can be done to keep the brain in top form your entire life.

Dr. Eric Braverman, director of the PATH Medical Center in New York, and author of *Younger Brain, Sharper Mind*, says that brain aging affects people differently and that brain health is a preventive process. "Even when you feel halfway decent in your fifties, sixties, and seventies, parts of your body may be breaking down," he cautions.

The part of the brain affected determines which symptoms manifest themselves. "Individuals age in all different shapes and forms, just as a face can have wrinkles on the brow or wrinkles under the eye," Dr. Braverman says. "The area of the brain that slows down can affect such things as general memory, concentration, and logic."

Another leading researcher in the field of antiaging, Dr. Ross Pelton of San Diego, author of *Mind, Food, and Smart Pills*, agrees that our brains do not have to deteriorate as we age. "It is simply poor nutrition and abuse that allows this condition to develop. Virtually everyone can enhance their memory, learning capabilities, and intelligence." Dr. Pelton helps his patients optimize brain functioning with two goals in mind: to slow down or stop the brain aging process and to optimize the function that they do have.

Dr. Dharma Singh Khalsa is president and medical director of the Alzheimer's Research and Prevention Foundation in Tucson, Arizona, and the author of *Brain Longevity*. "There are many simple things that we can do right now to improve our memories, to forestall any degeneration, to be at our highest mental potential no matter what age or what stage of life we are in," Dr. Khalsa says. "We just have to look at the brain as a physical organ. We have to give it the oxygen it needs, the blood flow it needs, the nutrients it needs. We have to eat right, lower our fat intake, take supplements, meditate or do something to lower the stress in our lives, get physical exercise, think positively, and use our brain. If we do all of these things we can improve our brains. Combine this with a knowledgeable doctor in the field of antiaging medicine and look at hormone replacement therapy. I think hormone replacement therapy is coming into its own now and there is no question that it is definitely beneficial."

Understanding Memory

The roots of memory have been studied and debated for centuries, yet many questions remain as to how the brain performs this basic function. What is known is that memories are constructed through a series of interactive steps triggered by exposure to new information. Your brain constructs memory from input from the entire neural network in your body. The practice of construction and reconstruction is critical to memory.

The two primary types of memory are declarative and procedural. The brain's medial temporal lobes, particularly the hippocampus, and the prefrontal cortex are responsible for maintaining declarative memory. Sometimes called explicit memories, these include facts, people, places, and things that we encounter frequently. The capacity to learn skills or procedures, including new motor skills, is governed by our nondeclarative, or implicit, memory. This memory function is governed by brain structures outside the medial temporal lobes, including the amygdala, cerebellum, and motor cortex.

Scientists are unclear as to the specific reasons for age-related memory loss. It may be that our brain becomes less agile as it ages, or that imbalances in the system of neurotransmitters that communicate within the brain cause memory loss, or that other types of chemical imbalances in our bodies, such as changing hormone levels, impact our ability to remember things. What is known is that it is normal for anyone at any age to have lapses of memory, but that older individuals may face a higher incidence of memory loss.

Researchers have speculated that changes may result from the subtly changing environment in the brain as it ages. Particular focus has been on the loss of brain cells and physical deterioration of the brain itself. But the role of an imbalance in the delicate systems of neurotransmitters that conduct all communication in the brain has been an area of recent study in relation to memory loss and brain function in aging.

It is important to understand the importance of the entire body's circulatory system in relation to the health of the brain. Blood carries nutrients to every part of the body, but the delicate tissues of the brain require a specialized security system. This tightly woven net of endothelial cells is called the blood–brain barrier (BBB) and acts as a filter, permitting only certain substances to travel from the blood to the brain. The BBB is responsible for providing neurons with glucose and other nutrients, maintaining proper neurotransmitter balance, and protecting the brain from foreign substances in the blood that may be toxic. Studies have shown age-related alterations in the blood–brain barrier transport function, including a decrease in choline transport and a decrease in brain glucose influx. Choline, one of the B vitamins, is critical in the manufacture of the neurotransmitter acetylcholine. Glucose is the primary fuel for the brain and supports many of the cognitive functions of the brain. It is important, therefore, that the blood circulating throughout your body and brain is nutrient-rich and full of antioxidants, such as NADH or N-acetylcysteine, and amino acids, such as acetylcholine.

Though memory loss affects both genders, it can be particularly devastating to women during and around menopause. In their book *Female and Forgetful: A Six-Step Program to Help Restore Your Memory and Sharpen Your Mind*, Dr. Elisa Lottor and Nancy Bruning explore the uncharted waters that link memory loss to menopause. Estrogen has a powerful influence on the brain, playing an important role in functions such as memory, language skills, moods, and attention. The authors describe case studies of women who, in the beginning of menopause, suddenly cannot remember simple things, such as their social security or phone numbers. The authors posit that the sharp decline in hormonal levels during menopause wreak havoc on memory. Fortunately, as the reported incidences of menopause-linked memory loss increase in scientific literature, so do the reported efficacies of treatment.

Diagnosis

It is difficult to know exactly when memory failure is a simple lapse on the part of the brain in processing known information, and when it is indicative of a more serious condition, such as dementia or Alzheimer's disease (see chapters 27 and 19). Many changes in memory or cognitive function in older adults are temporary and are linked to environmental factors, such as stress or poor nutrition, rather than to physiological processes. A doctor evaluating a patient who complains of memory loss will have to consider underlying factors, such as illness or medications, head injury or trauma, the possibility of stroke or heart disease, or drug or alcohol abuse. These factors can make it unclear whether their patient is suffering the "inevitable" memory decline associated with aging, or experiencing symptoms that indicate the onset of a serious condition such as dementia or Alzheimer's disease.

Your doctor should also consider a number of other factors, including essential fatty acid deficiencies; chronic inflammation of the brain, which can damage cerebral blood vessels or neurons; nutrient deficiencies; hormone imbalances, especially decreased levels of DHEA, thyroid, and testosterone; poor health habits, such as smoking, or drug or alcohol use, which can shortchange the amount of oxygen the brain receives; atherosclerosis or heart disease, which can affect the amount of oxygen the brain receives; brain neurotransmitter levels; and adverse side effects of prescription medications.

Generally speaking, a memory problem is serious when it affects your daily functioning. If you sometimes forget names, you should not be worried, and there is much you can do to correct this tendency. In fact, researchers suggest that people who are aware of their memory loss probably do not have a serious problem. If you have trouble remembering how to do things you have done many times before, or a place you visit often, or difficulty in understanding the order in which to do things (e.g., following a recipe), your doctor should be notified.

Natural Therapies

The good news is that the birth of new nerve cells in the brain is an ongoing process throughout our lifespans. Rejuvenating your memory or preventing decline in cognitive functions in the first place requires a holistic approach to a healthy lifestyle that considers proper nutrition and beneficial supplementation, mental and physical exercise, and stress management. We must reject the notion that memory decline is a natural consequence of aging. A person's memory should function at optimal levels well into old age.

Simple memory deficits, if not addressed, can worsen over time. Mental maintenance is a "use it or lose it" proposition. You must make a commitment to continually learn new information, to undertake new physical challenges, and to endeavor to remain open to new experiences. By concentrating on therapies and behaviors that improve circulation to the brain, rejuvenate brain cell metabolism, suppress free radical damage, and strengthen our mental muscles, we can boost neurological function and expect to maintain robust memory even as we age.

DIET

The nutrients present in the food you eat are the building blocks for neurotransmitters, the main network of communication in your brain. It's an easy correlation to make: if you don't nourish your brain with the proper foods, the health of the neurotransmitters will be compromised. When your mind suddenly goes blank, it may be that your lack of attention to diet has negatively impacted your brain's ability to do its job. It's a classic case of the domino effect, a perfect illustration of cause and effect.

A good maxim to remember is "What works for the heart, works for the head." When planning a brain-healthy diet, remember that, like your heart, your brain needs oxygen, it needs to be blood-rich in antioxidants and vital nutrients, and it needs glucose for energy. Processed sugars, simple carbohydrates, fast foods, alcohol, and artery-clogging saturated fats are as bad for your mind as they are for your body. Foods rich in the omega-3 fatty acids found in green leafy vegetables, walnuts, chia seeds, and flax seeds, as well as unrefined complex carbohydrates, high-quality proteins, and fruits rich in antioxidants, such as blueberries, blackberries, and prunes, are the basic ingredients for a diet that promotes a healthy body and a healthy mind.

SUPPLEMENTS

Certain vitamins and minerals may provide protection against memory loss. A longitudinal study conducted on nearly 3,000 people between the ages of 65 and 102 years concluded that vitamin E intake from foods or supplements is associated with less cognitive decline with age. I recommend increasing your daily vitamin E supplement from 400 to 800 units daily. Do not exceed 1,000 units daily. Vitamin C can reduce and reverse oxidative damage to tissues caused by free radicals, boost the immune system, and regenerate oxidized levels of vitamin E in the body, thus enhancing the potency of that vitamin. I recommend a daily dosage of 1,000 to 5,000 milligrams, taken twice daily.

A recent nationwide health and nutrition survey reported that grain products fortified with the B vitamin folate could help reduce memory loss in the over-sixty age group. Another study demonstrated that older adults with low vitamin B intake (in particular, folate) showed elevated blood homocysteine levels and suffered from a greater degree of memory loss than those with sufficient vitamin B intake. In fact, the participants in the study who had proper folate levels appeared to be immune to memory loss, even when their homocysteine levels were elevated. I recommend that your daily B-complex vitamin contain at least 1 milligram of methylated folic acid and 1 milligram of methylated vitamin B_{12}.

Lecithin is manufactured in the body and found in many animal- and plant-based foods, such as eggs, liver, peanuts, soybeans, wheat germ, and brewer's yeast. It is often found as an additive in processed foods, such as ice cream and salad dressing. Lecithin is a precursor to the neurotransmitter acetylcholine and has a positive effect on cerebral and memory functions. A key component of lecithin, phosphatidylcholine, is broken down in the body and becomes choline, a building block of acetylcholine, a key neurotransmitter that plays an important role in memory. Levels of acetylcholine are known to decline with age, and studies have shown that supplementation with choline—which can also be found in liver, egg yolks, peanuts, cauliflower, soybeans, cabbage, and grape juice—can improve memory and learning. For women, I recommend increasing your daily lecithin supplement from 1 gram to 2 grams maximum, in two divided doses.

Studies have shown that iron deficiency may be linked to problems with short-term memory. Iron is crucial in building brain neurotransmitter activity, and can be found in foods and supplements. Iron should be taken with vitamin C to improve absorption. Consult with your doctor about adding iron supplements to your daily regimen.

A number of other naturally occurring nutrients may have beneficial impacts on memory loss.

- DMAE (Dimethylaminoethanol). This nutrient, found in sardines, is a powerful stimulant that increases acetylcholine levels. Acetylcholine plays a role in memory, concentration, and focus. I recommend increasing your daily DMAE supplement from 150 milligrams to 300 milligrams. Consult your physician before taking heavy doses of DMAE.
- N-acetylcysteine (NAC). This amino acid protects the brain

from damaging free radicals by boosting quantities of glutathione, one of the body's most powerful antioxidants. I recommend a supplement of 500 milligrams taken three times daily.

- Nicotinamide adenine dinucleotide (NADH). NADH is present in all living cells and plays a critical role in energy production. It helps prevent cellular degeneration and may increase concentration and memory capacity. I recommend a supplement of 2.5 milligrams taken twice a day for two or three days of the week.
- Brain Shield (gastrodin) 50 mg
- cognitex as directed
- Magnesium L threonate 200 mg
- PQQ 20 mg
- Cytokine Supress with EGCG 300 mg
- grape seed extract 200 mg
- wild blueberry extract 200 mg
- ashwaganda 200 mg
- uridine 5 mono phosphate 50 mg
- decaffeinated green tea 1000 mg
- curcum 1000mg 5x day
- coconut oil 1tsp 2x day
- black cumin seed oil 1tsp 2x day
- Phosphatidylserine (PS). PS helps the brain use fuel more efficiently. By boosting neuronal metabolism and stimulating production of acetylcholine, PS may be able to improve the condition of patients in cognitive decline. For impact on memory loss, I recommend increasing your daily PS supplement from 300 milligrams to 400 milligrams. Do not exceed a daily supplement of 400 milligrams.

HERBAL REMEDIES

Some herbal extracts have properties similar to conventional medications, but are gentler and may lack the drugs' side effects. Always inform your medical practitioner of any herbal remedies you may be taking. Butcher's broom promotes healthy circulation to the brain, resulting in enhanced memory and clearer focus.

I recommend two to four 425-milligram capsules daily. Chamomile is widely recognized for its ability to reduce stress and anxiety, resulting in increased focus and concentration. I recommend two 325-milligram capsules three times per day, preferably with food. Eye bright is excellent for impacting inflammation; its cooling and detoxifying properties may help with memory loss. Take two 430-milligram capsules three times per day, preferably with food.

Garlic cleans clogged arteries and increases blood flow to the brain. Add to your diet or take prepared capsules as directed by the manufacturer. Ginkgo biloba enhances cerebral circulation, improves brain function and memory, and scavenges free radicals. Ginkgo can act as an anticoagulant, and individuals taking anticoagulant and antithrombotic drugs such as ASA, anti-inflammatories, and warfarin or Coumadin should consult with their doctors before taking ginkgo. If ginkgo is safe for you to use, I recommend taking 40 to 60 milligrams of ginkgo biloba extract three times a day.

Ginseng boosts energy and concentration and may help protect and strengthen the body against the damaging effects of chronic stress. Ginseng can interact with many medications. Talk to your health care provider before supplementing with ginseng, and follow your provider's instructions for use. Gotu kola improves memory and mental alertness. Do not use gotu kola if you take medication for diabetes or to control cholesterol. If gotu kola is safe for you to take, I recommend 200 milligrams taken three times daily. Huperzine A sharpens the mind, wards off memory decline, and improves cognitive and behavioral functions. I recommend 50 micrograms per day with meals. St. John's wort (hypericum) is very popular in Europe, so much so that it is actually covered by German health insurance as a prescription drug. The recommended dose for combating memory impairment is 300 milligrams twice a day. Vinpocetine, a derivative of an extract taken from the periwinkle shrub, enhances circulation to the brain and may improve mild, age-related cognitive impairment. I recommend taking 10 milligrams twice daily with meals.

HOMEOPATHIC REMEDIES

The following remedies may be of use for mild cases of short-term memory loss. When dealing with a chronic condition, homeopathic remedies must be utilized in conjunction with other therapies, as prescribed by a qualified health professional. Consult with your health care provider before taking any homeopathic remedy, and follow your provider's recommendation for the appropriate dosage. Always inform your medical practitioner of any homeopathic remedies you may be taking.

- Baryta carbonica is for memory loss of recent events and general difficulty comprehending.
- Lycopodium is for loss of memory due to anxiety.
- Argentum nitricum can help a generally weak memory.
- Anacardium is for impaired memory that seems worse after a hot bath and better after eating.

PHYSICAL EXERCISE AND STRESS REDUCTION

The brain is nourished by blood, so it should come as no surprise that physical activity that promotes circulation is beneficial in preventing memory loss and mental fogginess. The hippocampus section of the brain is vital for acquiring new memories. It is one of the select few areas in the adult mammalian brain that can grow new nerve cells. One study demonstrated that voluntary exercise increases neurogenesis in the hippocampus. Aerobic exercise, such as walking, gardening, swimming, tai chi, or dancing, has also been shown to sharpen memory skills.

Chronic stress—those day-to-day, irritating occurrences that continue to build up in our bodies—causes the body to release cortisol into the bloodstream. Cortisol then travels through the circulatory system to the brain, where it begins wreaking havoc on the hippocampus. As we age, our bodies find it more difficult to signal to the adrenal gland that it should stop producing cortisol. Prolonged exposure to stress then leads to the loss of brain cells in the memory center.

One should begin each morning in a positive way, with some form of stress reduction technique. Dr. Dharma Singh Khalsa calls it "Wake Up to Wellness." Simply put, instead of starting your day with coffee, turning on the news, or reading the paper, you should start your day off in a positive manner. Find a quiet place so that you can practice some form of relaxation meditation technique, which lowers cortisol levels, which in turn improves memory.

Quiet contemplation allows your body to relax completely. Meditation can be done at any time, in nearly any place. Simply sit comfortably with your spine straight. Let your gaze drop downward, allowing your eyes to rest comfortably while remaining open but unfocused. Allow your breathing to become rhythmic. If your attention drifts, or your eyes close, this is normal. Simply redirect your attention back to your relaxed, downward gaze. After taking several normal breaths, begin to breathe deeper with longer inhalations and exhalations. Breathe from your diaphragm—your chest will rise, your ribs will expand, and your belly will rise in sequence as you breathe. Breathe deeply and slowly, paying attention to each breath as you imagine tension draining from your body with each exhalation. Use your imagination to recall successful or positive life events and link the feelings of those events to your present state. Prayer can take the form of silent meditation, affirmations, chanting, or traditional words. Repeat calmly, quietly, and in harmony with your breath.

MENTAL EXERCISE

The best way to keep your memory skills strong is to use them. Memorizing dates, lists, and even telephone numbers can help keep your mind sharp as you age. The practice of construction and reconstruction of knowledge is critical to memory, so learning new skills stimulates your brain too. Keep your brain entertained and engaged by practicing crossword or jigsaw puzzles, doing word search and brainteaser puzzles, or playing board games or card games.

Here are some strategies to enhance learning and improve recall:

- Relax: Tension and stress cause short-term memory failure.
- Concentrate: Pay attention as you are receiving new information, you'll be surprised at how much more you retain.
- Focus: Reduce distractions when you are involved in new undertakings that require concentration.
- Slow down: It doesn't matter how long it takes you to learn something; it's the acquisition of new information, not the speed with which you acquire it, that's important.
- Follow a routine: Put important items, such as keys, in the same place each time.
- Organize: Knowing where important information is can reduce stress; storing vital information in a visible place may be enough to trigger your memory without even having to look.
- Write it down: Write down important things; keep lists.
- Repeat: Repetition improves recall; use it, especially when learning names.

■ Visualize: A strong link to a visual clue can improve memory; use landmarks to help you find places.

OTHER

Exposure to certain types of music, especially classical music, produces transient increases in cognitive performance. One report examined a group of healthy elderly people and Alzheimer's disease patients to determine the effects of listening to an excerpt of Vivaldi's *The Four Seasons*. The results of the study showed that listening to music enhanced the patients' ability to pay attention.

Essential oils can be used in baths, or inhaled, or mixed with a carrier oil, such as massage oil, and rubbed on the skin. Experiment with some of the following scents to see which are stimulating to you: rosemary, peppermint, frankincense, sage, and geranium.

A good night's sleep allows the entire body to recharge. If you get some quality sleep, you are better able to concentrate. Research shows that people who are awakened during dream sleep fail to process memories from the day before and thus forget more. Dr. Khalsa points out that "recent studies have shown that you don't need to sleep as much as you think because in the last two hours you have very weird dreams and the rapid eye movement sleep is very intense. This raises cortisol levels and can actually cause some problems. In fact, people who have heart attacks have them most often in the morning. High amounts of REM sleep produce high levels of cortisol, which is why many people awaken with morning stress and anxiety. This particular feeling has been found to lead to memory loss specifically and other illnesses perhaps as well."

For overall general improvement, Dr. Braverman also endorses chelation, electrostimulation, and Reiki. Chelation therapy pulls out aluminum and other heavy metals from the bloodstream, resulting in improved memory. Amino acids and neurotransmitter precursors are more effective when accompanied by electrostimulation of the brain. A transcutaneous electrical nerve stimulation (TENS) unit, worn on the forehead and left wrist, helps drive these substances along a good pathway. A cranioelectrical stimulation (CES) device also helps electrical fields and enhances the entire neurotransmitter system. In Reiki, a bodywork technique, pressure points are used to move energy through the body, achieving balance and harmony.

Gary Null's Protocol for Memory Loss

My baseline wellness protocol can be found in chapter 16. The following chart summarizes additional supplements I recommend for individuals who suffer from, or are specifically concerned about, memory loss. If you are concerned about additional brain conditions discussed in other chapters, consult with a health professional about how you can safely impact multiple conditions.

If you are taking medications—whether prescription or over-the-counter—or have any food restrictions, consult with your doctor before beginning any supplement program. Your health care provider should always be up-to-date on all vitamins, supplements, and herbal or homeopathic remedies you are taking. Supplement overdoses are rare, but possible, and certain combinations may affect individuals adversely.

SUPPLEMENT	DOSAGE	CAUTIONS
Lecithin	For men: increase daily dosage from 1 g to 2.5 g. Do not exceed a daily supplement of 2.5 g. For women: increase	Side effects may include nausea, bloating, vomiting, sweating, and diarrhea; extremely large doses can
cause	daily dosage from 1 g to 2 g. Do not exceed a daily supplement of 2 g.	a heart-rhythm abnormality; do not use if you have bipolar disorder.
DMAE (dimethylaminoethanol)	Increase daily dosage from 150 mg to 250 mg.	May be overstimulating for some people. Headaches, muscle tension, and irritability may occur. Do not take if you have epilepsy, a history of convulsions, or bipolar disorder. If you have kidney or liver disease, consult your doctor before taking this supplement.

Iron	Consult your doctor.	Have a blood test to determine true iron deficiency, as iron overload can cause health problems. Iron can interfere with a number of drugs, including thyroid hormone drugs, antibiotics, and drugs used to treat Parkinson's disease. Tannins found in coffee and tea can inhibit iron absorption.
NAC (N-acetylcysteine)	500 mg three times daily	Regular supplementation of NAC increases urinary output of copper. If supplementing with NAC for an extended period, add 2 mg of copper and 30 mg of zinc to your daily supplement regimen.
NADH (nicotinamide adenine dinucleotide, also called coenzyme Q1) insomnia.	2.5 mg twice daily, two or three times per week	High doses (10 mg per day or more) may cause nervousness, anxiety, and
PS (phosphatidylserine)	Increase daily dose from 300 mg to 400 mg. Do not exceed a daily supplement of 400 mg.	

Research Update

Research presented at the American Academy of Neurology's 64th Annual Meeting in April 2012 illuminated the association between overeating and memory loss. Measuring mild cognitive impairment among 1,233 seniors age seventy and above, the researchers discovered that those seniors who consumed between 2,143 and 6,000 calories per day more than doubled their risk of suffering from memory loss and other manifestations of mild cognitive impairment compared to those who consumed 600 to 1,526 calories daily. Sugar intake and brain function were the subject of a recent study by scientists at UCLA. The researchers found that rats given a diet high in fructose performed poorly in tests using mazes that were designed to assess memory and learning. In addition to being fed a fructose-enriched diet, some rats were fed omega-3 fatty acids in the form of flaxseed oil and docosahexaenoic acid (DHA); this group completed the tests much more quickly than did the rats not given omega-3s, suggesting that healthy fats may counteract the harmful effects of sugar on brain health.

In an article published in the *Journal of Applied Physiology* in 2011, researchers reviewed more than one hundred studies that investigated how aerobic and resistance training exercise influences brain fitness. The group found that aerobic exercise corresponds with improved ability to multitask and maintaining concentration over extended periods of time, while resistance exercise is associated with greater ability to focus in the face of distractions.

The relationship between a mentally active lifestyle and cognitive decline were the focus of a review published by the prestigious *Cochrane Collaboration* in early 2012. Analyzing the results of fifteen studies involving more than seven hundred patients with mild to moderate dementia, the authors found that those patients who participated in cognitive stimulation intervention programs performed significantly better on thinking and memory tests than did the individuals who did not undergo treatment. The benefits of the programs were observed to last at least one to three months after treatment ended. The patients evaluated in the review engaged in a variety of mentally stimulating activities, including discussion of past and present events, word games, puzzles, music, baking, and indoor gardening.

Chapter 43

Menopause

PATIENT STORY

My journey began when I was forty-five. I was going through what we now know as perimenopause. I was experiencing many symptoms that I didn't even realize were hormonally related. I had anxiety attacks in the middle of the night. I found that my mood swings were all over the place. I was fatigued a great deal of the time. My libido was really low, and I just found generally I didn't feel well. I noticed little dark hairs starting to appear on my chin. It wasn't until the night sweats arrived on the scene, which was occurring every night, I would wake up drenched. This really got my attention that something had to be done. As I began to investigate what were my choices and what was really going on I found myself exploring the world of hormones. This experience of perimenopause and the imbalance, which I have now realized was the result of many years of stress and poor diet, but it all culminated in this condition. Through the need to get to the bottom of this and through the need to find my health again I discovered a world of such deception and misinformation and propaganda relating to women and their hormones that it absolutely infuriated me.

So as I began to do my homework and investigate and read the medical journals and talk to experts around the world I uncovered the tremendous number of myths that are influencing women's choices these days. The number one myth is the fact that women's ovaries do not dry up and do not cease functioning. There is a prevailing belief out there that female bodies are dangerous, disease producing, and basically our hormones deteriorate and we become susceptible to all sorts of aging diseases and imbalances. This is not the case. In fact what happens at menopause is an amazing transformation. For years women in this country have been convinced that menopause is a downhill slide. We've been told that our ovaries fail. We cease to make estrogen and basically we are at greater risk of heart disease and osteoporosis and Alzheimer's and wrinkling, which is a very horri-fying picture and it's driven us into the arms of the doctors and the medical profession who told us that we could be rescued through using synthetic hormones.

The very basis for understanding menopause as defined by the medical model is actu-ally based on error. Nature endowed women with this divine intelligence to allow her body to remain healthy and vital and fit and functioning all the days of her life. Menopause is in fact not the end of her life. It's actually the beginning of a stage of her life cycle where she actually can step into the greater sense of power, inner authority, cre-ativity, and spiritual attunement, which is what has been known from many traditional cultures throughout time.

—Dr. Sherrill Sellman

Menopause marks the end of the female reproductive cycle, which typically occurs between the ages of forty-five and fifty but can happen anywhere from forty to sixty, or even earlier as a result of surgery, illness, or lifestyle. It is said to begin when a woman goes through one complete year without a period. The stage before menopause, called perimenopause, may last as long as ten years.

Menopause is not a disorder but rather a natural biomolecular process, a normal stage of life. We have a belief in this country that after menopause you're more apt to get breast cancer, heart disease, high blood pressure, arthritis, dia-betes, and other chronic degenerative diseases. But those things are not inevitable; they are all choices. It's true that after menopause they increase in incidence, but it is not because of menopause per se. It is about the fact that your body will no longer let you get away with the adverse lifestyle choices you've been making for decades. Armed with the right knowledge, menopause can be a time to flourish and be healthier, happier, and more positive than ever.

"The perimenopause is a crossroads," says Dr. Christiane Northrup, a board-certified obstetrician-gynecologist and pioneer in women's health and wellness. "One road says, 'Grow'. The other says, 'Die.' It is completely a choice. Are you going to continue doing the same old things that led you to where you are now? Or are you going to wake up and use your own power to truly flourish and move into what are the best years of your life?"

As Dr. Sherrill Sellman, naturopath, psychotherapist, and author of best-selling book *Hormone Heresy*, points out, many doctors and women alike harbor misconceptions about the nature and effects of menopause. Yet in cultures where menopause is less feared, symptoms are virtually nonexistent, and in fact menopause is anticipated as a rite of passage into a stronger, wiser time of life.

Symptoms

Menopause is a transition that manifests uniquely in each person. Nonetheless, there are a few common symptoms observed among perimenopausal women. One of the first changes is in the frequency of the menstrual cycle. The time between cycles may increase or decrease, or they may skip a month. Usually blood flow is reduced, but women may also experience heavy, irregular bleeding. Other common symptoms associated with menopause are hot flashes, dry skin, mood swings, depression, irritability, vaginal dryness, night sweats, bladder infection, fatigue, and sleep disturbances.

"Many changes appear in perimenopausal women, but the negative ones usually arise from stress, bad diet, pharmaceutical drugs, exhausted adrenal glands, and other things—not from lowered estrogen levels," says Dr. Sellman. "I believe, based on my own experience, that the symptoms of menopause—and also those of PMS, which are produced by the same imbalances—are really the result of poor health. When we can correct these imbalances, our hormones automatically go back into balance and we receive all the benefits. Women need to understand that a healthy liver, a healthy digestive system, a healthy adrenal system, and getting the colon working are the factors that contribute to healthy hormone production."

Among the factors that play a role in the timing and characteristics of menopause are genetics and overall health. Environmental influences also may be involved. Recent research has shown that exposure to certain chemicals is linked to early menopause. In a 2015 article published in the journal *PLoS One*, women with high levels of chemicals in the body from plastics, household products, personal care items, food, and the environment experienced menopause two to four years earlier than women with lower levels. Already associated with cancer, metabolic syndrome, heart disease, early puberty, and infertility, these endocrine-disrupting chemicals (EDCs) were found to interfere with hormone activity.

Estrogen dominance can be caused by hormone replacement therapy, the Pill, and even the hormones found in nonorganic foods. For example, most cattle are fattened with growth hormones, which we then ingest. Hormones can also be found in dairy products and nonorganic produce. Pesticides and herbicides are estrogen mimickers. They compromise liver function due to the toxins or other physical dysfunction, and they can increase estrogen levels.

The increase in estrogen in the environment is rapidly being acknowledged as a serious health problem affecting not only menopausal women but also men and younger women, and even children. People living in Western societies are now being flooded with a tidal wave of estrogen mimics. Even going into a health food store and having a glass of vegetable juice or buying the vegetables and making juice yourself can be cause for concern: if the vegetables are not organic, you're bringing in a concentrated amount of pesticides.

Among the problems associated with too much estrogen are weight gain, breast tenderness, mood disorders, brain fog, fibroids, endometriosis, and hypothyroidism. "The symptoms of too much estrogen out of balance with progesterone includes the gaining of weight, particularly on the abdomen, hips, and thighs, because the nature of estrogen is to turn food into fat," Dr. Sellman explains. "This happens to the animals in the feedlots. It also happens to us. As long as we have this imbalanced relationship we will continue to put weight on no matter how much we try to diet or exercise.

"Lumpy fibrocystic breasts are stimulated by high estrogen levels. Depression, mood swings, rage, anger are all caused by estrogen excess, as is food retention, bloating, fatigue, and headaches. Those migraine headaches that happen before your period or when your hormone levels are out of balance are all related to high estrogen levels. High estrogen also decreases sex drive, which is a major problem for women. It's not about menopause. It's really about these imbalances."

The liver is also affected by estrogen. "That's a problem that is not totally understood by medical doctors," Dr. Sellman says. "When we have compromised liver function, we cannot properly metabolize estrogen safely out of the body. So what happens with high levels of toxicity that overwhelm the liver is that the liver then metabolizes estrogen down a pathway that turns it into a more toxic form of estrogen. It then gets reabsorbed back into the body, putting women at risk of hormone dependent cancers like breast cancer."

Many women going through menopause experience anxiety, depression, or other types of mental difficulties, including mood swings, clouded thought, and increased irritability. There is a variety of potential causes of these symptoms. First, the hormonal changes that occur during menopause may have some effect. In addition, other menopausal symptoms—such as difficulty sleeping or vaginal dryness—may contribute to overall stress levels, leading to mental difficulties. Cultural expectations and perceptions of menopause may also play a role in provoking anxiety and stress during the perimenopausal years.

It is well known that there are cultures that do not associate the cessation of menstruation with negative consequences. Dr. Sellman explains, "The Japanese, for example, don't have a word for menopause or hot flashes. They look at it as just a transition period, but not one with a significant effect on a woman's life. So the symptoms we are told are inevitable, that all women must endure, are actually symptoms of imbalance. I've found that to be true in my own case. When I notice symptoms appearing, such as night sweats or cramp or fatigue, I get immediate relief when I work with natural healing methods."

Misconceptions about Menopause

Dr. Linda Ojeda, author of *Menopause Without Medicine*, says many women see menopause as the beginning of the end. "They believe that life is going to be downhill from this point on. They no longer think of themselves as youthful, as able to contribute to society. They fear that their behavior will become erratic, hysterical, and out of control. This is not true. When we reach fifty, we do not turn into raging maniacs, and we are not more susceptible to clinical depression. In some women, however, lowered levels of estrogen, endorphins, and serotonin, substances that affect mood, can create mood swings. Levels can be raised naturally in these women.

"We know that beliefs and attitudes affect the transition. In Asian countries, symptoms are virtually nonexistent. In these countries, menopause is looked at as an important event in a woman's life. She now has more prestige and is viewed as a wise, older woman. Women anticipate this time of life with relish. If you are approaching menopause with fear and trepidation, you need to examine your attitude."

According to clinical psychologist Dr. Janice Stefanacci Steward, society expects menopausal women to lose their sex drive, but this does not have to happen. "Many women fear that they are going to lose their passion and sexuality. Really, only a small portion of women who go through menopause have their sex drive adversely affected. For those women who lose their sexual desire or have difficulty becoming and staying aroused, help is available. But most women do not experience sexual arousal problems, and many report feeling more sexual because the risk of pregnancy is gone."

Dr. Christiane Northrup tells about her book, *The Secret Pleasures of Menopause*, which documents that women in their fifties and sixties are having the best sex of their lives. "You don't hear that because the mainstream culture would lead you to believe that after the age of forty you're pretty much washed up as a woman, and you're no longer desirable and that's the end for you. It is those messages that must be retooled in your brain so that when you hear one you turn off the TV, you stop reading the paper. You turn it around in your head, and you say today is a new day and I have everything I need to create the most pleasurable, fun life as possible from this moment forward."

To understand our society's misconceptions about menopause, we must go back at least a half century. "The beginnings of this whole myth that women lose their power and that the ovaries shrivel up and die as a result of menopause actually began in the 1960s," says Dr. Sellman. "It was the beginning of the era when cheap synthetic artificial hormones were readily available. Up until that point they were very expensive. Then there was this wonderful drug in search of a destiny. The menopausal woman was actually the focus, and it was the work of Dr. Robert Wilson who wrote a book called *Feminine Forever*, which was published in 1966—based on one study that he conducted over one year. The results of the study convinced him that the saving grace, the way we could keep women young forever, was to give them estrogen. He said in his book the ovaries shrivel up and die as a result of menopause, therefore necessitating the use of estrogen. He also had rather unflattering comments about the menopausal women, calling them the equivalent of a eunuch. So he painted this bleak picture where estrogen was the salvation, and he spawned the industry using estrogen replacement therapy for menopausal women with uteruses.

"As a postscript we need to say that he was discredited by the FDA as a researcher, and he also had received a large sum of money in his trust fund from the three leading manufacturers of estrogen drugs. Up until that time menopause was a psychiatric condition. Women were perceived as having psychological problems, but it wasn't a medical condition until these drugs became available."

Despite popular belief, the ovaries do not fail at menopause. Dr. Sellman explains, "We do not cease producing estrogen. At menopause we are going through a transition from our fertility years to our what I call wise women years. The body in its wisdom to conserve energy is reducing the amount of estrogen made by the ovaries by 40 to 60 percent. It's reduced because we don't need mature eggs in our menopausal years. So we have this reduction, this adjustment of hormones. We have this adjustment, and we also have a backup system to estrogen because our fat cells can be converted into estrogen. The World Health Organization has actually found through the use of saliva testing that an overweight postmenopausal woman has more estrogen running through her body than a skinny premenopausal woman.

"We have this condition of estrogen being made, in fact high levels of estrogen being made, in menopausal women and we also have a decline of progesterone, which is the other key hormone. Progesterone is made in our premenopausal years when we ovulate . . . We must ovulate to make adequate levels of progesterone. In our menopausal years we're not ovulating so that is not the source of the progesterone, but our adrenal glands become the primary support for producing progesterone. The fat cells become the primary areas that produce estrogen. So we actually continue to make these hormones."

Other changes are happening as well. "At menopause, the inner part of the ovary actually gets switched on for the first time in a woman's life, producing hormones that look after her heart, her blood vessels, her libido, her skin, and sense of well-being. This amazing organ the ovary actually is functioning the entire length of our lives and is supporting a woman in her health and well-being through the many, many years of her postmenopausal journey, which really is the prime of much heightened passion and purpose."

So actually what happens at menopause is not a deficiency in estrogen, but rather an imbalance in the ratio between progesterone (too little) and estrogen (too much). The symptoms of this imbalance, seen most prominently during perimenopause, are hot flashes, night sweats, weight gain, insomnia, headaches, loss of muscle tone, fatigue, and depression.

Hormone Replacement Therapy (HRT)

The natural medicine community has known about the dangers of hormone replacement therapy (HRT) for decades, but it took until 2002 for conventional doctors to finally take notice. That was when the US government abruptly stopped the hormone trial of the Women's Health Initiative citing evidence that HRT was not the panacea it was touted to be, and moreover was actually associated with an increased risk of breast cancer, heart disease, and blood clots in many women.

Dr. Sherrill Sellman provides some background on HRT. "In the 1970s, women turned their backs on supplementation with estrogen alone because it had been found to cause endometrial cancer. So the drug companies came up with hormone replacement therapy, which used a combination of estrogen and a synthetic progestin such as Provera. They used a synthetic because natural progesterone, which has no toxic side effects, cannot be patented. To sell HRT to women, who were scared of hormones after the revelations of the 1970s, the companies claimed that HRT reduced the risk of a condition most women were unaware of: osteoporosis. In the early 1990s, a new reason for healthy women to take this powerful carcinogenic steroid was introduced. HRT was said to be a way to protect the heart. So doctors began using HRT, originally supposed to be only a short-term treatment for relief of menopausal symptoms, as a long-term treatment to prevent other conditions, conditions that only might occur. A review of the research, however, even that which was used to back the use of HRT initially, revealed that instead of being beneficial, HRT actually increased the risk of serious complications and even death.

"We've been led to believe that hormone replacement therapy, the synthetic version that is found in whatever variety of pills or patches or implants, uses the same hormones that our body makes. The truth of the matter is that they are synthetic drugs, which have been listed by the National Institutes of Health as known human carcinogens."

According to Dr. Northrup, for the 10 million women still taking synthetic hormone replacement therapy today, synthetic progestin is one of the biggest worries. "For the life of me, I cannot understand why the medical profession still does not understand the difference between the progesterone that your body produces and progestin, which is a completely artificial hormone that your body has never seen before. Dr. Kent Hermsmeyer, at the Oregon Primate Center, has shown that in monkeys that are deprived of estrogen—so they're perimenopausal monkeys—when you actually give them Provera it will cause reactivity in the coronary arteries leading to heart attack.

"A synthetic progestin will actually cause the coronary arteries in a woman to become hyperreactive and many women when they go through perimenopause have chest pain. They actually have angina because their coronary arteries are not getting the blood flow they need. When you add Provera to that, you're making it much worse."

Natural progesterone or natural bioidentical hormone, as opposed to synthetic progestin, is the identical molecule that our bodies make. Although bioidentical hormones are frequently made in the laboratory, such as from soy phytochemicals, they are nevertheless identical to human hormones; therefore the actual biochemistry of the hormones is unchanged.

Natural Therapies

Natural therapies can make HRT unnecessary. A variety of options are available. Most women can start with lifestyle changes such as modifying the diet, taking herbs and supplements, getting more exercise and rest. Some use bioidentical hormone therapy, but this is not in itself a first line of defense, and its safety and effectiveness remain a matter of debate.

DIET

There is a lot of research out there on what we can do with our diets to rebalance hormone, turn off hot flashes, improve skin, hair, and nails, and boost immunity and energy. Scientists at Beth Israel Medical Center discovered a molecule in soy beans that can reduce the frequency and severity of hot flashes by as much as 50 percent in menopausal women. According to one of the researchers, Dr. Hope Ricciotti, "the chemical structure of this compound is very similar to that of our estrogen, allowing it to act as a regulatory mechanism if the body's natural levels decrease." Soybeans are rich in isoflavones and have the attribute of binding to estrogen receptors in the body tissue. By binding to these receptors, isoflavones block the mimicking estrogens from attaching themselves to tissue cells.

Soy is the food that has the highest content of estrogen, says Dr. Jane Guiltinan, a naturopathic physician from Washington. "Soybeans, tofu, tempeh—anything made with soy—will contain plant estrogens. Oats, cashews, almonds, alfalfa, apples, and flaxseeds contain smaller amounts of estrogen. A woman emphasizing those foods in the diet can experience significant decreases in her hot flashes."

A Mayo Clinic study has confirmed that dietary therapy including flaxseed oil twice a day (I prefer 1 teaspoon three times a day) will reduce hot flashes in post-menopausal women and menopausal women, and even in premenopausal women who are not taking estrogen supplements. In this study, flaxseed was shown to be more effective than black cohosh and vitamin E. One reason for this might be that flaxseeds have an important fiber known as lignan, which binds with the detrimental estrogens in the intestinal tract that can then be expelled from the body.

If these unwanted estrogens are not bound, they get absorbed into the body's tissues and promote disease. So flaxseed, the raw flaxseed in particular, will detoxify the body from these damaging mimicking estrogens.

Ann Louise Gittelman, author of *Before the Change: Take Charge of Your Perimenopause*, notes that weight gain, a common problem in perimenopausal and menopausal women, can be minimized by eating the right kinds of foods. These foods are incorporated in Gittelman's Changing Diet Plan.

"Low-glycemic, or slow-acting, carbohydrates will supply lots of energy for their calories. My favorites are those that are lower on the glycemic index, which is a list of carbohydrates ranked as to how they develop into blood sugar in your system. I like yams rather than white potatoes, and I like whole rye meal rather than wheat. I choose unprocessed carbohydrates that are moderate to low on the index, which also provide high-quality fiber to help eliminate excess estrogen from the system by lowering blood levels of this hormone."

Some fruits and vegetables are particularly high in phytochemicals and phytohormones. These include apples, grapefruits, lemons, pears, peaches, and a wide variety of vegetables that are also high in fiber.

"I have found that a diet with the right amount of proteins, fats, and low-glycemic carbohydrates not only helps regulate sexual hormone production but also helps to balance the hormonal response to food, which I think is critical in keeping blood sugar levels stable," Gittleman says. "A level blood sugar helps to prevent perimenopausal symptoms such as depression, mood swings, and hot flashes, and it leads to weight loss without any effort.

"Fats are important on the Changing Diet Plan. We need to add essential and beneficial fats, not take them away. These come in the form of the high-lignan flaxseed oil, olive oil, toasted nut seeds, and avocado. These fats stabilize blood sugar levels.

"So we're getting our blood sugar stable, we're assisting in long-term energy, and more importantly, we're providing the raw material for hormones, particularly progesterone, which is the key hormone in perimenopause."

Another natural source of phytohormones is the natural thickening agent kuzu. Several natural-foods recipes incorporate kuzu into sauces in place of flour, making this a way to both enjoy healthy foods and alleviate symptoms.

Sugar, which can cause hot flashes and other menopausal symptoms, should be avoided. Sugar, coffee, and alcohol adversely affect the blood sugar and can disturb the emotions. In addition, Dr. Northrup says, "excess sugar in the diet will cause increased insulin, increased cortisol, and that raises havoc with your own hormones. . . Decreasing sugar in the diet or eliminating refined sugar altogether will actually balance hormones in many women."

VITAMINS AND MINERALS

The following nutrients provide an additional boost to good health in the menopausal years. Always consult with a certified health care practitioner before taking any supplements.

MULTIVITAMINS—Women need a natural multivitamin/mineral supplement containing higher amounts of magnesium than calcium and high amounts of B and C vitamins. A good multiple vitamin helps build the adrenal glands, which lessens emotional symptoms.

VITAMIN E—This vitamin is known for its ability to rejuvenate the reproductive system and alleviate hot flashes. It also helps lessen vaginal thinning and dryness. Mixed (beta-, delta-, and gamma-) tocopherols are best, as they are found together in nature. D-alpha tocopherol is also preferred over synthetic vitamin E. Generally, 400 units per day should be taken in the beginning. The dosage can be gradually increased to 600 units, although some women may need up to 800 units.

ZINC—This mineral supports ovarian function. A good source is zinc picolinate. It can also be taken as an amino acid chelate or as zinc methionine. The recommended dosage is 25 to 50 milligrams per day.

B-COMPLEX—B-complex vitamins are important throughout life, but there is an extra need for these during menopause. They can be obtained from whole grains and green vegetables. B_1 and B_2 (25 milligrams/day), B_5 (300–400 milligrams/day) and B_6 (150 milligrams/day), and B_{12} (1,000 micrograms/day) are especially helpful during menopause. Folic acid, 800 micrograms per day, is also recommended.

ESSENTIAL FATTY ACIDS (EFAS)—EFAs, which are precursors to the natural hormones in the body, are very important for both men and women. People on low-fat diets should pay special attention to this. A diet too low in fats can lead to an increased risk of cancer and aging. Omega-6 fatty acids can be found in flaxseed, sesame, pumpkin, and safflower oils. Omega-3 fatty acids are found in fish oil capsules or fish. Both are needed. EFAs help prevent or treat vaginal dryness.

VITAMIN D—The best source of vitamin D is sunlight. It can also be taken in supplementation (400–600 IU/day), although caution should be taken not to get too much of this vitamin. Another source of vitamin D is salmon oil. People living in polluted environments need more vitamin D.

CALCIUM—Calcium is essential to prevent osteoporosis; supplementation should begin before the onset of menopause. There are many forms to choose from. Dairy is a poor source because many people have an intolerance to it. Calcium citrate is easy to digest, as it is already in an acidic medium. Calcium carbonates are alkaline and therefore more difficult to digest. Amino acid chelate is an excellent source of calcium. Calcium lactate is another good source. Calcium gluconate can be made into a powder and mixed into drinks. The recommended dosage is 1,200 to 1,500 milligrams per day.

GAMMA LINOLENIC ACID (GLA)—This is available as evening primrose oil, borage oil, or blackcurrant seed oil; 1,000 milligrams per day is recommended.

BORON—Research shows boron to be a precursor of both female and male hormones. You only need 5 milligrams a day.

HERBS

A number of herbs on the market help relieve perimenopausal and menopausal symptoms by restoring the progesterone-estrogen balance. They include alfalfa, black cohosh, blue cohosh, damiana, fennel, licorice root, motherwort, red clover, red raspberry leaves, sarsaparilla, and certain forms of wild yam. Flaxseed contains lignan, a phytohormone fiber that removes excess estrogen from the system. This is particularly important, since too much estrogen is believed to fuel breast cancer. Whole flaxseeds can be ground up or can be taken as flaxseed oil.

Vitex, or chaste berry, is commonly referred to as the menopausal herb because it alleviates many symptoms, including hot flashes, vaginal dryness, and mood swings. It works by raising the progesterone level. Ginkgo biloba has been shown to be effective in leveling mood swings.

The Chinese have been using herbs to treat women's problems for 5,000 years. Acupuncturist Roberta Certner says that Chinese medicine sees a woman as giving birth to herself at menopause, since she no longer has an obligation to her children. This philosophy thinks in terms of cycles of seven years. When a woman is forty-nine—often the age when menopause begins—it sees her lifespan as half-finished. "The next half of the lifespan is for self-growth."

Certner explains that "Chinese medicine is adamant that women shouldn't be suffering from night sweats, insomnia, mood changes, and other symptoms, and herbal formulas are good for this purpose. They help to rebalance the energies of the body so that a woman doesn't feel at the mercy of these tremendous moods and powerless over bodily changes."

According to Certner, one virtue of Chinese medicine is gentleness: "People aren't forced to take medications that reduce libido function and that set up terrain for heart conditions. It really addresses the mechanism itself and not just the symptoms. The reason Chinese medicine works is that it goes to the root of the problem. If progesterone is low, you enhance the progesterone, using something like dioscorea or leonorus, whose name itself means 'mother root.'" Many different herbs are available to the practitioner, who chooses the ones to use in a given case according to the nature of the particular person involved. As Certner says, "Chinese medicine doesn't really treat conditions—it treats people."

Important tonic herbs in Chinese medicine include astragalus, dong quai, her shou wu, ginseng, and licorice root.

HOMEOPATHY

The homeopathic remedy chosen should correspond to the symptoms described. According to the late Dr. Ken Korins, a classically trained homeopathic physician in New York City, only one should be used for best results. Sometimes it's a matter of trial and error; if one does not work, another can be tried. Here are some of the remedies Dr. Korins recommended for menopause.

The following remedies are recommended for hot flashes:

LACHESIS—Heat is felt all day long, while cold flashes may be experienced at night. Once the menstrual flow begins, all the symptoms disappear. Symptoms are worse with pressure and heat, and better with the onset of discharges or flows. Increased sexual desire is also associated with a need for lachesis.

BELLADONNA—There are many hot flashes. The face looks red and feels hot, and there is hot perspiration coming from the face and a pounding, throbbing, congested feeling in the head. Often there is dryness. Condition improves with resting quietly in the dark. Symptoms worsen with light, cold air, and sudden jolts. The emotional state can border on hysteria with rages.

GLONOINE—Hot flashes are focused, with pressure in the head and feelings of congestion. There may be an associated rise in blood pressure at the time of the flashes. Symptoms are worse with heat and better with cold air. Emotionally, there is a fear of death; there is mental agitation.

AMYL NITRATE—Flashes of heat are accompanied by headaches, often associated with anxiety and heart palpitations.

MANGANUM—Hot flashes are associated with nervous system depression. The body does not want to move. Symptoms improve when patient is lying down. Emotional state is peevish and fretful. There is a loss of pleasure in joyful music, but a profound reaction to sad music.

The term *flooding* refers to irregular periods that stop for a while but are very heavy when they return. The following remedies may also help younger women with extremely heavy periods:

CHINA—There is heavy bleeding, with dark, clotted blood, leading to debilitating fatigue. Symptoms get worse with drafts and light pressure, but better with strong pressure and heat. Emotional symptoms are apathy with a strong disposition toward hurting other people's feelings (not the normal state).

SABINA—The period is characterized by heavy, bright red, clotted blood. Expelling the clots is painful, and pain radiates from the sacrum to the pubis. Emotional symptoms are irritability and a dislike for music.

SECALE—Periods are profuse and prolonged. Blood is almost black. Symptoms worsen with heat and improve with cold.

PHOSPHORUS—There is easy, frequent bleeding of bright red blood, often with no clots. The patient is low-spirited, with multiple fears. Also, memory may decrease. Another symptom is constant chilliness.

Remedies for vaginal dryness and thinning include:

SEPIA—The vaginal area is itchy and dry. There is a sense that the uterus is falling out of the vagina. There is also a loss of libido. Symptoms tend to be worse with standing, cold, rest, anything that causes venous congestion. Symptoms are improved with anything that increases venous flow, such as motion. Emotionally, there is an indifference to loved ones, sadness, and a tendency to weep easily.

NATRUM MURIATICUM—Vaginal dryness makes sexual intercourse very painful. Discharges tend to be acrid and burning. There is often a loss of pubic hair. Emotional state is one of depression and irritability, which is worse with consolation. Symptoms also tend to worsen around ten o'clock in the morning.

BRYONIA—Vaginal dryness is accompanied by severe headaches. Any motion is painful and distressing. Condition improves with rest.

NITRIC ACID—Vaginal dryness reaches the point where the mucosa fissures, causing splinterlike sensations in the vaginal area.

BIOIDENTICAL HORMONE REPLACEMENT THERAPY: A DEBATE

In recent years, bioidentical hormone replacement therapy (also referred to as natural hormone replacement therapy, or BHRT) has gained popularity as a potential alternative to traditional hormone therapy. Following the Women's Health Initiative study results in 2002, many women, doctors, and scientists turned to bioidenticals hoping to find an effective replacement to HRT that did not carry the same harmful side effects. Today, it is still a matter of debate whether BHRT is safe and effective.

The terms *natural* and *bioidentical* refer to the chemical structure of these hormones. While the chemical compounds used in traditional hormone replacement therapy consist of hormones that are structurally similar to those found in the body, the hormones used in BHRT are chemically identical to what the body naturally produces. It must be pointed out, however, that bioidentical hormones are not obtained from humans but produced synthetically in laboratories.

Just as there is a wide range of hormones at work in our bodies, there are also a number of different compounds that fall under the category of bioidentical hormones. For this reason, the debate surrounding BHRT is often muddled, with voices arguing either for or against BHRT in general. Upon further inspection it seems that the answers are not so clear cut. To gain a better understanding of the safety and efficacy of this treatment, we must look at the effects of hormones and their bioidentical counterparts individually.

NATURAL PROGESTERONE

Progesterone is a hormone that plays a variety of functions related to the female reproductive system, including maintaining a balanced uterine lining, inhibiting overgrowth of breast tissue, and stimulating libido. Progesterone also works to balance blood sugar, produce new bone, normalize sleep, and moderate depression and anxiety in both men and women. By the time a woman has gone through menopause, however, her progesterone levels will drop significantly.

As a bioidentical hormone, natural progesterone is said to have a number of health benefits. Among the purported advantages of progesterone is its capacity to help counteract estrogen dominance in the body, thereby reducing the chances of developing fibroids, breast cancer, ovarian cysts, and other conditions linked with excess estrogen. Other proposed uses for natural progesterone include aiding bone formation, reducing the risk of stroke, and providing anti-aging effects through cortisol production. A non-bioidentical form of progesterone known as progestin is the added ingredient to the estrogen drug Prempro.

PREGNENOLONE

The hormone pregnenolone is synthesized in the body from cholesterol. Pregnenolone is essential to the formation of other hormones, including DHEA, testosterone, progesterone, estrogen, and cortisol. In addition to its role as a precursor hormone, it is believed to help maintain cognitive function and reduce anxiety. Pregnenolone levels tend to drop as a natural part of aging.

Because of the fundamental role played by pregnenolone in the endocrine system, many scientists see great potential for the use of this hormone in BHRT. Some researchers have concluded that replenishing pregnenolone levels in older individuals to those seen in younger people will have an anti-aging effect, allowing people to learn new information and aiding in new memory formation. Some scientists advocate using pregnenolone supplements to combat mental health disorders and chemical dependency.

Research proving these assertions and establishing the safety of using bioidentical pregnenolone, however, is still in its early stages. While associations between aging and lower levels of pregnenolone have been identified, there is not sufficient evidence to definitively assert the benefits and risks associated with its use as a supplement.

DHEA

Dehydroepiandrosterone (DHEA) has been used as a dietary supplement as well as a form of BHRT. Research points to the potential use of DHEA in anti-aging medicine. Studies have indicated that this hormone may help boost memory, preserve bone health, curb depression, and aid muscle development. DHEA is also a known precursor to other hormones.

Studies over the past few years have focused on the effects of DHEA in perimenopausal and postmenopausal women. A 2009 study at St. Louis University found that, when combined with vitamin D and calcium, DHEA resulted in increased bone density in older women. In another recent study published in *Climacteric*, Italian researchers discovered that menopausal symptoms and sexual function could be improved by DHEA.

There are reservations among scientists about the use of DHEA, especially when taken in high amounts. A number of side effects have been reported, including the growth of facial hair and deepening of the voice in women. Some experts contend that taking DHEA may also increase risk for endometrial and breast cancers.

ESTRIOL

Being the least potent of the three estrogens, estriol is often argued to be a relatively safe and mild hormone for use in bioidentical therapy. Estriol levels in the body increase greatly during pregnancy. As a bioidentical hormone, estriol is thought to have many uses, including reducing cardiovascular risk, improving bone mineral status in osteoporosis patients, and protecting urinary health. Estriol may also relieve more general menopausal symptoms, such as night sweats and hot flashes, as well as restore youthfulness in menopausal women. Certain studies have demonstrated that the relatively weak estriol does not raise the risk of developing breast and endometrial cancers in lab animals. Studies have also demonstrated estriol's efficacy in treating menopausal symptoms without carrying the same risks as the more potent estrogens, estrone and estradiol.

TRIPLE ESTROGEN

The triple estrogen formula commonly used in BHRT is composed of 80 percent estriol, 10 percent estradiol, and 10 percent estrone. It is believed that this concoction, which closely mimics the ratios seen during pregnancy, is potent enough to have significant effects on menopausal symptoms. This blend is used to treat common menopausal symptoms such as night sweats, hot flashes, forgetfulness, and others. It is also said to have a positive anti-aging effect, much like the desired effects of Premarin or other HRT drugs.

IN FAVOR OF BIOIDENTICALS

The majority of arguments in favor of BHRT revolve around the chemicals' natural composition. Again, while bioidentical hormones are not naturally produced, they are chemically identical to the hormones in our body and many argue that the body does not distinguish between the two. Those in the pro-BHRT camp maintain that bioidentical hormones are metabolized and excreted more easily than non-bioidenticals, reducing their overall stress on the body and thus being generally safer.

A second argument in favor of BHRT is, surprisingly, a lack of evidence of any dangerous side effects. Most studies showing links between hormone replacement and cancer, heart attack, and stroke have looked at the effects of non-bioidenticals. More long-term studies are needed to provide the necessary data for us to understand the true effects of bioidenticals. Proponents of BHRT also note that, because bioidenticals are usually available in topical cream form, they are not as likely to cause the liver problems associated with non-bioidentical hormone use. Bioidentical hormones can be applied to the skin because they can be absorbed by fats.

CRITICISM OF BIOIDENTICALS

The use of BHRT has drawn criticism from both those in the medical establishment and many alternative and complementary health authorities. In general, these criticisms tend to revolve around the lack of information surrounding bioidentical use as well as research showing the carcinogenic properties and adverse reactions associated with hormones, especially estrogen.

The first concern for many is that bioidentical hormones will have the same negative side effects as traditional HRT. It has been noted that some forms of bioidentical hormones are even more potent than synthetics. As a growth-stimulating hormone, estrogen is associated with cancer and tumor formation, particularly in the breast and endometrial areas. The worry here is that, although the chemicals used are not foreign to our bodies, excess hormone levels late in life may have consequences that are not yet fully understood.

Quality control is another area of concern for those critical of BHRT. Barbara Seaman and Laura Eldridge note in *The No-Nonsense Guide to Menopause* that "many natural hormones, prescription and otherwise, come from compounding pharmacies. . . But like many 'alternative' or 'natural' medicines, the products created in compounding pharmacies are often undertested." While compounding pharmacies are a necessary aspect of bioidentical creation—specific ratios of a drug can be tailored to a patient—this does imply a lack of standard dosage. In addition, bioidenticals are not regulated by the FDA, are often produced overseas, and usually come in the form of topical creams. Consequently, there can often be no way to know the exact purity or concentration present in one's bioidentical concoction.

Last, the long-term side effects of BHRT are still unknown. While BHRT's efficacy has been well demonstrated, its safety is still a matter of debate. Seaman and Eldridge conclude their argument by saying, "The bottom line, we believe, is that a natural hormone is made in your body, not in a lab, warehouse, or pharmacy. Once you take into account the risks inherent in less-tested products, we don't see a problem with using natural hormones. Just realize they probably carry the same risks as prescription HT and ET." Indeed, this gets to the heart of the matter: it is the choice of each individual to decide how she will deal with her health. No matter which side of the debate you may fall on, it is clear that more scientific studies, transparency, and accessible information are the keys to healthy decision making.

EXERCISE

Regular exercise can reduce the frequency and severity of hot flashes. For best results, it is a good idea to begin exercising before menopause begins. Other-wise, exercise may trigger hot flashes. Exercise also alleviates mood swings and depression by naturally raising serotonin and endorphin levels in the brain. The best exercises to engage in are dancing, brisk walking, running, swimming, biking, and tai chi. Additional benefit is derived from cross-training, doing dif-ferent exercises on different days. This prevents any one part of the body from becoming overdeveloped or overstressed.

"Exercise is absolutely crucial, especially after the age of forty," says Dr. Northrup. "Your body is not as forgiving."

Research has found that aerobic exercises as well as strength training are important for the body—and the mind. "Miriam Nelson at Tufts has shown that two forty-minute weight-training sessions per week increased bone density in women greater than they had with Premarin, which is a hormone replacement I would not recommend to anyone," Dr. Northrup says. "She found that the muscle mass itself and the ability to be more effective in the gym or more effec-tive with weights actually translated into being effective in the world. In other words, these women were then more apt to get out at night. They weren't afraid of driving into a strange city. Taking a night class or parking in a parking garage. . . We have some fascinating studies showing that when your body becomes more capable, your mind and your mood begin to feel more capable. You become more capable as well."

Dr. Northrup also tells about the recent research of Dr. Joan Vernikos, former head of life sciences at NASA, who says that the key to improved health is simply moving frequently throughout the day. She found that a lack of engaging with gravity causes aging and deterioration throughout the body. In menopausal women, this deterioration can affect the stabilizer muscles, including the core muscles and the muscles of the pelvic floor, leading to urinary stress incontinence and urinary problems. "Those problems are the number one reason why women get put into nursing homes," Dr. Northrup says, the inability to control their bladder. This results directly from loss of tone of the pelvic floor.

"When you just start to stand up and sit down, or really increase your G force by moving your body up and down through space, this dramatically decreases uri-nary stress incontinence because moving through that vector of gravity strengthens the core stabilizer muscles. Even if you exercise and you sit six hours a day, which is most people, those bits of exercise that you do will not counteract the adverse effects of sitting. You need to just stand up and sit down. It's so easy to do."

AROMATHERAPY

"Aromatherapy is truly holistic because it is a mind-body treatment," states Ann Berwick, author of *Holistic Aromatherapy and Women's Health*. "I think this is part of the secret of its power." Berwick uses essential oils to help alleviate a number of conditions, including hormonal imbalance in women going through menopause. "Cyprus, fennel, and clary sage are believed to have estrogen-like effects. For overall balancing, I recommend that my clients use these oils in a lotion or body oil, and apply it to their body two or three times a day. When women are experiencing hot flashes, I also suggest that they breathe in peppermint or basil on a tissue throughout the day. I find that a great help for most of my clients."

AYURVEDIC MEDICINE

Menopausal women report relief and rejuvenation from Ayurvedic formulas using herbal phytoestrogens and phytoprogesterones. Ayurveda believes that balance is the key to perfect health. It basically determines which mind-body type a person is and helps people choose the type of foods they should eat and the type of exercise that is best for them.

REFLEXOLOGY

Laura Norman, a certified reflexologist from New York City, says, "For menopause, in addition to working the reproductive organs, I would also encourage you to work your thyroid gland, as this will help take over when the ovaries produce less estrogen. This is how to find this point: the base of the toes reflects the neck area where the thyroid is located. Press your thumbs into the base of your toes and thumb-walk across that ridge, particularly in the base of the big toe.

"Another area to massage is the adrenal gland reflex point. You are on the big toe side of the foot. Go about a third of the way down your foot. You are under the ball of the foot, in line with the big toe. If you press your thumb into that area, it will provide energy when you feel fatigued.

"Also, the pituitary gland, which helps all the other glands to work, is located in the center of the big toe. Pressure applied there helps stimulate that area. Both feet should be massaged equally."

QI GONG

Tina Chunna Zhang, founder of the Qi Gong Center for Women in New York City and author of several books on the martial arts, says that qi gong has been used for 2,000 years in China to cultivate the body's energy and cure a variety of problems, including the hot flashes and night sweats associated with menopause. She recommends the following series of motions. "You do this in the morning and in the evening, at least twice a day. It's very simple. You stand up with feet parallel to the ground and keep both feet apart about shoulder width, and then you relax your body. You relax your mind as well. Your hands come up in front of you like you're holding a beach ball. Your palms face yourself in front of your chest. Then you start to take a deep inhale all the way through your nose while your arms rise upwards. Keep them moving upwards when you're inhaling. Then when you exhale, your arms go downwards from the side. You also exhale all the way through your nose. Repeat this about eight to sixteen times."

PATIENT STORIES

Prior to [Gary Null's] study group I had irregular and sparse cycles with extreme cramping and low energy. My body had turned into a pear shape. After I finished your program within a month or two I had my flow and regularity of the cycles was back to normal. I had my energy back and my happy attitude, and the pear shape just reversed itself completely. All signs from my blood work were extremely good. All that turned around in just those three months for me.

—Lisa

I had terrible acne. I was tired all the time. I was bleeding profusely. I had talked to a lot of people and they were saying, oh hysterectomy, hysterectomy. I was not wanting to go there. So that's what I was dealing with, and a lot of weight gain. As soon as I stopped eating meat, I think I dropped ten pounds in two weeks. My skin cleared up. I had so much more energy and I had a normal period for the first time in three years. There was none of the clotting or horribleness. For me, that was the biggest thing that could have happened. The lines around my eyes and on my face, they're much better. They sort of went away. My skin got firmer. I slept less. My LDL cholesterol went down.

—Diane

The worst thing that I had was a really terrible attitude towards the whole aging process and towards menopause. I'm a feminist in many ways and an activist. For some reason underneath all that I had a really bad attitude toward menopause. Seeing all these people just reverse their issues and their problems quite simply just by working with [Gary Null's] protocols was really inspiring. I tend to be inconsistent in my approach, like I'll be great with it for a month, and then I'll fall off again. One thing that happened that was interesting was that I was perfectly strict with it for two weeks and I just lost ten pounds with no discomfort and no trouble at all. I'm still working to create a consistent attitude toward my exercise. Having [this approach] under my belt allows me to go to the doctor and absorb what they say and go home and take care of things with a very balanced attitude. I use their information and then I'm usually able to completely avoid drugs and surgery. I see just incredible improvements in people and you're continually inspired. It's just a great protocol and I've really benefited from it overall.

—Elaine

Gary Null's Natural Solution to Menopause

In my eighteen-month study using a strict program of an organic plant-based diet, cleansing, and detoxifying, women who had been postmenopausal returned to a premenopausal state of health or improved their premenopausal symptoms. The women were eating no animal proteins, sugar, caffeine, or processed food; exercising six days a week for an hour; drinking lots of fresh organic juices; and taking certain herbs. Skin wrinkles were diminshed, energy restored, human growth hormone was back, hormones were balanced, and status was improved. The gray, thinning hair of one seventy-one-year-old woman grew back brown and thick. Another woman had had a low libido, and her mucous membranes had been dry, as was her skin. Her skin and mucous membranes regained moisture, and she enjoyed a level of health and energy that she hadn't experienced for years. Her toenails and fingernails, which had been brittle, yellow, and cracked, became pink and fresh. This was all without medication or any hormone replacement therapy. We just gave her body a chance to rebalance itself; we honored it by not giving it anything that would have led to an imbalance.

First and foremost, my program involved eliminating all dairy from the diet in every form. Women were told to read labels and make sure there was no casein in products because casein and whey are dairy. Women also eliminated wheat in any form. Then I had them eliminate all meat, sugar, fried foods, carbonated beverages, chicken, artificial sweeteners, and caffeine. They couldn't use the hydrogenated fats any longer.

Over the next six months, I introduced certain supplements. But the program was more than about supplements. It was about cleansing the system: taking the body burden of all these highly denatured foods and getting them out of the system. Once you stop something that is negative, it doesn't mean that the negative consequence is automatically gone. If you stop drinking fluoridated water and you've been drinking it your whole life, you still have all that fluoride built up in your body and with it a lot of lead as well. So first was elimination. Get rid of what's causing an assault on the body. Why? Many of these things are hormone disruptors. They can disrupt how the body creates hormones and utilizes them. Menopause is really about hormonal changes. So anything that could limit the radical shift in hormones could at the same time help the body.

Within three weeks, people talked about having more energy. Within two months, they were losing weight. They were sleeping better and having more energy. By four months people were talking about how their moods changed. They were feeling better. They no longer had the highs and the lows. They no longer had the anxiety and mania. They no longer had depression. By half a year, they were seeing changes in their skin. Aging spots were diminishing. Vision was improving. Body functions were working better. Localized joint inflammation was gone. They were breathing better. Their digestion was improved. We had people talking about their hair. There was one woman who showed everyone her hair. She had gray hair on the outside, but near the roots for about a quarter of an inch was natural black hair. She hadn't seen any black hair coming out of her head in twenty years. Here it was all over her head. So in effect the body was rejuvenating. It was de-aging. She was not the only one. One woman who was fifty-four said that she would be afraid to shampoo her hair because of how much hair would come out of her head. She had been going bald but it was filling back in again.

People started realizing that there was a rejuvenation process involved here. It was really doing something terrific. The weight across the room was just pouring off people. Why? I wasn't starving them. They were having plenty of food to eat, but it was the quality of the food. There were lots of live energy foods: fresh fruits and vegetables, fresh fish, fresh spices, grains, beans, legumes, and tubers. We had a class on making cooking more interesting using different types of oils: toasted sesame, garlic lemon, sweet basil, and black pepper oil. They started using more grains and more beans.

I heard about how their varicose veins went down, spider veins went away, and bruising was no longer the case. Receding and bleeding gums stopped. Teeth became firmer. All of this was accomplished without ever using new drugs or medications. It was just lifestyle. They were exercising using both weights and power resistance like power walking, jogging, or biking. They were also taking some time to deal with the stress in their lives. Most people don't realize how destructive stress is. Stress creates cortisol. Cortisol blocks progesterone. That allows estrogen no longer to have something that is blocking it and keeping it in check. That makes you more susceptible to breast cancer, endometriosis, and ovarian cancers.

I even showed them ways to make interesting juices. Get a bunch of your favorite fruit and throw it in a blender. Put in some soy or rice protein powder, and throw in a B-complex of 100 milligrams. Throw in some vitamin C. Throw in a banana and blend it all up with some juice, rice, or soymilk and you've got an energy shake that's filled with phytochemicals. The more phytochemicals you put in your body the more natural hormone rebalancing you're going to do. In effect every glass of fresh fruit juice and every glass of fresh vegetable juice is helping you remain younger longer. It has the phytoestrogens, the natural plant based ones, which protect you against cancer, and keep you more youthful.

Among the supplements I used was beta-1, 3-D glucan, which helps in marrow production and is great for the immune system. I don't believe there is anything you can put in your body that is as good for your brain and heart as coenzyme Q10. Then, of course, the mother of all hormones, DHEA, at 25 to 50 milligrams, helps your body protect you against cancer, heart disease, and diabetes. It is crucial on all levels. You're going to be less susceptible to fluctuations in insulin and cortisol, and all these other bad hormones. You're going to slow down the aging of the brain. It also helps raise the levels of circulating beta-endorphins known to decline with menopause, so quite simply you feel better.

I would also add in the essential fatty acids like primrose oil, borage seed oil, and flaxseed oil, generally about 1,500 milligrams. Start the day with some rice protein and folic acid at 800 micrograms, Vitamin E with tocotrienols at 400, boron at 3 milligrams, calcium magnesium at 1,000 milligrams, and quercetin generally 2,000 milligrams a day. Most women are deficient in potassium. They need potassium for energy.

You need vitamin C throughout the day. Remember you're creating free radicals all the time, twenty-four hours a day. Free radicals are what cause your cells to become inflamed and damaged. So the more free radicals you have, the more damage you're going to have and the more disease you're going to produce. Also, the quicker you're going to age, and the more you're going to be sick. Free radicals can be stopped or limited with antioxidants. Chinese green tea and bilberry extract, n-acetyl cysteine, and glutathione trap the free radicals. Alpha lipoic acid should be at the top of most people's list of things they should have in their system. Take melatonin at nighttime, generally 1 to 3 milligrams. Aloe vera is quite simply one of the five most important immune boosting, antiviral, antibacterial superstars of nutrition. Take two ounces of aloe vera twice a day. Additionally, the women took black cumin seed oil to assist in decreasing inflammation throughout their bodies as well as curcumin to help protect their DNA.

We also had the women take some things to enhance libido, like black cohosh, cramp bark, dong quai, and Siberian ginseng. Chickweed, dandelion greens, fennel, sage, and squaw vine are terrific at rebalancing naturally the hormones. Gotu kola and dong quai relieve hot flashes, vaginal dryness, and even depression.

The more of the red fruits you consume or the powdered concentrates of red fruits, the more repair to your DNA, and that's what we want to do. We want to repair the DNA. Now it's done slowly. It's done over a period of time, but yes it can be repaired.

These women also exercised every day. They dealt with stress every day. They focused upon positives and the things they could control. The results were amazing.

Research Update

An increasing body of evidence is showing the benefits of natural modalities to overall health and well-being. Following is a sample of recent peer-reviewed scientific studies in the area of menopause.

According to a 2014 article in *Life Extension Magazine*, among the most effective bioidentical hormones recommended during menopause are prenylflavonoid molecules in hops and lignans found in the Norway spruce. In 2015, researchers at the University of Georgia reported in the journal *Obesity* that a mix of phytochemicals and vitamin D may prevent liver damage caused by fat accumulated during menopause. The plant chemicals used in the study included reservatrol (from grapes), genistein (from soybeans), and quercitin (from apple peels and onions). In a 2010 study published in *Phytomedicine*, menopausal women who took a hops extract standardized to 100 micrograms/day of 8-prenylnaringenin (8-PN; a potent phytoestrogen) showed notable reductions in menopause symptoms such as hot flashes and low sex drive after eight weeks of therapy. A 2013 report in the *Journal of the American College of Nutrition* found that women who took supplements of either 36 or 72 milligrams of 7-hydroxymatairesinol (HMR) lignan per day for eight weeks experienced higher levels of the mild phytoestrogen in their bodies and had a 50 percent reduction in hot flashes. A 2012 study of ninety menopausal women published in the *Iranian Journal of Pharmaceutical Research* concluded that licorice root decreased the frequency and severity of hot flashes. A 2015 study published in *Menopause* found that a ten-week program of exercise training according to the Nordic walking model caused more significant changes in glucose and basic blood lipid levels than Pilates and dietary intervention alone.

Chapter 44

Menstrual Cramps and Irregular Menstruation

Painful and difficult periods are so commonplace in our society that some women have come to think of them as normal. However, they are not normal at all. Many experts feel that the symptoms of menstrual cramps (dysmenorrhea) are related to dietary practices as well as to unresolved emotional difficulties.

Causes

What factors contribute to menstrual cramps? Dr. Pat Gorman, an acupuncturist and educator from New York City, explains: "In addition to toxins found in foods with preservatives, additives, and caffeine, they are due to putrid proteins found in dairy and red meat. These foods contain a lot of hormones that upset the system. In addition, foods fried in heavy oils cause problems and should be cut out immediately by any woman interested in getting rid of dysmenorrhea."

Dr. Gorman adds that the Chinese attribute this condition in part to pent-up anger and frustration. "If you are not happy with your life, if you are angry with people, you must work this out. The liver, which stores blood and prepares it for the period, is also responsible for anger. That's not a Western concept, but with my patients I find that working out anger helps the liver relax. As a result, there is far less of a problem with dysmenorrhea."

Dr. Marjorie Ordene, a gynecologist in Brooklyn, New York, agrees that hormonal and psychological factors cause painful periods and explains the underlying factors. "What causes dysmenorrhea are exaggerated uterine contractions. These contractions are mediated by receptors in the uterine lining that are stimulated by hormonal and psychological factors. Hormonal factors that stimulate the uterine receptors have actually been isolated. They are chemical messengers called prostaglandins. Two things are clear: People with menstrual cramps have an excess of prostaglandins, and there is an imbalance in the types of prostaglandins they produce."

She adds that eating foods we are allergic to can increase prostaglandin production: "For example, many women are sensitive to yeast, and eating baked foods, breads, pastries, and processed fruit juices can cause an increase in prostaglandin production."

Clinical Experience

CONVENTIONAL TREATMENT

Medical doctors often prescribe medications such as ibuprofen to inhibit prostaglandins. While these agents work to relieve menstrual cramps and the accompanying symptoms, problems occur when drugs are taken month after month. The side effects can include gastrointestinal bleeding, decreased blood flow to the kidneys, and leaky gut syndrome, a condition that allows undigested food particles to enter the blood.

NATUROPATHIC TREATMENT

DIET

Changes in diet can decrease overproduction of prostaglandins and restore normal balance. Cool green foods help reduce hot, stabbing pains and inflammation. It is good to eat foods such as organic grains, legumes, oatmeal, and steamed green vegetables. Deep-sea fish such as salmon, tuna, and mackerel can be included, as well as flaxseed oil. Hot spices should be avoided, along with fried greasy foods, sugar, salt, alcohol, and stimulating foods such as garlic and onions. Foods that produce allergies should be eliminated as well.

Women who have nerve-related menstrual pain can benefit from tofu but should stay away from too many cold raw salads, hot spicy foods, and even white potatoes. Herbalist Letha Hadady suggests this soothing recipe: warm tofu cooked with sweet spices such as pumpkin pie spices and nutmeg. This quiets the nerves and helps a woman feel nurtured and relaxed.

SUPPLEMENTS

Taken throughout the month as a daily supplement, evening primrose oil prevents headaches and blemishes that occur just before the period. Magnesium deficiencies are common and result in the release of prostaglandins that cause spasm and pain. Magnesium citrate is antispasmodic and helps relieve the problem. You can take 500 to 1,000 milligrams daily and work up to bowel tolerance. Among the other supplements that have been found to help are folic acid, calcium with vitamin D, vitamin B_6, and vitamin E, black cohosh, evening primrose oil, and chasteberry.

HERBS

The following herbs may help alleviate menstrual problems:

GARDENIA AND PHILODENDRON—These are popular in Chinese medicine and can be obtained by prescription from an herbalist.

CORN SILK TEA—This tea helps get rid of the bloating that comes from too many hormones stored in the blood. Women's Rhythm also eliminates bloating.

XIAO YAO WAN—This is a wonderful remedy that can be purchased at pharmacies in Chinatowns in major cities. It helps digestive processes. Not only does this formula relieve painful periods, it also alleviates anger.

GREEN TEA—Green tea is cooling and satisfying, and has very little caffeine. A pinch of tea can be added to a pot of boiled water, steeped for five minutes, and sipped throughout the day. People experience an energy pickup from the digestion being activated, not from the nerves being stimulated. Green tea helps soothe sharp, stabbing pains.

ALOE VERA JUICE OR GEL—Aloe can eliminate headache, irritability, fever, stabbing pain, blemishes, and bad breath associated with menstrual cramps. Aloe also reduces acid from the stomach and liver and is slightly laxative. Just add to juice, tea, or water.

DANDELION—Dandelion helps break apart impurities in the system. It can be bought as capsules or tea.

SARSAPARILLA—Sarsaparilla helps hot, stabbing pains brought on by inflammation. It is anti-inflammatory, antiseptic, diuretic, and soothing.

VALERIAN—Valerian is a sedative herb that makes a woman feel quieter, more relaxed, and grounded. It is especially good for nervous women who experience insomnia, anxiety, crying jags and emotional upsets, and other nervous problems. Valerian quiets the nerves that go to the uterus.

YUNNAN PAI YAO—This combination of herbs helps reduce heavy bleeding and stabbing pain. Because it increases the circulation, internal bleeding is healed and swelling and pain are reduced.

HOMEOPATHY

Homeopathy was developed in Germany more than 200 years ago by Dr. Samuel Hahnemann. The word *homeopathy* means "like cures like." The same substances that cause a disease in a healthy individual can heal an ailment in a sick person when they are diluted and given in minute proportions.

The late homeopathic physician Dr. Ken Korins explained that the dilution process is what makes homeopathic remedies so safe: "Homeopathy is a vibrational medicine. We are dealing with very subtle energies. Substances are given in extremely small doses that cannot possibly have any toxic effects. In fact, if you were to analyze these substances, you would not find a trace of the original material in the final dilution."

The correct homeopathic remedy is the one that most closely matches the symptoms that manifest themselves. Dr. Korins recommended that dysmenorrhea sufferers choose from among the following:

COLOCYNTHIS—Colocynthis is a frequently indicated remedy that is useful when you have a severe onset of sudden cramps, particularly on the first day of menstruation. Emotionally, intense irritability and anger are associated with the menstrual cramps. A key indication is that you feel better when your knees are pulled up toward the stomach and held with firm pressure.

MAGNESIA PHOSPHORICA—Magnesia phoshorica helps spasmodic cramps with bloating. The key indication for this remedy is that you feel better from warmth. Magnesia phosphorica and Colocynthis help alleviate the symptoms in 85 percent of cases.

PULSATILLA—A key indication for Pulsatilla is variation; the cramps and the flow of bleeding are changeable. The pains themselves are typically cutting and tearing and may be felt in the lower back or kidney region. Generally, you feel worse in warm, stuffy rooms and better in the fresh open air. Emotionally, you tend to be mild, gentle, and weepy when entering the menstrual state and prefer the company of other people to being alone.

VIBURNUM—Viburnum is indicated when the menses are very scanty and often late. In fact, they may last only a few hours. When you get cramps, the flow of blood stops. Cramps tend to radiate to the sacrum and the thighs. You may feel faint or feel like passing out.

CIMICIFUGA—Cimicifuga is indicated for spasmodic, cramping pains. The pain radiates across the pelvis from one thigh to the other. It is often associated with a premenstrual headache. Increased flow results in more pain. Emotionally, you may feel nervous to the point of being scattered and are often somewhat depressed.

CHAMOMILLA—Chamomilla is helpful if you are either hypersensitive or insensitive to pain. Emotionally, you tend to be irritable and contrary. Someone brings you something that you ask for, and then you don't want it. During intense periods, you may become dependent on coffee and other stimulants and sedatives. Another symptom is anger. When you become angry, your symptoms become worse.

AROMATHERAPY

Marjoram, clary sage, and lavender are wonderful analgesics. Eighteen to 20 drops of oil added to a lotion or oil and massaged into the abdomen and lower back will help relieve menstrual pain. Breathing in the cooling fragrances of rose, lavender, or sandalwood can alleviate sharp, stabbing pain.

STRESS MANAGEMENT

Deep abdominal breathing, meditation, tai chi, and other mind-body disciplines can help eliminate frustrations and anger that bring on pain. Additionally, it is helpful to slow down the pace of life from the time of ovulation to the period.

Amenorrhea and Menorrhagia

Amenorrhea and *menorrhagia* are medical terms for abnormal blood flow. Amenorrhea refers to the cessation of bleeding or very light and infrequent periods, most often caused by an abnormally functioning hypothalamus, pituitary gland, ovary, or uterus as a result of drugs or surgery that removes the ovaries or uterus. "Bulimics and anorexics also exhibit this pattern," notes Dr. Pat Gorman. "Sometimes this is caused by excessive dieting and overexercise. Not accepting who she is, a woman thinks, 'I've got to make myself thin, beautiful, and perfect.' If this is going on at the end of the cycle, when toxins are being released into the system, the woman is aggravating her body to the point of saying, 'We're not going to give up this blood. We desperately need it. Forget ovulation, forget periods.'"

Dr. Ruth Bar-Shalom and Dr. John Soileau, naturopaths from Alaska, in an article on the website of the American Association of Naturopathic Physicians (www.naturopathic.org), list several other causes of amenorrhea. First, it happens normally after a woman stops using birth control pills, during pregnancy, and during all or most of the breast-feeding period. It is important to establish that pregnancy is not the reason for amenorrhea, since some of the remedies for this condition may harm the woman and her child while she is pregnant or nursing.

Malnutrition, crash diets, obesity, stress, intensive exercising, extreme obesity, abuse of antidepressants and amphetamines, and mental illness are other causes of amenorrhea, say Drs. Bar-Shalom and Soileau. When a young woman of 16 has not yet begun to develop sexually, when weight fluctuates dramatically, and when amenorrhea is accompanied by severe depression, drug use, or pain, consult a qualified health care professional.

With menorrhagia the opposite scenario occurs, and there is profuse bleeding. The condition can be debilitating, sometimes bad enough to warrant immediate attention in a hospital's emergency ward. "The Chinese say menorrhagia is caused by excess toxins and heat in the blood from foods containing preservatives, additives, and caffeine, especially coffee. It's like water in your car radiator becoming low," Dr. Gorman says. "The engine will overheat and explode. Alcohol adds more toxicity because it constantly removes water from the blood. As water diminishes, it heats up the blood. When the blood is what we call 'hot,' or fast-moving, it's very hard for the body to hold it in. It can't stop the bleeding."

The emotional profile of a menorrhagic individual is someone who sees herself as a victim. Dr. Gorman explains: "This person feels the need to serve everybody. She does not know how to set boundaries. Whatever anybody wants, they get. She keeps pouring out her energy and pouring out her blood."

Dr. Vicki Hufnagel, a gynecological surgeon and activist for women's health rights, adds that heavy bleeding is often a sign of an underlying problem in the female system, especially when it is accompanied by pain. The problem is frequently because of a hormonal imbalance. "Anything can throw off a cycle," she says, "including emotional stress, insomnia, too much estrogen in the system, or too little light, as in the winter. Other physical problems that can cause menorrhagia are fibroids, polyps, and a malfunctioning thyroid gland."

Before you can restore the blood flow in patients with amenorrhea or menorrhagia, you must discover the reason for the problem. Once the cause is addressed, periods should return to normal.

Asian medicine can diagnose amenorrhea and menorrhagia by examining the skin. Amenorrhea manifests as pale, sallow, slightly yellowish skin from a deep lack of blood and nutrients. Often this is accompanied by a great deal of emotional anxiety. With menorrhagia, the tongue has a red tip and tiny red dots. When the condition is long term, a woman can become anemic.

CLINICAL EXPERIENCE

HORMONAL BALANCING FOR MENORRHAGIA

Dr. Hufnagel says that hormonal dysfunctions in women with menorrhagia can be corrected with oral doses of natural progesterone. "Often the creams women use are not adequate because they don't cause a rise in the blood level. We often have to give what we call oral physiological levels of progesterone. I give women natural hormones in a cyclic manner, the way the body should be getting them."

Hormone balancing can also be accomplished through the diet. Fatty diets cause higher levels of estrogen in the system, which in turn can cause menorrhagia. Lean diets and exercising with weights produce more testosterone, which in turn helps balance hormones and put an end to menorrhagia.

DIETARY REMEDIES

The late Dr. Anthony Penepent said that amenorrhea is one of the easiest conditions to correct. He recommends a diet that includes two green salads daily, using romaine lettuce, fresh lemon juice, olive oil, and some brewer's yeast. You should also include two pieces of fresh fruit and two soft-boiled eggs in the daily menu. When amenorrhea is caused by a thyroid condition, a thyroid supplement is needed. Additionally, if stress is in the picture, the stressful situation must be remedied. For more serious cases, additional dietary intervention is necessary.

Usually, small changes in diet are all that is needed. Dr. Penepent said, "Even if the woman doesn't follow a completely natural hygienic regimen and is not vegetarian, she can still get tremendous results simply by increasing the amount of green leafy vegetables in the diet and providing concentrated nutritional sources, such as eggs and unsalted raw-milk cheese."

Drs. Bar-Shalom and Soileau add that women with amenorrhea need adequate protein, which means eating a number of grams per day equal to half your weight in pounds. They advocate fish and chicken instead of red meat, as well as nuts, seeds, and beans. Second, they advocate eating seaweed of all kinds.

SUPPLEMENTS

Drs. Bar-Shalom and Soileau recommend the following supplements: 400 international units (IU) of vitamin E a day, 25 milligrams of B-complex vitamins a day, 1,000 milligrams of vitamin C twice a day, and 1,200 milligrams of calcium a day.

HERBS

The following herbs are good for amenorrhea, say Drs. Bar-Shalom and Soileau:

GINGER TEA—Drink one to four cups of ginger tea each day (made from powder or grated fresh ginger).

BLAZING STAR, FALSE UNICORN, BLUE COHOSH, CHASTE TREE, AND ANGELICA—Mix together equal parts of these herbs and steep 1 tablespoon of the mixture in a cup of boiling water for twenty minutes. Drink three cups a day. You can also combine tinctures of these herbs. Drink 1 teaspoon of the mixed tinctures added to 1/4 cup of water three times a day.

The following Chinese herbs have specific effects on the blood and are needed at different times of the monthly cycle. Dr. Gorman recommends working with a health practitioner to create an individual protocol and monitor progress but offers these general guidelines.

At the beginning of the cycle:

DONG QUAI—High in vitamins A, E, and B$_{12}$, this blood builder can be taken most days of the month, up to the point of menstruation, or just before it begins if there are strong premenstrual symptoms. "You don't want to be building blood if you are having trouble moving that blood," Dr. Gorman warns.

WOMEN'S PRECIOUS—This formula is a tremendous blood builder that is taken for about three weeks after the period ends. Women's Rhythm is then used the following week.

At the end of the cycle:

GARDENIA—Gardenia is taken when the symptoms of premenstrual syndrome (PMS) arise. By moving blood that is stuck, gardenia helps relieve that heavy, bloated feeling.

WOMEN'S RHYTHM—Women's Rhythm helps release a woman's blood. It is usually taken a week before the period to help move toxins out of the organs. (Women's Precious and Women's Rhythm are Ted Kapchik formulas that can be found in some health food stores and ordered directly from Kahn Herbs.)

Can be taken every day:

FLORADIX WITH IRON—This wonderful product is available in most health care stores. Liquid Floradix is superior to the dry form because it contains more live nutrients.

PHYSICAL MEASURES

Drs. Bar-Shalom and Soileau stress the importance of focusing on deep breathing, consciously giving yourself periods of relaxation, and getting sufficient exercise to reduce stress as much as possible. Other suggestions include:

SITZ BATH—Make an infusion of a pound of oatstraw boiled for a half hour in 2 quarts of water and add it to warm bath water. Sit in the water, which should reach your navel, with your feet propped on a chair outside the tub. Cover your top so that you stay warm. Soak like this for ten to fifteen minutes once or twice a week.

CLAY COMPRESS—Sterilize clay by heating it in a low oven for an hour and then grind it and make a paste with water, or use the powdered French healing clay that you can buy in health food stores. Apply the paste to your abdomen, cover with a cloth, and leave until the paste dries.

CASTOR OIL PACK—Put a cloth soaked in castor oil on your abdomen, then cover with plastic and then a dry cloth. Rest for an hour.

HOMEOPATHY

Two homeopathic remedies are good for amenorrhea, according to Drs. Bar-Shalom and Soileau:

NATRUM MURIATICUM is for amenorrhea that occurs after extreme mental strain in women who have trouble expressing emotion. Use the 12c potency.

PULSATILLA is for a woman who misses her periods after stressful and emotional situations. Take it in the 6c potency three times a day for three weeks or until the period begins.

Toxic Shock Syndrome

Toxic shock syndrome (TSS) is a rare but serious and sometimes fatal disease. The victims tend to be tampon users under the age of thirty, especially those between fifteen and nineteen. The incidence of TSS has decreased over the past two decades due to manufacturing changes making tampons less absorbent, as well as education regarding prevention.

CAUSES

This sudden and serious disease affects persons with severely compromised immune systems who are poisoned by a strain of bacteria called Staphylococcus aureus, phage group I. This type of staph produces a substance called enterotoxin F, which can overpower and destroy a weak body.

Toxic shock syndrome is linked to the introduction of tampons with four new ingredients in the early 1980s. Before then tampons were made primarily of cotton. In the 1980s, though, highly absorbent polyester cellulose, carboxymethyl cellulose, polyacrylate rayon, and viscose rayon came into use. Three of these new ingredients were soon taken off the market; today only one of the new ingredients, viscose rayon, is in use. Today's tampons are either entirely viscose rayon or a blend of cotton and viscose rayon. In addition, the tampons on the market today may contain an assortment of chemicals, including pesticides used in growing cotton, chemicals used in the manufacture of viscose rayon (lye, sodium sulfate, and sodium hydroxide), and dyes (some of which have been considered carcinogenic since the 1950s).

One theory about the cause of TSS is that the vagina is normally an oxygen-free environment that limits the growth of dangerous bacteria. However, air is trapped between the fibers that make up tampons. When that air is inserted in the vagina along with the tampon, the possibility of toxin production increases. Even after the tampon is removed, some of its fibers may remain.

TSS was originally thought to affect only women who wore high-absorbency tampons, but now it is known to affect newborns, children, and men as well. The initial indications can include a high fever, headache, sore throat, diarrhea, nausea, and red skin blotches. These signs can be followed by confusion, low blood pressure, acute kidney failure, abnormal liver function, and even death.

A severe case of TSS is a medical emergency that may necessitate hospitalization. However, there are many natural ways to support the system once a crisis is over for quick recovery and prevention of recurrence.

CLINICAL EXPERIENCE

NATUROPATHIC PROTOCOL

Dr. Linda Page, author of *Healthy Healing: An Alternative Healing Reference*, developed a protocol for healing from TSS out of necessity. "I actually came close to death on an operating table from TSS. I had to bring my body back, and I did it herbally. It took a couple of years, and now I can speak from experience."

HERBS

Dr. Page's personal ordeal gave her a great deal of confidence in the power of natural remedies. The following herbs helped her overcome toxicity, restore immunity, and return to health:

GINSENG—Both Panax ginseng and Panax quinquefolius (American ginseng) varieties are general tonics that balance and tone all body systems as well as improving the circulation. Ginseng should not be used when there is a high fever.

CAYENNE AND GINGER—These nervous system stimulants can help the body recover from shock. They can be taken internally or applied to the skin in compresses.

HAWTHORN EXTRACT—Hawthorn speeds up and normalizes the circulation and restores a sense of well-being.

DIET

In addition to herbs, Dr. Page ate supernutritious foods that could be easily digested and quickly utilized by her failing system. These foods included high-potency royal jelly, bee pollen, wheat germ, brewer's yeast, and unsulfured molasses. The addition of green drinks, including chlorella, barley grass, spirulina, and wheatgrass, supplied her with high potencies of vital minerals. "All these go into the body very quickly and help it recover even from a near-death situation," explains Dr. Page. "By going on a program of concentrated nutrients, I was eventually able to create a state of health that was better than before."

PREVENTION

Limiting use of tampons, sponges, and diaphragms may prevent TSS. Tampons that are 100 percent cotton and thus present less risk than do modern superabsorbent tampons that may also contain added chemicals are available in many health food and natural goods stores.

Research Update

An increasing body of evidence is showing the benefits of natural modalities to overall health and well-being. Following is a sample of recent peer-reviewed scientific studies relating to menstrual cramps and irregular menstruation.

A review and analysis of randomized clinical trials published in a 2015 report in *Pain Medicine* provided suggestive evidence for the effectiveness of ginger powder (750–2,000 mg) during the first three to four days of the menstrual cycle in women with primary dysmenorrhea. According to a 2014 study in *Alternative Therapies in Health and Medicine*, acupuncture point injection of vitamin K_1 was useful in reducing pain associated with dysmenorrhea. The authors noted that this outcome was consistent with findings from the Chinese hospital where the protocol was developed.

Chapter 45

Migraines

Nearly 30 million Americans suffer from migraines. Lasting several hours to as long as a few days, these debilitating headaches are three times more common in women than men.

Causes

It is believed that migraine headaches occur when a sudden dilation of the blood vessels creates pressure on the brain. There are numerous triggers for migraines. Dr. Mary Olsen, a chiropractor from New York who specializes in craniosacral adjustments and applied kinesiology, tells about the most common reasons for their occurrence.

ALLERGIC REACTIONS

Allergies can be dietary or environmental. "Dietary triggers can be foods, food combinations, or additives in foods," Dr. Olsen says. "Alcoholic beverages, particularly red wine and beer, are among the most common causes of migraines. Tyramine, a chemical found in cheese, smoked fish, yogurt, and yeast extracts, may be involved. Monosodium glutamate (MSG), which is found in some preparations of Chinese cuisine and most processed foods, is often implicated, as is sodium nitrate, found in cold cuts and hot dogs. Aspartame, a commonly used artificial sweetener, may lower serotonin levels in the body. Some researchers believe that this contributes to severe headaches. Chocolate and other foods containing caffeine can also be dietary triggers. In addition, people can have allergies to such common foods as wheat, dairy products, corn, and eggs. A person can also have environmental allergies to toxic fumes emitted from modern products found in the home."

HORMONAL FLUCTUATIONS

Women suffer from migraines to a much greater extent than men. Dr. Olsen explains: "Among women who suffer from migraines, approximately 60 percent correlate headaches to their menstrual cycle. The major contributing factor is the hormone estrogen. We know that women who take oral contraceptives are more susceptible to severe migraines and that women experience a lower frequency and severity of headaches after menopause, when there is a sharp reduction of estrogen. Unfortunately, the widespread use of estrogen replacement therapy has resulted in many women having a return of these headaches. Although the exact relationship between migraines and estrogen is unknown at this time, we do know that estrogen affects the central nervous system, including the systems involving serotonin, which can be involved in the development of migraines."

CRANIAL FAULTS

"Malposition in cranial bones, or cranial faults, is another factor contributing to migraines," says Dr. Olsen. "Trauma to the head, such as striking the head on a car door or birth trauma, may be enough to lock a bone into a particular position. A whiplash injury may also result in cranial faults."

MERIDIAN IMBALANCE

Applied kinesiologists and acupuncturists check for a meridian imbalance. "Meridians are twelve bilateral electromagnetic channels of energy in the body identified within the Chinese science of acupuncture," says Dr. Olsen. "Blocked energy, or *chi*, within a meridian causes dysfunction, including migraine headaches."

UPPER CERVICAL SUBLUXATION

Cervical subluxation (partial dislocation) in the upper part of the neck is another common cause of migraine. Dr. Olsen says, "This is especially prevalent among people who use the telephone as a regular part of their work. The tendency to hold the phone between the neck and the shoulder forces the vertebrae in the opposite direction. You also see this with people who tend to read in bed. Propping the head up in one direction causes the vertebrae to shift, which puts stress on the nerves and contributes to the migraine."

LOW MAGNESIUM LEVELS

"A number of studies have noted that many people suffering from migraines have low levels of magnesium in their blood," Dr. Olsen says. "This is also true of people who suffer from fibromyalgia, a myofascial condition that can cause severe pain to the head, mimicking a migraine."

DRUGS

Medications may also cause migraines. Dr. Olsen explains: "If you use aspirin, acetaminophen, mixed analgesics, or other acute care medications to get rid of your headaches, you may actually be causing them. The use of these painkillers is the single most common reason for migraines. They are called rebound headaches, and this is why they occur: When you take a painkiller often, the body gets used to having a certain amount of that drug in the bloodstream. When the level falls below that threshold, the body begins to experience withdrawal symptoms. One of these symptoms is a headache. If this situation exists, any preventive treatment for migraine will be undermined."

STRESS

Finally, Dr. Olsen cites stress as a factor in migraines. "Although stress is not a cause in itself, it can exacerbate the effects of a headache or cause an increase in the frequency of headaches."

Symptoms

Migraines differ from regular headaches in that they usually occur on one side of the head. The pain can last from a few hours to a few days. The headaches can be accompanied by lightheadedness, nausea, vomiting, sensitivity to light and sound, fatigue, weakness, irritability, and vision problems. An aura sometimes precedes a migraine. Usually, this is a visual phenomenon that may appear as flashes of light or visual distortions. However, other sensory systems can be disturbed, causing the aura to manifest as numbness, tingling, odor hallucinations, language difficulties, confusion, or disorientation. A migraine attack can leave the sufferer listless, exhausted, and vulnerable to other mental or physical conditions.

Clinical Experience

CONVENTIONAL TREATMENT

Conventional treatment usually consists of taking pain-relieving medications and preventive medications, and avoiding triggers.

ALTERNATIVE TREATMENT APPROACHES

Complementary medicine offers a host of other remedies, including dietary and environmental changes; herbal, vitamin, and mineral supplements; homeopathy; acupuncture; and biofeedback.

DIETARY AND ENVIRONMENTAL CHANGES

One strategy is to fast for a few days to detoxify the body. A glass of water to which lemon juice and a half teaspoon of baking soda have been added can help eliminate waste in the digestive tract.

Certain foods tend to promote migraines and should be avoided. These include spicy foods; stimulating foods such as chocolate, tea, and coffee; alcohol; and fried food. Obviously, any food to which you personally have a bad reaction should be avoided.

"Since migraines don't necessarily follow immediately after ingesting a food, it may be difficult to make a connection between a particular food and the resultant headache," Dr. Olsen says. "We often have patients keep a food diary to record what is eaten and their physical reactions. That makes it easier to correlate foods with delayed reactions. If we suspect that a particular food is troublesome, the patient is asked to place a sample of that food under the tongue. If there is a sensitivity, a muscle that tested strong previously will weaken. The pulse is also evaluated for such changes as increases in intensity or frequency. Treatment can be as simple as removing the offending food."

If environmental exposure is suspected, houseplants may be helpful. "Different plants have the ability to absorb different toxins," Dr. Olsen says. "For example, spider plants absorb the formaldehyde released from particleboard, plywood, synthetic carpeting, and new upholstery, while chrysanthemum protects against the toxic effects of lacquers, varnishes, and glues."

SUPPLEMENTS

Certain vitamins, minerals, and herbs are very important in the prevention of migraine.

- **Magnesium.** About half of the people who suffer migraines are deficient in the free and active form of magnesium called ionized magnesium. Magnesium's role in fighting migraines is undeniable. It has the ability to relax muscles, including those that encircle the arteries. Magnesium also affects serotonin receptors. A double-blind study conducted to examine the effectiveness of magnesium on migraines showed that when given to patients on a daily basis, it reduced migraine attacks by 42 percent after nine weeks. If you suffer from migraines, I recommend a daily supplement of 1,000 milligrams of free-form magnesium from citrate. Be sure you are taking a daily B-complex vitamin along with the magnesium, as vitamin B_3 plays an important role in aiding the absorption of magnesium.

- **Vitamin B_2 (Riboflavin).** Vitamin B_2 is important in mitochondrial energy production. In individuals suffering from migraine, mitochondrial energy production may be low. To optimize this cellular energy production, I recommend increasing your daily supplement from 50 milligrams to 150 milligrams. Do not exceed a daily supplement of 150 milligrams.

- **Vitamin B_3 (Niacin).** Vitamin B_3 may aid in preventing migraine headaches by opening constricted arteries and increasing blood flow. At the onset of a migraine aura, I recommend taking a supplement of 100 to 150 milligrams.

- **5-Hydroxytryptophan (5-HTP).** 5-HTP is a form of the amino acid tryptophan that the body converts into serotonin and can be effective in preventing migraines. I recommend 50 to 100 milligrams daily.

- **Melatonin.** Research has shown that migraine sufferers are low in melatonin, a hormone produced by the pineal gland to aid in sleep and setting our circadian rhythms. Melatonin also has an anti-inflammatory effect and is a powerful antioxidant. To prevent migraines, I recommend a supplement of 300 micrograms to 1 milligram, taken a half hour before bed, two to three nights per week.

Some herbal extracts and homeopathic treatments have properties similar to conventional medications, but are gentler and may lack the drugs' side effects. Always inform your medical practitioner of any herbal remedies you may be taking.

- Butterbur, native to Europe, Asia, and Africa, contains petasin and isopetasin, which are believed to slow the body's production of leukotrines, substances that can cause an inflammatory response and constricted blood cells. I recommend a daily supplement of 75 milligrams.
- Feverfew is commonly used in Europe to impact migraine headache, especially the type with vomiting and sensitivity to noise and light. I recommend a daily dose of 250 milligrams.
- Ginkgo biloba enhances cerebral circulation and oxygen flow to the brain tissue. I recommend a daily dose of 120 milligrams, taken in two equal doses with meals. Ginkgo can act as an anticoagulant, and individuals taking anticoagulant and antithrombotic drugs such as ASA, anti-inflammatories, and warfarin or Coumadin should consult with their doctor before taking ginkgo.
- Valerian acts as a mild sedative and may play a role in helping lower blood pressure. For migraine relief, I recommend taking 300 to 500 milligrams.
- White willow bark is commonly used in Germany as an alternative to aspirin for headache pain. I recommend taking 60 to 120 milligrams per day for relief of headache pain.

Dr. Elizabeth Lipski recommends high-dose riboflavin (400 milligrams), vitamin B_{12} (1,000–2,000 micrograms), butterbur (25 milligrams twice a day), magnesium, and feverfew. To address hormone imbalance, Dr. Olsen suggests supplementing the diet with vitamin B_6 and evening primrose oil around the time of a woman's menstrual period. For migraine triggered by stress, Dr. Olsen recommends feverfew. "Studies in England suggest that the herbal remedy feverfew can reduce the frequency of migraines," she says. "Feverfew has sedative qualities and can be taken as a tea. One cup per day is usually effective. In addition, relaxation techniques such as meditation, progressive muscle relaxation, and yoga can help to reduce stress. Regular moderate exercise, such as swimming or walking, also lowers tension and creates a psychological sense of well-being."

According to Dr. Jennifer Brett, director of the Acupuncture Institute for the University of Bridgeport, where she also serves on the faculty for the College of Naturopathic Medicine, "When feverfew is taken with magnesium in doses of 250 to 500 milligrams daily, as well as with ginkgo biloba, most people notice a significant reduction in the number of migraines, even to the point of disappearance. This includes people who suffer daily migraines. Many people come to me who have had no success with more conventional treatments. After I start them on feverfew and magnesium, they get a significant reduction in the number of headaches and the severity of pain. Even when they have headaches, they tend to be less frequent and less painful." Feverfew should not be taken by pregnant women.

For migraines associated with poor digestion or depression, Dr. Emily Kane, in an article on the website of the American Association of Naturopathic Physicians (www.naturopathic.org), says that lavender, which calms the nervous system, can be added to your bath water or rubbed into your temples. She also suggests that the following herbal tea, by cleansing the system, can prevent or decrease migraines:

- 1 part hops
- 1 part chamomile
- 1/2 part oatstraw
- 1/2 part catnip
- 1/2 part skullcap
- 1/4 part peppermint leaf

Add a heaping tablespoon to a cup of water that has just boiled and steep for three to five minutes. You can add honey to sweeten. Drink this tea two to three times a day.

HOMEOPATHY

Many homeopathic remedies can help relieve migraines; the remedy must be matched to the particular symptoms. Some of those mentioned by Dr. Kane include the following:

ARNICA MONTANA—Arnica montana is for treating migraines that feel as though the head is burning but the rest of the body is cool. There is aching above the eyes that radiates to the temples. Sneezing and coughing cause shooting pains. Arnica is also used for migraines caused by head injuries such as concussion.

LACHESIS—Lachesis is for a severe congestive migraine, usually on the left side, that involves vomiting and loss of sight. There is throbbing and a sense of bursting. The headache is induced by sun (chronic). It is relieved by pressure on the top of the head and gets worse if discharges are suppressed (e.g., with antihistamines).

NATRUM MURIATICUM—Natrum muriaticum (table salt) is particularly effective for chronic headaches that involve intense pain accompanied by a feeling of bursting or of compression, as if in a vice.

NUX VOMICA—Nux vomica relieves migraines associated with stomach, liver, abdominal, and hemorrhoidal conditions. The migraine comes on when the person awakes or gets up, after eating, in the open air, or when the eyes are moved.

PHOSPHORUS—Phosphorus is used to treat congestive migraines in which the head throbs. These headaches are made worse by motion, light, noise, lying down, hunger, and heat; they improve with rest. The person feels cold but likes cold applied to the head.

PULSATILLA—Pulsatilla is used for congestive migraines in which the head throbs and is hot. The headache improves with applications of cold or walking slowly outside. It may be associated with overeating and menstruation.

RHUS TOXICODENDRON—Rhus toxicodendron is used in cases where the person feels intoxicated or stupefied, as though the head were being weighted down. When the person wakes and opens her eyes, a violent migraine comes on. Children may get this type of migraine when they get cold or damp or have wet the bed.

SEPIA—Sepia is used for migraines, especially in women, that are related to nervousness, indigestion, or heartburn, and may be violent or periodic and improve when the person lies quietly. This type is often cured by sleep, by strenuous activity such as dancing, or by long walks outdoors.

SILICA—Silica relieves chronic migraines involving nausea and vomiting that begin at the nape of the neck and move over the crown of the head to the eyes. The headache improves with pressure, lying down, heat, and urination.

THUJA OCCIDENTALIS—Thuja occidentalis is used for the person who feels as though a nail were being driven into the top of the head and who has severe stitches in the area of the left temple and pulsation in both temples. Thuja is effective for severe headaches that follow vaccination.

ACUPUNCTURE

Meridian imbalance can be addressed by acupuncturists or applied kinesiologists. Dr. Olsen states, "The task of the practitioner is to balance the energy by stimulating the meridians. There are various ways of accomplishing this. Three acupressure or acupuncture points are helpful in treating migraines. Lung 7 is located about two finger widths from the crease in the wrist, on the thumb side of the anterior part of the arm. Bladder 67 is found at the nail point of the little toe, and Gallbladder 20 is located between the mastoid and the occipital protuberance in the skull. These points are stimulated in a circular or tapping motion until there is an effective change."

BIOFEEDBACK

Using thermal control, a biofeedback technique, people may be able to control migraines by learning to raise their finger temperatures with a digital-temperature device. They learn the technique in the practitioner's office and from manuals and audiotapes at home. Generally people need about two months to learn the technique. It appears to work by increasing blood flow, which is decreased by nervous tension.

Another biofeedback technique places sensors on the temples, over the temporal arteries. People learn to change their pulse rates in order to diminish their migraines.

PHYSICAL MEDICINE

Aerobic exercise, says Dr. Kane, can lessen the frequency of migraines if it is performed regularly, three times a week for a minimum of twenty minutes.

There are many inventive forms of hydrotherapy that involve applying cold to the head and heat to the feet. For example, cold wet packs on the forehead, back of the neck, and head will constrict the blood vessels so that less blood flows into the head. Soaking the feet in a hot footbath in which peppermint and apple cider vinegar are added to the water will bring the blood away from the head and into the feet, and also cool and cleanse the blood. A hot hip bath will also bring the blood away from the head. When the headache is severe, try alternating hot and cold, using towels that are soaked and then wrung out and applied to the face and head. The last application should be cold. You can also alternate hot and cold hip baths.

An enema with cool water may give relief, since migraines are frequently related to wastes remaining in the colon.

ACUPRESSURE

Dr. Kane describes acupressure points that can be used to relieve different types of migraines. A point known as Wind Gate is effective for migraines related to the change of seasons. It is actually two points located at the highest point of the neck just below the hairline on either side of the muscles that run up the spine. You can press these points or put two tennis balls in a sock and lie on your back so that the balls press into these two points.

Another point is in the fleshy area between the thumb and forefinger. Squeezing it can reduce migraine pain and also stimulate a bowel movement, which itself often relieves the headache. A point below the bottom of the big toe can relieve migraines that affect the upper part of the face and the eyes.

A PSYCHOLOGICAL APPROACH

Dr. Kane suggests pondering some themes that make connections between migraines and a person's emotional or mental condition. Insight into hidden stresses that manifest physically as migraines may help you release the tensions that lead to the migraine. For example, Dr. Kane explains, some experts believe that migraines represent an attempt to live out one's sexuality through the head. On a physiological level, the pattern of tension manifested as constricted blood vessels releasing into relaxation when the vessels finally dilate and the pain is relieved can be compared to an orgasm. This type of migraine can frequently be relieved by masturbation, although it may require more than one orgasm to bring relief. Dr. Kane notes further that constipation and problems with digestion are often associated with migraines. This indicates a "closed-up" condition in the lower body.

COLORS

Dr. Kane describes the use of color to relieve migraines as well as other ills. You can wear certain colors or use gels placed over lamps or other light sources. The colors most effective during a migraine, she says, are purple and scarlet. Purple increases the ability to tolerate pain and makes a person drowsy when a purple light is shined on the chest, throat, and face. Scarlet can be shined on the face to raise blood pressure, though only for migraines caused by decreased blood flow. For migraines that affect the right side of the head, shine blue on the face or the liver for five minutes.

In between migraine attacks, use lemon (said to dissolve blood clots) and yellow (which works on the lymphatic system and motor nerves) for two weeks. Then use lemon and orange, which act as decongestants, for four weeks. Repeat this pattern for as long a period as required.

REFLEXOLOGY

Applying pressure to the feet can alleviate migraines because specific reflex points correspond to the head area. Reflexologist Gerri Brill says that the greatest benefit comes from a routine that encompasses all body systems. Here she gives a detailed description of her program:

CREATING A COMFORTABLE ENVIRONMENT—"I start off by getting you to feel relaxed. Sometimes I use a foot basin to soften and warm up the feet. Then I have you lie down on my massage table while I explain the anatomy of the foot and the idea that each part corresponds to an area of the body. The big toe relates to the head, and the little toes relate to the head and sinuses. Under the toes is a ridge that corresponds to the neck and shoulders. The chest-lung area corresponds to the ball of the foot. The narrow part is the waist area, and at the heel you have the small and large intestines, the sciatic nerves, and the lower back."

RELAXING BREATHING—"There is a special place on the foot that corresponds to the solar plexus. This is a little notch just below the ball of the foot. The solar plexus is the seat of the emotions. By placing my thumb in this little notch as you inhale and releasing as you exhale, I help you to let go of a lot of stuck feelings held inside. It helps promote relaxation and is good to do at the end of the session as well."

WRINGING THE FOOT—"As you lie down, I wring out your foot three times or so, as if I were wringing out a washcloth. That helps the foot relax."

LUNG PRESS—"This is where I press the fist of my right hand into your chest-lung reflex while holding your foot with my left hand. This area is on the pad of your foot, directly beneath the ridge of the toes. As I press, I slowly bring the flat of my fist down to the heel. I repeat this action three times. It is another relaxation technique."

FOOT-AND-TOE BOOGIE—"Next I do what is called the foot boogie. That means rocking your foot back and forth to loosen it up. Then I do the same with your toes. I place my hands around each toe as I shake your toes back and forth. It sounds silly, but it feels great."

ZONE WALKING—"Zone walking is performed with the outer aspect of the thumb. If you place your thumb on your lap, it is the area that rests on your lap. It's important to keep the fingernails short to avoid digging into anyone. Using the outer aspect of my thumb, I start way down at the heel. I mentally divide the foot into five zones, with each zone leading to a different toe. Starting at the outside portion of the foot, the fleshier part, I bend the working thumb at a forty-five-degree angle and apply pressure as I creep up the foot ever so slightly. Each move is no more than a sixteenth of an inch. There are a lot of nerve endings in the feet, and I want to hit all of them. Applying steady pressure, I work my thumb upward all the way to the tip of the toe. When I reach the top of the toes, I go back down to the heel again to repeat the process. These steps are repeated for all five zones. By covering the whole body in this way, I help to create an equilibrium."

SPINE REFLEX—"Now I am at the inside aspect of the foot. That's the spine reflex, and it is very important because the spine supports you and holds you erect. I start at the bottom by your heel with my thumb. Again, I work with the outside corner of my thumb held at a 45-degree angle and walk up your spine. I go all the way up to the big toe. Then I turn around and thumb-walk down, using little steps and steady pressure. I don't want to hurt you, but I do want to exert a good amount of pressure since this is pressure therapy."

SHOULDER AND NECK REFLEX—"Now I move to the ridge underneath the toes. This corresponds to the neck and shoulder line, and it is important for headache relief because when people have tension and headaches, their neck and shoulders are usually tense. Again, I use the thumb-walk. I start at the outside of the big toe and thumb-walk to the ridge. I bend the toes back slightly to get inside. This is repeated until I get to the little toe. Then I turn around and thumb-walk back."

HEAD AREA—"The big toe relates to the head, so of course I want to work this area. I place the fingers of my right hand over my left hand and thumb-walk down the fleshy part of the big toe. I divide the big toe into five zones and work down each area using very, very tiny bites or steps. My aim is for twenty-five bites on that big toe. That covers the whole area. I do that five times. This is very important."

BRAIN REFLEX—"Rolling my index finger over the top of the big toe stimulates the brain and relieves aches caused by migraines. Often this area feels sensitive because of crystal deposits that accumulate. These deposits need to be broken up."

HEAD AND SINUSES—"After finishing the big toe, I move to the little toes. Again, using my thumb, I divide each toe into three zones and thumb-walk, using little bites. This is repeated three times on each toe. This is another place where I feel tiny grains of sand. Breaking them up is the main way to relieve migraines."

CLOSING THE SESSION—"Just to make the session complete, I go back to the top of the foot while supporting the heel with the fist. I finger-walk with the right hand between the little bones on the top of the feet. This area helps the lymphatics, chest, breast, and part of the back. Massaging here helps you to achieve a state of balance. Then I work around the ankle areas. The ankles relate to the reproductive organs and alleviate headaches caused by PMS. That's just one foot. Now I wrap up the foot that was worked on and start over on the other side. Afterward, I massage both feet at the same time, which is very soothing. At this point, you know that the session is coming to an end. Once again, I massage your solar plexus area and have you take a deep breath. Finally, I do a nerve stroke to soothe the feet. This is where I ask you to imagine taking in peace and balance with each breath. This promotes a profound sense of relaxation. At this point the session is over, but you should rest a few moments instead of getting up quickly. Just relax and acknowledge how great you feel. Be sure to drink some water after the session to flush out the deposits."

OTHER

In some cases, correcting cranial faults is crucial to treatment. Dr. Olsen says, "Since migraines involve the cranial nerves, patients suffering from migraines should always be examined for cranial faults. These faults are extremely difficult to evaluate, due to the subtle movement of bones, but correcting them can be key to healing.

"One of my patients responded only partially to treatment after we corrected other findings that contributed to her headaches. Although the frequency decreased, she still reported migraines. At first, she had a general examination for cranial faults; there were no positive findings. Finally, after examining every single sutral point (or area of articulation) along the frontal bone in the forehead, we found the problem and corrected it. Her headaches stopped. In this case, the patient had an internally rotated frontal bone. Applied kinesiologists find this to be the most common cause of migraines from a cranial fault. This is particularly true if the patient reports eye pain with the migraine.

"The correction for this is done in three steps. First, pressure is applied to the posterior aspect of the palate on the side of internal rotation. Then light pressure is applied on the lateral pterygoid muscle, located behind the upper molar in the mouth. Next, pressure is applied to the medial pterygoid on the opposite side. That completes the treatment."

Neurofeedback, also known as brainwave training or EEG biofeedback, is being used as a safe, drug-free alternative to impact stress, migraines, chronic pain, seizures, and more. Painless electronic sensors are placed on the scalp and earlobes. These sensors record the brain's activity, registering relaxed and focused brain waves with a video game–like pattern on a computer screen. When the mind drifts, the screen goes blank. Neurofeedback is being used to reset particular brain patterns associated with certain illnesses or conditions, so that the brain is able to perform at optimal levels. The effects that are experienced with the computerized biofeedback device are practiced and learned until the exercise and its effect on the brain can be reproduced at home without the device.

Gary Null's Additional Supplements for Headache

The following chart summarizes the supplements I recommend adding to the protocol for overall brain health from chapter 16. In some cases, I recommend increasing the dose of a particular vitamin or supplement to specifically impact headache. In these cases, you should increase the daily dosage from chapter 16 to the level recommended for this specific condition. This protocol is designed for individuals who suffer from or are specifically concerned about headache. If you are concerned about additional conditions discussed in other chapters, consult with a health professional about how you can safely impact multiple conditions. If you are taking medications, whether prescription or over-the-counter, or have any food restrictions, consult with your doctor before beginning any supplement program. Your health care provider should always be up-to-date on all vitamins, supplements, and herbal or homeopathic remedies you are taking. Supplement overdoses are rare, but possible, and certain combinations may affect individuals adversely.

SUPPLEMENT	DOSAGE	CAUTIONS
5-hydroxytryptophan (5-HTP)	50–100 mg	Several months of 5-HTP treatment may be needed for maximum benefit. Nausea is the main side effect, but if it occurs, it usually dissipates within several days. Do

		not combine with prescription antidepressants. If you are taking prescription medication for depression, you should consult with your doctor before taking 5-HTP. Excess levels of serotonin in the blood can be dangerous in case of coronary artery disease.
magnesium	Up to 1,000 mg	May take six weeks or more for effects to be felt.
melatonin	1–5 mg two to three nights per week	Tolerance may develop with regular use. Long-term effects of nightly use are unknown.
vitamin B2	Increase daily dosage from 50 mg to 150 mg	May build up to a therapeutic level. May not show results for several months. Do not exceed a daily supplement of 150 mg.
vitamin B3	At the onset of migraine aura 100–150 mg	High doses of niacin may cause a "hot flash" sensation. Some varieties are advertised "flush free" to prevent this.

Research Update

An increasing body of evidence is showing the benefits of natural modalities to overall health and well-being. Following is a sample of recent peer-reviewed scientific studies relating to migraines.

According to a 2015 report in *BioMed Research International*, vitamins could play an important role in migraine prevention given the association of the headaches with deficits in mitochondrial energy and increased homocysteine. Vitamins B_6, B_{12}, and folic acid are potentially useful for treating migraine with aura. Vitamin E can help with menstrual migraine, which is linked with increased prostaglandin levels in the endometrium, and vitamin C can be used as a scavenger of reactive oxygen for treating neurogenic inflammation. A 2015 study in the *Journal of Headache and Pain* reported that participants in a randomized, placebo-controlled, multicenter trial who took a proprietary supplement containing riboflavin, magnesium, and coenzyme Q10 experienced a significant reduction in intensity of migraine pain, as well as fewer days per month of symptoms. In the journal *Headache*, researchers administered a homeopathic blend of ginger and feverfew to patients suffering from migraine headaches, and found that 63 percent experienced a reduction in pain, while only 39 percent in the placebo group noticed improvement. According to a 2011 study in *Headache*, 4.5 percent of adults with migraines/severe headaches reported using complementary and alternative medicine specifically to treat those ailments. Mind-body therapies such as deep breathing exercises, meditation, and yoga were used most often.

Chapter 46

Multiple Sclerosis

Multiple sclerosis (MS) is a progressive and deteriorating muscular disability in which there is a loss of the protective covering of nerves in the brain and spinal cord, causing fatigue, numbness, mobility problems, visual disturbances, and more. According to the Multiple Sclerosis Association of America, MS affects some 400,000 people nationwide, twice as many women as men. Most people are diagnosed between the ages of 15 and 50. The most common types of MS are relapsing-remitting, secondary-progressive, primary-progressive, and progressing-relapsing.

Dr. Michael Wald, who holds degrees in nutrition and chiropractic, and has authored five books about health, explains, "Multiple sclerosis is a syndrome of progressive nerve disturbances. What we have is a gradual loss in myelin, which is part of the outer covering of the nervous system. The nervous system breaks down."

MS is a condition that can present itself quite suddenly. A young woman could be quite healthy and then one day have problems moving the limbs. Muscle weakness, dizziness, and problems with perception and touch may appear. Vision may be blurred.

"Generally the person will go to a neurologist and the neurologist will take an MRI," Dr. Wald continues. "Maybe he will take some of the patient's cerebrospinal fluid and look for things. The doctor says, 'You've got the disease.' Then the person is put on one of several steroids and that is the end of that.

"That's really not enough. There is enough nutritional and medical literature to support the use of a whole host of dietary and nutritional changes in the lives of these people. What we want to do in natural medicine is slow down and reverse the degeneration of myelin. When myelin breaks down, it's called demyelinization. In about two-thirds of the cases of MS, the onset is between twenty and forty. We are talking about the most fit people in the prime of their lives being struck with this condition."

Possible Causes

The etiology of MS is still unknown. Among the studies attempting to pinpoint the cause are those involving the immune system, genetics, and environment. Most likely, there is a combination of factors.

Multiple sclerosis is classified as an autoimmune disease. An autoimmune disease is one in which the immune system fails to recognize a component of the body's systems as "self" and mounts an attack on that component. For example, says Dr. Wald, "the body may be breaking down the myelin, causing symptoms of MS. So anything we do to slow that down or reverse it should theoretically help."

"In autoimmunity, the problem with immune breakdown occurs eventually to everyone as aging happens, so we are really talking about a situation that will affect everyone."

Some experts postulate that MS may be due to a virus. Often, a woman will have a viral problem and will get MS shortly thereafter. So that may be a cause or a trigger. The theory that MS is caused by a virus is based on animal studies. "Certain viruses can be given to certain animals, for example, which will cause every single symptom of MS," Dr. Wald says. The common viruses that might be involved in causing MS are the Epstein-Barr virus, herpes simplex virus, and the parainfluenza virus.

The National Multiple Sclerosis Society reports that scientists in Australia are studying the relationship between vitamin D and the disease. Vitamin D, produced by the body when exposed to sunlight, helps improve immune function and may protect against MS. People who live closer to the equator, where there is more exposure to sunlight, have a lower risk of MS.

Nutritional factors also have been implicated. Excess consumption of fats and insufficient omega-3 fatty acids may play a role in increasing the risk of MS. Smoking also increases the risk of developing the disease.

Dr. Wald cautions, "Human beings are complicated, as we well know, so even if we knew the cause, we would still want to approach it from a natural medicine perspective by giving the body whatever it needs to help whatever it wants to correct. Whether it's MS or a headache or some other problem, the natural healer strives to give the body what it needs."

Clinical Experience

NATURAL TREATMENTS

DIET

In terms of diet, the first thing is to identify and eliminate food allergies. Dr. Wald remarks that allergies also indicate problems with the immune system. "An allergy means that the immune system becomes hyperresponsive. We already have that going on in MS, so we don't want to create any other hyperresponsiveness with foods."

A number of foods are associated with a higher risk of allergies, including gluten-containing foods such as barley, rye, oats, and wheat. "These are common offenders," Dr. Wald says. "Milk products also fit this category. In fact, the intake of milk in adolescents is correlated with a far higher MS incidence. That much has been proven."

How would a person determine if she were allergic? Dr. Wald says, "You can do what is called an IgG4/IgG1 combination test for allergy, which is a blood test. Ninety foods can be checked, and you can determine quite quickly how your immune system hyperresponds to some of them. Then you eliminate the foods and use substitutes. Another way to approach this would be to look at your diet for the top ten or fifteen foods that you eat most often or that are your favorite and eliminate them, because those best-loved foods tend to be the allergy foods. Even allergists recognize this."

Dr. Wald adds, "Most people find it strange that their favorite foods are what are getting them into trouble. A person will say, 'But I eat the food all the time.' Yes, but you are also causing some disruption of the immune function by doing that, particularly if you have a weak immune system to begin with." By eliminating these foods, "you will reduce overall stress on the immune system. That means healing has a chance to take place."

Aside from allergens, other foods to be avoided in relation to this disease are animal fats. "A high intake of saturated fats in the diet, animal fats, is definitely linked to MS."

Dr. Wald notes that some studies have supported vegetarianism as a positive path for MS sufferers. "Dr. Roy Swank, professor of neurology at the University of Oregon Medical School, did one of the longest studies of MS ever done, which was about twenty-six years in duration. People who had MS symptoms were put on an essentially vegan diet, cod liver oil, and several other similar things. Over time he noticed that those on this diet who had initially had symptoms had fewer exacerbations and less worsening of their condition over the years or had no exacerbations, and did very well or better in comparison to those who had had an initial MS diagnosis and were given the standard drugs."

SUPPLEMENTS

Another important avenue to explore is supplementation. Dr. Wald told me about an unusual supplementation therapy developed at Harvard. "One practical suggestion is something called myelin basic protein. This is something that you or anyone can buy in the health food store. Harvard has investigated reactions with MS patients, using oral myelin from a cow, actually. Basically, if you eat myelin, the stuff in the nervous system will attack the myelin you are eating, leaving your nervous system alone and giving it a chance to repair. The technical term for that is molecular mimicry. You are mimicking your myelin, so it's a distraction technique. That's very important."

Less experimentally, there are certain supplements of proven effectiveness, particularly the omega-3 and omega-6 fatty acids. Dr. Wald notes, "Most of the readers probably know something about these. Evening primrose oil is an example of an omega-6. We get that from grains and seeds. The omega-3s can be obtained from such things as flaxseed oil and fish oil. There are dozens of other types of fats that are important. I do recommend that those with MS have what is called an essential fatty acid blood test done, so that you can find out exactly what oils you need and then simply put them back."

These oils control inflammation in the body and immune function. They are also needed for vascular function—in other words, all the things we need for healing MS. Dr. Wald says that even if you don't have these special tests done, you certainly would want to at least purchase a supplement that contains a reasonable balance of omega-3 and omega-6 oils. Probably, you should look for one that is heavier on the omega-3 oils, the flax and fish oils.

"I myself find that MS patients have difficulty metabolically breaking flaxseed oil down into what they need. So, rather than flax, I tend to recommend what is called ephedra, a supplement. For dosage, you should follow the directions on the bottle unless you are seeing a health care practitioner who can individually tailor the dose."

Another very important nutrient for MS is glutathione. This amino acid is the major immune booster in the body. If you are going to help your health, regardless of what the concern is, you have to somehow raise glutathione levels. Dr. Wald recommends anywhere from 250 to 500 milligrams orally.

Selenium helps the body utilize the glutathione. The recommended dose would be in the 200 to 400 micrograms range.

Vitamins D and B_{12} are extremely important. Dr. Wald says, "Alcoholics, for example, can have the shakes, which are caused by degeneration of their myelin, due to a B_{12} deficiency. This seems very similar to the problems of MS. So, though a B_{12} deficiency is probably not the cause of MS, many MS sufferers have a B_{12} imbalance, one that doesn't necessarily show up on a blood test. So every MS patient we see gets a B_{12} shot. Oral supplements might do it, but it really depends on the level of disability."

Enzymes also may be recommended. As Dr. Wald puts it, "Any conversation about autoimmune disease would not be complete without speaking about them. Bromelain and papain are plant-derived enzymes. They are pancreatic enzyme supports."

Dr. Wald notes that these enzymes are key to defending the body against autoimmune chemicals in the blood, which irritate and break down tissues. Enzymes that you eat, such as bromelain, papain, and others found in fresh fruits or vegetables, as well as pancreatic enzymes, get into the blood and literally digest some of these irritating chemicals. It's a must to include lots of those enzymes.

"Lastly," Dr. Wald says, "some other supplements should be mentioned. One is N-acetyl-cysteine (NAC). Cysteine and methionine are sulfur-containing amino acids that help liver detoxification and overall body detoxification. So any anti-autoimmune approach should contain generous amounts of NAC, between 250 and 1,000 milligrams orally. It works really well orally. The NAC increases glutathione levels. As we said earlier, glutathione is the single most important immune-boosting chemical in the body."

HERBS

Dr. Wald also uses extracts of herbs that are standardized, meaning they have been assayed for the active ingredient. "In other words," he says, "what the bottle says is in there, is in there." The herbs goldenseal, astragalus, and echinacea are the ones most often recommended for autoimmune disorders. Green tea may also be useful.

He mentions a common criticism of herb use. "I do want to recall a question I often field about herbs. A person will ask, 'If MS is a case of the ultrasensitization of the immune system, would you want to take herbs that would bolster the immune system?'

"Well, the wonderful thing about how nature has worked this out is that these supplements will not enhance immunity. They are what are called biologic response modifiers. They work to balance what is wrong. If your immunity is too high, they will work to bring it low. If your immunity is low, they will bring it up. Of course, you can abuse these things to a certain point. But almost no one, if she follows the general directions on the bottles, will be caused any harm. The most the person will experience is a little gastrointestinal upset, and once she experiences that, she will naturally decrease the dose." In taking herbs, no matter which ones, Dr. Wald recommends a four-day on, four-day off cycle so that the body doesn't become insensitive to the herbs, which could result in the herbs losing some of their effectiveness.

OXYGEN

Work has been done with oxygen in aiding sufferers from this illness. Dr. Wald says, "Something not commonly talked about in MS is hyperbaric oxygen. It is possible—and there are many studies on this with MS—for a person to get into a chamber and be exposed to clean, purified oxygen under pressure for health reasons. The purpose of the pressure is to increase oxygen levels in the blood so that healing can take place. As we age—and you can think of MS as accelerated aging of the immune and nervous system—we do not use oxygen well, so tissues break down, producing lots of free radicals. Anything that helps prevent or reverse that has to be healthy just in general. So for those with less severe cases of MS, hyperbaric oxygen will be quite valuable."

EXERCISE

In Dr. Wald's experience, the effectiveness of exercise for those with MS depends very much on the individual. "Sometimes exercise worsens MS and sometimes it helps it. I think the reason is that if someone's nutritional status is lousy, and the person is exercising, she is only increasing her stress. So you want to have a complete holistic program where supplements, diet, exercise, and stress reduction are all combined intelligently."

Gary Null's Protocol for Multiple Sclerosis

The following chart summarizes the supplements I recommend adding to the protocol for overall brain health from chapter 16. In some cases, I recommend increasing the dose of a particular vitamin or supplement to specifically impact headache. In these cases, you should increase the daily dosage from chapter 16 to the level recommended for this specific condition. This protocol is designed for individuals who suffer from or are specifically concerned about multiple sclerosis. If you are concerned about additional conditions discussed in other chapters, consult with a health professional about how you can safely impact multiple conditions. If you are taking medications, whether prescription or over-the-counter, or have any food restrictions, consult with your doctor before beginning any supplement program. Your health care provider should always be up-to-date on all vitamins, supplements, and herbal or homeopathic remedies you are taking. Supplement overdoses are rare, but possible, and certain combinations may affect individuals adversely.

The pathology of MS consists of the partial destruction of the myelin sheaths around the spinal cord, brain, and optic nerves, with its root in an autoimmune type of reaction from the body. The lesions are disseminated at intervals and symptoms are based on the location of the lesions. The course of illness takes on the form, then, of relapse and remission.

IN CHINESE MEDICINE, PATHOLOGY IS CAUSED BY

- Invasion of internal dampness from the environment, which gives a feeling of heaviness in the legs

- Greasy, fried, or cold foods in the diet, plus dairy and gluten, causing internal dampness
- Excessive sexual activity, which weakens overall body energy
- Shock from trauma, which depletes heart and digestive energies, leading to poor circulation

OTHER THEORIES OF CAUSATION INCLUDE

- Chemical poisoning by pesticides, industrial chemicals, and heavy metals
- Mercury poisoning
- Viral infection

Take the following daily as directed:

Brain and Nerve Support

Phosphatidyl serine	1,000–1,500 mg
Phosphatidyl choline	1,000–1,500 mg
Alpha GPC (glycerol phosphoryl choline)	
(go to www.LEF.org)	500 mg
Vitamin B12 (sublingual or via	
IM injection Methylcobalamin)	1–3 mg as directed
Vitamin B complex	100 mg daily total
Vinpocetin	10 mg
Acetyl L-carnitine	500 mg twice a day
Ginkgo biloba	200 mg twice a day

Healthy Oils and Fats

Coenzyme Q10	200–400 mg daily
Fish Oil	
EPA	1,000–2,000 mg daily
DHA	750–1,500 mg daily. An excellent anti-inflammatory. Consider testing inflammation status via blood level of Cardio CRP. If the level is above 1.5, then higher fish oil is required.

GLA from evening primrose
oil or borage oil 300–900 mg daily
Eliminate butter, milk, cheese,
and all saturated fats.

Anti-Oxidant Support

Vitamin C individualized as tolerated
Vitamin E 400–1,200 IU daily
NAC 1,200 mg daily
Alpha-lipoic acid 500–1,000 mg in split doses
Selenium 200–400 mcg daily
Beta-carotene 15,000–25,000 IU daily

Anti-Inflammatory

Quercetin 1,000–3,000 mg daily.
Also an immune supporter.
Curcumin 1,500–3,000 mg daily
Nexrutine (Cox 2 inhibitor) 500 mg
5-Loxin 50 mg

Check homocysteine blood level to determine inflammation status. If above
8.5, then add the following:

Folic Acid 1 mg daily
Vitamin B_6 up to 150 mg daily from
all sources or more
Vitamin B12 1 mg daily
Vitamin B complex 100 mg daily
TMG (trimethylglycine or
described as Betaine, but
not Betaine HCL) 500 mg daily or more.
Then retest homocysteine levels to determine if your doses are adequate.
Cardio CRP blood level: a measure of inflammation elevated above 1.5
Homocysteine: a measure of inflammation elevated above 8.0

Hormone Supplements

Vitamin D3	2,000 IU daily or more. Consider monitoring blood levels via lab test code CPT 82306 (25-OH).
DHEA	25–50 mg. Consider monitoring blood levels via lab test code CPT 82626.
Pregnenolone	10 mg or more. Consider monitoring blood levels via lab test code CPT 84140.
Melatonin	2–10 mg per night. Consider monitoring blood levels via lab test code CPT 83519.

General

NADH	5–10 mg daily for energy
AHCC (mushroom complex)	individualized dose
MSM	individualized dose
Plant-Sprout sterols/sitosterolins	500 mg four times a day
Magnesium citrate	600–1,000 mg as tolerated
Calcium citrate	600 –1,000 mg as tolerated

Research Update

An increasing body of evidence is showing the benefits of natural modalities to overall health and well-being. Following is a sample of recent peer-reviewed scientific studies relating to multiple sclerosis.

In a 2012 article in the *Townsend Letter*, Dr. Marianne Marchese reviewed the alternative therapies for MS that have proven effective. Reports published in the *Journal of Ophthalmology* in 2010 and *Frontiers in Neurology* in 2012 found that resveratrol given to mice with an animal model of MS prevented neuronal loss during optic neuritis. A 2011 *PLoS One* animal study showed that a combination of green tea extract with a common conventional medication for MS, glatiramer acetate, positively affected disease onset, inflammatory infiltrates, and severity of clinical symptoms. A 2011 study published in the *British Journal of Pharmacology* concluded that cannabidiol inhibits pathogenic T cells, decreases spinal microglial activation, and decreases multiple sclerosis-like disease in mice. Other substances that have been found to possibly play a role in MS are lipoic acid, omega-6 fatty acids, omega-3 fatty acids, and gamma-aminobutyric acid (GABA).

Chapter 47

Musculoskeletal Injuries

According to the US Department of Labor, musculoskeletal disorders accounted for 33 percent of all injury and illness cases requiring days away from work in 2013. Among the conditions that are particularly concerning to women are repetitive strain injuries and temporomandibular joint (TMJ) dysfunction.

Repetitive Strain Injuries

In all the hoopla that has accompanied the manifestations of the computer revolution, not much attention has been paid to how the installation of computers in offices has physically affected the people using the devices. What is talked about is how jobs that were grimy, dirty, and physically grueling, such as those in steel mills and automobile plants, are being replaced by jobs in service industries, including many that involve sitting in offices at terminals processing and moving information. Those who are infatuated with the world of computers see this transition as all for the good. However, although there are undeniable benefits to workers from this exchange, they do not necessarily fall in the area of occupational health and safety. The owners and managers of plants that manufactured heavy industrial equipment were notorious for disregarding toxic chemicals and other dangers in the workplace, but it is also true that the managers of many light industries have exposed people to years of looking into computer screens and rattling out numbers on keyboards without ever taking a look at the possible health effects of this labor.

Repetitive strain injuries affect hundreds of thousands of American workers at a cost of more than $20 billion a year in worker's compensation alone. Among the causes of repetitive strain injury are repeated movement combined with physical stress; chronic tension; faulty biomechanics; inappropriate ergonomics; and previous injuries or surgeries.

SYMPTOMS

Dr. Timothy Jameson, author of *Repetitive Strain Injuries: Alternative Treatments and Prevention*, is a graduate of Los Angeles Chiropractic College and a certified chiropractic sports physician. He says that a number of overuse injuries can affect the neck, back, chest, shoulders, arms, and hands. He describes the symptoms that typically occur: Most people start off with simple muscle fatigue due to overexertion. Putting stress on an already fatigued muscle eventually leads to problems with the connective tissue, or fascia, that forms a sheath around the muscle. The fascia responds to repeated stress by becoming harder and thicker. It may get "sticky" and begin to bind to the muscle and other neighboring tissues. The muscles and fascia also become tight and restricted. Nerves and blood vessels get squeezed, causing tingling and numbness. Eventually, the nervous system gets involved, setting off pain signals throughout the body.

Dr. Jameson adds that repetitive strain injuries can be extremely serious. "You can become very limited in your ability to do any type of work, especially repetitive work. In severe cases, people cannot work at all, cannot even get dressed in the morning. They cannot do the things they normally would do."

CLINICAL EXPERIENCE

Anti-inflammatory drugs and surgery may be recommended. There are a variety of less invasive natural options as well.

DIET

If you are engaged in activities that can lead to repetitive strain injury or are already suffering from this disability, there are foods you should cut out of your diet. The number-one item to avoid, which is a major precursor of joint pain, is refined sugar, particularly high-fructose corn syrup. It increases sugar within the body, which sets off the whole process of the insulin reaction, with release of prostaglandins, which starts the inflammatory reaction.

Dr. Jameson recommends the book *Enter the Zone* by Barry Sears as a good source of information on proper nutrition. The book "goes into depth on how to prevent an inflammatory reaction. If you look through the aisles of the grocery store, you'll see that something like 50 percent of the products sold there use high-fructose corn syrup as an ingredient. The body has a lot of trouble digesting that. I know of cases where people cut it totally out of their diet, and their repetitive injury subsided within a few days."

Processed meats, such as corned beef, salami, and hot dogs, are very tough for the body to digest and can trigger an inflammatory reaction. Some of the more saturated oils, such as corn oil, palm oil, safflower oil, and butter, should also be avoided. Margarine, too, is bad. Many people think margarine is better than butter. However, margarine, because of its trans-fatty acids, is actually worse for the body than butter.

VITAMINS AND MINERALS

Dr. Jameson advocates use of supplements. "I would recommend vitamin C, which is very important for tissue healing, starting out with about 1 gram and going up to about 3 grams a day. Also very important are the B-complex vitamins. These are used for nerve regeneration and nerve healing."

Minerals also can help in cases of repetitive strain injuries. "You should never underestimate the power of minerals to rejuvenate cellular tissue," Dr. Jameson says. He puts his patients on a complete mineral regimen, with either colloidal or chelated minerals.

"A lot of people—especially people in jobs that involve heat and a lot of sweating in the summer—are sweating out many of the minerals in their body. So if they are doing a lot of cumulative work and sweating, they are depleting their body's mineral's resources." A list of the minerals and vitamins that Dr. Jameson finds useful for preventing and treating repetitive strain injuries follows. "I usually prescribe these substances in pill form," he notes, "but you can also get all these things in food."

CALCIUM—Calcium is very important for muscle activity and for bone growth; it is also a muscle relaxant. Take about 800 milligrams a day of calcium, a little more if you are pregnant or postmenopausal.

MAGNESIUM—Magnesium is important for muscle relaxation and is required for the functioning of about 80 percent of the enzymes in the body. Good sources of magnesium are vegetables and whole grains. Dr. Jameson recommends starting out with about 200–300 milligrams of magnesium a day. "That's a small amount, considering that magnesium is not well absorbed," he says. "However, I always like to start my patients out with small amounts to see how they react."

ZINC—Zinc is needed for enzyme function and cellular healing. Dr. Jameson recommends about 20 or 30 milligrams a day. Zinc is found in fish, meat, and poultry.

SELENIUM—Selenium, another valuable substance, is found in fish, wheat germ, and garlic. Take 50–200 micrograms a day in the pill form.

VITAMIN E—Vitamin E is a potent antioxidant; Dr. Jameson recommends 200 to 400 IU a day.

BETA-CAROTENE—"Beta-carotene," Dr. Jameson remarks, "is a compound found in vegetables of a yellow-orange or dark green color. Carrot juice is a great source of beta-carotene. I recommend that patients drink carrot juice to get a natural, fresh form of the compound."

COENZYME Q10—Coenzyme Q10 is particularly important for patients with underlying heart disease. It helps to maintain cellular energy, which is vital in cases of repetitive strain injuries.

PROTEOLYTIC ENZYMES—These enzymes "scavenge around the cells and rake up any cellular debris, aiding the healing process," Dr. Jameson explains.

CARTILAGE GROWTH FACTORS—"There is also some good research now on the cartilage growth factors glucosamine sulfate and chondroitin sulfate," Dr. Jameson says. He recommends them for patients with joint pain or irritation of the elbow, spine, or hands and fingers.

HERBAL REMEDIES

Certain herbs help the body relax, which is important in overcoming repetitive strain injuries. "Valerian root can be used for reducing muscle spasms," Dr. Jameson says. "It should be taken toward the end of the day, because it's a relaxant. You wouldn't want to take it throughout the day, because it might affect your ability to perform. Garlic is a natural antibiotic as well as antifungal. Some of these muscular problems can stem from an underlying fungal problem, something we also see in fibromyalgia. A third valuable herb is ginkgo biloba, which increases circulatory function and brain function and enhances memory. It helps the blood flow get down to the extremities. Cayenne has also been found to help increase circulation. And ginseng is great for stress relief."

HOMEOPATHY

In addition to vitamins, minerals, and herbs, homeopathic remedies can be of service. Try the ones you find in health food stores that are recommended for muscle and joint injuries and for rheumatoid arthritis.

CARPAL TUNNEL SYNDROME

Carpal tunnel syndrome, a widely recognized type of repetitive strain injury, is a common disability affecting office workers who sit at computer terminals. It is important that people at risk for carpal tunnel syndrome not only follow the suggestions we make here but also learn to sit and type with the correct posture and to use ergonomically designed chairs and keyboards.

In 2010, an estimated 3.1 percent of employed American adults had carpal tunnel syndrome in the past year, according to the Centers for Disease Control and Prevention (CDC). Women in every age group had higher rates than men. Some cases of carpal tunnel are pregnancy-related, and resolve on their own after the woman gives birth.

CAUSES

The carpal tunnel is a bony canal in the wrist through which the median nerve as well as nine tendons of the hand pass. Carpal tunnel syndrome occurs when the nerve becomes compressed in this narrow space, causing numbness, tingling, and/or pain that gradually increase over time. The symptoms often appear at night because of the way people position their wrists when sleeping. Although the cause of carpal tunnel syndrome is often unknown, many people report increased hand activity or day-in, day-out use of the same muscles and nerves to perform a repetitive task.

The late Dr. Ray Wunderlich, author of many books including *The Natural Treatment for Carpal Tunnel Syndrome*, said that when treating a patient, he started by looking for contributing factors. For women, he asked immediately, "Is she taking birth control pills?" The Pill, in essence, "puts you in a simulated state of pregnancy, and we know that pregnancy is one of the risk factors for carpal tunnel syndrome. Birth control pills also diminish the nutrients in the body, some of the water-soluble vitamins. Moreover, many women who take them become bloated. They develop minor degrees of fluid retention." Women who are taking birth control pills and who perform tasks likely to lead to carpal tunnel syndrome should consider some other form of birth control.

Two other contributing factors, said Dr. Wunderlich, are hormone replacement therapy (HRT) and thyroid deficiencies. With regard to HRT, Dr. Wunderlich said, "If the estrogen preparations are not in balance with the progesterones, this can cause problems."

Dr. Wunderlich found that 75 to 80 percent of his patients had some kind of thyroid disorder. He said, "On top of the repetitive movement of their jobs, many people have thyroid disorders, which contribute to the syndrome and may be hard to diagnose. To pin this down, look for a pale, puffy person, edematous, which is to say retaining fluid. When there is swelling, especially in connective tissue and in the nine tendons that run through that carpal tunnel, that medial nerve in the tunnel is often screaming for more room."

Low adrenal states, which may occur for a variety of reasons, may contribute to carpal tunnel syndrome. People who overwork themselves, who consume a lot of caffeine and/or sugar, and who are now faced with repetitive tasks and sedentary living, may wind up with low-functioning adrenals. In the workplace, they develop various allergies, sometimes combined with low blood pressure. These people often have swollen tissues, which contributes to the problem.

Type 2 diabetes is often accompanied by edematous conditions. This may not be readily observed, Dr. Wunderlich cautioned. "It may be microedema rather than pure edema. The ankles may not be swollen, for example, or the lungs congested, but the tissues may be slightly swollen.

"When the blood sugar is too high, osmotic pressure rises. As we know from high school, osmosis is what controls the body's fluid pressure. The fluid should be in the blood vessels and in the lymph tissues. When it's outside in the body tissues, as happens in high blood sugar states or after we eat a lot of candy or, sometimes, fruits or juices in excessive quantities, the tissue may become water-logged. This, too, can cause problems in that narrow carpal tunnel. The medial nerve is numb and irritable, and we have pain every time we move our fingers."

Food allergies are another potential factor in the development of carpal tunnel syndrome. The monotonous diets that so many people consume, especially with high-protein antigens—such as milk, cheese, and sometimes eggs—often produce food allergies. And a hallmark of the allergic response is swelling. Although the swelling is on the microlevel, the cramped carpal tunnel reacts, causing pain.

Even if you are not allergic to what you're eating, if you're on a typical American diet, you may have problems. "The 140 pounds of sugar per person, per year, that the average American still eats is one problem," Dr. Wunderlich said. "We're not talking about a long time ago. It's still happening. And there are also the salt-laden diets, which could be improving as people are counseled by alternative nutritionists to take high-potassium foods over high-sodium foods. There are animal foods, which are high on the inflammatory scale—they tend to accentuate the inflammatory cascade, or series of chemical reactions through which inflammation develops. Animals are on top of the food chain, and that is where all the refuse accumulates, all the toxic chemicals that get into the animals' fat. This is especially true if the animals are domesticated and not wild, which is the case with most of our animal food sources."

Finally, Dr. Wunderlich said, there are "the chemicals in the workplace. When you are sitting at your computer, you may be bombarded with pesticides they have sprayed around your place—every month they come in and do that, or every two weeks if they see a lot of roaches. All of this adds to the toxic load as background factors."

CONVENTIONAL TREATMENT

By the time a person with carpal tunnel syndrome consults a physician, the condition is often quite advanced. According to Dr. Wunderlich, "The person often has atrophy of the muscles and irreversible or nearly irreversible nerve damage. The doctors operate, often with excellent results. So it's very appealing." However, this is a drastic therapy and will result in a life with further impaired function.

For less severe cases, conventional medicine's procedure is less felicitous. "What ordinary medicine does is give pain relievers—aspirin, Tylenol, ibuprofen, and other nonsteroidal anti-inflammatory drugs—which in the long term are all counterproductive, damaging the gastrointestinal system, producing leaky gut, as well as actually destroying cartilage. But those are the standard therapies that are offered."

ALTERNATIVE TREATMENTS

Dr. Wunderlich's program was short, sweet, and sensible. "The number-one approach in treating this problem," he stated, "is detoxification. We do a vitamin C bowel flush. That's the first step for bowel tolerance." The vitamin C flush gets accumulated toxins out of the body. Follow this up with the second step, taking your favorite bulking agent, rice powder or psyllium, for example. "Number three," he mentioned, "is to support the liver. I like artichoke and thistle compounds. Maybe 100 milligrams of thistle, three times a day, and 500 milligrams of artichoke leaf three times a day. Those are basics, plus water.

"I also use infrared heat to have people sweat, carefully monitored, of course, so there is exchange of body fluids. Also, exercise is important. I do running."

In his program, then, he emphasized detoxification of the body, shifting to a sensible vegetarian diet, exercising, and improving stress management.

It is a question of priorities, Dr. Wunderlich concluded. "Many people have kids, two jobs, and so forth, so they think they do not have time. But you have to sort out the priorities, which we are not doing. You have to have good air and an appropriate amount of sleep. You need to avoid toxic foods. It is also important to have regular bowel movements, and you have to use your body appropriately for you."

The advice that Dr. Wunderlich gave about carpal tunnel syndrome also applies to people who have any type of repetitive stress syndrome. Ultimately, we need to make our workplaces more livable. This will involve the improvement of human interaction and of the machines we surround ourselves with. If we upgraded our environments as obsessively as we upgrade our computers, we might have very few occupational disorders with which to cope.

Temporomandibular Joint (TMJ) Dysfunction

The temporomandibular joint (TMJ) is a hinged joint that opens and closes the jaw. There are two such joints at either side of the head. The jaw is part of a wider system, the craniosacral system, which extends from the skull to the lowest segment of the spine. Disruption at any level of the craniosacral system can result in TMJ dysfunction.

According to 2014 data from the National Institutes of Health, more than 10 million Americans have TMJ dysfunction. Women are affected more often than men.

CAUSES

The two most common causes of TMJ problems are poor bite and stress. Poor bite may be the result of new dental work that affects tooth alignment. Sometimes braces shift the palate, which affects the jaw.

TMJ dysfunction affects larger numbers of women than men due to stresses brought on by hormonal changes. Dr. Deborah Kleinman, a chiropractor who works with TMJ patients, explains. "There are various stress factors we can talk about that are specific to women. First, we have premenstrual tension. This further weakens an already weakened system. I know women who only have a problem with their jaw three days before their period. As soon as their period comes, their pain goes away. This tells me that there is a weakness in the system and that hormones push the body past the point of being able to compensate for it."

Hormonal changes also occur during pregnancy. "Hormones loosen the pelvis so that the woman is more flexible during delivery. And pregnancy creates structural changes through weight gain and the loosening of ligaments. These changes can further aggravate TMJ dysfunction.

"With nursing, postural changes can play a big role. Nursing places stress on the upper back muscles, especially if the woman doesn't use the proper pillows or if she gets lazy and slumps over while feeding her baby. These upper back muscles insert into the occiput, which is part of this craniosacral system. The occiput is the bone at the bottom of the skull. Tightening or pulling on the occiput can affect the head, neck, and TMJ."

The hormonal changes that occur during menopause also play a role in TMJ dysfunction.

SYMPTOMS

Pain can be isolated in the joint itself or it can radiate to the face, neck, ear, and shoulder. Headaches may be a part of the picture. There may be a nagging toothache, even though the tooth is healthy. A person with TMJ problems may find it difficult to open the mouth all the way. Inflammation of the muscles around the joint may cause a spasm in those muscles, locking them open. Clicking, grinding, or popping noises may accompany chewing or movement of the joint.

CLINICAL EXPERIENCE

CRANIOSACRAL THERAPY

Cranio means "skull" and *sacral* refers to the sacrum, which consists of the lowest five vertebrae of the spine. Craniosacral therapy is founded on an understanding of the relationship between these structures and several points in between, including the TMJ. Dr. Kleinman, who uses a specific form of craniosacral therapy called the sacro-occipital technique, explains: "A chiropractor like myself who uses this technique understands that there is a balance between the nervous system and the musculoskeletal system, and a relationship between the pelvis and the sacrum and then the head and the cranium. Between both structures rests the spine, the shoulders, the neck. All of these structures react to shifts in the pelvis and the cranium. The TMJ is part of that." She adds that a stable pelvis balances the body and works in harmony with the cranium. This allows information to flow to the brain smoothly.

Dr. Kleinman says that with TMJ the first step is to have a doctor perform a series of tests to determine whether structural stresses exist, and, if so, where. Once the structural stresses are identified, treatment can begin. Dr. Kleinman explains: "We place wedges or blocks under the pelvis. The muscles will relax and contract around these levers in an unforced way, based upon what these levers tell the brain. Then we incorporate breathing techniques to assist the brain in making musculoskeletal changes. This reestablishes the proper craniosacral flow." Sometimes secondary manipulations are necessary to readjust parts of the spine that lie between the pelvis and cranium that get knotted up as a result of compensating for the pelvis and the cranium. Cranial adjustments, made specifically to the temporomandibular joint, also help to reestablish proper balance.

OTHER PHYSICAL THERAPIES

Isotonic exercise, done regularly, can help in some cases of TMJ dysfunction. In addition to jaw exercise, self-treatment for TMJ problems may include jaw awareness, in which the patient tries to notice and avoid clenching and grinding the teeth, as well as biting on gum, ice, or fingernails. Eating soft foods and avoiding resting or sleeping on the stomach can also help, as can learning to rest the jaw and to adopt proper jaw posture. Other potentially helpful techniques include self-massage; relaxed rhythmic opening and closing of the jaw; alternating moist heat (fifteen minutes) with ice (two to three minutes) to increase circulation; cool sprays and cryotherapy; bite guards; and splints. Surgery should be a last resort when dealing with TMJ problems.

Another physical therapy that can help relieve TMJ problems is body rolling, a technique developed by bodyworker Yamuna Zake, author of *Body Rolling: An Experiential Approach to Complete Muscle Release.* "Many of the muscles that run up the back and insert in the skull, as well as the muscles in the front of the neck, have attachments between the head and the chest. Thus the amount of tension in the muscles of the back, front, and sides of the neck can affect the level of contraction of the sutures (joints) and muscles of the cranium, and specifically the TMJ," she explains.

In body rolling, a six-inch-diameter ball is used to apply traction that lengthens and releases muscles. "The degree of tension in the TMJ is controlled by the tension maintained in the neck," Zake explains. "By working the neck muscles with the ball to keep them at maximum length and minimum tension level, you can help reduce the buildup of tension in the TMJ." Zake has designed specific routines that use the ball to release the front and back of the neck, as well as an around-the-neck routine that helps break the holding pattern of tension that distorts head and neck alignment.

NUTRITION

Nutritional supplements may help in treating TMJ problems. Some of the most useful are listed here:

CALCIUM AND MAGNESIUM—These minerals are essential for proper muscular function and have a sedative effect.

B-COMPLEX VITAMINS—Take 100 milligrams of B-complex vitamins three times a day. B-complex vitamins are essential for combating stress.

PANTOTHENIC ACID—The appropriate amount of pantothenic acid to take is 100 milligrams, twice daily. B-complex vitamins, such pantothenic acid, are for combating stress.

COENZYME Q10—Coenzyme Q10 is another stress fighter.

OTHER SUPPLEMENTS—L-tyrosine and vitamins B$_6$ and C will improve sleep quality and alleviate anxiety and depression. It is also important to take a multi-vitamin and mineral complex.

Chapter 48

Obsessive-Compulsive Disorder

Obsessive-compulsive disorder affects an estimated two to three million American adults. It is characterized by repetitive thinking and the inability to control or put a stop to this thinking process. As orthomolecular psychiatrist Dr. José Yaryura-Tobias explains, these thoughts become urges that are so demanding that it appears to the person who has them that they *must* be carried out. OCD can have a significant impact on daily living. Two of the main compulsions are double-checking and hand washing.

CAUSES

According to Dr. Yaryura-Tobias, "As to why this condition exists at all, we don't have a sure answer to that question. The behavior may result from a learning process that takes hold during childhood. It may relate to changes in neurotransmitters—the chemical substances in the brain that build bridges between nerve cells so that they can transmit signals from the outside into our system or, in the reverse direction, direct us to act to affect the outside world. The key neurotransmitter that is being studied in this regard is serotonin."

SYMPTOMS

Dr. Yaryura-Tobias tells about some of the peculiar characteristics of obsessive-compulsive behavior: "It usually takes about seven years or so for a patient to come in for a consultation, which tells us that the condition tends to occur gradually, becoming part of the patient's behavioral system in a very, very slow manner. It occurs with equal frequency in males and females. Fifty percent of obsessive-compulsive patients manifest their sickness during childhood or adolescence. Later on—primarily after the age of forty—it fades away, and it becomes very rare after age fifty.

CLINICAL EXPERIENCE

CONVENTIONAL TREATMENT

According to the late Dr. Robert Atkins, there is some common ground here between conventional and alternative medicine. "Both orthodox medicine and complementary medicine recognize that if a certain neurotransmitter is in short supply, certain syndromes will result. A classic example is that a serotonin-deficient person will often be an obsessive-compulsive. These are the people who can't get out of the house because they've got to make sure the light switches are off or the gas jet isn't on, the people who have to wash their hands twenty times a day, and the people whose desks have to be perfectly neat. These people are serotonin-deficient."

The difference between the conventional and the alternative medical communities lies in how they address the problem. Dr. Atkins described the conventional approach: "Now there are drugs that block the degradation of serotonin and allow the serotonin level to lift, but those drugs do a lot of other things: they poison a lot of enzyme systems, and that's why so many people got into trouble with Prozac and drugs like that." In addition to Prozac, other drugs used to treat obsessive-compulsive disorders are Anafranil, Luvox, and Paxil.

ALTERNATIVE THERAPIES

To treat obsessive-compulsive disorders, Dr. Yaryura-Tobias uses conventional behavioral therapy and an amino acid approach, along with some other nutrients.

"We basically treat with behavioral therapy. We try to use thought-stopping, exposure (flooding), and response prevention to prevent the brain from repeating the same thought. That is difficult, so we also use cognitive therapy to explain the reasons we think the things we do and try to modify the thoughts."

Behavioral therapy is most effective in dealing with compulsions. Dr. Yaryura-Tobias explains that it's important to expose the patient in some way to her fears. "If you have fears of AIDS or of blood, you are exposed to blood or taken to the hospital where there might be patients with AIDS. Or you will read articles on the condition.

"If it is contamination from dirt the patient is afraid of, we teach that person how to touch objects and not be afraid of them. Then we prevent the patient from washing her hands; in other words, she must remain unclean for a while. I'm talking about patients who, when they are seriously ill, might completely use up one or two bars of soap per day. They might engage in rituals of washing for many hours. They may wash their hands sometimes a hundred or more times a day. Some of these patients will also clean their hands with alcohol or other substances. Sometimes their skin becomes extremely raw. I've seen cases where patients require plastic surgery.

"Overall, the treatment takes about six months. With medication there is improvement up to 60 or 70 percent of the time."

People with obsessive-compulsive and anxiety disorders often improve on the amino acid tryptophan. Dr. Yaryura-Tobias says, "My colleagues and I were the first to use tryptophan, and with it we were able to reduce and almost eliminate completely the use of drugs for this condition, and we obtained very good results. We were using between 3,000 and 9,000 milligrams per day.

"Then we used vitamin B_6, 100 milligrams, three times a day. Vitamin B_6, pyridoxine phosphate, is a vitamin that is very important for the breakdown of tryptophan into serotonin. The idea behind this was that these patients didn't have enough serotonin in their brains or were very dependent on serotonin or that the normal conversion of tryptophan into serotonin was not occurring.

"When we found by measuring that there was a lack of serotonin, this could be reversed by the administration of L-tryptophan with niacin and vitamin B_6. Some medications also accomplish this result, but with medications we face many types of side effects."

Not all patients see good results. "About 30 percent of patients do not respond to any form of therapy," Dr. Yaryura-Tobias says. "But it is not a closed chapter for these patients either. An investigation has to be conducted. Now that we have brain imaging, we are able to visualize the brain. We can measure, for instance, the metabolism of sugar in the brain. We find, for instance, that the frontal and temporal lobes and the basal ganglia, which are related to Parkinson's disease, are disrupted. We see the metabolism of the breakdown of sugar and also images of an abnormal brain. The same can be seen with some electrophysiological measurements of brain wave tests and so forth.

"Interestingly, work has been going on using pure behavioral therapy before and after measuring serotonin. With just behavioral therapy, we were able to modify the levels of serotonin in the body. In other words, we may not need medication to change or challenge the presence of a neurotransmitter such as serotonin. Behavioral techniques alone may have an effect."

Research Update

An increasing body of evidence is showing the benefits of natural modalities to overall health and well-being. Following is a sample of recent peer-reviewed scientific studies relating to obsessive-compulsive disorder.

A pilot study reported in 2015 in *Cognitive Behaviour Therapy* found that adding a twelve-week structured physical exercise program to cognitive behavior therapy for people with OCD had significant positive effects. A 2011 report in the *Indian Journal of Psychological Medicine* found that OCD may be one of the first signs of vitamin B_{12} deficiency.

Chapter 49

Osteoporosis

More than eight million American women have osteoporosis, and another twenty-seven million are at risk due to low bone mass, according to 2014 data from the National Osteoporosis Foundation. The disease is responsible for more than 1.5 million fractures a year. Osteoporosis (the word means "porous bones") is a serious problem in which the skeletal system weakens and fractures easily. It may be accompanied by pain, especially lower back pain, loss in height, and body deformity.

Eighty percent of those affected are women, with postmenopausal women being at greatest risk. Osteoporosis is attributed to the gradual loss of calcium. In women, this loss begins in the mid-thirties at a rate of 1 to 2 percent a year, and can increase during menopause to a rate of 4 to 5 percent a year.

In the past, osteoporosis was thought to be an inevitable part of the aging process, particularly in women. Now most of us know that it is treatable and, more important, preventable.

Causes

According to naturopathic physician Dr. Jane Guiltinan, the most likely candidates for osteoporosis share a number of characteristics:

- Northern European ethnic origin
- Small frame
- Family history of osteoporosis
- Diet high in meat, caffeine, sugar, refined carbohydrates, and phosphates (found in sodas and processed foods)

- Cigarette smoking
- Alcohol use
- Sedentary lifestyle

Contrary to what we've been told, large quantities of calcium rich dairy products in the diet can actually contribute to the condition of osteoporosis. If you asked your physician or your dietician or your nutritionist what would help prevent or reverse osteoporosis, the answer would be dairy products. Not true. It's just the opposite. Dairy products cause osteoporosis. Acid blood is a condition induced by the consumption of acidic foods. Extra quantities of protein from animals or stress with the accumulation of hazardous waste products within the body creates osteoporosis because the parathyroid glands are forced to balance the pH levels of the blood by releasing excess calcium from the bones. So the moment that you eat anything even though it makes you feel good and even though it's a comfort food and even though you're used to it, your bones are releasing calcium to balance out the high levels of acid to correct the pH.

A lot of women suffer from faulty calcium assimilation due to a deficiency of silica or phosphorous, while others may have a malfunctioning of the thyroid or parathyroid glands, which are responsible for calcium metabolism. The parathyroid glands control the level of calcium in the blood by secreting hormones that can be balanced, if you understand the right way of taking calcium in. During a calcium shortage, excess calcium, which is stored in the bones, joints, and soft tissues, is discharged in the bloodstream, and that reduces the bone loss. So you see it's not just in what you do, but it's also what you don't do.

Registered nurse and acupuncturist Abigail Rist-Podrecca notes, "When I was in China, we noticed that no dairy was used. We expected to see a high incidence of osteoporosis, rickets, and other bone problems. In fact, we saw the lowest incidence. In the west, dairy is used a lot and osteoporosis is rampant. Something is not quite right here." Three main factors responsible for the Chinese not getting osteoporosis, she learned, are diet, weight-bearing exercise, and acupuncture.

Dr. Sangeeta Pati, a board-certified physician who has practiced traditional and holistic medicine for two decades, explains that several hormones are responsible for bone health. As we age, hormone production declines, and this in turn can contribute to osteoporosis.

Progesterone is actually the first hormone in the body to decline. "The time to really look for this is the late thirties and early forties because that's when we start losing most bone," Dr. Pati says. Among the other hormones that may decline are testosterone, which promotes bone formation; estradiol, which prevents bone loss; DHEA, a precursor to testosterone; thyroid; and growth hormone.

Diagnosis

In the past, osteoporosis was not diagnosed until the condition was so advanced that patients began to break their bones. Today, however, bone mineral density testing is being used to detect the disease and those at risk for developing it. New guidelines issued by the National Osteoporosis Foundation in 2014 recommend that every woman over the age of sixty-five have a bone density test. For postmenopausal women, the test is recommended if there are risk factors for fracture, such as excessive thinness, cigarette smoking, a previous fracture in adulthood, or a family history of fractures.

Bone density testing is noninvasive and takes only a few minutes to perform. It provides a measurement known as a T-score. T-scores can indicate normal bone density, low bone density, or osteoporosis.

Because progesterone starts to decline in the thirties and forties, Dr. Pati suggests that bone density testing be conducted much earlier than is currently recommended. "I find that the best way to know whether there is bone loss is to look at the urine bone markers," she says. "There are a number of urine bone markers, but one of the common ones is Urine N Telopeptide. It's called Urine NCX, and it's literally a measure of how much bone you are leaking out in the urine. If that number is under thirty-five, you know that you have that process under real good control."

Clinical Experience

CONVENTIONAL APPROACH

Conventional treatment often involves the use of prescription medications. Synthetic estrogen was the traditional drug of choice for postmenopausal osteoporosis and its prevention, but controversy surrounds its safety and effectiveness. Among the other drugs that are used are biophosphonates, selective estrogen receptor modulators (SERMs), calcitonin, teriparatide, and tamoxifen.

Dr. Saralyn Mark, an endocrinologist and women's health specialist, is often asked whether estrogen prevents osteoporosis. "It's an important question," she says. "I think with a lot of the results from the Women's Health Initiative that came out over the last few years there has been a lot of concern about estrogen therapy and the risk for heart disease, stroke, and cancer. What we did see in the study was that estrogen did decrease the risk of hip fracture and overall bone fractures. Those women who select to go on estrogen for whatever reason need to talk to their doctors about checking their bone mass before they go on it and then for a period of time after they go off it because the effects of estrogen after you go off it don't continue for years and years."

NATUROPATHIC PREVENTION AND TREATMENT

The first step in osteoporosis prevention is noting whether or not you are at high risk for the condition, says Dr. Guiltinan. Obviously, certain risk factors cannot be changed, but many can be addressed, and will prevent the destructive effects of the disease.

DIET

A diet that is low in animal products and high in plant foods promotes bone growth and repair. Green, leafy vegetables contain vitamin K, beta-carotene, vitamin C, fiber, calcium, and magnesium, which enhance the bones. Other calcium-rich foods include broccoli, nuts, and seeds. Sesame seeds have high calcium content. The Chinese, who as mentioned earlier have low rates of osteoporosis, use sesame often in their foods, and cook with sesame seed oil.

Foods to avoid include sugar, caffeine, carbonated sodas, and alcohol, as these contribute to bone loss. Chicken, fish, eggs, and meat are also contraindicated. These are high in the amino acid methionine, which the body converts into homocysteine, a substance that causes both osteoporosis and atherosclerosis.

The official recommended dietary requirement for calcium for people at risk of osteoporosis is 1,200 milligrams per day for women aged 51 and older. I recommend that women over twenty-five take approximately 1,000 milligrams in supplement form and an additional 500 to 1,000 milligrams from the diet. For those over forty, supplements of 1,500 to 2,000 milligrams are needed. Women on estrogen replacement therapy require about 2,000 milligrams.

Vitamin D is also important. You can get this from food, supplements, and sunshine. "I often recommend to patients that if they have problems with their diet they can get a little bit of vitamin D from just going outside fifteen minutes a day," says Dr. Mark. "I know that causes a lot of concern for people because we've done such a good job getting the message about sun protection to prevent skin cancer. But again, ten to fifteen minutes a day shouldn't be much of a problem, and we know that it's very helpful to allow your body to make its own vitamin D." The official recommendation for vitamin D is 800 to 1,000 IU per day, including supplements if necessary for people aged 50 and older.

In addition, the following nutrients are critical for keeping bones strong:

- Magnesium (800–1,200 milligrams in citrate form)
- Vitamin C (5,000–20,000 milligrams)
- Vitamin K (100 micrograms)
- Beta-carotene
- Selenium (200 micrograms)
- Boron (5 milligrams)
- Manganese (25 milligrams)
- Folic acid (800 micrograms)
- Silica (20 milligrams)
- Copper (2 milligrams)
- Zinc (30 milligrams)

A balanced vitamin/mineral supplement will provide most of these nutrients. It is best to take zinc separately, however. Otherwise, it can have an adverse effect on vitamin and mineral absorption. Also recommended are black cumin seed oil (1 tsp, 2x day), coconut oil (1 tsp, 2x day), emulsified cod liver oil (1 tsp), and Cytokine Supress with EGCG (300mg).

NATURAL HORMONES

Research indicates that natural progesterone from wild yams is safer and more effective than estrogen in that it builds strong bones and has no harmful side effects. Dr. Jane Guiltinan notes, "Estrogen minimizes calcium loss from bones, but progesterone can actually put calcium back into bones." Natural progesterone can be taken in pill form. It also comes in a cream form. Half a teaspoon should be rubbed into the skin over soft tissue and the spine, twice a day, for two weeks out of every month.

DHEA is important in the prevention of numerous chronic conditions associated with aging. As we get older, there is often a drop in DHEA. I recommend that you increase the DHEA to 25 to 50 milligrams a day unless you have breast or pancreatic cancer.

Dr. Pati explains that bioidentical hormones should be used. A hormone interacts "like a lock and a key with a receptor site on any organ that it's going to affect," she says. "A bioidentical hormone would be a hormone that is molecule per molecule identical to the human body. It could be made from soy or yam, or even synthetically, but the end product one is something that is molecule per molecule identical."

This distinction is important and sometimes difficult to detect. For example, Dr. Pati says, "there are some over-the-counter creams that are yam derived, but we have to remember that these are literally wild yam progesterone, which means molecule to molecule they do not bind with receptors exactly the same way as human progesterone." To remedy this, the product can be modified in a compounding pharmacy by essentially "cutting off all the extra molecules that don't match the human body."

To protect the bone, the progesterone level should be between 5 and 10 nanograms per deciliter, Dr. Pati says. "That's the level that you're looking for. I usually find that women who are progesterone deficient are also complaining of other things like anxiety and sleep issues, so I generally use the progesterone orally and it gets converted in the liver to 5 alpha pregnenolone."

HERBS

Some herbalists recommend horsetail, taken as a tea every day, to restore bone strength and density. They add that dandelion root tincture will promote absorption of calcium. The micronutrients important for bone flexibility and strength are found in the greatest abundance in seaweeds, dandelion, and nettles, and in organic vegetables and grains.

EXERCISE

Dr. Howard Robins, former director of the Healing Center in New York City and coauthor of *Ultimate Training* and *How to Keep Your Feet & Legs Healthy for a Lifetime*, stresses the importance of weight-bearing aerobic and weight-lifting exercises for osteoporosis prevention.

Aerobic exercises use major muscle groups in a rhythmic, continuous manner.

Weight-bearing aerobic exercises such as brisk walking, jogging, stair climbing, and dancing produce mechanical stress on the skeletal system, which drives calcium into the long bones. Non–weight-bearing aerobic exercises such as biking, rowing, and swimming are not as helpful in osteoporosis prevention, but they do promote flexibility, which is useful for people prone to arthritis.

People "need to perform aerobic exercises anywhere from three to five or six times a week," says Dr. Robins. "You need a day off every third or fourth day so that the body can heal and reenergize."

"Most women stay away from weight training because they are afraid of developing huge muscles like Arnold Schwarzenegger," says Dr. Robins. "The good news is, that won't happen. No matter how hard she trains, a woman will never get huge muscles unless she takes steroids to alter her body's metabolism."

Not only is weight training safe, it is important for preventing osteoporosis. As muscles are pulled directly against the bone, with gravity working against it, calcium is driven back into the bones. It also stimulates the manufacture of new bone. This adds up to a decrease in the effects of osteoporosis by 50 to 80 percent. People need to do weight training two to three times per week for fifteen to thirty minutes. All the different muscle groups should be worked on. Twenty-four hours should lapse between sessions to rest muscles. For women, an exercise program should be started long before the onset of menopause.

A complete routine is more than aerobic and weight-training exercises only. It incorporates warm-ups at the beginning and cool-downs at the end of a routine. Warm-ups are not to be confused with stretches. Rather, they are gentle exercises that produce heat by getting blood to flow into the muscles. To warm up leg muscles, for example, one could lie down on one's back and move the legs like a bicycle, or walk gently in place. Moving the arms and joints gently in all their ranges of motion will warm up the upper body. Warming up the body helps prevent injuries.

After exercise, when the body is loosest, stretching is performed. Stretches are long, continuous pulls, not bounces. Bouncing only tightens the muscles and can lead to injury. Dr. Robins's book *Ultimate Training* describes a holistic workout in detail. Aromatherapist Ann Berwick adds that essential oils enhance a warm-up and cool-down routine. "Before exercise, use warming and stimulating oils, such as black pepper, rosemary, ginger, and sage. Additionally, eucalyptus helps to deepen breathing. After exercise, you can apply a blend of lemon, rosemary, and juniper. These help to carry away waste products and ease any stiffness."

Dr. Saralyn Mark also stresses the importance of exercise, and says that a lot can be done without even going to the gym. "What we need to understand is that what you do to your bones affects every part of your life. You can do just what you need to do in your daily life to maintain bones. For example, just walking up stairs or doing housework. People often complain about doing housework. Well try to look at it as if you're doing something great for your body."

YOGA

Yoga prevents osteoporosis by building and fortifying bone mass, keeping muscles strong and flexible, improving posture, and helping balance and coordination. Physical therapist and yoga teacher Bonnie Millen explains why this is important: "With yoga, the old adage 'Use it or lose it' applies. Building and maintaining bone mass is most important for preventing osteoporosis. Remember, bone is alive. Yoga is unique in that it incorporates weight bearing on the upper extremities. This is important because many wrist, forearm, and upper arm fractures occur when people reach forward with outstretched arms as they are falling.

"Also important is building and maintaining muscle strength and flexibility. Let's keep the muscles strong so that they can receive the stress before the fracture happens. Also if the body is strong and flexible, it can cushion falls when they occur."

What about posture? "Good posture improves overall functioning and prevents osteoporotic fractures of the spine," Millen says. "I teach yoga to a lot of older women who tell me they are afraid of getting a dowager's hump. This is where the body slouches forward and there is a hump on the back. Just take a moment to get into that posture where your chest caves in and your shoulders slump forward, with your head looking down toward the floor. Try to raise one arm up as if you wanted to touch the ceiling, and see how high the arm comes up. Now let the arm down and come into a nice seated posture, as if someone were going to take your picture. Sitting very tall, raise your arm up and see how high it goes. You can see from that little exercise that the slouched posture really decreases your range of motion. That makes it difficult to function. This is why you want to keep a good posture."

The dowager's hump can create additional problems. Millen explains: "By placing great pressure on the spinal vertebrae, the dowager's hump often leads to compression fractures of the spinal column. This is very painful, as you can well imagine, and you do not have to do anything special for it to happen. Just going up and down stairs or taking a step can cause breakage."

Yoga also helps to improve balance and coordination. "When you are balanced and coordinated, there is less chance of your falling in the first place," Millen says. "You are quicker to respond. And that can help prevent fractures."

Millen points out that there are several styles of yoga, but that all systems have foundation poses that address the above needs. Here she outlines a few basic postures:

DOWNWARD-FACING DOG—This posture strengthens bone mass in the wrists and arms. In this pose, you stand and bring your hands to the floor so that the space beneath you is triangular. One part of the triangle is from your hands to your hips, and the other part is from your hips to your heels. The space on the floor between your hands and your feet is the third part. As you hold the position, you will feel that you are bearing weight on your arms.

WARRIOR POSES—These poses increase muscle strength and flexibility as well as balance. Here you are standing with your legs three to four feet apart, depending on your height. With your legs apart, you work at the hip to turn one leg out to the side. The other leg is turned slightly inward. That really works the hip muscles, which is important in helping to prevent the all-too-common osteoporotic hip fracture. The arms are either held out to the side or up over the head, depending upon which warrior posture it is.

COBRA—This is a back-bending pose that helps posture and gives flexibility and strength to the paraspinals, the muscles of the back of the spine. To begin, lie facedown on the floor. Using the back muscles, sequentially lift the head and chest away from the floor.

SIMPLE STRETCH FOR CHEST MUSCLES—This is another exercise for improving posture that is especially helpful for women who tend to slouch forward. Take a blanket and fold it to resemble a box of long-stemmed roses. Lie down on this bolster, making sure that your head and your entire spine are completely supported. Place your arms out to the side or up to form a V-shaped position with the palms facing up toward the ceiling. Just allow gravity to relax the shoulders down to the floor. Shoulders should not be on the blanket. Breathe deeply. That will expand the intercostals, the muscles between the ribs. This is important because the intercostals become constricted with slouching. That, in turn, decreases lung capacity and causes all the organs to become compressed. This is a wonderful pose where you don't have to actually do anything. You just allow gravity to work for you and your breath to move through you.

Millen says that the best time to begin yoga is before osteoporosis sets in. "The time to begin a yoga practice, or any exercise, is not when you've gotten to menopause, and all of a sudden you realize, 'Oh my gosh! I'm at risk for osteoporosis.' You need to build bone mass throughout your whole life so that you have bone stored up. It's like preparing for retirement. You build up bone mass through exercise, you eat right, you maintain a healthy lifestyle. Then, when you reach your menopausal years, you've got a good store of bone mass to help protect you."

BODY ROLLING

This technique, developed by Yamuna Zake, a bodyworker in New York City, uses a six- to ten-inch ball in a series of routines designed to elongate muscles and increase blood flow in all parts of the body. As you relax your body weight onto the ball, the ball applies pressure onto bone, stimulating even bone that has begun to ossify to "wake up." "To me," says Zake, "bone is like dried fruit. Just as a raisin plumps up after you put it in water, when bone is stimulated and becomes alive, it undergoes a subtle change, acquiring a supple quality.

"Studies have found that, by stimulating bone, weight-bearing exercise can prevent and possibly reverse osteoporosis. Weight bearing is nothing more than pressure exerted on bone. Body rolling is actually a mild form of weight-bearing exercise in which the pressure is never more than the person's own body weight."

ACUPUNCTURE

As mentioned earlier in this chapter, in China, osteoporosis is the exception rather than the norm. When it is present, acupuncture is used. Acupuncturist Abigail Rist-Podrecca explains how this works: "The Chinese use an electrical stimulus along the spine. The electrical impulse actually helps the bone stem cells, which are the reproductive cells of the bone, to reproduce, thereby strengthening the bone mass. It was very exciting to see this because we have some Western studies proving that peripheral stimulation by electricity, especially in the long bones in the leg, help this process also." She adds that women low in calcium need to take this supplement so that the body has the raw materials for making bones denser. When weight-bearing exercises are added, the benefits are remarkable.

HOMEOPATHY

Homeopathy can be used as an adjunct to the nutritional and lifestyle factors discussed above. Among the remedies to consider are the following:

CALCAREA PHOSPHORICA—This may help where the bones are weak, soft, curved, and brittle. It can be given for a long period of time.

CORTICOID—Homeopathic corticoid is for painful posttraumatic osteoporosis, especially when it affects the hip. Consider this remedy for an elderly person who has fractured her hip because of osteoporosis.

PARATHYROID—For diffuse pain in the bones, especially the long bones. Walking is very painful. Often, there is pain in the ankles, hips, and knees.

Regarding the appropriate potencies for these substances, the late homeopathic physician Dr. Ken Korins said, "For acute conditions, meaning they come on suddenly, and they are very intense, use a 200c potency. That is a very dilute potency, but energetically speaking, it is very powerful. For more chronic conditions, where you will be giving the remedy for a longer period of time, you might want to start with 12c or 30c. In general, the remedies should be taken as three to four pellets placed under the tongue. Take them on an empty stomach. Wait fifteen to twenty minutes before or after eating. Avoid coffee and aromatic substances, such as mints, perfumes, and camphors, which can interfere with the remedies' effectiveness. Also, it is a good idea not to touch remedies with your hands because any residues from perfumes or other substances can interfere with their energetic properties."

Research Update

An increasing body of evidence is showing the benefits of natural modalities to overall health and well-being. Following is a sample of recent peer-reviewed scientific studies relating to osteoporosis.

A 2011 study published in the *British Medical Journal* examined the effect of dried plum on bone loss in osteopenic postmenopausal women. When compared with a control group that received dried apple, the participants who received dried plum (100 grams/d) experienced significantly increased bone mineral density of the ulna and spine. In response to a 2010 analysis indicating that calcium supplements increased the risk of heart disease, Dr. Alan Gaby wrote in the *Townsend Letter* in January 2011 that although the results should be interpreted with caution, it would not be surprising if long-term monotherapy with calcium caused imbalances with other nutrients. This has occurred with other substances, including zinc, magnesium, and alpha-tocopherol, and the problem can be avoided by supplementing calcium with magnesium and silicon. Food sources of silicon include bananas, wheat bran, green beans, root vegetables, soybean meal, and beer.

Chapter 50

Parkinson's Disease

Although he attempted a comeback, Michael J. Fox, the television and film actor, has had his career cut short by Parkinson's disease. He seemed to be a young, healthy, happy, and active person. How could this have happened to him? It raises all kinds of questions as to what Parkinson's disease is and how we can prevent it. He is devoting his life now to raising awareness of Parkinson's disease.

Dr. Michael Wald describes the condition, also known as PD: "It is characterized by tremors and muscular tightness and problems with posture and reflexes. It is one of the most frequently encountered disorders and is a predominant cause of disability in those older than fifty years of age. Its prevalence is estimated at one million to two million cases in the United States, and the incidence increases with age. There are different types of Parkinson's, primary and secondary.

"Particular to PD is a loss of cells in the area of the brain known as the substantia nigra, locus cerleus, and substantia innominata, and a formation of abnormal bodies called Lewy bodies. Basically we don't know the cause, but the most likely mechanism of the cellular damage is oxidation by toxic free radicals. In particular, this oxidation might break down a certain amino acid we need for normal health and normal motor function that leads to dopamine depletion.

"Someone with PD has what is called a 'resting' tremor or 'pill-rolling' tremor, as if they were rolling something between their thumb and their first finger and their hands are moving. During sleep it fades away. If you try to move their arms and legs, the muscles are very rigid, called 'lead pipe' rigidity, and the muscles move with a 'cogwheel phenomenon.' These individuals walk very slowly and often shoot forward and fall down and hurt themselves because their motor function is skewed. Infrequency of blinking is one of the early signs and a loss of overall facial expression, a loss of voice volume, with a poverty of body movement. Reflexes are diminished."

This lack of movement is called bradykinesia, and the shuffling gait with poor arm swing is very characteristic of Parkinson's patients. One key is that the incessant tremor disappears with intentional movement and then returns as soon as the arm is at rest. There is also a very strong association between PD and depression and eventual dementia.

These clinical signs are due to the nerves in the brain starting to degenerate and are a strong clue in the diagnosis. MRIs sometimes show atrophy, or wasting, in advanced cases, but mostly the CT scan and MRIs of the brain do not show anything. The diagnosis is usually made based on the clinical picture.

Parkinson's is mostly a disease of the elderly, but it can sometimes be seen in younger people, such as Michael J. Fox. Younger people tend to develop the motor and muscle problems first. In the older population there is a much higher incidence of dementia. Other kinds of dementias can also have features that look like Parkinson's disease, and many times there is an overlap of different causes for the dementia.

Signs and Symptoms

As mentioned above, signs and symptoms of Parkinson's include shaking (tremors), stiffness and rigid limbs (generally asymmetric), extremely slow movement (bradykinesia), and impaired postural reflexes (extended arm tremor or trouble with handwriting). When two of these symptoms are present, it is probable that the patient is suffering from Parkinson's. When three or more symptoms are evident, the patient is positively considered to have Parkinson's disease.

Frequently, tremor of a hand or a leg, particularly when the person is resting, is the first indication of Parkinson's disease. The tremor often begins on one side of the body (asymmetric). Eventually, a person's voluntary movements become increasingly difficult. For example, a once-simple task such as walking becomes stiffer and slower. This is followed by speech difficulties (speaking in a hushed tone). Then the face becomes expressionless because of increased muscular rigidity. Because the person cannot control his or her facial muscles, there is often drooling. There may also be numbing of the hands and feet. Also, the person's handwriting becomes small (known as micrographia) and is illegible. Although the person's thinking processes remain normal, they are stuck inside a debilitated body. For this reason, as symptoms worsen, a great depression may set in and lead to a shortened lifespan.

Potential Causes

The cause is unknown, but there is a lot of speculation. A current theory is that PD may be caused by a toxic environmental agent or chemical compound. This is because there were reports of greater prevalence in rural areas. The herbicide Parquat is a likely culprit. Dieldrin and DDT have also been implicated. Another study by Scheider and colleagues in 1997 found that the antioxidant lycopene (found primarily in tomatoes and related products) was not associated with higher PD risk, but intake of sweet foods, including fruit, was. They theorized that pesticide residues in the fruits and vegetables may have contributed to the development of PD.

"There have been a number of studies of pesticides and insecticides," Dr. Wald says. "If you are genetically susceptible and are exposed to toxins in the soil or air, they can break down or oxidize the dopamine. In the *Journal of Neurology* they reported causing PD with pesticides, and they were able to reverse it. It is our liver that detoxifies toxins. They also say that ongoing exposure to manganese and copper of greater than twenty years will cause PD. A diet higher in mono- and disaccharides, the simple sugars, is associated with a higher risk of PD."

Dr. Jay Lombard, a neurologist who blends traditional and complementary medical approaches, has seen and treated many Parkinson's patients. He has this to add about the causes of Parkinson's: "Environmental toxins have been implicated in the etiology of Parkinson's disease, particularly pesticides. It appears that patients who have Parkinson's disease have an inability to detoxify these very common pesticides found in the environment because they lack a particular enzyme."

It is also known that certain drugs can cause a reversible form of PD. These drugs are the phenothiazines and butyrophenones, drugs that affect the central nervous system. Carbon monoxide poisoning has been known to induce a Parkinsonism.

There is widespread belief that Parkinson's is caused at least partially by a deficiency of dopamine, as well as free radical damage.

Clinical Experience

CONVENTIONAL TREATMENT

Parkinson's is generally managed with drugs, physical therapy, and surgical interventions. As of now, we do not have a way to prevent the loss of nerve cells that produce dopamine or to restore those that have already been lost. Thus, effective treatment of Parkinson's would seem to rest on the ability to halt the damage to, and death of, the nerve cells that manufacture dopamine. In fact, many individuals suffering from Parkinson's are prescribed the drug levodopa (L-dopa), which can be converted into dopamine in the brain. Levodopa is often used in combination with other drugs that appear to have protective effects on brain cells. Treatment with these drugs, however, does not completely alleviate the symptoms of Parkinson's, although the disease may progress slower. Long-term treatment with these drugs may result in neurotic or psychotic symptoms.

Research is ongoing on the effects of other drugs and methods of treating Parkinson's, including a new generation of drugs that work to mimic levodopa and inhibit the enzymes that break down levodopa in the brain. Research is also progressing on surgical options, including a brain "pacemaker" that blocks brain signals that cause tremors. In late stages of the disease, some patients are treated with a surgical option called pallidotomy, in which a small section of the globus pallidus is destroyed. Some patients also undergo thalatomy, another surgical procedure that destroys a specific group of cells in the thalamus (the brain's communication center).

Neurotrophic proteins and neuroprotective agents are also being studied, along with neural tissue transplants and genetic engineering. Obviously, Parkinson's is a serious condition, and professional medical management and prescription drugs are crucial in staving off the progression of the disease and maintaining quality of life. Recent advances in molecular science, however, are beginning to alter the diagnostic approach to Parkinson's and the ways in which we approach treatment of the condition. Prior to these recent developments, the chief focus—and rightfully so—was on oxidative damage. Now, other causes—mitochondrial damage, excitotoxicity, and inflammatory cytokines—are being examined for the part they play in the death of brain cells. At some point in the future, the chief cause of Parkinson's may be determined to have come from this group. But, as of now, any of these can lead directly to Parkinson's. Hence, the treatment modality should be multifaceted.

NATURAL THERAPIES

Although full-blown Parkinson's can be crippling or disabling, early symptoms of the disease may be so subtle and gradual that patients attribute them to other causes. Even if your doctor is fairly certain you are suffering from Parkinson's, there is much you can do in the early stages that may help to slow the progression of the disease. Exercises involving weight training have been linked to increasing testosterone levels that, in turn, elevate dopamine levels. Hence, exercising is crucial in fighting Parkinson's. Exercise also reduces stress, which has been found to aggravate the symptoms of Parkinson's. Specific exercises, such as those taught by the Alexander Technique, which focuses on ridding your body of harmful tensions through improving the mechanics of moving your body in day-to-day activities, may offer particular benefit to individuals suffering from Parkinson's.

When a person first exhibits these symptoms, it is traumatic. From a physical perspective, doctors generally treat the problems associated with motor functioning, for they are extremely alarming to someone who has never had sluggish movement of their limbs or rigidity. Though the patient is being treated for these physical symptoms, the doctor should also address the anticipated cognitive decline, for this greatly affects quality of life.

Older adults commonly develop drug-induced Parkinson's disease after having been prescribed antipsychotic drugs, such as Haldol, Thorazine, Mellaril, and Stelazine. These antipsychotics are used to sedate nursing home patients with dementia and chronic anxiety, two nonpsychotic disorders. When these drugs are discontinued, most newly diagnosed Parkinson's patients return to normal.

DIET

Your diet should incorporate mostly alkaline foods, with green drinks, such as chlorella, spirulina, barley grass, or wheatgrass, once or twice a day. Eat fruits and vegetables that provide a good supply of antioxidants, which are critical for overcoming oxidative damage to the brain and slowing down progression of the disease. Research has shown that a combination of antioxidants can mimic chelating agents. (A chelating agent is a water-soluble molecule that can bond tightly with metal ions, keeping them from coming out of suspension and allowing them to be flushed from the system.) For maximum results, I suggest trying a combination of the C and E vitamins, polyphenols (found in green and black tea), bioflavonoids, proanthocyanidins (in grape seed extract and pine bark extract), and curcumin.

Foods such as red peppers and onions that contain glutathione (a metabolite of the essential amino acid methionine) are thought to be beneficial, as are broccoli, cauliflower, brussels sprouts, and cabbage, which are rich in cyanohydroxybutene (a naturally occurring chemical that helps increase glutathione levels).

It is important to choose organic foods. Unheated extra virgin olive oil and herbs for flavoring should be used. Sugar and fat should be avoided, as research has shown diets high in sugar triple the risk of developing Parkinson's, while diets high in fats result in a fivefold increase in the odds of developing Parkinson's. You should also avoid wheat, dairy, and gluten products, margarine, fried foods, polyunsaturated oils, artificial sweeteners, processed food (e.g., deli meats), monosodium glutamate (MSG), alcohol (except red wine), and water containing chlorine or fluoride. (Remember, this not only applies to the water you drink but also the water you bathe in; for best results, purchase a water filter, or be sure to keep your mouth closed while showering.) Do not use microwave ovens to cook your foods. Individuals who are taking the prescription drug levodopa should limit protein intake to one meal per day, eaten late in the day, because protein hinders the absorption of levodopa.

SUPPLEMENTS

Certain vitamins and minerals may be beneficial in preventing and impacting the symptoms of Parkinson's disease.

Vitamin B_6 is essential in the synthesis of dopamine. When taken with zinc, it can help stimulate the production of dopamine. While adding foods rich in B vitamins to your diet is fine at any time, when you use vitamin B supplements in combination with levodopa, the vitamin B may act to stimulate production of dopamine in other areas of the body, with less reaching the brain. Therefore, if you and your health care provider decide to try supplementing with vitamin B, you should take it either at the end of the day after the last dose of levodopa, or at intervals between doses of levodopa. I recommend increasing your daily vitamin B_6 supplement from 75 milligrams to 150 milligrams. Do not exceed a daily supplement of 150 milligrams.

Vitamin C may help to slow the progression of Parkinson's symptoms and counteract severe side effects of levodopa. It appears to be even more effective when paired with other antioxidants, such as vitamin E. I recommend increasing your daily vitamin C supplement from 500 to 1,000 milligrams to 3,000 milligrams, taken in three divided doses. For Vitamin E, I recommend increasing your daily supplement from 268 milligrams to 536 milligrams. Do not exceed a daily supplement of 536 milligrams.

Zinc, a cofactor of vitamin B, may help with control of symptoms, such as tremors and rigidity, and may improve walking skills and bladder control. I recommend a daily supplement of 30 milligrams.

A number of other naturally occurring nutrients have beneficial impacts on the symptoms of Parkinson's disease. Coenzyme Q10 (CoQ10) is the most important nutrient for people over thirty. Because the cells of our bodies need CoQ10 to produce energy and to combat mitochondrial free radical activity, a CoQ10 deficiency can result in a greater incidence of many degenerative diseases associated with aging. It should be taken with the fattiest meal of your day. When consumed in an oil-based capsule, the CoQ10 can be absorbed through the lymphatic canals for better distribution throughout the entire body. I recommend increasing your daily supplement from 100 to 300 milligrams to 1,200 milligrams.

Glutathione, a metabolite of the essential amino acid methionine, is an important part of the body's antioxidant defense system. Studies of the substantia nigra after death in Parkinson's disease sufferers have shown the depletion of glutathione. To impact the symptoms of Parkinson's, I recommend a supplement of 200 milligrams taken twice daily.

Melatonin, a hormone manufactured by the pineal gland in the brain, is released into the bloodstream and is involved in synchronizing the body's hormone secretions and setting daily biorhythms. In a study conducted at Thomas Jefferson University, researchers showed that melatonin was effective in blocking the oxidative damage in dopamine-producing cells, thereby reducing or blocking Parkinsonian effects. To help ease the symptoms of Parkinson's disease, I recommend supplementing with 300 micrograms to 1 milligram, taken a half hour before bed two or three nights per week.

N-Acetylcysteine (NAC), an important amino acid that enhances the production of glutathione, can help protect the brain from free radicals and minimize age-related deterioration of the nervous system. I recommend supplementing daily with 1,500 milligrams taken in three doses of 500 milligrams.

Nicotinamide Adenine Dinucleotide (NADH) is an enzyme that helps improve neurotransmitter function. It helps prevent cellular degeneration, and may increase concentration and memory capacity. I recommend a supplement of 2.5 milligrams taken twice daily.

Proanthocyanidins (chemical relatives of bioflavonoids) serve to benefit the brain in a twofold manner: They are antioxidants, and they protect collagen. Research has shown that proanthocyanidins are fifty times more powerful antioxidants than vitamins C and E. Intricate tests prove that proanthocyanidins are great killers of the hydroxyl radical—the free radical that is responsible for the most damage—and lipid peroxides (rancid fats). Although proanthocyanidins can be found in the diet, the levels in food are generally insufficient to help fight the symptoms of Parkinson's disease. I recommend increasing your daily supplement from 80 milligrams to 380 milligrams, taken in three divided doses. Do not exceed a daily supplement of 380 milligrams.

Fish oil is abundant in omega-3 fatty acids that have been shown to support neurological health in Parkinson's patients. I recommend taking 2,000 to 4,000 milligrams daily of a purified fish oil concentrate. Consult with your doctor if taking anticoagulant or antiplatelet medications or have a bleeding disorder.

HERBAL REMEDIES

Some herbal extracts have properties similar to conventional medications, but are gentler and may lack the drugs' side effects. Always inform your medical practitioner of any herbal remedies you may be taking.

- Atmagupta (Mucuma pruins) is an Ayurvedic herb that contains the natural form of L-dopa. Ayurvedic herbs are commonly taken in combination to neutralize toxicity. Do not take this without consulting with your doctor.
- Gotu kola has been historically used in the treatment of Parkinson's disease. I recommend taking it as a tea once daily. Do not use gotu kola if you take medication for diabetes or to control cholesterol. If gotu kola is safe for you to take, I recommend 200 milligrams taken three times daily.
- Ginkgo biloba is an extract of the ginkgo plant used in Europe to help fight dementia and Alzheimer's disease. It is a circulatory stimulant and an antioxidant. Ginkgo can act as an anticoagulant, and individuals taking anticoagulant and antithrombotic drugs such as ASA, anti-inflammatories, and warfarin or Coumadin should consult with their doctor

before taking ginkgo. If ginkgo is safe for you to use, I recommend a supplement of 120 milligrams per day, taken in three equal doses.

- Hawthorn acts as a circulatory stimulant and potent antioxidant. I recommend a supplement of 2 to 5 grams per day.
- Lady's slipper may help provide relief from tremors. I recommend 10 to 30 drops of tincture taken three or four times daily.
- Milk thistle can provide liver support and detoxification. I recommend a supplement of 30 to 60 drops of tincture per day.
- Skullcap acts to strengthen the brain. I recommend 10 to 30 drops of tincture per day.
- Curcumin, derived from the turmeric spice popular in Indian cuisine, is a beneficial phytochemical that has been shown to shield against oxidative stress and inflammation related to neurodegenerative illness. I recommend taking a daily supplement of 400 to 4,000 milligrams. Do not take if you have gallbladder problems or gallstones. Consult with your doctor if taking anti-coagulant or anti-platelet medications or have a bleeding disorder.
- Also recommended are Cytokine Supress with EGCG (300 mg), resveratrol (200 mg, 2x day), black cumin seed oil (1 tsp, 3x day), coconut oil (1 tsp, 3x day), Brain Shield & Cognitex (as directed).

HOMEOPATHIC REMEDIES

The following remedies may be used for relief from the symptoms of Parkinson's disease. When dealing with a chronic condition, homeopathic remedies must be used in conjunction with other therapies, as prescribed by a qualified health professional. Consult with your health care provider before taking any homeopathic remedy, and follow your provider's recommendation for the appropriate dosage. Always inform your medical practitioner of any homeopathic remedies you may be taking.

- Anthimonium tartaricum may help with trembling head and immobile hands.
- Gelsemium may provide relief from trembling and drooping eyelids.
- Agarius is for limbs that are stiff but tremble and twitch; your back and spine may be especially sensitive.
- Rhus toxicodendron is good for mild tremors and stiffness that feels better after movement but worse with damp weather.

DETOXIFICATION

Chelation therapy eliminates metals from the brain, as well as other toxic agents that encourage free radicals development. A hair analysis can determine whether high levels of metals need to be chelated out of the body. Studies indicate that to properly impact Parkinson's disease, effective treatments must reduce oxidative stress. Chelation therapy plays an important role in eliminating iron as well as other toxins from the brain. These toxins infuse the brain with free radicals. Some think that chelation can only occur through chelation therapy. Antioxidants can also play the role of chelators, however. The C and E vitamins, bioflavonoids, polyphenols (from black and green teas), grape seed extract (specifically, the proanthocyanidins), and tocotrienols from curcumin also serve as chelators.

AROMATHERAPY

Essential oils can be used in baths or inhaled to provide rebalancing effects. Do not apply essential oils directly to the skin; they must be mixed with carrier oils. Though massaging with fragrant essential oils will not cure Parkinson's, it can provide temporary relief. Experiment with various scents to see which brings you relief: clary sage, marjoram, and lavender.

SPECIFIC TREATMENT APPROACHES

Dr. Lombard follows three general strategies in attempting to prevent progression of the disease. He remarks, "These strategies are useful for other neurodegenerative conditions as well. We know the immune system is overactive in particular ways that are destructive to the brains of Parkinson's patients. We know that patients with Parkinson's have an inability to handle a particular metal found in our diets called iron and we know that Parkinson's patients may have a deficiency of a part of the cell called the mitochondria that is responsible for the manufacture of ATP [adenosine triphosphate, which is involved in the storage and transfer of cellular energy]. Using these three evidences, a comprehensive program can be drawn up that addresses each of these issues separately.

"In regard to excessive inflammation, certain types of white blood cells make a compound called nitrous oxide, which is a free radical. It is very destructive to areas of the brain in Parkinson's disease. There are certain antioxidants that are effective in quenching or inhibiting the effects of this free radical. These include an extract of green tea that has profound antioxidant properties. Dihydrolypoic acid, which is a glutathione precursor, increases brain glutathione levels and is very effective as an antioxidant. Lycopenol is another antioxidant that crosses the blood-brain barrier and inhibits excessive free radical activity.

"Second, we know Parkinson's patients have too much iron in their brains, and iron acts as a free-radical inducer. So we try buffering the effects of increased iron with a protein called lactoferrin. This prevents excessive iron absorption from the intestinal tract into the bloodstream.

"Finally the mitochondria, the energy-producing units of the cell that make ATP, are also deficient in Parkinson's patients. Ways of increasing the mitochondria include coenzyme Q10, serotonin, and two other compounds: NADH, which is also called ignatia, and ubiquinone, which is a coenzyme Q10 analog. They dramatically increase brain ATP levels. These three things are a very worthwhile strategy for treating a Parkinson's patient."

Dr. Wald has devised a detoxification program that he feels is worthwhile for PD. "Beta-carotene has been fairly well studied in PD. It is an antioxidant, and I use about 50,000 units. It helps protect the liver and other cells and the nervous system from premature degeneration. Vitamin C helps protect dopamine, an important neurotransmitter that is low in those with PD."

"Essential fatty acids, such as omega-3 and omega-6, are important for protecting the nervous system. Toxins in our environment known as zenobiotics are fat soluble, meaning they love to hang out in the nervous system. We need to take all the antioxidants . . . with essential fatty acids such as omega-3 and omega-6. So we want to get vitamin E, 400 to 800 IU a day, and vitamin C to balance tolerance. Some of the studies show PD patients have low levels of vitamin B_3, niacin. There is a nonflushing form called hexaniacinite, 250 milligrams a day. Melatonin is a very important hormone not just for sleep and repair but also as an important antioxidant in the nervous system. It slows down the breakdown of dopamine. Another important amino acid is N-acetyl cysteine or NAC. It is used by the liver to convert fat-soluble toxins into water-soluble toxins so that we can excrete them in the urine. The body must be able to eliminate toxins once they are mobilized. Any detoxification program needs to focus on the liver and intestine and the lymphatic system and so on to get these things out."

Dr. Wald adds, "Glutathione has been found to be low in PD. The most effective way to increase it is with Vitamin C. Glutathione is not only an immune booster but helps fight degenerative changes. It tends to become lower as we age."

Gary Null's Additional Supplements for Parkinson's Disease

The following chart summarizes the supplements I recommend adding to the protocol for overall brain health from chapter 16. In some cases, I recommend increasing the dose of a particular vitamin or supplement to specifically impact Parkinson's disease. In these cases, you should increase the daily dosage from chapter 16 to the level recommended for this specific condition. This protocol is designed for individuals who suffer from, or are specifically concerned about, Parkinson's disease. If you are concerned about additional conditions discussed in other chapters, consult with a health professional about how you can safely impact multiple conditions. If you are taking medications, whether prescription or over-the-counter, or have any food restrictions, consult with your doctor before beginning any supplement program. Your health care provider should always be up-to-date on all vitamins, supplements, and herbal or homeopathic remedies you are taking. Supplement overdoses are rare, but possible, and certain combinations may affect individuals adversely.

SUPPLEMENT	DOSAGE	CAUTIONS
Brain Shield and Cognitex	as directed	
black cumin seed oil	1 tsp, three times daily	
coconut oil	1 tsp, three times daily	
coenzyme Q10 (coQ10)	Increase daily dosage from 300 mg to 1,600 mg.	Do not exceed a daily supplement of 2,000 mg. Take with

		fattiest meal of the day. If going higher, do so under medical supervision. Dosage should be gradually increased, with 300 mg daily added over a six-week period until the daily dose reaches 2,000 mg. Individuals supplementing with coQ10 at high doses should be monitored closely by their doctors.
Cytokine Suppress with EGCG	300 mg	
glutathione	200 mg two times daily	Glutathione levels may also be elevated through supplementation with cysteine, N-acetylcysteine, or L-cysteine.
melatonin	300 mcg–1 mg two to three nights per week, a half hour before bed	Tolerance may develop with regular use. Long-term effects of nightly use are unknown.
N-acetylcysteine	1,500 mg in three . divided doses	Regular supplementation increases urinary output of copper. If supplementing for an extended period, add 2 mg of copper and 30 mg of zinc daily.
Nicotinamide adenine Dinucleotide (NADH)	2.5 mg twice daily	High doses (10 mg per day or more) may cause nervousness, anxiety, and insomnia.

proanthocyanidins	Increase daily dosage from 80 mg to 380 mg, taken in three divided doses. Do not exceed a daily supplement of 380 mg.	
resveratrol	200 mg twice daily	
vitamin B$_6$	Increase daily dosage from 75 mg to 150 mg. Do not exceed a daily supplement of 150 mg. Take with zinc (30 mg).	Contraindicated for use with levodopa. Discuss with your health care provider.
vitamin C	Increase daily dosage from 500–1,000 mg to 10,000 mg, taken in three divided doses.	
vitamin E	Increase daily dosage from 400 mg to 800 mg. Do not exceed a daily supplement of 1,000 mg.	If you have high blood pressure, limit your supplemental vitamin E to 268 mg daily. If you are taking blood thinners, consult with your doctor before taking vitamin E.
zinc	Up to 30 mg daily	Large doses (50 mg or more) can interfere with the body's absorption of essential minerals, impair blood cell function, and depress immune system.

Research Update

An increasing body of evidence is showing the benefits of natural modalities to overall health and well-being. Following is a sample of recent peer-reviewed scientific studies relating to Parkinson's disease.

An article on the *Life Extension* website provides an in-depth look at

Parkinson's disease, citing numerous research studies on alternative treatment methods. A 2011 report published in the *American Journal of Psychiatry* revealed that symptoms of depression improved in 56 percent of patients with Parkinson's disease who participated in cognitive-behavioral therapy as compared with 8 percent who were monitored clinically. A 2011 report in the *European Journal of Neuroscience* showed in an animal model that eighteen weeks of treadmill exercise offered neuroprotective effects, including improvement in movement and balance coordination. Mucuna seed extract was shown in a 2010 study published in *Parkinsonism & Related Disorders* to provide long-term relief of symptoms similar to traditional treatment, but without the side effects such as drug-induced dyskinesias (movement disorders). In 2012, a report in *Neurology* concluded that intake of some flavonoids may reduce Parkinson's disease risk, particularly in men. The researchers examined five major sources of flavonoid-rich foods: tea, berry fruits, apples, red wine, and oranges/orange juice. Other useful treatments and preventive substances include vitamin B_6, coenzyme Q10, carnitine, and resveratrol.

Chapter 51

Pregnancy

What we in the United States accept as the safest, most acceptable way to give birth is a historical anomaly—something that has existed for some hundred years and is not practiced in the rest of the world. Suzanne Arms, an independent researcher and activist who has published seven books on pregnancy and women's health, including *Immaculate Deception*, *Breast Feeding*, and *Seasons of Change*, explains.

"In other parts of the world," she says, "childbirth is seen as a natural process. The only exceptions are areas where American obstetrics and neonatal approaches have been aggressively promoted and marketed. Many European countries and a growing number of third world countries are gradually adopting these practices as they buy our wares, such as neonatal monitoring devices."

In the US, the vast preponderance of women give birth in hospitals. They are led to believe, Arms explains, that the larger the hospital, the better the care. They are told that the more narrow the subspecialization training of their doctors, the safer the birth will be. So women don't want to go to a general practitioner (GP), but instead go to a perinatologist with a subspecialty in obstetrics. Says Arms, "Although we do have midwives in hospitals and birthing centers outside hospitals, and we do legally permit home births, fewer than 5 percent of births are done with these resources, even if we count births done with midwives in hospitals."

Most of the world—the US being a large exception—sees the natural way of giving birth as the sanest and healthiest way to bring a child into the world. After examining the issue of natural childbirth and American attitudes toward it, this chapter will turn to the stages of pregnancy, certain things you must avoid to have a safe pregnancy, and the many things you can do to make pregnancy as healthy and uncomplicated as possible.

Natural Childbirth

One reason for the greater American preference for hospital births as compared to the rest of the world is that Americans have been led to believe you are risking the baby and the mother if you choose not to have a hospital birth. But, Arms points out, "If we look at the facts, we see this is not true." In the United States, there has been very little comparative study of the benefits of home delivery versus hospital births. "Therefore, to actually compare the safety of hospital and home births," she says, "we have to go to a place like England, where they have very good national statistics on births and they have commissioned studies to see which are the safer methods."

Back in the 1970s, a controversial study appeared called the Peel Report. It was used to support a belief among politicians that home birth should be outlawed. At the time, Marjorie Tew, a statistician who was not involved in the controversy but happened to be analyzing statistics in a number of epidemiological areas, noted flaws in the report. She restudied the statistics on home births and found these births were as safe as hospital births. This was true not only for low-risk women—those who enter the process in a healthy state—but even for those with problems.

As a result of these findings, England has reversed its policy, which had been focused on eliminating home births and getting rid of midwifery. The country has gone back to supporting midwives, birthing centers, and local home births. They are finding that hospitals are not the best place to give birth. "In fact," Arms concludes, "there is no study that shows a hospital is a safer place than alternative venues for giving birth."

One aspect of women's fear of birth is that they think it will be unendurably painful. So, in many cases, they fill themselves with painkillers before the process even begins.

Arms recognizes this tendency. She says, "Those who advocate natural childbirth are often asked, 'Why should modern women experience painful childbirth rather than benefit from the painkillers modern medicine provides?'"

The issue of pain is a complex one, in her view. "Our media tell us that we should be free of any pain and discomfort in our lives. If you look at TV advertising, billboards, and so on, you see there are a tremendous number of products geared to the elimination of the pain that occurs in pathological conditions. We are taught we shouldn't have to experience pain. Since we are used to taking drugs for everything else, why not for labor? But childbirth is not a pathology and the cause of pain during birth is not a disease."

In addition, the potential problems caused by drugs and anesthesia need to be addressed. Drugs and anesthesia can distort and warp the birth process and make it harder for the baby to do the work he or she is supposed to do. They can complicate labor and make birth a pathological problem, something that we do, in fact, need to treat in the hospital.

Midwifery

The most important difference between midwifery and traditional medicine is that medicine treats disease, whereas midwifery is about preventing complications while going through a natural process. Obstetrics, a subspecialty of medicine, seems to consider birth "too unwieldy." Doctors need to get in and out of the hospital quickly, so they want to control the length of time a woman is in labor and how long it takes to give birth. However, the natural variability of giving birth does not conform to their standard. Each human body is unique, as is each human psyche. A four-hour labor may be normal. A thirty-six-hour labor may also be normal. But under a physician's management, a day and a half is too long.

Medicine focuses on giving drugs and doing surgery. Midwifery concentrates on following through the process normally, spotting problems as they arise and treating them as simply as possible before they become complications, while teaching people how to handle contingencies.

Midwife Jeanette Breen is a great enthusiast of using water during labor. "It has a wonderful analgesic quality, which is much better than an epidural. Being immersed in water provides tremendous relaxation. It does not take the pain away, but women do report feeling less pain in the water. They feel less effect from the pull of gravity. Their movements are very easy, and there is much better tissue relaxation, which means there is almost no tearing in a water birth. It is also easier for the baby because the mother is more relaxed and moving freely. She is not stuck in one position. It is easier for the baby to negotiate the pelvis and to slip out into a warm, moist environment that is quite familiar.

"Two keys to a normal healthy pregnancy and birth are a healthy diet and good social support," says Breen. "Those seem to be overlooked, especially in traditional maternity care in this country. The focus is on diagnostic testing, but not a lot of emphasis is placed on healthy diets, other than prescribing prenatal vitamins and iron. There is no question that a high-quality diet rich in all the nutrients can make a woman's whole body work more efficiently and effectively.

"Social support creates an environment of love that is all-important, but too often overlooked in hospital birthing environments, which focus solely on technology. No one can have the baby for the pregnant woman; she has to do it herself. But if she is surrounded by love and support rather than fear and technology, she is able to give birth in a very intuitive, instinctual way which is satisfying and safe."

Stages of Pregnancy

A woman's body undergoes numerous changes during each stage of pregnancy. These physiological changes are described by nurse practitioner and massage therapist Susan Lacina.

FIRST TRIMESTER

"The fetus grows rapidly, and the mother's body changes to support this swift development. Hormonal balance changes. Human chorionic gonadotropin hormone (HCG) is needed for development. As it is released, it causes many discomforts, such as breast tenderness, digestive problems, nausea, and vomiting. Progesterone levels increase and may cause mild hyperventilation, heartburn, indigestion, and constipation. Increased blood flow and its change in composition contribute to fatigue, overheating, and sinus congestion."

SECOND TRIMESTER

In the second trimester, the placenta becomes responsible for hormone production, and the levels of HCG drop. "Along with that, the discomforts of nausea and vomiting ease up," Lacina says. "Physical growth of the fetus crowds the abdomen, and a woman's body expands to accommodate the growth. Fetal production of thyroid stimulating hormone (TSH) begins in the fourteenth week and causes the mother's thyroid level to increase. This can lead to irritability, mood swings, mild depression, increased pulse rate, and hot flashes. Adrenal hormones become elevated and remain that way until delivery. This may cause impaired glucose tolerance and swelling.

"Skeletal structure becomes softer and more flexible to allow for expansion. If a woman doesn't have enough muscle flexibility, she will have some pain, for tight muscles do not allow for these adjustments. She may experience sciatic nerve pain from the lower back down the back of her legs due to the extension of the pelvis, especially at the joint of the sacrum and the pelvic bone. The growing baby puts pressure on the inferior vena cava, which can cause light-headedness, nausea, drowsiness, and clamminess. Prolonged reduction of blood flow can cause backaches and hemorrhoids. Lying on the side decreases this problem."

Starting at week twenty, abdominal muscles and ligaments stretch to support the uterus. "There may be abdominal pain," Lacine says. "There is an increase in melanin production, causing darkening of the nipples and a line called the linea nigra down the abdomen. If the lymph drainage system is not functioning well, an excess of melanin in the skin can cause brown spots. A well-functioning lymph drainage system is believed to keep melanin levels down so that brown spots do not occur. Increased progesterone causes sinus congestion, postnasal drip, and bleeding gums. Increased capillary permeability may cause the hands and feet to swell."

THIRD TRIMESTER

During the third trimester the expectant mother changes posture to shift her center of gravity. "Heavier breasts can cause shoulders to slump forward," Lacine says. "The spine is pulled out of alignment, and this commonly causes backaches. The growing fetus also compresses the veins and the lymphatic system. That can cause ankle edema and varicose veins. There is increased pressure on the intestines and bladder, causing frequent urination and constipation. Pressure on the sciatic nerve can cause more lower back and leg pain. As the diaphragm starts to rise, breathing becomes more difficult. Insomnia is common."

Miscarriage

Surprisingly, two-thirds of all pregnancies end up as miscarriages. One reason is that many women miscarry before they even know they are pregnant. Most commonly, genetic abnormalities precipitate the problem. The embryo develops wrongly, and the woman's body naturally aborts the fetus. Endocrine system imbalances are also associated with miscarriages. Women in their late forties have an especially difficult time carrying to term because of hormonal changes that accompany aging. Poor thyroid gland functioning can also interfere with pregnancy, as can intercourse during pregnancy.

Another cause of miscarriages is low-grade infections, which are often the result of sexually transmitted diseases. The woman is not conscious that a problem exists, but the body knows, and rejects the fetus. Bladder infections are also common; as the uterus enlarges, it places great pressure on this organ. Miscarriages may also occur when women are too hard on their bodies. Women who push themselves to the limit by overexercising and undereating to the point of anorexia are risking miscarriage. They are not getting enough nutrition for their own bodies, much less for the fetus.

When a miscarriage occurs more than once, a woman needs to have a thorough medical workup. Once the problem is understood, it is often correctable. If a woman is having intercourse during pregnancy, for example, she may simply need to take precautions. Using a condom during intercourse can prevent a miscarriage because it keeps male prostaglandins out of the female system, which, in turn, prevents premature uterine contractions. Low-grade infections must be cleared up, and increasing the intake of liquids and vitamin C can sometimes do the trick. Mixing 4 ounces of strawberry juice with 4 ounces of water is an especially good source of vitamin C, which acidifies the urine and helps prevent bladder infections. More serious infections should be cultured and treated appropriately. Sometimes, this means taking antibiotics. Older women who are having a difficult time holding on to a pregnancy due to hormonal changes may need low doses of progesterone, about 25 milligrams, in suppository form.

Some herbs seem to prevent miscarriage. Midwife Jeanine Parvati Baker uses the following formula. She mixes together 1 ounce wild yam root, 1 ounce Mitchella repens (also called partridgeberry, twinberry, squawvine, or partridge root). Baker also adds 1/2 ounce false unicorn root and 1/2 ounce cramp bark. She puts them together in a half-gallon jar, fills it to the top with boiling water, and lets it sit for about four hours. You can sip this brew slowly until you are over the symptoms of miscarriage or, if you are just worried about your pregnancy, drink a half cup each day.

Healthy Pregnancy the Natural Way

WHAT TO AVOID DURING PREGNANCY

Before describing the positive steps you can take to make your pregnancy, labor, and time after delivery as healthy as possible, I want to note some things, a few of which are normally benign, that you should avoid.

According to natural childbirth educators, it is well known that the health of a baby's parents affects the health of the baby. If the mother has an overgrowth of candida, so may the child. If the father is a heavy drinker, this may cause liver problems for the child. During the first two months after conception, women and their fetuses are the most sensitive to toxins, hair dyes, aspirin, and so on. Thus it is of paramount importance that a woman be aware of what things can have a detrimental effect on her growing fetus.

CERTAIN VITAMIN SUPPLEMENTS

Women must also be careful about taking vitamin supplements. Women who take 10,000 units of vitamin A during the first six weeks of pregnancy are five times more likely to have a child with birth defects than women who don't take the vitamin. "I believe that during her fertile years a woman should be quite cautious about taking supplements," Weed says. "Of course, we want to get those good vitamins, but we want to try to get them from our fruits, our vegetables, our beans, and so on."

It is not only vitamin A that can lead to birth defects; vitamins D and E are also potentially dangerous. "Those three are oil-soluble vitamins," says Weed, "and they tend to be quite detrimental to fetal development when taken in pill form."

CERTAIN MEDICATIONS AND HERBAL THERAPIES

Avoid aspirin and certainly antihistamines. This last is a hard one, especially for women who are dealing with hay fever. Antihistamines have a fairly tarnished record when it comes to causing birth defects, Weed says. "I don't just mean drug antihistamines but herbal ones as well, such as ma huang or ephedra."

Laxatives are not the way to go. Unfortunately many people use them and, even worse, many misguided herbalists even suggest women use them to clean out. Of course, there's nothing to clean out. All laxatives, Weed believes, should be avoided by all people, but especially by women during their fertile years, or at least if they are having a baby or trying to get pregnant. This includes herbal laxatives like senna, aloe, castor oil, rhubarb root, buckthorn, and cascara sagrada. Even a bulk-producing laxative like flaxseed should be taken with some caution. To use it, buy the whole flaxseed, grind it up, and sprinkle a small amount into foods.

Generally, you should stay away from diuretics. A woman in her fertile years usually doesn't take them anyway, but anyone inclined to take diuretics should be aware that they could cause problems. Herbal diuretics such as juniper berries and buchu can also cause problems. Avoid hair dyes, all kinds of chemical stimulants and depressants, antinausea drugs, sulfa drugs, vaccines, and anesthetics, especially at the dentist's office.

Weed notes, "There is some question about what happens if we take steroid-like herbs. The more we look into steroids, the more widely we find them spread across the herbal kingdom. As a matter of fact, carrots, the regular carrots you find in the supermarket, contain so many phytohormones that generous use of carrots may prevent conception. We know that wild carrot seed, in fact all parts of the carrot plant, act to prevent contact between the egg and the sperm and prevent that egg from attaching to the uterine wall. So we often advise pregnant women to avoid drinking any carrot juice at all and to cut back on the amount of carrots they are eating."

There are a few other herbs that you need to avoid only if you have miscarried frequently. They include many herbs in the mint family, such as basil, thyme, sage, rosemary, marjoram, savory, and peppermint itself.

OTHER THINGS TO AVOID

It won't surprise you to learn that smoking and drinking are not good for your fetus. Radiation is not good, so even a mammogram should be avoided during pregnancy or if you think you are going to get pregnant. Caffeine in any form should be avoided. Coffee and lattes, tea, and many soft drinks contain generous amounts of caffeine, and all can cause birth defects. Nutritionist Gracia Perlstein also says to avoid chemical exposure to toxic household cleansers, as well as fumes from paints, thinners, solvents, wood preservatives, varnishes, glues, spray adhesives, benzene, dry cleaning fluid, anything chemically based and questionable. A 2014 study found high levels of the commonly used herbicide glyphosate (Roundup) in the breast milk of 30 percent of women tested. It had already been found in urine and drinking water.

Perlstein also counsels women to avoid a toxic psychological environment. "As much as possible, avoid stress, negative people, and aggravating situations. Instead, try to spend quality time alone and with loved ones, people who are supportive. Spend time in nature. Read inspiring literature. Listen to beautiful music. This has a beneficial effect on your mental and emotional state. That, in turn, affects your baby's biochemistry."

DIET

The best insurance for a well baby is to follow a highly nutritious whole-foods diet. What you eat now will impact the health of your child later, according to nutritionist Gracia Perlstein. "When a woman is considering pregnancy, it is important that she address her diet to see how healthful it is, as many difficulties have their root in prenatal deficiencies. Scientific studies reveal that birth defects, and even problems that develop much later in life, can be prevented when the mother has excellent nutrition. I would like to include the father there too, because the quality of the sperm is also very important." Since the most crucial stage of embryonic development occurs in the first few weeks, before a woman realizes that she is pregnant, good-quality foods should be eaten all the time.

Eating properly means selecting unprocessed or minimally processed foods. A wide assortment of whole grains, legumes, vegetables, fruits, nuts, and seeds supplies multiple nutrients. "So many people eat the same ten or twenty foods over and over again," Perlstein says. "In traditional cultures, people have much more variety. I would like to emphasize that supplements should only enhance an excellent diet. Make the effort to eat high-quality, nutrient-dense foods. That means whole foods, the way nature produced them."

The body intuitively knows what it needs to support new life, and paying attention to its messages can be a helpful guide. "A woman's body is very wise when she is pregnant. Many women can't stand the look or smell of coffee or cigarettes, even when they used to smoke or drink coffee several times a day," states Perlstein. She adds that worrying about eating the right foods all the time is stressful and can produce more harm than good. But nutrition education can benefit women with highly processed diets, who need to learn about better food choices. "Vegetarian women may crave animal foods or be drawn to dairy when they are pregnant. Usually it is good to pay attention to these cravings, but to respond in the most wholesome way possible."

Wholesome means organically grown. Pesticide-free fare is better for everyone, of course, but vitally important for young children and developing fetuses, according to recent research. Dairy and other animal products should be from creatures naturally raised. One reason for this is that pesticides and other contaminants tend to concentrate in an animal's tissues. The higher up the food chain, the higher the concentration of toxins. Fortunately, many health food stores, and more and more supermarkets, sell the healthful varieties.

Animal products, when a part of the diet, should be eaten in moderation.

Although protein needs increase during pregnancy, they can be easily met from vegetarian sources, which are less toxic than their animal counterparts. Excellent vegetarian protein sources include fortified soy milk, tofu, tempeh, beans, nuts, and seeds, for example.

The increased need for calcium is similarly fulfilled in such a diet. "Many women do not realize that there are excellent sources of calcium other than milk and dairy. There are green leafy vegetables, fortified soy milk, tofu, almonds, and many other calcium-containing foods. If you eat a diet rich in fresh vegetables and fruits, you tend to get quite a bit of calcium. If you want a supplement, calcium citrate is easiest on the stomach. Other forms sometimes cause digestive upsets or constipation. Definitely avoid calcium-depleting foods: coffee, chocolate, and sodium."

Perlstein adds that eating several small meals throughout the day offsets common complications: "Hunger, not calorie counting, is the most reliable guide to eating during pregnancy. Five to six small, nutrient-dense meals per day is a sensible ideal. This is a good habit to develop in the last trimester of pregnancy, when the organs in your stomach are somewhat constricted, and good in the early stages to prevent nausea. It keeps the blood sugar from falling, and nausea has a lot to do with low blood sugar."

Water should be pure and taken in adequate amounts. Eight to twelve glasses are recommended to help flush out toxins from the liver and kidneys: "Many people do not drink enough fluids," notes Perlstein. "This is especially important during pregnancy because the woman is filtering the waste for two bodies."

VITAMIN SUPPLEMENTS
Perlstein recommends the following daily nutrients for pregnant women: multiple vitamin and mineral supplement, vitamin C, B_{12}, zinc, and folic acid. Folic acid, which is also contained in green leafy vegetables and whole grains, is especially important in pregnancy because science has shown it to prevent neural tube defects. Even when included in the diet, extra folic acid should be taken in supplement form, since it is fragile and easily damaged by heat. Additionally, acidophilus helps prevent constipation and other types of colon problems.

Extra iron may be needed, but a woman should have her hemoglobin tested first, just to be sure it is really needed. Research shows that excess iron in the system can have damaging effects.

HERBS

There are a number of herbal recommendations for pregnant women.

RED RASPBERRY TONIC—Tonics are herbal preparations that keep your body in good trim, up and running for optimum performance and healthy living.

This tonic increases fertility in both men and women. It helps prevent miscarriage and hemorrhaging during the birth. It's one of the best herbs to ease morning sickness, and it helps provide a safe, fast birth, reducing pain during labor. It reduces afterbirth pains, helps bring down undelivered placenta, and increases the amount and quality of breast milk. The rich concentration of vitamin C, vitamin E, carotenes, vitamin A, calcium, iron, the B-complex vitamins, and the large amounts of phosphorus and potassium make taking red raspberry well worth it.

STINGING NETTLE TONIC—Another tonic for early pregnancy is stinging nettle, which is one of the most nutrient-rich substances available. It is loaded with carotenes, from which we make vitamin A; vitamins C, E, and D; the B vitamins; vitamin K; and calcium, potassium, phosphorous, and immune-strengthening sulfur.

Make a tonic the same way as for raspberry. Weigh out 1 ounce of the dried herb, put it in a jar, fill the jar with boiling water, then tightly lid it and steep overnight. You can drink it warm, cold, or in between, up to four cups a day. The chlorophyll in this brew is so high that the infusion will actually look black rather than green.

Nettle is tremendously nourishing. It eases leg cramps and any other muscle spasms during pregnancy. Because of nettle's high calcium content, it diminishes labor pains and birth pains. It is such a superb source of vitamin C that it is one of the world's most highly favored herbs for preventing hemorrhaging after birth. It's a wonderful way to reduce hemorrhoids. It can increase the amount and richness of your breast milk. Stinging nettle tonic can also help pregnant women who have fatigue, moodiness, and preeclampsia.

DANDELION AND OTHER HERBS—Dandelion is also good for mood swings. You can take it in any form. You'll probably find dandelion root tincture in any health food store. The usual dosage is 5 to 15 drops, taken before meals.

Dandelion leaves, especially when eaten as a cooked green, provide potassium, calcium, and sodium. They can even be used as a remedy for a woman who already has preeclampsia.

Here are a few more suggestions about herbs: Ginger is one of the best natural remedies for nausea. Ginger works best when the person taking it eats small, frequent meals and gets plenty of fresh air and rest. Ginger can be taken as a capsule or tea. A washcloth soaked in ginger or comfrey tea and applied to the area where an episiotomy has been performed promotes healing. Rosemary added to bath water relieves tension and back pain. Finally, adding jasmine and clary sage to a bath has an uplifting effect and prevents postpartum depression.

MASSAGE

Susan Lacina tells why a pregnant woman and her unborn child benefit greatly from massage. "We tend to think of a baby in utero as being cut off from the world," she says. "In reality, the child within is a conscious being who responds to sounds, emotions, and the inner environment that its mother creates, either through her sense of well-being or through her lack of it." Here Lacina describes how maternity massage promotes a comfortable and healthy pregnancy:

"Research shows that prolonged stress builds up abnormal levels of toxins and chemicals in the bloodstream. These are passed through the placenta to the baby. Minimizing the buildup of toxins can be achieved by periodic deep relaxation. Relaxation increases the absorption of oxygen and nutrients by the cells of the muscles. When oxygen and nutrition increase, the woman has more energy. Some doctors also believe morning sickness and nausea are eliminated by lowering stress levels.

"Massage assists the lymphatic system in eliminating excessive toxins and hormones. Unlike the heart, the lymphatic system has no pump. It moves freely until muscles tighten up, but when muscles become too tense, either from the fetus or from stress, lymph movement decreases and the concentration of toxins rises. In the lower extremities, the growing uterus can inhibit lymph drainage, leading to swelling, varicose veins, hemorrhoids, and fluid retention. By relaxing the muscles, massage helps stimulate lymphatic drainage of toxins. It decreases the development of varicose veins by its draining effect and helps reduce swelling in the legs."

Massage also helps with overall muscle tone and elasticity. "A woman's body must expand to accommodate the growing fetus," Lacina says. "Hips widen and abdominal, lower back, and shoulder muscles stretch. Legs must accommodate increased weight. Massage promotes flexible muscles, joints, ligaments, and tendons. It also helps decrease muscle spasms and leg cramps by getting rid of lactic acid buildup, and can alleviate the pain caused by sciatic nerve pressure. Added flexibility helps the muscles that are needed for labor."

In addition, massage assists in hormonal balance. "Massage balances the entire glandular system. An overactive thyroid gland becomes less active, thereby decreasing irritability, mood swings, and hot flashes. An underactive thymus gland is stimulated, which increases its ability to fight infection. The alternating relaxation and stimulation that massage provides helps a woman's body function in a more balanced manner."

Lacina describes the benefits of a peroneal massage. "This is a gentle stretch of tissues in the area between the vagina and rectum. Learning peroneal massage increases the mother's awareness of the muscles she needs to relax during the actual delivery and decreases her chances of having an episiotomy, an incision made to enlarge the vaginal opening at the time of birth.

"The actual procedure is as follows: Using warm vitamin E or vegetable oil, the mother places clean, oiled thumbs or index fingers an inch to an inch and a half inside the vagina and applies firm, gentle pressure downward and outward. Stretching continues until a burning sensation is felt. This is held for a few minutes. Performing this once or twice a day, up until the time of delivery, can result in an easier birth."

What about during labor and the postpartum period? "Massage during labor helps to reduce pain and anxiety by offering relief from muscle contractions." Lacina says. "The stimulation of certain acupressure points can speed up labor.

"*Postpartum* is the name given to the six-week recovery period after birth. During this time, hormones readjust and the uterus involutes (returns to its prepregnancy size). Massaging the abdomen in a circular motion helps the uterus to contract and helps to expel blood. Massage also helps to stimulate milk flow. The following techniques can be applied for this purpose: The pressure point at the base of the sacrum can be held for about fifteen seconds, and then released. Breast massage is another technique that can be used. Using some light oil, a woman circles her breasts with her fingertips. She places the hands flat on the breasts, starting at the nipple, and moves outward and up. That helps the glands to release milk. Additionally, there is an acupressure point at the top and middle of the shoulder. Holding it for fifteen seconds helps milk production. Pressing the point between the sixth and seventh ribs at the nipple level on the breast bone helps to release milk."

ACUPRESSURE POINTS

Thumbs can be applied to the sacrum, at the bottom of the spine, and walked up the spine to the waist. Each point is held for about five seconds.

The point in the center of the buttocks is pressed in as the mother exhales and released as she inhales.

Thumbs can be pressed along the shoulder blades between the spine and the scapula.

On the legs, pressure can be applied to Spleen 6, an acupressure point located approximately three inches above the ankle, on the inside of the leg right below the tibia bone. Holding this spot for ten seconds and then releasing it helps to stimulate uterine contractions and speeds up labor.

The uterus point is on the inside of the foot, just under the ankle bone. The ovary point is on the outside of the foot, under the ankles, near the heel. Squeezing these points at the same time for about ten seconds and then releasing them helps to speed up labor.

Breast and nipple stimulation helps create oxytocin, the hormone that helps the uterus to contract.

ALEXANDER TECHNIQUE

The Alexander technique differs from massage in that the pregnant woman is actively engaged. Kim Jessor, an Alexander teacher, makes an analogy to a piano lesson: "We talk about being Alexander teachers, the people who come to us are students, and the context is a lesson. So while the results are very therapeutic, I don't think of the work as a therapy but rather as a learning process. This is significant in that it empowers students to take charge in changing their movement habits."

The Alexander technique is based on the concept that all of us know how to move comfortably as children, but lose that natural flexibility over time. The method teaches people how to move freely again, which is especially valuable for women undergoing the stresses of pregnancy.

Jessor describes some of the ways the Alexander technique helps women during and after pregnancy: Lower back pressure is relieved, breathing improves, rest is enhanced, labor is eased, stamina increases after delivery, and breastfeeding is easier. In addition, there are less tangible, but equally valuable, benefits from working with the Alexander technique during pregnancy. "Women begin to realize that they can make different kinds of choices about the kind of birth they want to have, where they want to have it, and who they want to use for labor support. In the same way that they begin to find freedom in movement, they find greater options in terms of the choices they make about their pregnancy."

EXERCISE

The benefits of exercise during pregnancy are many, and extend to the baby as well as the mother. For the mother, it helps with weight gain, strength and stamina, moodiness, back pain, and sleep. A 2015 review published in the *International Journal of Obstetrics and Gynaecology* showed that exercise reduced the risk of gestational diabetes. Two studies presented at the Society for Neuroscience found a link between exercise during pregnancy and the baby's neurological development. The *American College of Gynecologists and Obstetricians* (ACOG) endorses physical activity during pregnancy and has created specific guidelines for the dos and don'ts of exercise:

Pregnant women derive health benefits from a mild to moderate exercise routine. Exercising sixty minutes, three times per week, is preferable to intermittent activity, but some benefit can be derived from shorter durations as well. Sometimes little oxygen is available for aerobic exercise due to the body's increased oxygen demands. Therefore, a woman should begin an aerobic activity slowly, and gradually build to capacity. She should not push too hard, and certainly not to the point of breathlessness. Pregnant women should not exercise in the faceup position after the first trimester. This position limits blood supply to the baby.

Avoid standing for prolonged periods of time, doing heavy work in the standing position, and exercising at high intensities. These activities are associated with diminished birthweight in newborns. It's better for women to engage in non–weight-bearing activities such as cycling and swimming, rather than exercises like running. Non–weight-bearing exercise minimizes the risk of injury and allows activity levels to remain closer to prepregnancy levels, right up to delivery. A woman should be aware that her center of gravity is different, and that she might lose her balance when exercising. Anything that could involve falling over, or even mild abdominal trauma, should be avoided.

Pregnant women require an extra 300 calories per day in order to maintain their normal metabolic rate. Exercise increases the need for more calories.

A pregnant woman must be careful not to raise her body temperature with vigorous workouts, especially in the first trimester. Excessive body heat in the mother can adversely affect the development of brain tissue in the baby. The threshold for this is a body temperature of about 39.2 degrees Celsius, which is 100 or 101 degrees Fahrenheit.

When should a pregnant woman not exercise? "Basically, every pregnant woman can benefit from starting an exercise program at any point in pregnancy. However, there are certain exceptions to this rule. When any one of the following conditions is present, a pregnant woman should limit or avoid exercise: pregnancy-induced hypertension, premature rupture of membranes, incompetent cervix, persistent second- or third-trimester bleeding, premature labor during the prior or current pregnancy, and intrauterine growth retardation."

Other medical contraindications include thyroid, heart, vascular, or pulmonary conditions. Women with medical problems need a physician's evaluation to determine whether an exercise program is appropriate.

AROMATHERAPY

Ann Berwick reports that in Europe, where aromatherapy is scientifically studied and widely prescribed, hospital maternity wings utilize essential oils for their soothing and uplifting mind-body effects: "There is a report of one woman who had severe anxiety throughout her pregnancy. They gave her neroli oil, which helped to keep her blood pressure down and allowed her to go into delivery in a more relaxed state. During delivery, she was given lavender and clary sage to relax her uterus. Clary sage is also slightly euphoric, so it helped her to cope mentally with the birth." Here are some formulas to try before, during, and after birth:

- As an antidote for nausea and vomiting, peppermint oil is effective when a very diluted amount is rubbed into the stomach or inhaled.
- For relaxation, 8 ounces vegetable oil, 13 drops lavender, 2 drops geranium, and 10 drops sandalwood can be massaged into the skin or used as a compress.
- To clear nasal congestion, a teaspoon of eucalyptus oil can be added to a cold-air humidifier or pan of hot water. The steam inhaled reduces congestion.
- To help heartburn, place 2 to 3 drops of diluted peppermint oil on the back of the tongue.

- A good massage oil to use during labor consists of 5 drops rose, 12 drops clary sage, and 5 drops ylang-ylang in 2 to 3 ounces vegetable oil.
- To prevent stretch marks, massage 2 ounces wheat germ oil, 20 drops lavender, and 5 drops neroli oil into the thighs.
- To soothe sore nipples, mix 1 pint cold water, 1 drop geranium, 1 drop lavender, and 1 drop rose oil.
- After an episiotomy, a sitz (shallow) bath is helpful, especially when 2 drops cyprus and 4 drops lavender oil are added. Soak for 15 to 20 minutes.
- To promote milk production, take 2 drops fennel oil with some honey water, every 2 hours.
- Hemorrhoids will be helped by 5 drops cyprus oil added to the bath.
- The astringent action of cyprus and lemon oil constricts varicose veins. A few drops can be added to a body lotion and applied to the veins morning and evening.

HOMEOPATHY

Homeopathic physician Stephanie Odinov Pukit lists a variety of remedies for all stages of pregnancy. She begins with treatments for morning sickness.

SEPIA—Ambivalence is the key word here. There is a conflict between self-preservation and the urge to procreate, which makes wanting a child questionable. The woman becomes angry and irritable and feels as if a black cloud hovers over her. Although her appetite is insatiable, heavy pains worsen with smells or thoughts of food.

PULSATILLA—This is the opposite scenario. Pulsatilla is an excellent remedy for the woman who is cheerful, sweet, and somewhat helpless. The person is warm and may throw the covers off at night. She becomes worse with emotional excitement. Nausea comes and goes and is characteristically worse in early evening.

NUX VOMICA—This is a wonderful remedy for soothing the nerves after a woman has abused her body with alcohol, drugs, or coffee. She tends to be constipated. She tends to wake up at night to think about business because she is ambitious and driven.

ARSENICUM—The picture here is a person constantly anxious about her state of health. She always runs to the doctor fearing that something is wrong. The woman tends to have burning pains. She has great thirst and takes little sips. Symptoms are usually exacerbated at midnight.

COCCULUS INDICUS—This remedy specifically helps motion sickness. The woman tends to lose sleep and to be constantly exhausted. She may be nursing children or caring for someone. The woman feels dizzy standing and better when lying down. She feels worse in fresh air.

PETROLEUM—Petroleum may be indicated if there is a voracious appetite followed by persistent vomiting.

BRYONIA—The person has strong sensitivity to smells and may have connective tissue and arthritic problems. Nausea becomes worse with motion.

Dr. Odinov Pukit suggests the following remedies for problems that occur in the latter stages of pregnancy:

SEPIA OR PULSATILLA—In the third to sixth month, the fetus presses high up in the abdomen, causing heartburn, shortness of breath, and indigestion. These remedies also help hemorrhoid problems. The one chosen depends on the other symptoms manifested. Sepia is for a gloomy disposition, while pulsatilla is for a sweet nature.

CARBO VEGETABILIS (CARBO VEG)—The woman is slightly heavy and tends to have indigestion and shortness of breath due to poor oxygenation. Although she tends to be chilly, she prefers open windows with the air directly on her.

BELLIS PERENNIS—As the baby drops into the pelvis, pressure is felt on the organs in the lower part of the bladder. Pain and arthritis may occur as a result. Bellis perennis is specific for pain in the uterine area or groin. The woman might be walking when all of a sudden her legs weaken from a sharp nerve pain. After childbirth, once arnica has done its job (see below) and there are still some lumps remaining in the tissues, bellis perennis is also excellent.

KALI CARBONICUM—Kali carbonicum is for women with back pain, especially those who tend to wake up between two and four o'clock in the morning. This individual's personality is somewhat crabby and closed. She is vague and evasive about answering questions. Pains are better with pressure and rubbing. The person tends to be anxious and chilly.

ACONITE—High-potency aconite is wonderful to use at any point in pregnancy when there has been shock or fright. Arnica and calendula may be useful for this purpose as well.

Midwife Jeanette Breen finds homeopathy useful during labor and after birth:

ARNICA—Starting a month before delivery, regular application of arnica cream directly to the nipples prevents later tearing and cracking with breast-feeding. After birth, arnica quickens recuperation. Calendula can be used in the same way.

CALIFILUM—Califilum may help a stalled labor. This is specific for a weak uterus or a uterus running out of steam. The woman often experiences weakness, exhaustion, trembling, and shivering. Sharp, brief, unstable, and painful lower uterine contractions fail to completely dilate the cervix and push the baby out.

GELSEMIUM—Gelsemium may be indicated as a follow-up to califilum. It is also good for neuralgia, rheumatic discomfort, and pains in the bladder and vaginal area. The person tends to be thirsty and chilly.

CIMICIFUGA—Cimicifuga is good for stalled labor, especially when the woman is becoming fearful, hysterical, and exhausted, and the pains are becoming erratic. This tones the uterus, calms it down, and helps it to become more coordinated.

Breast-feeding

For many of today's working mothers, breast-feeding is difficult because they can't be at home enough to be with their infants. However, women are further encouraged to neglect breast-feeding by the growth of fallacies about it, as well as a lack of full knowledge of its benefits.

The first major benefit of breast-feeding is the mother's milk itself: It gives the baby the appropriate nutrients. For the first nine months, Arms notes, the baby doesn't need any other food at all other than breast milk, which helps establish and nourish the baby's immune system. Feeding the baby from the breast creates in the mother a feeling of calm, relaxation, and deepening love for her child. For the baby, just being there, skin to skin, with the mother, affords immune protection.

The components of breast milk actually change from feed to feed, and, for a mother who has more than one child, the milk changes from child to child. This is why formula can never mimic breast milk. Nor can the container that breast milk comes in ever be duplicated. There's a real difference between providing pumping stations at work and giving working mothers access on their job time to day care where mother and baby can be together when the baby wakes up—not to mention allowing mothers to be home with their babies until the babies are old enough to be without milk for more than four hours at a time.

Breast-feeding does many things for the baby and the mother. It causes the mother's gut to secrete twenty-three hormones (that we know of), which bottle feeding does not do. These hormones cause a woman to lose weight as well as help her sleep better and feel calmer. If a mother is malnourished and underweight, breast-feeding helps her to get as much nutrient value out of her food as possible. More nutrient value is absorbed in her gut than would be if she were not breast-feeding.

Arms tells us, "All babies need to be breast-fed and almost all mothers, even those who have had breast surgery, can breast-feed, if we give them three months to get settled before we even think of having them go back to work. And then we need to create work situations where they can breast-feed during the day.

Corrective Vaginal Surgery (Episiotomy)

In the United States, about 80 percent of women who give birth have an episiotomy performed. This is an incision that is made during birth when the vaginal opening does not stretch adequately. Of those operations, most are improperly performed. "Doctors are just not instructed in how to do this surgery," says Dr. Vicki Hufnagel. "All you have to do is go to your local medical school, get out the textbook on obstetrics, and look at what an episiotomy is. It will have a drawing and a discussion that says to put one or two sutures here, and one or two there. They are teaching physicians to close an entire organ system in just one or two layers. If you were to close a laceration on your face in one or two layers, your muscles wouldn't work, your face wouldn't work. You'd be a real mess. We are teaching students how to close the vaginal vault area in a manner that is not allowable in other places. That is the standard of care that we have, and it is completely unacceptable."

Incorrectly performed episiotomies result in problems down the road. Without the support of the vaginal muscles, the cervix pushes through the vagina. It appears that the uterus is being forced out, when really it is not. Doctors mistakenly diagnose a prolapsed uterus and commonly recommend a hysterectomy. Tragically, 100,000 to 200,000 women with this misdiagnosis receive this operation each year.

Corrective surgery easily ameliorates the problem. Repairing the vagina is a simple procedure that can be performed in a doctor's office. It takes all of forty-five minutes, and patients can go home the same day.

Postpartum Depression

Depression after childbirth affects thousands of women each year. Although the exact cause is unknown, hormonal shifts after birth, particularly drops in progesterone, may play a large role. Research also links the condition to low levels of the neurotransmitter serotonin. Emotionally, it is often connected to difficult labor and disappointments after birth.

Symptoms range in degree, but are generally worse than a temporary feeling of the blues immediately following childbirth. Dr. Marjorie Ordene, a complementary gynecologist from New York, explains: "Postpartum depression is defined as a gradually increasingly sullen mood and a loss of interest and enthusiasm starting around the third postpartum week. This is different from the 'baby blues,' which is a common occurrence in the normal population. The blues happens the first week postpartum, and basically goes away by itself. We are talking about something much more severe." In the worst-case scenario, women can become sick for years and lose touch with reality.

HOMEOPATHIC REMEDIES

Homeopathic physician Dr. Jane Cicchetti recommends that women try the 30c potency of the remedy that best addresses their symptoms. If this does not help, a visit to a homeopathic physician can provide more individual support.

SEPIA—Sepia may be needed after an exhausting delivery, after giving birth to two or more children at once, or after having several children. The woman feels completely worn out and depressed. Physically, she feels as if her uterus might fall out, and finds herself crossing her legs a lot. Often there is an actual prolapse of the uterus. Emotionally, a woman who loves her husband and children suddenly has an aversion to them. In fact, she has an aversion to everyone and wants to be alone. She becomes irritable and angry if anyone bothers her, and has an aversion to sex. The woman cries often but cannot understand what is wrong; in fact this problem is caused by a hormonal disturbance rather than an emotional one.

NATMUR (NATRUM MURIATICUM)—Natmur is for chronic grief. The woman is introverted and dwells on past, unpleasant memories but keeps them to herself. She tries to put on the appearance that everything is fine, and becomes aggravated if someone tries to comfort her.

IGNATIA—Ignatia is for postpartum depression brought on by emotions. It is needed when disappointment follows childbirth. A woman imagines an ideal pregnancy and birthing situation. When that does not work out, she feels extremely let down and depressed. These feelings may occur after a stillbirth or a miscarriage. There is uncontrollable sobbing and sighing, and a rapid change of emotions, which are often contradictory.

ARNICA—This commonly needed remedy is useful for depression, upset, and malaise brought on by bruising, soreness, and pain that lasts a long time. Arnica helps heal the physical trauma and improves the mother's energy and emotional state.

PULSATILLA—Pulsatilla is given when a woman cries a lot and wants to be taken care of. She needs to attend to her newborn baby, but feels as if someone should be attending to her. This individual will eat sweets and other goodies to alleviate overwhelming feelings of sadness and loneliness. The woman is often warm-blooded and enjoys the fresh air. She is happier walking around outside, and much happier if she can be with people.

CIMICIFUGA—This remedy is used less often, but is very important for those who need it. Cimicifuga is derived from black cohosh, a powerful herb for treating hysteria and female complaints. It is needed when a woman feels as if a dark cloud of gloom has settled over her. She fears losing her mind. Often this stems from a very difficult delivery. She may have had a mini-nervous break-down, feeling at one point as if she was going insane. This leaves her with a great fear of ever having a baby again. Often she alternates between different emotional states. When she is not under this dark cloud of gloom, she becomes excitable and talkative, jumping from one subject to another in an almost hysterical fashion. Cimicifuga heals the nervous system.

KALI CARBONICUM—This deep mineral remedy is indicated for women who become anxious and irritable after a delivery that leaves them feeling weak. Easily startled, they want to be left alone, and have an aversion to being touched. They tend to be chilly and to have insomnia from two to four a.m. Further, they are reg-imented and have trouble going with the flow of caring for a new baby. Often these symptoms follow a delivery that primarily consists of back labor. Sciatica develops to some degree, which can lead to an emotional state like this.

PHOSPHORIC ACID—Homeopathic phosphoric acid is helpful when a woman is extremely disappointed from physical or emotional shock. She may have lost the baby, or something might be wrong with the baby. A loved one may have died at the time of birth, or she may be affected from the loss of much bodily fluid during delivery. Indifferent to everything, the woman lies in bed with her face to the wall. It is as if her emotions have completely disappeared. She doesn't want to talk, think, or answer questions.

COCCULUS—This is a remedy for fatigue and emotional depression brought on by loss of sleep. The woman feels drunk and may go through the day feeling dizzy and staggering. These feelings are brought on by sleep deprivation.

AURUM METALLICUM—Aurum metallicum is for profound depression characterized by total hopelessness, self-destructive behavior, and a longing for death.

OTHER REMEDIES

"Studies show that postpartum depression can be prevented by treating women with progesterone," reports Dr. Ordene. "Companies that make natural progesterone cream recommend using a half teaspoon twice daily, starting a month after delivery. Since postpartum depression is supposed to start three weeks after giving birth, it makes sense to begin using natural progesterone at that time."

According to research, this vitamin raises serotonin levels. Patients given B_6 for twenty-eight days after delivery did not have a recurrence of postpartum depression.

Abortion Aftercare

Although most women who have abortions do not have any serious medical complications from the procedure, the period after an abortion is a time for a woman to focus on herself; she may have a variety of physical and emotional needs that require attention.

It's particularly important to remember that after an abortion your body's hormone levels have to readjust to the sudden change from a pregnant to a nonpregnant state. Dr. Susanna Reid, a naturopathic physician, describes the physical changes in a woman's body after an abortion.

"Hormone levels are elevated dramatically during pregnancy, so the body has to readjust itself to its prepregnancy state," Dr. Reid explains. "One way to help the body to do that is by focusing on dietary factors that would be beneficial in regulating hormone levels. As well, you want to increase the circulation in the lower abdomen so that the body can heal itself. The more circulation in an area and the more nutrients that are in that area, the easier it is for the body to remove the toxic waste products. You'd also want to strengthen liver function, since the liver is essential to the balancing of hormones in the body; it functions to promote excretion of hormones. So if the liver isn't functioning correctly, you can have an imbalance of hormones."

To strengthen liver function, she suggests eating foods that contain fiber, particularly fruits, vegetables, and whole grains. The gut needs fiber to prevent the reabsorption of hormones. "If there isn't enough fiber in the diet, the hormones are reabsorbed through the intrahepatic circulation. So fiber is very important. In the springtime, one can strengthen liver function by eating large amounts of fresh dandelions and other greens such as cleavers. In other seasons, use yellow dock, nettle, dandelion, and cleavers with some red raspberry to make a tea. Red raspberry is a uterine tonic, so it helps to heal the uterus. You can put some peppermint in the tea to make it taste better and aid in digestion."

About two weeks after the abortion, she suggests using cold friction on the lower abdomen for ten minutes at a time before going to bed or first thing in the morning.

PREVENTING INFECTION

One of the more common complications from an abortion is infection. It's important not to put anything into the vagina for several weeks after the abortion and to refrain from intercourse. Dr. Reid suggests several natural remedies to help prevent infections.

"If we enhance the immune function, we prevent infection. You can use an immune-enhancing diet that focuses a lot on fruits and vegetables. Fruits in particular are immune-enhancing." She also recommends echinacea, goldenseal, astragalus, and ligustrum to help immune function.

Dr. Allan Warshowsky, a board-certified obstetrician and gynecologist who practices holistic gynecology, recommends taking vitamins C, A, and E and other antioxidants to enhance immune function.

Dr. Reid also emphasizes fluid intake. She explains that an abortion creates many by-products, and one way the body can help eliminate them is through the exchange of fluids, so you should drink a lot of fluids. Although each woman experiences abortion in her own way, it can sometimes create a strong emotional response, either positive or negative. "If it is a desired pregnancy and it's a spontaneous abortion," Dr. Reid says, "then people are dealing with grief. Even if it is a therapeutic abortion, there can be many reasons for the abortion. It may be because the pregnancy isn't viable or wouldn't be viable, or maybe it isn't the right time. So there are just a lot of grief issues for some women around abortion."

Dr. Warshowsky believes it is very important to deal with any negative feelings. He suggests that women who experience grief and other emotional and psychological consequences after an abortion may be helped by using meditation or visualization techniques.

Is Circumcision Necessary?

Sixty percent of babies born in hospitals in the United States are circumcised. Suzanne Arms, an independent researcher and activist who has published books on pregnancy and women's health, including *Immaculate Deception*, *Breast Feeding*, and *Seasons of Change*, sees this as a wasteful and counterproductive practice. "The difficulty with circumcision," she believes, "is that it touches some of the most sensitive tissue on the human male body and takes a large amount of material from the penis. You are taking away all the natural protection of the penis, the tissue that keeps it from getting infected and getting diseases and that makes sexuality more exquisite."

She also says that in Europe, circumcision has never been routinely performed on infants, as it is in the United States. She believes that the US practice of routine circumcision is one aspect of a cultural attitude that grew, in part, out of seventeenth-century Puritanism, which viewed sexual pleasure, including masturbation, as sinful, and advocated tying babies' hands to their cribs to keep them from touching their genitals, which might provide pleasure. In the 1920s and 1930s, for the same purpose, clitoridectomies were performed on little girls in some parts of the country. She regards circumcision as an outgrowth of such attitudes: it was done to prevent male babies from using their penises as organs of pleasure.

Arms says, "We can contrast this with the reason for circumcision under Judaic law. In that tradition, circumcision was done on the eighth day as part of a convenant with God. Many Jews now believe that circumcision can be done without cutting the boy."

She also argues that the medical reasons once given for this operation—for example that it prevents cancer—have turned out to be false. Circumcision has no medical value at all and has a lot of risks associated with it, including bleeding and other effects of surgery. "It exposes newborn babies to what is for them excruciating pain," Arms says. "Some babies feel it less than others, but, by and large, it puts the baby into shock and trauma."

Many advocates of circumcision apparently feel it is a way to harden the boy. In the past, children to be circumcised were tied down on boards, six in a row. A baby would lie there unable to move, listening to the screams of the little boys next to him. This was considered a way of preparing boys to be ready as adults to give up their bodies in war.

"I think it's very important that we begin to understand the shock and trauma from this process that we have called normal in the United States," Arms concludes. "And we don't even acknowledge this trauma, so how can we heal it? People are running around with the long-term effects in their nervous system of an unresolved trauma. Believe me, that is what we are seeing in this culture."

Chapter 52

Premenstrual Syndrome (PMS)

According to 2014 data from the National Library of Medicine, up to three out of every four women experience at least one symptom of premenstrual syndrome (PMS) as part of their monthly cycle. PMS refers to the symptoms that begin during or after ovulation and end with the conclusion of the menstrual flow. Because of diet and lifestyle, PMS is more widespread in Western societies than in Asian and less developed countries. Dr. Jesse Hanley, in an article in *Alternative Medicine* magazine, says that PMS is an indication of imbalance in the body, which can be psychological, nutritional, or hormonal. Dr. Hanley sees PMS as "a wake-up call" signaling us to pay attention to these imbalances and fix them before they turn into a more serious condition.

Causes

Dr. Hanley points out that menstruation does not create pain and discomfort when a woman is healthy. However, we live in an environment full of synthetic chemicals, including herbicides and pesticides, which mimic estrogen once they get inside the body, enhancing the effects of natural estrogen and disturbing the hormonal balance. Further, an excess of estrogen in relation to progesterone causes problems of hormonal imbalance.

Symptoms

The effects of PMS range from mild to severe, and they vary from woman to woman. They may include bloating, cramps, headaches, swelling, fluid retention, low back pain, depression, abdominal pressure, insomnia, sugar cravings, anxiety, irritability, breast tenderness, mood swings, and acne.

Clinical Experience

DIETARY REMEDIES

Dr. Michael Janson, an orthomolecular physician and author of *The Vitamin Revolution*, says, "Sugar, caffeine, and alcohol precipitate or worsen symptoms and should be avoided. This is because a lot of patients with PMS have overt hypoglycemia. Their sugar levels fluctuate up and down. Eating sugar sends blood sugar levels way up, and the body responds by dropping sugar levels way down. Additionally, caffeine, even when taken in small amounts in the morning, can aggravate symptoms such as breast tenderness and sleep disturbances."

According to Dr. Janson, the best diet for lessening the symptoms of PMS is high in fiber and complex carbohydrates; meals should be small, with snacks in between. This helps to regulate blood sugar, and in many cases is enough to reduce or eliminate PMS symptoms. Herbalist Letha Hadady recommends eating a lot of cool green foods such as salads; avoiding hot, spicy, and acidic foods; and eliminating coffee from the diet. Some people, however, need more help and can benefit from vitamin therapy, exercise, and a stress management program.

Dr. Hanley recommends that a woman who suffers from PMS should completely avoid milk and milk products, for milk has a high concentration of pesticides and other estrogen-mimicking chemicals.

NUTRITIONAL SUPPLEMENTS

When symptoms are severe, diet alone may not be enough. The following nutrients may prove useful:

VITAMIN B_6 (PYRIDOXINE)—Pyridoxine has a number of helpful properties for alleviating PMS. As a smooth muscle relaxant, it can decrease cramps. As a diuretic, it reduces fluid retention, swelling, and breast tenderness. Fifty milligrams should be taken three times daily, and vitamin B_6 can be taken throughout the month, rather than just premenstrually. For the first two weeks of the cycle, take 100 milligrams a day in a B-complex vitamin; take an additional 250 milligrams the last two weeks of the cycle. Note that the more B_6 you take, the more magnesium you need.

MAGNESIUM—Magnesium calms the nervous system and relieves anxiety, depression, irritability, nervousness, and insomnia. As an antispasmodic, it alleviates cramps and back pain. Magnesium also helps reduce cravings for sweets. Between 500 and 1,000 milligrams may be needed.

GAMMA-LINOLENIC ACID (GLA)—GLA is a precursor of prostaglandin-E1, a hormonelike substance that helps to regulate neurological and hormonal functions. Prostaglandin-E1 helps reduce muscle spasms, cramping, sugar cravings, mood swings, depression, anxiety, irritability, acne, and to some extent breast tenderness. It also reduces inflammation and decreases the stickiness of the platelets, which prevents blood clotting. One 1,000 milligrams capsule of borage oil provides a daily dose of 240 milligrams of GLA.

EICOSAPENTAENOIC ACID (EPA)—EPA, which is found in fish oil and flaxseed oil, produces prostaglandin-E3, which helps to alleviate breast tenderness. Flaxseed oil is fragile and should not be used for frying. It can be used in salad dressings or over cooked foods.

VITAMIN E—Vitamin E, 400–800 IU, can reduce cramps, breast tenderness, and fibrocystic breasts, which often swell up before a woman's menstrual period.

OTHER—Also recommended are Cytokine Supress with EGCG (300 mg), evening primrose oil (as directed, 2x day), Vitamin B$_6$ (50 mg, 3x day).

EXERCISE
Exercise helps to improve mood, reduce cramps, eliminate excess fluid, and control sugar cravings. Aerobic exercises should be performed three to four times per week.

HERBS
Naturopathic physician Dr. Janet Zand, in an article on the HealthWorld Online website (www.healthy.net), suggests the following herbal program, which builds blood and balances hormones during the first two weeks, then decongests the liver during the second two weeks.

For the first and second weeks, or until ovulation occurs, take a combination of red raspberry leaf and dong quai, taken as tablets, capsules, tinctures, or tea, three times a day.

For the third and fourth weeks (starting when ovulation occurs, until the menstrual flow begins), take the following: magnesium and vitamin B_6, two to three times a day; choline, methionine, and inositol, two to three times a day; bupleurum and dandelion, taken as tablets, capsules, tinctures, or tea, two or three times a day.

Herbalist Letha Hadady offers the following recommendations for PMS pain. "We must approach the pain of PMS from both the emotional and the physical sides. Emotionally, there are two types of PMS. One is the angry type. Aloe leaf is recommended for this. It cleans the system and cleanses the liver. It may taste a little bitter, but it is easy to take when added to a little apple juice. A stronger gallbladder and liver cleanser that lessens the impact of 'angry' menstrual pains is the Chinese preparation lung tanxieganwan. Twenty percent ginseng, it aids digestion and reduces anger. It also calms and quiets headaches and other pains.

"The second type of PMS is weepy. It comes from sadness and excess phlegm brought on by eating foods that are too rich, sweet, and oily or by drinking too much milk. Eating radishes, parsley, or barley soup will cut down on the phlegm. (A homeopathic remedy for this type of pain is Pulsatilla.)"

To treat both types of menstrual pain, Hadady says, warming herbs such as cinnamon and myrrh are invaluable. Capsules or drops taken in tea will increase blood circulation and clean the uterus, inducing a more complete period that does not start too early, stay too long, or finish early only to begin prematurely. A warming and cooling remedy for the pain is as follows: 1/2 cup aloe vera gel, 10 drops or one capsule myrrh, and apple juice. This combines the cleaning action of myrrh with the cooling of aloe.

In addition, xiao yao wan helps relieve PMS symptoms of depression, poor circulation, indigestion, and bloating; and Women's Harmony increases circulation.

HOMEOPATHY

The homeopathic remedy chosen should correspond to the symptoms described; only one should be used for best results. Sometimes it's a matter of trial and error; if one does not work, try another.

The late Dr. Ken Korins, a classically trained homeopathic physician in New York City, recommended the following remedies for PMS and lists the type of PMS symptom for which they are most useful.

LACHESIS—Lachesis helps most physical and emotional symptoms that accompany PMS, such as headaches, right ovarian pain, and breast tenderness. It may be indicated if PMS symptoms stop once menstrual flow stops. It is also indicated when symptoms get worse with heat and with constricted clothing around the abdomen. Emotional indications are restlessness, paranoia, and a tendency to be talkative.

LACANINUM—Think of lacaninum when the only symptom is a painful, swollen breast, the pain leaves once the menstrual flow begins, and there is a tendency to be irritable.

BOVISTA—Bovista is indicated when gastrointestinal symptoms, such as diarrhea, occur before the period begins. There may also be traces of blood before the actual flow begins. Subjective and objective feelings of swelling occur throughout the body, even through the hands, resulting in a tendency for the woman to feel clumsy.

PULSATILLA—Pulsatilla is good for emotional symptoms of PMS involving a weepy disposition and a need for consolation from others. It helps curb a strong craving for sweets.

NATMUR—Natmur is good when the woman's emotional state is melancholy and sad and worsens when others attempt to console her. Headaches occur before, during, or after the period, and there is a craving for salty foods and an aversion to sex at the time of the period.

SEPIA—Sepia is indicated in the presence of symptoms such as sadness, depression, indifference, and feelings of discontent and discouragement about life. Often a colicky pain is felt before the menses. There may also be a sensation of the uterus dropping, as if it would fall through the vagina due to congestion in that area.

FOLLICULINUM—This is a new French remedy that can be given on the seventh day of the cycle in a 30c–200c potency.

Homeopath Dana Ullman, in an article on the HealthWorld Online website (www.healthy.net), suggests some additional remedies. Take each one in the 6c,

12c, or 30c potency every two hours while symptoms are strong, then every four hours after symptoms diminish. When symptoms become mild, stop the remedy. If you experience no clear improvement within twelve hours, try another remedy.

BELLADONNA—Use belladonna when the major symptom is "bearing down" pains or cramps that appear and disappear suddenly. It is also useful when cramps are made worse by motion, a draft, or being jarred, and when they are associated with a headache.

MAGNESIA PHOS—Magnesia phos is recommended for cramps made better by warmth, by simply bending over, or by bending over and at the same time firmly massaging the abdomen, and made worse by cold and by being uncovered.

COLOCYNTHIS—Colocynthis is indicated for cramps like those just described when those cramps are accompanied by feelings of extreme restlessness and irritability.

IGNATIA—Ignatia is good for bloating accompanied by strong emotional downs, such as hysteria and grief, and when the woman experiences conflicting feelings.

CIMICIFUGA—Cimicifuga is used for bloating accompanied by sharp, labor-like pains shooting across the body, perhaps accompanied by sciatica or back pain, difficulty tolerating pain, hysteria, talkativeness, and a sense of everything being just too much to bear.

NUX VOMICA—Nux vomica is used for Type A personalities who are often highly stressed, who experience bloating and nausea along with irritability, and who become quarrelsome and critical.

PROGESTERONE

To restore hormonal balance, Dr. Hanley advocates natural progesterone, preferably in the form of cream made from wild yam, which is rubbed into the skin. This is because only 10 percent of hormones taken by mouth actually reach the bloodstream; the liver filters out the rest, which stresses the liver and gallbladder and increases the risk of gallstones, gallbladder disease, and liver cancer. Progesterone cream is used between ovulation and the day before the menstrual flow starts.

Progesterone promotes youthfulness, and is beneficial against cancer and fibrocystic breast disease. Dr. Michael Janson says additional progesterone is especially important for women exposed to estrogens from pesticides, food additives, drugs, and other chemicals in the environment. These lead to an overload of estrogen and a deficiency of progesterone. Progesterone is extremely helpful for treating PMS symptoms when such an imbalance exists.

Dr. Hanley also cautions that women taking herbs to relieve PMS symptoms should be sure to include herbs that promote progesterone production. Dong quai, alfalfa, licorice root, ginseng, anise seed, garlic, fennel, papaya, red clover, and sage are all estrogenic herbs. They may relieve symptoms, but they may also lead to fibroids, tumors, and cancers. They should be balanced with progesterone-precursor herbs, including wild yam, sarsaparilla, and chaste berry.

LIVER DETOXIFICATION

According to Dr. Hanley, detoxifying the liver can relieve many female health problems. The first step is to reduce fat in the diet; and the second is to use a detoxifying formula that contains herbs and plant enzymes that work to remove toxins from the liver. The herbs and enzymes must be used together; neither should be used by itself. Dr. Hanley recommends a liver detoxification program two or three months out of each year; women who suffer from severe PMS can do the program for longer time periods and more frequently.

REFLEXOLOGY

Reflexology is a science and an art based on the principle that we have reflex areas in our feet that correspond to every part of the body. Massaging specific reflex areas in the feet helps to improve the functioning of specific organs and glands.

Laura Norman, a certified reflexologist from New York City, describes three reflexology techniques:

"Thumb-walking can be used on the bottom, tops, and sides of the feet, although it is most often used on the bottom. The procedure entails bending the thumb at the first joint and inching along the bottom of the foot like a caterpillar, pressing from the heel up to the toe. The right hand is used on the right foot. Taking little tiny bites, press, press, press the whole bottom of the foot.

"Finger-walking is similar to thumb-walking, but is done by bending the finger at the first joint and using the tip of the finger on the outside edge.

"Finger-rotation is where you rotate the finger into the foot."

Massaging the feet with thumb-walking, finger-walking, and finger-rotation using a nongreasy, absorbent cream warms the feet and helps promote overall relaxation. For addressing specific problems, reflexology must be applied to specific areas.

Reflexology for PMS helps most when performed three or four days before and then during menstruation. First the right foot is worked on, while resting on the left leg. Then the same actions are repeated on the left side.

A Final Note: Premenstrual Dysphoric Disorder (PMDD)

In the early 2000s, pharmaceutical giant Eli Lilly introduced a new drug, claiming it would change the lives of hundreds of thousands of women by treating a condition known as premenstrual dysphoric disorder (PMDD). The symptoms of PMDD, as described by the company, were exactly the same as those of PMS. So why the new name? The story of PMDD and the drug designed to treat it provide yet another cautionary tale about the unholy alliance between the drug companies and the medical world. Dr. Sherrill Sellman explains.

"Eli Lily, the maker of Prozac, which has been grossing over $2 billion a year, lost the patent on Prozac. So they can't really make their profits off of Prozac and in fact they expect their profits to plummet to $645 million. That is a pretty big drop. So what they did was convince the FDA to create a new condition for which their drug and their drug only is the solution. This new drug is called Seraphim and it is actually made as a pink and purple pill. It is very sweet and feminine. This drug is designed to take away PMDD. It's Prozac. It is the exact same drug. It has been colored differently. It has been given a name change and it has been increased in price. When I checked with my local pharmacy here, I actually found out that a prescription of Seraphim costs $10 more than Prozac.

"Why is Prozac a problem? Well, we know that Prozac is highly toxic to the liver. It can cause brain damage. It can cause huge mood swings. It can cause greater types of suicidal thinking. It is a drug that puts women at greater risk of breast cancer. Some of the other side effects of Prozac include depression, anxiety, insomnia, loss of libido, and mood swings, which sound pretty much like the very condition it is supposed to treat.

"The massive amount of advertising that is going on through the TV, through women's magazines, doctors seminars and conferences, convincing everyone, doctors and women alike, that they have a solution to this new disease is a marketing ploy of the highest degree. It is designed to push a drug that cannot be pushed in the old way. They have created a new disease. They have created a new market. I'm really concerned about the long-term consequences of basically healthy women needing to adjust some of the issues going on in their life to heal their PMS, but why are we putting them on this toxic antidepressant drug? Women need to wake up to the fact that again they are being sold a bill of goods, that this is not the solution, and that the motive behind it is purely profit."

Research Update

An increasing body of evidence is showing the benefits of natural modalities to overall health and well-being. Following is a sample of recent peer-reviewed scientific studies relating to PMS.

In a 2014 study published in the *Global Journal of Health Science*, women with PMS who took vitamin B_1 reported a 35 percent reduction in mental symptoms and a 21 percent reduction in physical symptoms, without any side effects. According to a 2010 report in *CNS Drugs*, 900 milligrams per day of *Hypericum perforatum* (St. John's wort) for two menstrual cycles was more effective than placebo treatment for the most common physical and behavioral symptoms associated with PMS. The researchers noted that further study is needed to determine whether pain- and mood-related PMS symptoms benefit from longer duration of treatment. A 2013 report in the *Archives of Women's Mental Health* suggested that complex carbohydrates may help with PMS symptoms during the luteal phase by increasing serotonin levels. Chasteberry extract was found to be more effective than placebo in seven out of eight published clinical trials as reviewed in *Planta Medica* in 2013, and nearly 70 percent of participants who took chasteberry in a study published in 2012 in the *Journal of American Science* reported that their PMS symptoms resolved fully. A 2013 report in *Complementary Therapies in Medicine* showed decreased levels of depression, anxiety, bloating, headaches, and breast tenderness in women who took 2 grams of omega-3 fatty acids per day for a period of ninety days. Ginger has proven beneficial as well; a 2014 study published in *ISRN Obstetrics and Gynecology* found that 66 women who took 250 milligrams ginger tablets twice a day experienced improved mood and behavioral symptoms of PMS.

Chapter 53

Sexual Dysfunction

Psychologist Dr. Janice Stefanacci Steward says that sexual dysfunction stems largely from a society that offers people no models of normal, healthy sexuality. "If we look to the media, we see things that are totally aberrant in terms of frequency and potency. We see relationships portrayed between males and females where there is power and domination, or submission and seduction. Role models of healthy sexual communication and actualization are virtually nonexistent. People need a sense of what is normal.

"They also need time to think about sexuality as an integrated part of their personality. Our culture is very fragmented in this regard. Many, many people, men and women alike, never spend time thinking about their sexuality. In fact, if you were to take an informal survey and ask people, 'What is sexuality?' a good proportion of them would say, 'It's sex. It's something you do, maybe in the bedroom, maybe at night.' Nobody is really sure how often you are supposed to have it or how long it is supposed to last. Most people don't realize that sexuality is a completely integrated part of their personality, as much as actualizing in education or interpersonal relationships. Sexuality is very much a part of who we are, how we present ourselves in the world, what we do, and how we think of ourselves. Our adequacy and our self-esteem are tied up in our sexuality."

Causes

Some sex researchers question the whole concept of sexual dysfunction, promoting broader and less rigid definitions of sexual response and pleasure. "The Masters and Johnson model of sexual response—excitement, plateau, orgasm, and resolution—is very performance-oriented," says Rebecca Chalker, a women's health activist whose book, *The Clitoral Truth*, explores ways in which feminists are redefining male standards. "After desire and willingness, the only other compulsory element is pleasure," Chalker points out. "Pleasure and intimacy are the real goals of sexual activity, and if you look at it that way, the concept of sexual dysfunction simply collapses."

Nevertheless, women may worry when they have difficulty achieving orgasm, especially with a partner, and men become concerned if they have difficulty controlling ejaculations and getting or maintaining erections. Both women and men are also distressed when they don't feel sexual attraction. In fact, most people who seek out counseling do so for difficulties with sexual communication and the lack of sexual desire.

Early on, through regular masturbation, boys learn what feels good and how to reliably get orgasms. Girls often wait to begin sexual exploration until they engage in sexual activity with a partner; they miss out on the benefits of self-exploration. "Learning about sex from boys or men isn't the best thing for women," Chalker says.

Many sex therapists recommend that women explore their sexual response through masturbation, using a vibrator, sex toys, and sexy videos to stimulate sexual fantasies. You may also want to experiment with things like aromatherapy, oils, and herbs. After sufficient homework, you can try integrating these changes into sex with your partner. Another important change heterosexual couples can make is to try rewriting the "intercourse script." That is, plan to have sexual sessions where intercourse will not take place.

Chalker points out that there are two powerful aspects of our sexuality—the physiological and the psychological—and that "neither can live without the other." Unfortunately, it is the psychological problems that are the more difficult to deal with. Psychological problems manifest themselves in various ways. "Today, we have enormous resources that we didn't have a few years ago to help with sexual problems," Chalker notes. "I've reviewed some of the herbal aids and remedies here, and I encourage the reader to explore the wide range of resources available in book stores or by mail order."

Of course, sexual dysfunction can also have physical causes. One, Dr. Vicki Hufnagel reminds us, is "improperly performed episiotomies." In *Prevention* magazine, Dr. Tori Hudson lists a number of other factors that can affect the sex drive. She says that sexual problems can be related to menopause, non-menopause-related hormonal changes (often following pregnancy), medications

(Prozac, Zoloft, Sertraline, and others), depression, relationship issues, a chronic health problem, fatigue, and others. "In order to diagnose the cause correctly, your health professional would have to ask you many specific questions," she says. Hormonal factors may involve low levels of testosterone or DHEA, although it is not known precisely what effect these hormones have on the libido. If blood tests show that levels are low, supplementation may be in order.

Clinical Experience

NUTRIENTS, HORMONES, AND SUPPLEMENTS
Studies show that a heightened libido and orgasmic intensity are related to blood levels of histamine. Women who have low histamine levels tend to experience low sexual excitement, while those with a high level are more able to sustain orgasms. Nutrients that increase histamine levels include vitamin B_5 and the bioflavonoid rutin. Broccoli, parsley, cherries, grapes, peppers, melons, and citrus fruits are good food sources of vitamin B_5 and rutin.

Dr. Tori Hudson says that oral testosterone (available only by prescription), and/or a testosterone cream applied two to three times a week or rubbed into the external genital area before sex have been used to stimulate sexual responsiveness. DHEA, the B-complex vitamins, adrenal extracts, and the herbs ginseng and damiana may also help improve sexual response. Dr. Hudson notes, however, that remedies that focus on sexual drive without addressing general health and emotional issues will not have a consistent effect.

Dr. Janson offers an example of a general supplement program that can be an initial step in treating sexual dysfunction:

- Multivitamin, three capsules twice a day
- Vitamin C, two 1,000 milligrams capsules twice a day
- Vitamin E, 400 IU mixed natural, twice a day
- Ginkgo biloba tincture, 60 milligrams twice a day
- Gamma-linoleic acid, 240 milligrams in the form of borage oil, once a day
- Magnesium aspartate, 200 milligrams twice a day
- Coenzyme Q10, 100 milligrams once a day

AROMATHERAPY

"Aromatherapy is fantastic for helping women regain their sense of sensuality," declares aromatherapist Ann Berwick. Following are her recommendations.

Rose is wonderful for enhancing feminine qualities. It brings out the loving, tender side of us that wants to surrender. Clary sage heightens sensation. It takes you out of your body and into a different realm, allowing you to relax and enjoy the romance. Sandalwood is a wonderful oil for people not in touch with their physical side. It is very earthy and very deep. Jasmine restores self-confidence in people who have been through traumatic sexual experiences. It can help women who have been abused or who are emotionally closed off from damaging relationships.

"By blending different oils, you can create a formula that enhances the sensual side of your nature," says Berwick. She suggests adding them to the bath or using them while massaging a partner or in self-massage. A personal perfume can be made and used daily. "Surrounding yourself with these glorious scents is a wonderful help."

CHINESE MEDICINE

Registered nurse and acupuncturist Abigail Rist-Podrecca explains sexual dysfunction from an Eastern point of view: "Chinese medicine looks to the root of the cause rather than just the symptoms, and the root seems to be the kidney. The kidneys are called the roots of life. Everything stems from the kidney, they say."

Weak kidney function can be diagnosed in Eastern medicine in multiple ways, including facial diagnosis: "Under the eye is the thinnest tissue in the entire body," explains Rist-Podrecca. "You can see through the skin there. If the blood is not being cleared by the kidneys and detoxified, you will see a darkness under the eyes. People will say, 'I haven't had enough sleep,' but it goes beyond that. In Chinese medicine, that darkness signals that the kidneys are not functioning optimally, so the blood isn't being cleansed."

She goes on to describe various factors that can drain the kidneys. "Cold can deplete the kidneys. Many people can't tolerate cold. This is so because in the winter, the kidney's function becomes suppressed, much the same way as the sap in a tree runs to the core and into the roots. When people have a compromised kidney situation, where it isn't functioning optimally, they can't stand cold weather.

"Overwork and tension can also weaken kidney function because the kidneys and the adrenal glands (the adrenal sits on top of the kidney) are considered one and the same in Chinese medicine. So too much stress, and too many chemical toxins, deplete kidney functioning." Hundreds of Chinese herbs nourish kidney function. Here Rist-Podrecca names a few:

HAR SHAR WOO—This is an essential herbal formula for nourishing kidney function. It is also said to darken the hair. Hair, bone, teeth, joints, and sexual functions are tied up with the kidney energies. When you energize the kidneys, you affect all these different areas. When combined with dong quai, har shar woo helps the type of kidney dysfunction that causes low back pain.

ROMANIA—Romania is a dark black herb that is high in iron and helps to nourish the blood and improve kidney function.

DONG QUAI—Dong quai resembles a cross-section of the uterus, and has an affinity for this area of the body.

Research Update

An increasing body of evidence is showing the benefits of natural modalities to overall health and well-being. Following is a sample of recent peer-reviewed scientific studies relating to sexual dysfunction.

A 2013 article in *Life Extension Magazine* cites research indicating that three complementary botanical-based compounds are useful for improving a woman's sexual function: *Cordyceps sinensis* extract, *Lepidium meyenii* (maca) extract, and EstroG-100TM three-extract blend. *Cordyceps sinensis*, a medicinal mushroom, balances levels of estrogen and testosterone, promotes normal vaginal lubrication and sexual function, and reduces inflammation, among other things. Maca helps achieve the optimum balance of nutrients utilized by the body's neuroendocrine system. The third compound contains three plant extracts—*Phlomis umbrosa*, *Cynanchum wilfordii*, and *Angelica gigas* Nakai (*Korean Angelica*)—which act to regulate estrogenic activity. Following up on research showing that saffron benefited men who experienced sexual dysfunction as a side effect of taking Prozac (fluoxetine) for depression, a 2013 study in *Human Psychopharmacology* revealed that women who took 30 milligrams/day of saffron extract in combination with their antidepressant medication had similarly improved sexual function.

Chapter 54

Sexually Transmitted Diseases

Although sexually transmitted diseases (STDs) are better understood and more treatable than in the past, they remain a major health concern in the United States. In 2013, the Centers for Disease Control and Prevention (CDC) reported that there were nearly 20 million new infections annually, with direct medical costs totaling nearly $16 billion. While many people realize that there has been progress in the conventional medical treatment of STDs, what they may not know is that there has also been progress in using alternative, particularly herbal, treatments.

Gonorrhea

Gonorrhea is caused by the bacterium Neisseria gonorrhoeae. Women are far more likely to become infected than men. Carol Dalton, a nurse practitioner, says that because gonorrhea can cause pelvic inflammatory disease (PID) and other illnesses, as well as infertility, she believes in treating it by conventional means. "We don't want women who have the infection to pass it on. Gonorrhea can occur without any symptoms for a long time, so that you might be passing it on without being aware of it. We treat this very aggressively."

The first recourse is antibiotics. However, Dr. Allan Warshowsky cautions that antibiotics must be carefully monitored. Dr. Warshowsky is a board-certified obstetrician-gynecologist whose specialty is holistic gynecology. He says, "Most of my treatment of this disease is fairly conventional. I use antibiotics unless patients specifically ask me not to use them. But it is also important to maintain and restore gut bacteria while treating a patient with antibiotics. I use bifidum, acidophilus, and some of the Saccharomyces strains of beneficial yeast to maintain normal gut biosis. I think this is paramount."

He combines this with herbal treatment and psychological counseling. "It is also important, especially if a patient is having recurrent problems with STDs, to look at her relationships, because whatever is going on physically is a manifestation of a deeper energy problem in the individual. If the patient is amenable to examining these deeper problems, it can really help lead to a much more lasting cure than just taking antibiotics.

"There are certainly people I see who prefer not to have antibiotics and, then, as long as the patient is a willing partner in her own therapy and not just looking to me to cure the disease, I use some herbal products, such as echinacea and goldenseal, and other herbs and supplements that can be helpful in enhancing immunity and fighting off infection."

Dr. Linda Page, a doctor of naturopathy who is the author of *Healthy Healing*, has found a variety of herbs useful in treating STDs, including gonorrhea. She uses a combination that includes goldenseal, myrrh, pau d'arco, vegetable acidophilus, ginkgo, and dandelion. Another combination she uses is burdock, juniper, squawvine, bayberry, dandelion, gentian, and black walnut.

She adds, "You can see where we are going with these herbs. This is obviously a broad-spectrum approach—antifungal, antiviral, and antibacterial. This is because these categories of STDs seem to exhibit symptoms of all these types of infections: fungal symptoms, such as discharge; bacterial symptoms, such as inflammation; and viral symptoms, in that these infections can migrate to other parts of the body."

Chlamydia

In 2013, 1.4 million chlamydia diagnoses were reported in the United States. Because many cases go undetected, it is estimated that there are actually many more new cases annually. Amanda McQuade Crawford, health expert and author of *Herbal Remedies for Women*, provides some background: The infecting organism, Chlamydia trachomatis, is a one-celled parasite with a rigid cell wall. Chlamydia is harder to clear up with herbal agents than some other one-celled organisms, such as bacteria and yeast, which respond very well to herbal treatment. "It often goes undiagnosed and can cause an inflammation of the cervix in women. This is why it is one of the leading causes of more serious pelvic diseases, particularly PID."

SYMPTOMS

"Usually the first symptom is a painless bump that goes unnoticed, followed by swollen lymph glands and headaches," Crawford says. "Some women get strange fleeting pains in their joints and muscles, as well as chills, and even weight loss, one to four weeks later.

"There will be a vaginal discharge that feels like mucus but has a bad odor. There may also be pain with sexual intercourse and some spotting after intercourse. If there is spotting between menstrual periods, a woman should see a licensed practitioner to look for signs of redness on the cervix.

"Other signs that women might experience are urinary frequency and painful urination, as well as some lower abdominal pain, although these symptoms may be caused by some other conditions as well."

Carol Dalton emphasizes that chlamydia often leads to PID. "It can go up into the uterus, the fallopian tubes, and the ovarian area and cause very serious infections and scarring and, therefore, infertility." As with so many diseases, early detection is essential. It can also cause problems in pregnancy, including premature or difficult delivery.

TREATMENT

In conventional drug treatment, antibiotics are used. "Which antibiotic is chosen, if any, will depend on whether a woman is pregnant or not," Crawford explains. "There are often secondary infections with bacteria or viruses, and that can complicate the picture. That's another reason why chlamydia is difficult to treat with simple remedies."

In Dalton's practice, she uses antibiotics. "We use antibiotics because of the risk factor. I think in health care you always weigh the risks versus the benefits of treatment. In this case, you see that the risk is great. Even if someone isn't concerned about fertility, you still weigh the risk of damaging the woman's immune system because you have an active infection that could become very serious. So chlamydia is one of the things that we don't really fool around with. We treat it with antibiotics; and we recheck it to make sure it's gone."

Crawford has looked into herbal treatments for chlamydia. One is the anti-inflammatory herb calendula, or marigold—not the garden variety but the medicinal single-flower kind. Demulcents such as plantain are also useful and are often combined with herbs that help normalize the hormones. As she puts it, "Sometimes a hormonal imbalance will have led to a change in the reproductive tissues, so these rectifying herbs are needed to make it possible to clear up this infection."

Herbal douches can also be of some help with reproductive infections, though, according to Crawford, they really can't get to the source of the problem. While the douche is rinsing out the infectious agent, it is also rinsing away the helpful bacteria, which is why you should be cautious about using herbal douches with any kind of infection. Still, the antimicrobial herbs used in the douches can help reduce the infectious organisms. "What we normally do," Crawford explains, "is follow each douche with a rest period, because these douches can dry out the tissue, making the irritated vaginal walls more susceptible to other infections. Even plain water douches will have that effect."

Crawford describes a douche formula that uses 2 ounces of organic grape root, also know as barberry bark root, and 1 ounce of calendula flower. Steep 1 ounce of this mixture in a pint of boiling water for about forty-five minutes. Strain it and let the tea cool to a comfortable temperature for vaginal use. To this mixture add about 7 drops of essential oil of tea tree. You can use a wire whisk to help mix them together. Make sure all the containers used are sterilized. Use this as a douche twice a week for up to three weeks. It's not necessary to rinse the herbs out of the vaginal canal afterward, but Crawford says that it feels very comforting to get rid of some of the bad-smelling discharge from chlamydia.

Dr. Page uses vaginal ointments to treat chlamydia. She suggests a combination of berberine-compound herbs: goldenseal, barberry, and Oregon grape. Mix this with vitamin A oil and apply directly to the cervix via a tampon.

Pelvic Inflammatory Disease (PID)

Pelvic inflammatory disease generally originates from an infection, such as chlamydia, that spreads out of control. Dalton says that chlamydia is the primary cause of PID. Because PID can be a "silent" infection, someone can have it for years without knowing she is infected. "So, it's easily transmitted. It can fester in the cervical canal, and then, when the immune system is low, can creep up into the other pelvic organs and cause a major infection."

She adds that it was a shift in birth control methods that played a big part in the rise of PID. "We really saw a lot of this disease when IUDs became popular, particularly when the Dalkon Shield was still being used. The Dalkon Shield had a multifilament string; there were multiple threads within this string, and bacteria could climb up the threads more easily, and into the uterus. The problems with the Dalkon Shield brought about a greater understanding of PID: how to develop cultures for it, how to study it, and what treatment to use knowledge of the damage that PID could do."

SYMPTOMS

PID symptoms vary; some women have very severe symptoms, other women have symptoms so mild that they are unaware they are infected. The most common symptom is pain, which ranges from a dull ache to pain so debilitating that walking is impossible. Other symptoms are bleeding, a foul discharge, cramps, swelling in the abdominal area, fever, and chills.

In addition to damaging the internal organs, PID can also result in scarring, particularly of the fallopian tubes. As Dalton explains, "This is how PID causes infertility. Even after you have cleared the infection, even if it hasn't blocked the tubes completely with scarring, the wavelike, hairlike projections that sweep the sperm through the fallopian tube to the egg and that sweep the egg up into the fallopian tube to meet with the sperm are often damaged and flattened. So that even though you may have a good, clear tube, the system isn't working properly. When this happens, it's a very serious problem, particularly for young, fertile women. It's probably one of the major causes of infertility. That's why we have to be really aggressive in testing for chlamydia and in treating it. We can clear the infection. We can give women antibiotics, but if we don't catch it soon enough, it can do all of this damage and may result in infertility."

TREATMENT

Dalton explains that once a woman is at the point where PID has really taken hold, there is severe swelling and inflammation in the entire pelvic area. To heal properly, the woman has to rest her body completely, which means bed rest. "Because whenever we are standing or walking, just because of gravity and the weight of the body, the pelvic area is impinged upon and there is a lot of pressure. So we encourage a woman to go to bed and rest while she is being treated. We get a much better response, much better healing, quicker healing, and less recurrence when this is followed.

"The other thing we advise patients to do is to use diet and supplements to encourage healing. We use zinc and vitamins C and E to encourage good oxygenation and tissue repair. We have to remember that the antibiotic just kills the bacteria, it does not cause healing to take place. Those tissues have to heal on their own, and if you give them a little extra encouragement with extra nutrients they are going to do that in a quicker and better fashion."

Human Papillomavirus (HPV)

According to a 2015 fact sheet from the Centers for Disease Control and Prevention (CDC), HPV is the most common sexually transmitted infection in the US, affecting nearly all sexually active people at some point in their lives. In 90 percent of cases, it resolves on its own without causing any health concerns. However, persistent infection can cause problems ranging from genital warts to cancer. Among the cancers that may be associated with HPV are cancer of the cervix, vulva, vagina, penis, anus, tonsils, and tongue.

HPV is particularly hazardous, says Carol Dalton, because it often goes undetected. "People often have no idea that they have it because it's microscopic, so it's easily transmitted during sexual intercourse. One study showed that 75 percent of a group of women and men who were tested were positive for HPV, and most of them did not realize they were infected." HPV is diagnosed in women most frequently by a Pap smear. The Pap smear results come back as "atypical, suspicious of HPV" or "dysplasia, suspicious of HPV," Dalton explains. She also underlines the possible consequences of getting HPV. "It's the primary cause of dysplasia. Probably over 90 percent of the time, dysplasia of the cervix or, eventually, cervical cancer, is caused by HPV. That's why it's so important to get a proper diagnosis."

The condition of the immune system is related to the health of a woman's vaginal and cervical cells. "Clearly, a woman can be infected with this, and we know it is in her system, but she is not having any problems. It's not invading the cells and growing and changing them into abnormal ones. Whether or not a woman will develop HPV depends on the response of the immune system.

"Once a woman develops abnormal cells, we diagnose it by doing a colposcopy and biopsy of any abnormal cells. A colposcope is an instrument we use to look at the cervix, vagina, and labia. It magnifies these areas so that we can actually see the cells to identify the areas where abnormal cells are present. After we have identified the abnormal cells, we do small biopsies—pinhead size or smaller. The biopsies are sent to a pathology lab where they section them and examine them under a microscope to identify the cells and see what is going on there."

PREVENTION AND TREATMENT

Although HPV cannot be cured, the cell changes that arise from infection can be treated. "The typical treatment can be to do nothing and watch for a while to see if the body can heal itself and reverse the process," Dalton says. "Cryotherapy, freezing of the cells, may be used, as well as laser therapy or a procedure called LEEP (loop excisional electrosurgical procedure), which uses an electrical wire to cut out abnormal tissue. All of these destroy the abnormal cells.

"The fortunate thing," Dalton continues, "is that the vagina and cervix produce a new surface of cells about every six to eight weeks. So if we can remove the cells that are abnormal, new, healthy cells will hopefully grow in. One reason it is important to remove the abnormal cells is that new cells tend to be like the cells next to them, so if abnormal cells remain in the body, the new cells will grow into abnormal cells too."

Unfortunately, just removing these abnormal cells often does not end the problem. As Dalton notes, "You can't kill off the virus completely, since it is in the surrounding tissue. You can't cauterize or remove the whole lining of the vagina. We only remove the cells that have become abnormal. There is a very high recurrence rate, with HPV causing the same abnormal cell growth all over again, unless you improve the woman's immune system and strengthen those normal cells."

Oral supplements of zinc, vitamin C, beta-carotene, folic acid, and general B-complex, along with a multivitamin-mineral, may aid in this process. Dalton says, "We recommend larger than usual doses of these because we have found that the new cell growth responds well to these nutrients. Moreover, many of these are antiviral nutrients. They help the woman's body fight the virus more readily and more systematically.

"We also use vitamin A suppositories. There's been a fair amount of work done on how cervical dysplasia can be treated with topical vitamin A. There are also suppositories we use called papillo suppositories that are made to fight the HPV virus topically. With these, we are treating the whole vaginal area and not just the cells that have become abnormal. We also use something called formula W, for wart virus, that contains herbs that help fight the HPV virus."

Her clinic uses both oral and topical treatments. They also examine patients' stress levels, their diet, and their lifestyle issues. This seems to be a successful approach, since, she maintains, "We have about a 1 to 2 percent recurrence rate with HPV, while the national average, when conventional methods are used exclusively, is 10 to 15 percent recurrence. So we feel that treating the whole person has made a huge difference in our ability to prevent recurrence, which is really the issue. HPV is not so hard to treat initially, but it's keeping it from coming back that is really the problem. I would encourage women who have this problem to look at the whole person."

HIV and AIDS have created a further difficulty in treatment. "We've had to be very careful about screening for HIV and AIDS and treating those patients," Dalton points out, "because the immune system with HIV is so compromised that if a woman with HIV does contract HPV, it seems to grow at a very rapid rate. The cells can turn into cancerous cells much more easily on the vulva, labia, cervix, and vagina. Practitioners treating patients who have HIV and AIDS need to be extremely cautious in doing colposcopies and biopsies. Even more than with the average patient, be aggressive with treatment and in building the immune system. Because having these other problems will greatly increase the risk factor of the abnormal cells turning into cancerous cells."

CAUTION ABOUT THE VACCINES

Every parent desires only the best for their children, which is why most insist that their children, primarily girls but now also boys, receive the three-shot series of HPV vaccines. Parents do this because there is the unchallenged assumption that vaccine public mandates and physician recommendations are founded upon sound scientific and medical principles of safety and efficacy. This is not only true for the HPV vaccines—Merck's Gardasil and Glaxo's Cervarix—but for all childhood vaccines.

When we investigate the vaccines rationally and objectively what is discovered should shake the pro-vaccine paradigm to its very foundations. What we find is a trail of permanent injury, neurological disorders, and death. And behind that we discover political and private obfuscation, cover-ups, lies, distortions, and no apologies from either government or the pharmaceutical industry. There is no desire by any government agency, corporation, or leading medical institution to seek the truth. In an article posted on my blog (http://blog.garynull.com), I shed considerable light on this topic. Here I will briefly summarize.

Relying upon the data from the CDC's Vaccine Adverse Events Reporting System (VAERS), the vaccine watch organization Sanevax determined that, since Gardasil's launch in 2006 until November 2012, the HPV vaccine was linked to

121 deaths and over 27,485 medical injuries of young girls, some as young as eleven years old. Unfortunately, only a fraction of vaccine adverse events reported by pediatricians, physicians, medical clinics, and hospitals make their way into the VAERS database. Few parents even know such a reporting system exists.

From the start, a vaccine against the human papillomavirus was completely unnecessary. Aside from the unreasonable health risks that come with this vaccine, Gardasil is also the most expensive recommended vaccine on the market at $120 – $150 per injection and three required doses. If this vaccine becomes mandated for school attendance, how are underprivileged people and the uninsured to come up with the money? And as funding for government programs dries up, does it make any sense to allocate state health care dollars to vaccinate Medicaid-eligible girls with Gardasil instead of using the money for something that actually might be of benefit?

In the US and the UK, the health agencies are ruled and dictated by the drug makers. Merck, Pfizer and a handful of other pharmaceutical firms are the CDC and FDA and vice versa. If we wish to find more accurate official views and policies regarding the HPV vaccines, we must look at other nations that care more about the public health of their populations rather than the revenues of private corporations. Today there is a growing concern among many nations' health ministries and physicians about the serious health risks associated with these vaccines.

So why hasn't the FDA, the CDC, the American Academy of Pediatrics, or Merck itself responded to the VAERS reports that Gardasil is not a safe vaccine? The argument, which is the same defense used by all the drug companies and government agencies against any adverse reaction to any vaccine, is that since the VAERS system uses voluntary, passive reporting, it does not prove that a sudden health problem—or even death—occurring after vaccination was in fact caused by the vaccine.

The only causal relationships acceptable to the powers that be are those that result from scientific studies. But these are often unacceptable to the rest of us since the majority of these studies are funded by the pharmaceutical companies themselves. So the fix is in. What can any injured child or concerned parent do in the face of this hard line—should they be required to set up their own scientific study? Obviously, neither Merck nor our government willing to spend money to prove that Gardasil is dangerous—it is much simpler and infinitely more lucrative to just ignore the allegations and try to portray the victims as conspiratorial whiners.

The CDC and the FDA maintain that Gardasil is an important cervical cancer prevention tool that could protect the health of millions of women. But the facts show that the opposite is true. In point of fact, Gardasil vaccination is not justified by the health "benefits" nor is it even economically feasible. Nevertheless, the lure of huge profits appears to cloud the thinking of everyone in a position to say no to the promotion of Gardasil. It is up to us, the victims, the parents, and the concerned friends and neighbors to get the message out to as many people as we can. We must flood our legislators with notice that this vaccine is dangerous, should not be given to anyone, and at the very least, should not be mandated for school attendance.

Genital Warts

Genital warts are caused by HPV. Symptoms of genital warts can take as little as three weeks and as long as eight months to develop after exposure to the virus. Genital warts are contagious, even before they become symptomatic.

Dr. Page treats genital warts successfully with vitamin C therapy. "Up to 10,000 milligrams daily is used to enhance white blood cell activity and boost immune interferon. We use a mix of carotenes up to 200,000 IU daily." She also uses aloe vera gel as a topical application for genital warts. She particularly recommends an aloe vera/garlic mixture. "You steep garlic cloves in the aloe vera gel, so you have a very high sulfur mix. We ask patients to drink two glasses of aloe vera juice daily. We also use a 'vag-pack' for genital warts, which includes goldenseal, burdock, chaparral, and sarsaparilla. Blend the herbs and put them on a tampon and insert into the vagina. This is an internal poultice to draw out the infection. It is very effective, especially when you add B-complex with extra folic acid. Both these supplements help normalize those abnormal cells."

She adds, "This is a virus, so you would want to take antiviral herbs. The ones I use regularly are lomatium, St. John's wort, and bupleurum. Occasionally, I also use myrrh. Any combination of these works. It's best to use them in an extract if you want antiviral activity."

Dr. Warshowsky notes that genital warts should be treated creatively and holistically. "When a woman is willing to do an entire body-balancing protocol, where she is looking at what is going on in her life that is making her susceptible to infection, balancing out her gut bacteria, eating a nutrient-rich diet, and employing some of these beneficial herbs and supplements, I think there is good success in restoring order, restoring balance, and getting rid of infection."

Research Update

Following is a sample of recent peer-reviewed scientific studies on sexually transmitted diseases.

A 2011 study in *Gynecologic Oncology* found that twice weekly intravaginal infusions of zinc citrate solution containing CIZAR (zinc chloride and citric acid anhydrous), administered for twelve weeks, resulted in elimination of high-risk HPV in nearly 64 percent of patients tested. A 2014 article on the *GreenMedInfo* website called more attention to the safety of the Gardasil vaccine, following recent studies showing its link to nervous and immune system disorders. Two cases of Postural Orthostatic Tachycardia Syndrome (POTS), a rare autonomic nervous system disorder, are described in 2014 reports in the *Journal of Investigative Medicine High Impact Case Reports* and the *European Journal of Neurology*. "Both studies raise questions about the safety of the HPV vaccine," the author says. "But more significantly they point to a body of recent evidence that links vaccination not just to POTS but to a much wider range of autoimmune sicknesses including multiple sclerosis, systemic lupus erythematosus and rheumatoid arthritis."

Chapter 55

Stroke

In a 2015 update, the American Heart Association reported that nearly 800,000 Americans have strokes annually. Although it is the third leading cause of death in women, many females are still unaware of the signs and symptoms that could get them the early help they need.

Causes

There are two different types of strokes: hemorrhagic stroke, which is a rupture in a blood vessel, and ischemic stroke, which is caused by a blockage in the blood vessels. The result of both types is a lack of blood flow to the brain and consequently insufficient oxygen for brain function.

Symptoms

Symptoms of stroke include dizziness, blurred vision and loss of sensation, slurred speech, loss of bladder control, and partial loss of hearing. A person should seek medical help immediately if she experiences one or more of these symptoms. Often a stroke will be accompanied by paralysis of an arm or leg on one side of the body. Strokes can cause swelling of the brain, stupor, and coma.

Clinical Experience

Traditional treatment may involve surgery, medication, hospital care, and rehabilitation.

ALTERNATIVE APPROACHES

DIET

Maintaining a healthy diet is crucial to overall health. Research from the Harvard Medical School and elsewhere has found that eating five or more servings a day of fruits and vegetables can reduce the risk of ischemic stroke by up to 30 percent. Among the most beneficial foods are cabbage, bok choy, brussels sprouts, broccoli, cauliflower, collard greens, spinach, citrus fruits, and citrus juice.

HERBS

Herbal remedies may be useful in preventing blood clots and increasing blood flow to the brain. They also can help to prevent complications of stroke. The following herbs are recommended by a variety of practitioners: garlic, ginkgo biloba, ginger, turmeric, willow, onion, evening primrose oil, astragalus, hawthorn, horsetail, and kava kava. Some of these should not be used if you are pregnant or nursing.

ENZYME THERAPY

Dr. Anthony Cichoke is a leading medical researcher in the field of enzyme therapy. He has taught at the University of Minnesota and the University of Rochester Medical School, and is the author of hundreds of articles and seven books, including *The Complete Book of Enzyme Therapy.*

Dr. Cichoke uses enzyme therapy to boost the immune system and detoxify the body. "Enzymes are catalysts," he explains. "Anything that is alive has to have enzymatic activity—whether it is in the grass outside or whether it is in your body. Enzymes are critical for every cell of our body. Nothing can go on in the body without enzymatic activity. Without enzymes there would be no breathing, no digestion, no growth, no blood coagulation, no reproduction." Enzymes, he says, fight strokes by acting "as a sort of 'Roto Rooter' that helps break up cholesterol and toxins in your body.

"Strokes can be treated systemically with enzymes. They are used as digestive aids; they improve the absorption of other nutrients, herbs, health foods, whatever. Enzymes aid absorption and metabolism at the cellular level."

Dr. Cichoke has his patients take enzyme supplements orally between meals. He recommends enzymes such as bromelain, papain, trypsin, chymotrypsin, pancreatin, and microbial proteases, all of which have primarily proteolytic enzyme activity. Dr. Cichoke describes how enzyme supplements pass through the gut into the small intestine, where they are absorbed into the circulatory system. "These are all enzymes that work in the bloodstream and the various organs as well as at the cellular level of the body."

Enzymes aid in detoxification at the cellular level in various organs and in the bloodstream and digestive tract. He explains why it is important to have a well-ordered circulatory system: "The blood must get to the cells in order to bring nutrients to the body, and blood needs to help take the waste products away from the cells. Further, enzymes help break up the cholesterol and fibrin in the blood vessels." Dr. Cichoke pictures a blood vessel as a stream or river, with little curves and eddies. These curves fill up with fibrin and cholesterol, which clog blood vessels so that the blood and oxygen can't get through.

"Proteolytic enzymes help to break up the fibrin and cholesterol and allow the body to eliminate these waste products. Enzymes also improve circulation. They help keep the bloodstream normalized." He explains that it is important to have a balance between blood coagulation and blood thinning. "Enzymes help to keep this critical equilibrium in order."

Enzymes also help break up free radicals. "As part of the aging process, and also as a result of stress and illness and injuries, the cells of our body tend to oxidize—they rust. Think of the body's tissue as if it was like a lovely leather jacket. When you first buy that leather jacket, it's soft and pliable. But then, as it gets older, the leather oxidizes and it becomes cracked and hard. As we go through life, our body tends to oxidize. When you take antioxidant enzymes, such as superoxide dismutase, catalase, glutathione, and peroxidase, they fight free radical formation and work as antioxidants."

Enzymes can also dissolve large blood clots, which can cause strokes. Dr. Cichoke says that enzymes are currently being used both in and out of hospitals to break up blood clots and also to break up fibrin formations. "In hospitals, some enzymes used for this purpose are brinase, which comes from Aspergillus oryzae; streptokinase, which is of bacterial origin; and urokinase or prourokinase, which is actually from human urine."

Dr. Cichoke tells a story about a stroke patient in Portland, Oregon, who was treated with these enzymes. "They had given up on him. But as a last-ditch effort, nine hours after the stroke, they began to give him urokinase. Not only did he regain consciousness, he also regained the ability to move his arms and his legs. After six weeks of rehabilitation therapy he went home."

Dr. Cichoke cites an article in the *New York Times* that stated, "Enzymes offer hope for reducing devastation from strokes." Currently, Dr. Cichoke notes, the Cleveland Clinic in Cleveland, Ohio, is using prourokinase to fight strokes. He stresses the importance of proteolytic enzymes as well as antioxidant enzymes. "I suggest taking 200 micrograms of antioxidant enzymes three times a day between meals and eight to ten tablets of combination enzymes three times a day, also between meals. If you take bromelain, take four to six tablets of approximately 230 to 250 milligrams every day.

"I know this can be fairly expensive," he goes on, "but how much does health mean to you? We eat too much fat and too many refined carbohydrates, we smoke too much, we get virtually no exercise, and we overeat. For this reason, exercising, having a positive mental attitude, and eating fresh fruits are all very important. And enzyme supplementation is critical."

Research Update

An increasing body of evidence is showing the benefits of natural modalities to overall health and well-being. Following is a sample of recent peer-reviewed scientific studies regarding stroke.

A 2013 study published in the *Journal of Stroke and Cerebrovascular Disease* concluded that Gingko biloba has protective effects after a stroke. A total of 102 patients with acute ischemic stroke received either the herb or placebo tablets for four months. Nearly 59 percent of the gingko group achieved a 50 percent reduction on the National Institutes of Health Stroke Scale (NIHSS), used to measure functional outcome, as compared with 19 percent in the placebo group. In 2011, researchers reported in *Stroke* that greater consumption of white fruits and vegetables was inversely associated with incident stroke. Each 25 gram per day increase in consumption of foods such as apples, pears, bananas, cauliflower, and cucumber was associated with a 9 percent lower risk of stroke. Research reported in *Angiology* in 2012 found that adherence to a Mediterranean diet decreased the risk of ischemic stroke regardless of cholesterol levels. Results from a 2011 study in *Neurology* indicated that high olive oil consumption in older people was associated with a 41 percent lower risk of stroke when compared with those who never use it. Among the other nutrients that have been proven effective are nattokinase (an enzyme extracted from fermented soybeans), L-carnitine, acetyl-L-carnitine, propionyl-L-carnitine, vinpocetine, vitamin D, vitamin

B, omega-3 fatty acids, garlic, and DHEA. Additionally, the following nutrients have been found to be beneficial: vitamin C, vitamin E, magnesium, calcium, resveratrol, arjuna, hawthorne, cayenne, L-carnotine, and ubiquinol.

Chapter 56

Thyroid Disease

According to the American Thyroid Association, approximately 20 million Americans have some form of thyroid disease, a large percentage of whom are not even aware of their condition. Women are affected five to eight times more often than men. One in eight women will develop a thyroid disorder during her lifetime. Thyroid disease is at once a hot-button issue and one of the most misunderstood illnesses facing us today. A 2013 study published in the *Journal of Clinical Endocrinology and Metabolism* indicating that low or high thyroid levels present risks for pregnant women and their babies is just one example of the effects of thyroid conditions on overall health and well-being.

The thyroid gland, a critical component of the immune system, is a small, butterfly-shaped organ at the base of the neck. It produces thyroid hormone, which basically controls the metabolism of all the cells in the body—from our hair follicles to our toenails and everything in between. The thyroid can be implicated in just about any condition involving any part of the body, including the liver, brain, heart, kidneys, gut, reproductive system, and more.

Thyroid disease is called the great masquerader because it can deceive both doctors and patients alike. "It has such a wide range of effects that it can literally imitate or mimic so many diseases," says Dr. Raphael Kellman, author of *Gut Reactions* and *Matrix Healing*. "And that's one of the reasons why it's so terribly often overlooked."

Among the types of thyroid disease are hypothyroidism, hyperthyroidism (overactive thyroid), thyroiditis (inflammation of the thyroid), and thyroid cancer.

Hypothyroidism

In *Solve the Riddle of Illness*, Dr. Stephen Langer, a preventive medicine specialist in Berkeley, California, says that more than 40 percent of the population may have subclinical hypothyroidism that is not detected by the traditional blood chemistry done at their general practitioner's office. The symptoms of low thyroid include tiredness; lethargy; weakness; slow speech; dry, coarse skin; coarse hair; hair loss; weight gain; difficulty breathing; problems with menstruation; nervousness; heart palpitations; brittle nails; and severe chronic fatigue and depression. "A patient with a constellation of symptoms like that is going to be sick and tired of feeling sick and tired," Dr. Langer says. "Plus they're going to feel depressed all the time because they're going from one doctor to another, sometimes with two or three or four pages' worth of complaints, and the doctors tell them it's all in their head, or that they should go home and learn to live with it."

According to an article in the online magazine *Alternative Medicine* (www.alternativemedicine.com), hypothyroidism can also aggravate many female problems, including miscarriage, fibrocystic breast disease, ovarian fibroids, cystic ovaries, endometriosis, PMS, and menopausal symptoms.

CAUSES

Hypothyroidism is linked to hormonal imbalances, particularly an excess of estrogen over the other female hormone, progesterone. Normally, a woman's ratio of progesterone to estrogen is ten to one. If she has too much estrogen, this is bad for the thyroid, since estrogen inhibits thyroid production while progesterone promotes it. The connection between thyroid production and female hormones indicates that a disruption in one sphere will affect the other.

Dr. Mark Lader, from the Natural Wellness Center in New York, believes that nutritional deficiencies and stress are the two major keys to hypothyroidism. He says that although iodine deficiency or excess has been fully documented as a causal factor, it is not significant in the United States because most of the salt consumed here is iodized.

Micronutrient deficiencies are important. Some of the major nutrients involved in thyroid metabolism are selenium, glutathione, and zinc, which are known to be required for proper conversion of T4 into T3, the form of thyroid hormone that is active in the tissues. Dr. Lader says that we also should examine protein, fat, and carbohydrate consumption to really get an idea of what's happening with the thyroid gland. With hypothyroidism, as with so many other chronic illnesses, excess carbohydrate intake can be a major contributing factor. Too much carbohydrate can push blood sugar up and stimulate cortisol production, leading to hypoglycemia, and this increases thyroid production.

Dr. Lader also notes that suboptimal intake of calories, especially in women, may contribute to hypothyroidism. Diets high in caffeine may also adversely affect thyroid function. In addition, Dr. Lader notes, "Food allergies affect our thyroid glands, and that is why we see so many people with allergies who commonly have other systemic endocrine problems in their bodies. You also have to stop and look at chemical and medical toxicity. People whose cholesterol rises year after year may have hypothyroidism."

The gut is another place where problems can start. Our bodies detoxify and eliminate thyroid hormones through the gut, where certain enzymes in a healthy intestine help to break apart the soluble thyroid hormones so that we can reabsorb them through our intestines. Many people have had a lot of antibiotic therapy, and poor diet or intestinal problems have led to imbalances in microflora. This imbalance decreases the body's ability to reuptake active thyroid hormone. It's very important to establish a healthy environment in the intestines in order to maintain normal levels of thyroid hormones.

"We also have to look at the liver," Dr. Lader continues, "which is probably the most abused, overworked, and stressed organ in the body. Our liver is exposed to a number of toxins, which we have to make soluble so that we can excrete them out of our bodies. The same enzymes that break down many environmental toxins also break down thyroid chemicals. If our livers are overworked due to exposure to toxins, and those enzymes speed up, we are also going to be moving lots of thyroid hormone out of the body. This is really the X factor in thyroid illness."

Dr. Lader says that many drugs that people take also interfere with thyroid function. These include antidepressants and interferon, which is taken to treat hepatitis C but can affect thyroid function.

DIAGNOSIS

In conventional medicine, hypothyroidism is diagnosed by serum testing of the hormones thyroxine (T4), triiodothyronine (T3), and thyrotropin or thyroid-stimulating hormone (TSH). The textbook explanation is that low T4 and T3 levels along with high TSH indicate hypothyroidism. Dr. Lader comments, "On the face of it, hypothyroidism seems to be a real simple illness. The symptoms and blood values seem to correlate very well to a hypothyroid case, and then when we give levothyroxin, the symptoms seem to go away."

However, these tests are not as accurate as they might seem. An *Alternative Medicine* article points out that "most of the standard thyroid tests (for T3, T4, and TSH levels) often fail to pinpoint an underfunctioning thyroid, leading physicians to make erroneous diagnoses." The article goes on to say that doctors diagnose by symptoms, even while they remain unaware of the medical cause. So a patient with depression gets Prozac; one with weight gain is prescribed a weight loss drug; and one who is continually tired is said to suffer from chronic fatigue syndrome and gets no treatment.

In Dr. Lader's opinion, the standard blood tests do little to pinpoint the actual cause of the thyroid problem. Instead, he looks at the patient's overall environment to locate key problem sectors. The first step is ascertaining the patient's body temperature.

"For my own diagnosis, I ask the women about their symptoms and also use something called a basal temperature test, which is a very simple way to learn if the body is running cold. [Basal body temperature is a person's resting temperature upon waking up in the morning.] We ask the woman to use an oral thermometer. She shakes it down before she goes to sleep at night. First thing upon arising in the morning, she puts it under her armpit for about seven minutes.

"The temperature should be above 97.8. If it's below that level, many doctors will say that is diagnostic for hypothyroidism. However, we must remember that some people have a lower body temperature than others. They tend to run a little cool but don't have the hypothyroid symptoms. Some people's underarm temperature doesn't even rise after they have a significant improvement in their symptoms."

Dr. Lader looks at the whole body and a person's whole environment. In his experience, most of the symptoms that people with hypothyroidism come in with are lethargy, weakness, dryness, and cold intolerance. By studying both the temperature and the patient's whole history, he is able to assess the patient's condition. Among the other symptoms of hypothyroidism are insomnia, anxiety, forgetfulness, muscle and joint pain, reflux, constipation, and hair loss including thinning of the eyebrow.

Dr. Raphael Kellman tells about other useful tests. He has used the TRH stimulation test in the diagnosis of thousands of his patients. "It's a challenge test that can really help us when we suspect hypothyroidism and yet the routine blood tests come out normal," he says. TRH (thyrotropin-releasing hormone), which is the hormone that stimulates the pituitary gland to release TSH, is injected into the body, and the blood is tested twenty-five minutes later. "If the thyroid is low," Dr. Kellman says, "the pituitary is going to start producing a lot of TSH, and it's going to start building up in the pituitary gland."

In addition, Dr. Kellman suggests testing for heavy metal toxicity, as well as vitamin and mineral levels. "Very few people know that there are blood tests that we can do that can assess your vitamin levels: your vitamin C level, your vitamin E level, your beta-carotene level, your vitamin A and vitamin D, etc., and we can see which vitamins and nutrients one might be deficient in. A selenium deficiency can adversely affect the thyroid. You need selenium to produce an adequate amount of thyroid hormone. Amino acid deficiencies can also impact on the thyroid. You can also do an amino acid profile and see which amino acids one might be deficient in."

CONVENTIONAL TREATMENT

Conventional treatment relies on prescription thyroid hormone replacement drugs. They include levothyroxine (Synthroid), a synthetic form of the T4 thyroid hormone, the most common drug; liothyronine, a synthetic form of the T3 hormone, sometimes used with levothyroxine; and liotrix, a synthetic combination of T3 and T4. There are also natural thyroid hormone replacement drugs, which are made from the desiccated thyroid glands of pigs.

According to Dr. Lader, on the surface, it would seem reasonable to treat the symptoms of hypothyroidism with hormone replacement drugs. "These drugs make the symptoms disappear in a high percentage of cases," he says. "But, are we really getting to the true causes of the problem?"

Dr. Lader tells about the drawbacks to these medicines. "We know that in conventional treatment the patient will be on the medication for her whole life. Natural doctors believe we don't need to medicate people that long. Moreover, the increasingly larger doses these people are getting over the course of a lifetime cause more and more adverse symptoms."

It's important to treat the whole body, Dr. Lader says. "One of the true hallmarks of an alternative, natural practitioner is that she or he believes that eliminating symptoms is not really enough to determine if a successful therapy has been carried out." He adds, "Probably most readers realize that we have a medical tradition in this country of relegating hypothyroidism to the idiopathic trash heap. *Idiopathic* is a term used when traditional medicine does not know what the cause is. In my opinion, though, it means we are not asking the right questions. Saying that this problem has unknown causes or ones that cannot be addressed nutritionally is really a cop-out. At the same time, many doctors just whip out the hormone replacement therapy prescription pad in order to treat the symptoms while ignoring the cause. To me this is sad, a sad commentary on our whole health care system in this country."

Dr. Lader notes that there are many different agents in our environment that decrease thyroid function, ranging from stress to food. And, he says, treating environmentally induced hypothyroidism by using hormones or drugs is an excuse for those who are not willing to do the right work to get people well. He argues that to treat hypothyroidism, we have to use a natural approach to make the body stronger and healthier. "To really give optimal treatment for hypothyroidism, we have to treat the ultimate cause of the illness. So we will have to deal with diet, nutrition, and all the environmental factors that can affect our thyroid gland."

ALTERNATIVE TREATMENT

There are several dietary recommendations for hypothyroidism. A healthy, balanced diet is important. Among the foods to include are fresh fruits and vegetables, whole grains, and lean protein. "One thing I urge my patients to try to avoid is the Brassica family foods—cabbage, broccoli, cauliflower," Dr. Lader says. He acknowledges that these foods have many health benefits, but says that they are considered goitrogenic (goiter-causing), especially in their raw form. Other foods in this category that should be avoided or limited include kale, spinach, brussels sprouts, peaches, pears, and strawberries.

Another aspect of alternative treatment is nutritional supplementation. The creation of a supplement program has to be handled carefully, Dr. Lader explains. "It comes down to the fact that every hypothyroid patient is different and requires a different approach. Supplemental programs need to be customized so that they address all the factors that have been ascertained during the diagnosis and workup. In general, we have to make sure people are taking in adequate amounts of selenium, glutathione, and zinc."

Stress management is also important. One of the major problems of hypothyroidism, as noted, is inadequate conversion of inactive thyroid (thyroxine) into active thyroid (triiodothyronine). Stress elevates cortisol, which inhibits this conversion process. Heavy activity, exercise, and different stress-reduction methods are needed.

Dr. Langer describes his treatment approach using case examples. "Recently I treated a patient who was the wife of a doctor and the mother of two young children. She basically came in and told me that she didn't want to go on living. She was so tired all the time and so depressed that she couldn't keep her head off the pillow after two in the afternoon. If she didn't go to bed, she would just fall apart. I did a history and physical on her and we made some dietary changes, but basically this woman was profoundly hypothyroid. We put her on a quarter of a grain of thyroid, which is what I start my patients with before building them up very gradually. A quarter of a grain is the smallest dose available. It's such a small quantity that most pharmacies don't even carry it, because when doctors order thyroid they don't even think to order so small a dose. But a quarter of a grain of thyroid was enough. Within a three-week period, this woman not only regained her mental health, but she was out taking tennis lessons, which was shocking even to me because although the treatment usually works it usually takes a longer period of time. So, just that amount of metabolic support was enough to turn this person's life around.

"Another person I treated was a sixty-two-year-old woman who was a member of the Catholic clergy. She had been a nun for at least thirty years when I met her and I will never forget this woman. She came in bloated, profoundly depressed and fatigued. The only thing that kept her going was basically overworking her adrenal glands. She came in and told me that when she was twelve years old, she went under a dark cloud. When I saw her it was fifty years later, and by that time she had been through thirty or forty different doctors, including internists, endocrinologists, psychiatrists, and psychologists of various sorts.

"One of the first things that showed up in her—which I thought was a very positive sign—was that she was freezing all the time. When we did a basal body temperature, it never went above ninety-five degrees. Basal body temperature is a person's resting temperature when she wakes up in the morning. However, when I did a blood work-up on her, all her thyroid hormone levels were within normal limits. I empirically placed her on a dose of thyroid that we gradually built up to about four grains a day, which is quite a high dosage. She's one of the few people I've treated who has needed that high an amount. Within three months her depression of fifty years' duration was totally gone. Now, obviously she was bitter and angry that she had been suffering for all that time. But the organic feeling that she had of overwhelming fatigue totally disappeared within a three-month period of time, and I've seen that response in thousands of patients over the years. A small dose of thyroid, combined with things like nutritional support and eliminating food allergies, can really turn a person's life around."

Dr. Kellman, who outlines his approach to natural treatment in *The Microbiome Diet*, says that "first and foremost, you have to heal the gut. . . We have to rethink the overuse of antibiotics. We have to clean up our diet. We have to eat healthier foods, no processed foods, no trans fats. Eat more organic foods and say no to genetically modified foods. Take probiotics and prebiotics." There are many herbs that can improve thyroid function, including ashwagandha and gugulipid. Selenium may also be used.

Hyperthyroidism

Hyperthyroidism is a condition in which there is overactivity of the thyroid gland in producing thyroid hormone. It is about ten times more common in women than men.

Dr. Saralyn Mark, an endocrinologist and women's health specialist, describes some of the most common symptoms. "Women who have overactive thyroid glands may feel very restless. They may feel like they're having hot flashes. They feel warm. They might find that they can't keep weight on. In fact, I've had some patients say please don't treat my thyroid problem. I like it because it allows me to keep my weight down and have all this energy. Well, unfortunately, too much thyroid hormone in the body can be very toxic to many cells, including the heart as well as your bones. So we really want people to be what we call euthyroid thyroid in a normal thyroid state."

Some people with hyperthyroidism have thyroid enlargement caused by nodules or masses in their thyroid gland. "That can be part of the thyroid gland that is overactive, and fortunately we can treat that," Dr. Mark says. "We can take these nodules out. We can also give medications that can suppress the thyroid glands so that your body is in a normal state."

Causes of hyperthyroidism include Graves' disease, excessive intake of thyroid hormones, abnormal secretion of thyroid-stimulating hormone (TSH), and thyroiditis. Diagnosis typically involves physical examination and blood tests. Conventional treatment includes drugs to inhibit the production of thyroid hormones; beta-blockers to reduce symptoms such as heart palpitations, tremor, and anxiety; surgery to remove all or part of the thyroid; and radioactive iodine to destroy the thyroid.

Natural approaches to hyperthyroidism emphasize diet, exercise, and alternative therapies. Diet should consist of nutritious foods including papaya, mango, green leafy vegetables, and fish. Vitamins A, B-complex, C, calcium, and phosphorus should be increased via food or supplements. Omega-3 and L-carnitine may help in regulation of the thyroid. Among the herbs that have been found to decrease thyroid activity are bugleweed, motherwort, and turmeric. Homeopathy, acupuncture, and massage also are beneficial.

Thyroiditis

Thyroiditis is inflammation of the thyroid gland. The most common type of thyroiditis is Hashimoto's thyroiditis, or autoimmune thyroiditis. Thyroiditis is a root cause of a variety of emotional and physical problems. According to Dr. Hyla Cass, a holistic psychiatrist, "When the thyroid isn't working properly, the immune system is impaired, and this sets up a vicious cycle. You have a person whose immune system is depleted and who is anxious; they're told by regular doctors that the problem is all in their head, that there's nothing physically wrong with them. So then they feel worse."

CAUSES

What triggers the autoimmune response associated with the most common type of thyroiditis? Dr. Stephen Langer explains: "Imagine autoimmune thyroiditis to be like rheumatoid arthritis of the thyroid gland. A person can have rheumatoid arthritis, which is an autoimmune condition where the body puts out antibodies to the joints. Frequently people with rheumatoid arthritis can experience long periods of remission. When they are under a great deal of stress, the body puts out antibodies to the joints and all their joints swell up. A similar thing happens with thyroiditis; if a person gets stressed out for any reason whatsoever, the body can start pumping out antibodies to the thyroid gland. The thyroid becomes acutely inflamed, and thyroid hormone, which under normal circumstances would not be released, starts escaping. It's almost like pumping speed into your system."

CLINICAL EXPERIENCE

Dr. Langer notes, "There is a very precise blood test that any doctor can order called the autoimmune thyroid antibody test, and most of the people who I suspect have thyroid conditions and have normal thyroid hormone levels will have an elevation in their antithyroid antibodies. If they have an elevated antithyroid antibody level, they have the symptoms that go along with low thyroid, which can be any one of 125 symptoms that we enumerate in *Solve the Riddle of Illness*."

Like hypothyroidism, thyroiditis can cause a number of psychological symptoms. Dr. Langer explains: "With thyroiditis people get anxiety attacks and panic attacks for no apparent reason. They could be sitting and reading a book. All of a sudden they will develop a cascade of heart palpitations and fearfulness.

"I've had a number of patients who have been rushed, almost on a monthly basis, to the emergency room to be worked up by cardiologists because their heart was pounding over 200 beats a minute. Cardiologists would do EKGs and echocardiograms and then tell them to go see a psychiatrist. The psychiatrist would work them up, not find anything, and then put them on an antidepressant or a tranquilizer, and actually make the condition worse. When you have an undiscovered organic basis for a psychological problem, being put on psychotropic medication is like sitting on a thumbtack and being put on pain pills for the rest of your life. It has about the same effect. It wears the system down, and as a result the patient's condition not only does not improve but will in fact deteriorate, because the underlying cause is not being treated."

A large number of Dr. Hyla Cass's patients also have thyroiditis. "I really can't emphasize the importance of this problem enough," she says, "because thyroiditis often accompanies the mixed infection syndrome, which can consist of any combination of the following: parasites, candidiasis, and the viral syndromes, including Epstein-Barr virus and cytomegalovirus. Psychological components include depression, anxiety, and even panic attacks.

"To treat thyroiditis, I've done nutritional consults on people who were under the care of other physicians. When I suggested that they had thyroiditis and that it was to be treated with low doses of thyroid hormones, I was met with skepticism from the other doctors."

Depression is common in these patients. "When people have these long-standing chronic conditions, they can become extremely depressed," Dr. Cass says. "They feel like they can't go on anymore, particularly when their body has been so racked by the continuing illness. Also, some of the mixed infection of thyroiditis and the parasites or other viruses can actually affect the brain directly. Thyroiditis and its accompanying infections affect the central nervous system along with every other organ of the body. So people come in extremely depressed, both as a reaction to their prolonged illness and as a primary symptom of the illness, and this is usually totally overlooked. That's why it's crucial to do a good medical workup on a patient whose disorder may at first appear purely psychological in origin."

"There is one more connection to be drawn between depression and thyroid dysfunction," Dr. Langer adds. "Poor libido. One of the classic symptoms of depression is a loss of interest in sex. Those people who in the past were sexually active but who all of a sudden or gradually started to lose interest in sex will be diagnosed as being depressed right away. Men come into my office by the score— many of them young—who have potency problems, and they can't figure it out because they have no apparent organic illness. As a result, they get performance anxiety, and if that continues long enough, they wind up getting severely depressed. But I have found that if you go to the root cause of their depression, very often it's the thyroid that's malfunctioning.

"If a person develops an acute depression that leads to a sexual dysfunction— which it frequently does—a doctor would be remiss if he or she didn't look for an imbalance in the thyroid. Patients have got to start taking their health destinies into their own hands and demanding that doctors do thyroid testing and look for autoimmune thyroid disorders and nutritional imbalances, which are frequently the underlying causes of sexual dysfunction and depression."

ALTERNATIVE THERAPIES

Dr. Langer describes his approach to treatment. "The question for holistic clinicians to ask themselves regarding each individual patient is where they're going to intervene," he says. "Different physicians will intervene at different places, depending upon their background and interests. I try, to the best of my ability, to get to the root cause of what's going on. If I am having difficulty figuring out the cause, then I try to intervene at a point in a person's imbalance that will cause the least disruption to their lifestyle and give them the best results for the least amount of money in the quickest period of time. Frequently, that turns out to be treating with small doses of thyroid and altering eating habits. In my clinical experience, I have found that with the thyroid and nutritional support, very often a person will get better. The thyroid is not a lifetime treatment and can be removed after the person's condition has been stabilized. Thyroid treatment is inexpensive, works rapidly, and when done properly is absolutely nontoxic."

Dr. Allan Spreen, a general practitioner who specializes in nutrition-based medicine, reminds us that while thyroid supplementation is an important modality, it is not fail-safe. "I'd love to say that correcting thyroid function is a panacea. While it doesn't work 100 percent of the time, if a patient comes in complaining of fatigue and depression that is linked with the physical findings of foods not digesting well, and cold extremities, then an underactive thyroid may be the root cause. People come and say, 'Oh, my husband says, 'Don't touch me with your feet at night because they're just ice cold.' These are the same people who are comfortable in a room when everybody else is boiling and who are freezing in a room when everybody else is comfortable. Their thinking seems to have slowed down. They just don't seem to be able to concentrate like they used to, and they don't remember lists the way they used to."

Dr. Spreen says that when a patient's blood levels of thyroid are normal, he then keeps track of body temperature. "I go back to the old school of Broda Barnes, who, 40 or 50 years ago, did axillary temperature testing. I ask my patients to keep a record of their early-morning basal body temperature. If their basal metabolic rate based on early-morning body temperatures is really low, then I consider them to be candidates for thyroid supplementation. In axillary testing, Broda Barnes talked about temperature ranges between 97.8 and 98.2 degrees Fahrenheit, which is lower than the 98.6 people think of as normal. But the axillary temperature is taken in the armpit first thing in the morning, using a mercury thermometer that stays there for ten minutes before they get up. If their temperature is, much of the time, down in the 96.8, 96.7, 96.5 range, I at least consider the possibility that the person needs low doses of natural thyroid, which is still available.

"Thyroid is a prescription drug. Some doctors who use this type of testing use synthetic thyroid. I prefer to prescribe natural thyroid in very low doses. If a person responds—either their temperature rises or their symptoms lift—then I retest them to see if their blood levels of thyroid have changed. Many times a person with this profile of symptoms who takes thyroid begins to feel better, but their blood tests remain unchanged, including levels of thyroid stimulating hormone (TSH) and actual thyroid hormone. This means that the blood testing has missed the diagnosis, and yet the person feels well with the increased, but undetectable, dose of thyroid hormone."

PATIENT STORIES

I came to be treated by Dr. Spreen only after first following the conventional route in medical treatment. I was in my fifth year of infertility treatments, had taken multiple infertility drugs, and wound up severely depressed, which caused me to lose thirty-five pounds in two months. I couldn't sleep, I had panic attacks, the whole horrible group of symptoms associated with depression. The doctors put me on the conventional Xanax treatment for three years before I met Dr. Spreen, who was helping me with some other related medical problems. I had hair loss, skin problems, nail-biting problems. I had aches all over my body, especially in my legs. Dr. Spreen got me on a vitamin regimen, which made me feel somewhat better.

Then Dr. Spreen put me on very low doses of thyroid and immediately—within two to three weeks—all the problems I just mentioned were gone. Now, I had had thyroid checks three times during the whole time when I was being treated for infertility, and the blood tests had always come up negative. But I knew that in my family there were thyroid problems. There are at least six members of my family I can think of who have thyroid disorders, but mine just never showed up on my tests. After taking these very low doses of thyroid, my skin problem cleared up, I stopped biting my nails, and my legs stopped aching. The mild depression I was still suffering from all of a sudden in August vanished. I felt great. I slept like a normal person again. I had energy. People started commenting on how I seemed to be like my old self again. It was like getting a new lease on life!

I feel rather fed up with the original doctors I went to see. They treated me like I was a hysterical woman who needed to get a grip on things. I have never told them about my recovery using alternative methods because I don't think they'd be receptive to it.

—Jenny

■ ■ ■

I had hives, some kind of an allergic response, about five years ago and it progressed to the point where I had hives on my vocal cords. It was a pretty serious allergic reaction, for which I was first treated with antihistamines. Later, I was treated with prednisone. When small doses of prednisone given every other day didn't help, my doctor began increasing the dosage until I was taking 70 milligrams every day. After about six weeks I started declining physically from taking this tremendous dose. I gained about fifty pounds. I had conjunctivitis in both of my eyes. I had open sores.

I was so weak I was almost bedridden. I did find another doctor who slowly weaned me off of the prednisone. But when it was all over, my immune system had been damaged. I had a lot of viral illnesses that are usually associated with chronic fatigue syndrome. I could scarcely get out of bed, and I couldn't lose all the weight I had gained. So I went from doctor to doctor. I was living in the Midwest at the time, and many of these doctors said, "Your metabolic system has been altered by prednisone. Too bad, but you will never lose that weight. And prednisone can damage the immune system. Too bad, but your immune system has been damaged." No one could offer me any help at all.

I first went to Dr. Atkins in New York and he was a lot of help. It was through Dr. Atkins and his association with Dr. Huggins that I learned about dental amalgams, because when your immune system is depleted, you are much more susceptible to any kind of toxins, including mercury leaching from mercury amalgam fillings. It was causing me a great deal of trouble and I did have those removed.

Then I moved to California and I had heard, previous to my moving, about Dr. Slagle and her work with depression. In fact, I referred friends to her, friends I had made in California, and they had these miraculous cures from depression after two weeks of taking B-complex vitamins and amino acids. But I didn't think of going to her myself for quite a while because I thought of her as someone who only treated depression. In fact, like many alternative physicians, she treats the whole person. She had worked with fatigue a lot, and she first tested me thoroughly and found that my thyroid and, in fact, my whole endocrine system, was not functioning properly, most likely as a result of prednisone. She picked up subtleties in the test that other doctors ignored. She has the philosophy that a body should be healthy and whole. She doesn't need gross parameters of unusual test results to say something is wrong here. So she was able to discover that I had a rather unusual problem in my thyroid and she was able to treat it.

When I began seeing her, I still had very limited energy. Even though Dr. Atkins had helped me lose weight so I looked normal, I still didn't feel normal. In one day, I could either go to the grocery store or go to a doctor's appointment. That was all I could do. The remainder of the day I had to rest. I went to Dr. Slagle and after she began treating my thyroid, I had a leap of improvement. I regained my energy. She also gave me amino acids, which heightened my mood. Even though I hadn't thought I was depressed—and I still don't think I was—generally the amino acids made me feel healthier. And while I don't have the energy of a lot of people around me, I can pretty much function normally, which is a miracle. It has been a five-year struggle and I'm finally living practically a normal life.

Here's what I have learned from my experience: You simply cannot go to a traditional physician and carelessly allow that doctor to treat your symptoms with drugs. Traditional physicians tend not to look at the whole person, but to give drugs to ameliorate the symptoms, or to treat individual problems without regard to what that treatment does to the rest of the body. I learned to use tremendous caution when entrusting my body to someone. If you're going to trust your body to someone, you should know a lot about the physician. You should know whether the physician treats the whole person and sees you as more than an allergy or a gallbladder.

—Helen

Research Update

An increasing body of evidence is showing the benefits of natural modalities to overall health and well-being. Following is a sample of recent peer-reviewed scientific studies regarding thyroid disease.

A 2012 report in the Russian journal *Likzars'ka Sprava* concluded that the herb *Polentilla alba*, used in traditional Russian medicine for centuries, "could be recommended for monotherapy and for combine conservative therapy of diffuse and mix benign euthyroid goiter, and also for complex treatment of toxic and hypothyroid goiters."

Chapter 57

Urinary Incontinence

Causes

Eighty-five percent of the 13 million people who are incontinent are women. This is because urinary incontinence is often related to childbirth and menopause. Gynecologist Vicki Hufnagel explains, "In many cases, women are given episiotomies after delivery, without proper closure. Since muscles are not put back together correctly, the whole area is unable to provide support." Dr. Hufnagel adds that during menopause, urinary incontinence occurs when a woman is not making enough estrogen. Too little estrogen enters the vaginal tissue, causing the area to become thin, inelastic, and weak.

Urinary incontinence can also be the result of brain and spinal cord lesions, trauma, multiple sclerosis, and allergies.

There are many causes of transient incontinence. Some common ones are infection, strophic urethritis or vaginitis, certain medications (sedatives, hypnotics, diuretics, anticholinergics, alpha-adrenergic agonists or antagonists, and calcium-channel blockers), psychological disorders (especially depression), endocrine disorders, hyperglycemia, restricted mobility, and stool impaction.

Smoking has been found to be the cause of 28 percent of cases of urinary incontinence in women. Smoking increases the odds of both stress and motor urinary incontinence, and with increased daily and lifetime cigarette consumption, the odds for genuine stress incontinence rise. A study of 600 women showed that genuine stress incontinence was twice as common for both former and current smokers as for nonsmokers.

Symptoms

Urinary incontinence is a partial or total loss of control over one's bladder and urinary sphincter muscles. Sometimes, incontinence is accompanied by a feeling of urgency. This is usually the result of a person's inability to empty the bladder completely. Coughing and other stressors can set off urinary incontinence. Overflow can occur when bladder capacity is small.

Clinical Experience

Women with urinary incontinence are often advised to get bladder surgery, even hysterectomies. But this drastic approach may be completely unnecessary, according to Dr. Hufnagel, who says that women need to be educated about more conservative treatments for this common problem.

OUTPATIENT SURGERY AND HORMONE REPLACEMENT

Women need to repair their failed episiotomy, or to receive hormones, Dr. Hufnagel explains. Often, they simply need outpatient surgery to put the muscles and tissues back the way they should have been restored at the time of delivery.

Regarding menopause, Dr. Hufnagel adds, "We can treat this locally, without surgery, by simply putting hormones into the vagina. One or two months later, we see normal, healthy tissue."

ELECTRICAL STIMULATION

This treatment became popular in Europe after it was learned that high voltages of electricity to the vaginal area caused muscles to contract. However, the effects were short-lived, and the technique was not without problems. Voltages had to be applied constantly, which sometimes resulted in tissue burning and nerve damage.

In the United States, electrical stimulation is being performed with lower voltages and a pulsing sequence of one second on and one second off to prevent muscle fatigue. The objective is to strengthen the urethral muscles and the puborectalis muscle, which control the opening and closing of the bladder muscles. This form of electrical stimulation, combined with pelvic floor exercises, has produced favorable results in trial studies. It allows for a retraining, toning, and strengthening of muscles so that a patient can regain continence. One electrical product that looks promising is called Cystotron, put out by a company called Biosonics.

HOMEOPATHIC REMEDIES

Dana Ullman suggests in an article posted on HealthWorld Online (www.healthy.net) that homeopathic medicines can help prevent involuntary urination. He advises consulting a homeopathic practitioner who can individualize the treatment and work on strengthening the overall immune system, rather than just treating the bladder symptoms.

But there are homeopathic medicines that you can use on your own. One new, inexpensive homeopathic medicine he recommends is EnurAid, which is nontoxic and nonaddictive. Other homeopathic remedies that he recommends are listed below. Ullman recommends that someone who has not used homeopathic remedies before should start all the remedies suggested at the sixth potency and take the medication three or four times a day. If there is no improvement after taking a medication for a week, a different homeopathic remedy should be tried.

ARNICA (LEOPARD'S BANE)—Arnica is good for involuntary urination after surgery.

BELLADONNA (DEADLY NIGHTSHADE)—Belladonna is helpful for people who dribble urine and who sometimes have a burning sensation when they urinate.

CAUSTICUM—Causticum may help if involuntary urination gets worse in the winter and better in the summer. Often people with these symptoms lose urine when they cough or sneeze.

EQUISETUM (SCOURING RUSH)—Equisetum is a general remedy for anyone who loses urine or is a bedwetter, with no apparent cause.

FERRUM PHOS (IRON PHOSPHATE)—Ferrum phos works best for people who tend to lose urine during the day. Often people with this symptom have the strongest urge to urinate when standing; lying down lessens the urge.

KREOSOTUM (BEECHWOOD)—Kreosotum is recommended for people who cannot control sudden urges to urinate. Ullman says that these people tend to wet their bed during the first part of the night, and may dream that they are urinating.

Research Update

An increasing body of evidence is showing the benefits of natural modalities to overall health and well-being. Following is a sample of recent peer-reviewed scientific studies regarding urinary incontinence.

A 2014 study published in *Female Pelvic Medicine & Reconstructive Surgery* found that incontinent women aged forty years and older who participated in a six-week yoga therapy program experienced a 70 percent reduction in frequency of leakage, as compared with a 13 percent improvement in a control group. Other research has shown that pumpkin seed oil and soy isoflavone extract have similar beneficial effects.

Chapter 58

Urinary Tract Infections and Inflammations

Urinary tract infections and inflammations are quite common, accounting for approximately 6 million office visits per year in the United States. Dr. Jennifer Brett, a naturopathic physician from Stratford, Connecticut, says only 60 percent of people with symptoms of urinary tract infections have true infections; the other 40 percent have inflammations. The types of infections and inflammations that Dr. Brett commonly sees are true urinary tract infections, urinary tract inflammations, and interstitial cystitis, a more distressing form of inflammation that can last for months or even years.

Causes

The cause of urinary tract inflammations is unknown, but some doctors believe they may be caused by viruses, food allergies, Candida in the colon, hormonal changes, new sexual partners, or vigorous sexual activity. Interstitial cystitis may result from infection by Candida or allergic reactions to foods and additives. "These irritants inflame the pelvis and bladder, and the body responds by increasing blood flow to the area," Dr. Brett explains. "Pelvic congestion causes further irritation and pressure on the bladder. Again, the body responds by sending more blood. This becomes a vicious cycle."

Dr. David L. Hoffman, in an article posted on the HealthWorld Online website (www.healthy.net), adds that microcrystals of calcium phosphate in the urine may cause mechanical irritation to the bladder walls, resulting in inflammation.

HIGH-RISK GROUPS

Dr. David Kaufman, a specialist in women's urological problems, says that there are basically four types of women at high risk. "The most common patients are young, sexually active females. Another large group at risk are postmenopausal women. In fact, 8 to 10 percent of all women over sixty will get a bladder infection at some point. We also see a lot of patients who are hospitalized. The risk of bladder infection increases about 5 percent per day for every day that a catheter is in place. For this reason, medical doctors try to get catheters out as quickly as possible. The last high-risk group is patients with neurological problems. An example would be multiple sclerosis; patients with MS do not completely empty their bladders."

Dr. Kaufman says, "Many sexually active women get cystitis as a result of intercourse because the bacteria that normally live in the vaginal vault area get pushed up into the urethra. A woman's urethra is only about an inch and a half long, while in men it is much longer. In females, it doesn't take too much for bacteria to migrate from the outside of the urethra to the inside of the bladder. That's why we see so many more young women than men with bladder infections.

"It is very important for women to know that their partners are not giving them infections. The bacteria are already in the vaginal area and simply get pushed into the bladder during intercourse."

Dr. Hoffman mentions several other risk factors. One is being diabetic or eating a lot of sugars. Another is use of products such as douches, feminine deodorants, antibacterial soaps, and certain contraceptive creams or jellies that irritate vaginal tissue, making it vulnerable to infection. Using a diaphragm can also irritate the urethra. Excess use of antibiotics will promote growth of bacteria resistant to those drugs, which can make cystitis more likely. Finally, he says, eating foods containing pesticides can cause some types of interstitial cystitis.

HORMONAL IMBALANCE

Dr. Kaufman says there are many reasons that not all sexually active women get bladder infections. "One of the more interesting ones has to do with the woman's hormonal balance. We know that there are estrogen and progesterone receptors on the lining cells of the urethra. In some women bacteria sticks to these receptors, a condition that is related to hormone levels. Imagine bacteria as little organisms with Velcro hooks. Picture the lining cells of the urethra with the opposite kind of hooks. Bacteria hook on to the Velcro on the receptor sites. In most women, the urinary stream washes away most bacteria. But in women who have specific hormonal environments, the bacteria are not expelled that easily. These are the women we see in our office with recurrent bladder infections."

Dr. Kaufman adds that postmenopausal women tend to get urinary tract infections for this reason as well. Their low estrogen levels cause their urethral linings to be "stickier" for bacteria. "One way to treat that is simply to insert low-dosage estrogen cream into the vaginal vault, about once a week," he advises. "Many women are on estrogen pills, but that does not have the same protective influence on the urinary tract as does estrogen cream."

WEAKENED IMMUNITY

Dr. Linda Wharton, a naturopathic physician and acupuncturist from New Zealand and author of *Natural Woman Health: A Guide to Healthy Living for Women of All Ages*, says recurrent bladder infections reflect a state of lowered immunity and weakened vitality. "Remember that cystitis is an infection. As with all infections, individuals with lowered nutritional status, poor cellular health, and lowered immunity are much more susceptible to infection. Women don't always develop acute cystitis each time a stray bacterium finds its way into the bladder. Often, women play host to these potentially problem-causing bacteria for weeks or months or even a lifetime without ever experiencing acute symptoms. It is only when the health of the whole body is reduced that an explosion of this bacterial population takes place. This may occur, for example, when a woman goes through a period of great stress, such as a divorce or the death of a loved one."

STRUCTURAL PROBLEMS

Dr. Wharton adds that other causes of cystitis are often overlooked. "Pelvic floor muscles can weaken as a result of pregnancy and childbirth. When these muscles are weakened, the bladder may prolapse and bulge forward into the wall of the vagina. If the back part of the bladder droops below the neck of the bladder, it becomes virtually impossible to empty the bladder properly. This leaves an almost permanent reservoir of urine in the bladder. In time, the stagnant urine becomes a haven for bacteria to multiply, should they be present." Dr. Wharton also says that a prolapsed transverse colon—due to childbirth, age, abdominal fat, poor posture, or spinal problems—can eventually cause bladder problems.

Over time the prolapsed transverse colon—which lies across the abdomen—sags, compressing the organs beneath it, including the bladder. Blood flow is impeded, and the oxygen-starved bladder becomes ripe for infection. She adds, "This same downgrading of tissue health can occur as a direct result of a chronic back problem. All the pelvic organs receive nervous impulses from the spine, and a chronic lower back problem can interfere with those nervous impulses from the spinal cord." Dr. Wharton advises women with chronic back problems to see an osteopath or chiropractor.

CONSTIPATION

Dr. Wharton says, "Waste materials are excreted from our bodies through several different channels. The bowels excrete in the form of feces; the lungs gets rid of toxins in the form of carbon dioxide; the skin eliminates toxins as perspiration; and the kidney and bladder pass toxins out in the form of urine. If any one of these waste disposal systems is functioning inadequately, it places an excessive load on the others. If you only manage a half-hearted bowel movement every two or three days, you are placing undue stress on your kidneys and bladder, as accumulated toxins are passed out this way instead. In a sense, then, there is actually a direct link between chronic constipation and repeated urinary tract infections."

Symptoms

Typical symptoms of urinary tract infections and inflammations are frequent urination, a sensation that the bladder is never quite empty, and a burning sensation upon urination. Often women get up at night to urinate. There may be cramps, and the urine may be dark and foul-smelling. In severe cases, there may be blood in the urine as well.

Clinical Experience

A diagnosis of cystitis is usually made by collecting a midstream urine sample and testing for the presence of bacteria. If the problem stems from an inflammation, no pathogenic bacteria will be found in the urine, nor will bacteria be found on a vaginal culture.

The conventional treatment for cystitis is a course of antibiotics. Standard therapy for chronic cystitis generally consists of repeated rounds of the same therapy.

In the long term, this practice may actually exacerbate the condition rather than cure it. It is well known that broad-spectrum antibiotics are indiscriminate killers that destroy colonies of friendly gut bacteria along with problem-causing organisms. Once the delicate balance of the normal gastrointestinal microflora has been disrupted, less desirable organisms proliferate, virtually unchecked. These include *Escherichia coli*, the prime cause of cystitis, and candida overgrowth, a suspected cause of inflammations.

Dr. Kaufman says that antibiotics should be a last-ditch effort, used only when various holistic protocols fail to achieve results. Even then, mild medicines should be used: "What of women who do all the right things, and still come back with bladder infections? In these cases, we need to turn to more traditional medical approaches. The gold standard for treating patients who do everything right and still get infections is a very gentle, bacteriostatic antibiotic. A bacteriostatic antibiotic does not kill the bacteria, but limits bacterial growth. It is gentler on the system, and generally does not cause yeast infections or gastrointestinal problems. I am not big on taking antibiotics, but this is a better alternative than constant infections."

Dr. Brett reports that radical therapies are sometimes used for persistent cases. "Treatments I have read about in recent medical journals include surgery to cut nerves to reduce irritation to the bladder, hormonal therapy, and even antidepressive medications to help women sleep better, even though this doesn't get at the root cause of the problem."

NATUROPATHIC TREATMENTS

DIET

It is important to drink plenty of pure water, about one 8-ounce glass each hour. "If you are in agony and you don't know what to do, start drinking water and don't stop," advises Dr. Wharton. "Stay away from tea, coffee, soft drinks, and alcohol, but drink plenty of water."

Cranberry, either in the form of unsweetened juice or capsules, changes the pH of the urine, making it more acidic and less hospitable to bacteria. Cranberries also contain powerful antibacterial substances. In fact, studies reveal that as little as 15 ounces of cranberry juice results in an 80 percent inhibition of bacterial growth. Bacteria lose the ability to cling to the bladder wall and must exit the system along with urine. Other research indicates that cranberry juice combined with vitamin C acidifies the urine further. The effect is therefore much greater when both are taken together.

Other drinks useful for temporarily acidifying the urine include lemon juice and water, buttermilk, and 2 teaspoons of apple cider vinegar stirred into a glass of water. Drink any of these substances three or four times a day.

VITAMIN C

Any time the body is fighting an infection, it tolerates large amounts of C, sometimes as much as 10,000 to 15,000 milligrams orally each day (and even more intravenously). For cystitis, or for any infection, take vitamin C to bowel tolerance. (Bowel tolerance is where the stool becomes quite loose, almost to the point of diarrhea.) Vitamin C should be taken every two to three hours since it is water-soluble, which means that it is rapidly excreted from the body. According to Dr. Hoffman, recent studies indicate that ascorbic acid irritates the bladder. For this reason it is best to take vitamin C in the buffered form of calcium ascorbate. Aspartate also irritates the bladder, so avoid vitamins that contain it.

Dr. Wharton says that vitamin C fights infections in several ways. "Vitamin C concentrates in very high levels in the urine and exerts a direct bactericidal effect. It also supports systemic immune system function by helping to activate neutrophils, the white blood cells most involved in the front line defense against infection. It also works to stimulate the production of lymphocytes, which are important for coordinating immune function at the cellular level."

VITAMIN A

In addition to vitamin C, think about vitamin A. An easy way of supplementing with this vitamin is to use halibut or cod liver oil capsules, up to 25,000 IU a day, during acute phases of infection. Vitamin A helps protect the mucous membrane lining of the bladder and urethra from irritation during infection. It also improves antibody response and white blood cell function. Just a word of warning here: if you are pregnant, do not use such high doses of vitamin A, as they have been associated with birth defects. Beta-carotene, with which the body can make vitamin A as it is needed, is a safer alternative.

ZINC

Zinc is essential for increasing white blood cell activity in response to infection. For acute cystitis, approximately 50 milligrams elemental zinc is needed daily.

BLACK CUMIN SEED OIL

One teaspoon daily.

COCONUT OIL

One teaspoon daily.

HERBS

The classes of herbs used to treat cystitis include antiseptic herbs, demulcents, and diuretics. Antiseptic herbs for bladder infections include uva-ursi, buchu, goldenseal, juniper berries, and garlic. "Think garlic whenever you have any type of infection, including cystitis," says Dr. Wharton. Demulcents soothe inflamed mucous membranes inside the bladder and urethra, and include marsh mallow root, juniper berry, and corn silk. Diuretic herbs stimulate the production and excretion of urine, which helps to wash out bacteria. Common diuretics are parsley and goldenrod.

Dr. Wharton recommends the following old naturopathic herbal remedies for treating burning urine: "Mix together equal parts of fennel, burdock, and slippery elm. Steep a teaspoon of this mixture in a cup of boiled water for about twenty minutes. Have one cup before each meal, and one before bed."

She also recommends flaxseed tea or a combination of uva-ursi and buchu: "For either tea, use 1 teaspoon of the dried herbs to a cup of boiling water. Again, let it steep for fifteen to twenty minutes. Then drink one cup, three or four times a day. The results more than compensate for the awful taste.

Dr. Hoffman recommends the following formula for cystitis: Combine two parts corn silk, two parts uva-ursi, and one part buchu. Take 5 milliliters of this tincture three times a day. At the same time, drink an infusion of yarrow, another antiseptic herb, throughout the day.

Dr. Tori Hudson, a naturopath in Portland, Oregon, in her column for *Prevention* magazine recommends the following combination of herbs, either as capsules or in tinctures: pipsissewa, uva-ursi, echinacea or goldenseal, and buchu.

For two days, take two capsules or 20 to 30 drops every two hours. For the next seven days, take the capsules or tincture three times daily.

Dr. Joseph Pizzorno adds this bit of advice: "After sexual intercourse, women should wipe the opening to the urethra with a dilute solution of Betadine or a strong solution of goldenseal tea to wash away any bacteria that may have been forced up into the urethra."

OTHER THERAPIES

Judyth Reichenberg-Ullman and Robert Ullman, naturopathic and homeopathic doctors in Edmonds, Washington, in an article posted on the HealthWorld Online website (www.healthy.net), recommend Cantharis (Spanish fly), a frequently used remedy in cases in which extreme pain in the bladder occurs very suddenly and there is blood in the urine. Staphysagria (stavesacre) is the remedy to use when a bladder infection has developed after having sex ("honeymoon cystitis"). When cystitis is associated with pain in the kidney area, especially on the right side, they suggest Berberis aquifolium (Oregon grape).

Hydrotherapy is another traditional naturopathic method for helping people overcome the discomforts of cystitis. Sitz baths or hot compresses stimulate blood circulation and remove toxins from the pelvic area. Dr. Wharton explains how this is done: "You can use a hot compress by dipping a small hand towel into a basin of water, as hot as you can possibly tolerate it. Wring out the water and quickly apply the cloth to the area just above the pubic bone. As the cloth cools, repeat the process. In total, apply the compress eight or nine times. Repeat this process two to three times throughout the day. It actually feels wonderful and gives quite a bit of local relief to the symptoms.

"Alternatively, you can try making a sitz bath. Fill a small tub with water, once again, as hot as you can bear it. Add 6 drops bergamot oil, and sit in the bath so that water actually covers your pelvis and lower abdomen. Stay there for around half an hour. As the water cools, keep replenishing with fresh, hot water to keep the water up to a hot, even temperature. Just a word of warning: If you have a problem with a weak heart or high blood pressure, hot sitz baths aren't really for you. You are better off just using a local compress."

Dr. Wharton reports impressive results in the treatment of chronic cystitis with acupuncture when it is accompanied by lifestyle and dietary changes: "Usually an acute attack of cystitis responds to two to four acupuncture sessions, spaced two or three days apart. Chronic cystitis sufferers often benefit from an extended course of acupuncture treatment to prevent the recurrence of their problem."

Essential oils can enhance any treatment program, according to aromatherapist Ann Berwick. To help clear up a urinary tract infection, 18 to 20 drops of juniper and cedarwood can be added to 1 ounce of lotion and massaged into the lower abdomen. Also, 6 to 8 drops of juniper, bergamot, or sandlewood can be added to a sitz bath or full bath.

Judyth Reichenberg-Ullman and Robert Ullman caution further that it's important not only to rest but to pay attention to whatever message your body is giving you with this bladder infection, in order to avoid recurrences. Therefore, consider what might be its underlying cause. They add that breathing into the pain and relaxing can be remarkably effective: "We had one patient who cured a bladder infection solely through visualization and meditation."

Urinary Tract Inflammations

For urinary inflammation not caused by bacteria, Dr. Brett says it is important to avoid foods that encourage the growth of candida, such as wheat, simple sugars, white flour, pastries, candies, alcohol, aged cheeses, vinegar, and even fruit. Avoid known food allergens. It is a good idea to get a test to determine if there are any other foods in the diet that are acting as irritants.

As with bacterial infections, you should drink one 8-ounce glass of water every hour. It is also a good idea to drink a glass of water and to urinate immediately after sexual intercourse. This tends to reduce the bladder irritation that sexual intercourse may cause.

Clothing is important too. Avoid tight-fitting pants, nylon underwear, and pantyhose. They encourage the growth of candida in the vaginal tract, which irritates the bladder and urethra.

Vitamins and herbs may also be useful. For vitamins, take 2,000 to 6,000 milligrams of buffered vitamin C and 100 to 200 milligrams of vitamin B_6. Also take four to six capsules of evening primrose oil. Herbs that soothe the bladder include althea or marsh mallow, corn silk, slippery elm, and goldenrod. Finally, as with bacterial infections, the homeopathic remedy Cantharis (Spanish fly) is often effective in reducing bladder and urethra irritations.

Interstitial Cystitis

"The basic way to treat interstitial cystitis," says Dr. Brett, "is to remove congestion from the pelvis." The therapies she suggests in cases of interstitial cystitis are listed below. "If you follow these basic guidelines," says Dr. Brett, "within three to four weeks, you are likely to notice that your ability to sleep through the night is improved and that your cramping and pain during the day is significantly lessened."

TESTS

It is a good idea to be tested for food allergies to see if some food is causing an antibody-antigen reaction and irritating the bladder. It is also important to test for candida in the colon because candida can cause irritations and antibody reactions that irritate the bladder. Next, check to see that the hormones are in balance. If they are not, use vitamin B_6, evening primrose oil, and herbs to restore hormonal balance.

EXERCISE

The two types of exercise that help in cases of interstitial cystitis are aerobic exercise and inversion exercise. Doing aerobic exercise every day helps to remove blood congestion from the pelvis. *Aerobic* means anything that gets the blood moving, such as walking briskly, jogging, swimming, and bicycling.

Specific exercises for moving the blood involve turning upside down. In yoga, this is accomplished with the headstand or shoulderstand. It can also be achieved by lying on the back, raising the legs up, and performing cycling rotations with the legs. If there is a back or neck problem, however, a simple solution is to use a slant board, which can be made simply with an old door or a couple of one-by-four boards. One end can be placed on the couch, and the other end on the floor. Once it is stable, the person lies upside down, that is, with the head near the floor and the feet near the couch. The blood is automatically pulled out of the pelvis by gravity, and moved into the chest and head. Remaining too long can cause dizziness; five or ten minutes works for most people.

HERBS

The soothing herbs previously mentioned are useful here as well: marsh mallow, corn silk, slippery elm, and goldenrod.

DIET

A low-acid diet decreases irritations. High-acid foods to omit are red meat, dairy, shellfish, and citrus fruits. The diet should include whole grains, beans, and vegetables. Essential fatty acids, such as those found in flaxseed oil, evening primrose oil, and fish oils, can help reduce inflammation. In interstitial cystitis, they are key for reversing the cycle of irritation and blood congestion.

PREVENTION

Long-term preventive changes obviously make a lot more sense than simply dealing with each acute infection as it arises. Here are some simple personal-hygiene measures to reduce the likelihood of reinfection:

- After a bowel movement, wipe from front to back, away from the vagina, and wash area thoroughly with soap and water.
- Encourage your partner to wash thoroughly before any sexual contact.
- Avoid the transfer of bacteria from the anus to the vagina during lovemaking.
- During a period, change pads and tampons frequently.
- Do not wear tight-fitting jeans or nylon pantyhose or pants. Cotton pants and stockings with garters allow more airflow and ventilation.
- Make a habit of drinking lots of water. Aim for seven to eight glasses each day. This keeps the urine dilute so that bacterial proliferation is less likely. It also prompts frequent urination, which washes out problematic bacteria.
- Reduce the intake of coffee and tea.
- Make a habit of emptying your bladder frequently. Research shows that women who ignore their urge to urinate for long periods of time are much more likely to develop cystitis. The motto here is: When you need to go, go right away. Also urinate after sexual intercourse. This will help to wash out any of the bacteria that may have been pushed up into the urethra.
- Try not to urinate before sex so that more bacteria are pushed out after sex.

- A glass of water right before intercourse will further increase the volume of liquid in the bladder for the washout of bacteria later on.

- If infections are an ongoing problem, try this: Take a detachable shower head, or use a bidet, and direct a stream of water into the vaginal area before sex. This will dilute the bacteria and decrease their numbers so that fewer bacteria get pushed up into the bladder during intercourse.

- Avoid chemical irritation to the urethra by staying away from perfumed or colored personal hygiene products. Diaphragms and birth control pills, as a means of contraception, often promote urinary tract infections and should not be used by women who tend to get the condition. Condoms or a properly fitted cervical cap are better.

- See a registered osteopath or chiropractor if you think you may have a spinal problem that can be contributing to your recurring cystitis.

Dr. Hudson suggests drinking one glass of cranberry juice (or the equivalent in capsules) and taking vitamin C every day to reduce the frequency of recurrent attacks of cystitis by creating an acidic environment in which bacteria cannot easily grow.

"Remember that your bladder health reflects your overall health," says Dr. Wharton, "so take a good look at your lifestyle. Ask yourself, 'Do I eat a nutritious, balanced diet? Do I get enough relaxation and sleep? Am I under stress?' Maybe you drink too much coffee or alcohol or smoke or use recreational drugs. If your lifestyle is unhealthy, your body will be too."

ASIAN PERSPECTIVE

Dr. Brett explains that traditional Chinese medicine views cystitis as the end result of an accumulation of damp and heat in the bladder: "Often there is a weak flow of chi (energy) in the kidney and the spleen meridians. Weakness of spleen energy leads to the formation of damp in the body, which, in turn causes a stagnation of energy. As in nature, whenever anything builds up, there is friction. A stagnation of chi eventually leads to the development of heat, what we in the West interpret as cystitis.

"Spleen chi is easily disrupted through dietary indiscretion. Spleen chi can be damaged by any of the following: overeating; drinking with meals; overconsumption of damp-forming foods, such as dairy products, chilled foods or drinks, and raw fruits and vegetables; and eating greasy foods, such as takeout foods.

"What you do with your mind actually affects spleen energy as well. An overuse of the mind, particularly through chronic anxiety and worry, or through many years of overstudying, also tends to deplete spleen energy.

"When the cooling yin energy of the kidneys is weakened, cystitis becomes much more likely as well. Kidney yin is consumed naturally as we age, but it can also be prematurely diminished as a result of lifestyle. The long-term overwork, stress, and exhaustion that form a part of many American lives these days, along with an overconsumption of alcohol and too much sex, all deplete the vital kidney energy." Acupuncture, combined with lifestyle changes, can help to balance energy and eliminate cystitis.

Research Update

An increasing body of evidence is showing the benefits of natural modalities to overall health and well-being. Following is a sample of recent peer-reviewed scientific studies regarding urinary tract infections and inflammations.

In a 2014 study published in *World Journal of Urology*, researchers determined that D-mannose, a naturally occurring sugar, significantly reduced the risk of recurrent urinary tract infection (UTI), and that its effectiveness was similar to that of the antibiotic Nitrofurantoin but without any side effects. The women in the study received 2 grams of D-mannose powder in 200 milliliters of water daily for six months. Although many studies have examined the use of cranberry juice for UTIs, a 2012 report in the *Cochrane Data of Systematic Reviews* concluded that its benefits were minimal. However, as reported in 2015 in the *International Journal of Molecular Science*, cranberry phenolic compounds were found to have anti-adhesive activity against *Escherichia coli*, which indicates that they could work against bacterial colonization and progression of UTI. Other substances shown to be effective against UTI include ascorbic acid, probiotics, berberine, hibiscus, and pumpkin seed extract.

Chapter 59

Vaginal Inflammation and Infection

According to Amanda McQuade Crawford, a medical herbalist and author of *Herbal Remedies for Women*, "there are many causes of vaginitis, which simply means an inflamed vagina. There's not always an infection. Many women use the term to refer to any number of situations where there's an irritation of the vagina. When it is caused by bacteria, it's called bacterial vaginosis. So we are talking about a number of different conditions.

"Though vaginitis isn't always caused by an infection, there are various microbes that commonly cause it. One of the microbes most commonly involved in nonspecific vaginitis is *Gardnerella vaginalis*, a bacterium that doesn't like oxygen. When men have *Gardnerella*, they don't show many signs or symptoms, so it may unsuspectingly pass to a female partner."

Some other common causes of vaginitis are candida (a yeast), *Trichomonas vaginalis*, a parasite, and a number of sexually transmitted diseases, such as gonorrhea, genital warts, and herpes. When an infecting agent is not the cause of vaginitis, it may simply be caused by a hormonal imbalance.

Vaginitis can occur at many stages of a woman's life; for example, it is common when a woman's body adjusts to a lower level of estrogen at menopause. Vaginitis can be aggravated by stress, nutritional imbalance, a foreign object such as a diaphragm or a tampon, and problems that originate in the vulva, which can lead to a vaginal irritation.

Crawford points out, "Vaginitis is not a punishment. It is the body's way of signaling an irritation of the most tender gateway to the interior that leads all the way up to our heart, and of our relationship to the person we love and let into our body."

Symptoms

One common vaginal symptom is a discharge, which can be of different types and colors. These differences can help determine the necessary approach for healing. If the discharge is clear and has a normal smell, it may well be due to ovulation and does not require treatment. If the color is a milky white, and the discharge has a creamy texture but smells normal, this can also be a sign of ovulation. If the discharge is white but sticky, it might be simply postovulation or an effect of taking the birth control pill.

When the discharge is brown and watery or sticky but has a normal odor, it can be spotting from the end of the menstrual period or, occasionally, spotting in between periods. If that is the case, it might be a good idea to consult a licensed practitioner to see why this is occurring.

When the discharge is watery and white, with almost a buttermilk quality, and smells fishy or foul—and especially when there's itching or other symptoms, such as fever—then you may have a case of BV (bacterial vaginosis), possibly from Gardnerella, which requires treatment.

Sometimes the discharge is white and flecked, like curds, smells a bit like beer or rising bread dough with a yeasty smell, and is accompanied by itching. This could be from a yeast infection, which also requires treatment with antifungal, antiyeast herbs or other remedies.

When the discharge is yellow and frothy, sometimes with dots of red, has a very foul odor, and is itchy, it may be from Trichomonas. See a medical practitioner to ensure that the infection is adequately treated, because this can be persistent.

Crawford notes, "Be careful if the discharge is yellow to green, and there's a heavy, thick mucous discharge, with or without a bad odor, that may be accompanied by other symptoms, such as abdominal cramps or pains, painful urination, and a fever. It could be evidence of PID [pelvic inflammatory disease] or possibly gonorrhea. Even if there's no discharge, it still might be gonorrhea if the other symptoms are present. So go to a medical practitioner for a clear diagnosis."

Clinical Experience

TREATMENT

In treating vaginitis, some very simple herbs can be used, such as the soothing, anti-inflammatory calendula flowers. Crawford also likes licorice root, which can be used as a douche externally. Another herb that is quite good is plantain (sometimes called ribwort). These should be used with an astringent herb. They will help pull the inflamed vaginal tissues together so that the natural forces of your body can fight off whatever the infection or inflammation might be.

Crawford details, "An astringent herb which I use internally is anemone pulsatilla, or pasqueflower. Take 3 ounces of that and combine it with 1 ounce of licorice root and 2 ounces of plantain. Mix those together. Over 1 ounce of the mixture, pour a pint of boiling water. Let that stand, then take a teacup full of this tea, strained, three times a day. Alternatively, a woman can take extracts or tinctures of these herbs. The relative amounts would be the same. Take a teaspoon, diluted in 1 cup of water, three times a day."

Treat vaginitis for one or two weeks, then stop treatment and see if the condition is gone. "If there is a more deep-seated infection that doesn't resolve in that time period," Crawford says, "then I usually add 2 ounces of echinacea root to the other ingredients. Steep an ounce and use it in the same way as you did the previous tea, three to four times a day for at least ten days. If that doesn't clear things up, it is necessary to reassess."

"There's always nutritional advice that goes along with herbal treatments," Crawford adds. "Avoid sugar, including honey, maple syrup on your pancakes, or fruit juice–sweetened cookies, even if they are from the health food store. Lots of sugar is not going to help a woman fight off an infection."

Vaginal Yeast (Candidiasis)

Carol Dalton is a nurse practitioner who helped found the clinic Wellspring for Women. She explains that yeast infections are actually a general gathering of bacteria, a multiplicity of them, not just one organism. "Many of these organisms live normally within the vagina. If they are in the right balance and there are small amounts of them, they really don't cause any problem. But if they get out of hand and if the partner has a lot of bacteria as well, then it can really start to cause a lot of inflammation, itching, redness, and a foul-smelling discharge. Then it is obviously a problem."

She adds that just as we can be around someone who has a cold but not catch the cold if our immune system is good, a woman can come into contact with yeast but will not necessarily begin to grow it herself if her cells and immune system are healthy. On the other hand, if her immune system is depressed, she will pick it up and it will turn into a raging infection very easily.

CAUSES

A vaginal yeast infection has multiple causes, according to Dalton. She notes that the type of birth control you use will influence whether you can be infected. You may get the yeast infection from a partner, "if you are sexually active and particularly sexually active without any barrier protection or any spermicide—spermicide helps to kill off all of these things. So it may be passed more easily to women who are using the Pill or the IUD, for example, and not using female or male condoms or a diaphragm. They will be at higher risk, because everything that comes into contact with the genital area can pass way up into the vaginal canal. That's one of the reasons we are seeing more of this and have been for the last fifteen or twenty years: women are using more different kinds of birth control than we used to have. Women are tired of using the older methods, so they have switched to hormone injections (Depo-Provera), IUDs, and oral contraceptives, and those methods don't really offer any protection against yeast infections."

The late Dr. William Crook, author of *The Yeast Connection and Women*, said that taking antibiotics can lead to yeast overgrowth and that women are especially susceptible. "The yeast we're talking about normally live in the body of every man, woman, and child. When you are healthy, there are no problems, but when you take a lot of antibiotic drugs, you begin to get complications. Antibiotics knock out the normal, friendly bacteria. As a result the yeast overgrows, and a woman may get a vaginal yeast infection, a child may develop thrush or diaper rash, and a man or woman may get bloating, constipation, and digestive symptoms.

"But that's not the major problem. This yeast puts out toxins that weaken the immune system. It so disturbs the interior membrane of the intestinal tract that you absorb food allergens that would normally be excreted. People truly become sick all over."

"There are several reasons why a woman is more susceptible to yeast infections than a man," said Dr. Crook. "Since her genitalia are internal, yeast is able to grow on the warm interior membranes of the body. The little tube going from the urinary bladder to the outside is only an inch and a half long in a woman, whereas in a man it is many inches long. This allows the bacteria to get up into the woman's bladder much more easily. Women have 50 times more urinary tract infections than men, and they are given antibiotic drugs as treatment. Birth control pills further promote yeast growth. So does pregnancy. And teenage girls with a few pimples on their face are much more likely to run to the dermatologist and get tetracycline, an antibiotic that makes yeast grow."

Nutritionist Gracia Perlstein adds these causes to the list: "Some women are susceptible at the end of each month's menstrual flow. There are low estrogen levels present at menopause, and also pregnancy, when the rate of infection can be as high as 20 percent toward the end. Also women who have diabetes have an increased risk.

"Stress is another factor. Many people have two or three jobs. They are running around, eating on the run, not really paying attention to their diet. When people do that, they also tend to overdo sweets and processed foods, which weaken their immunity and set up a perfect environment for the candida overgrowth."

Complementary physician Dr. Robert Sorge says Candida is the result of drug pollution. In addition to antibiotic overuse, mentioned earlier, he adds, "The most likely candidate for overgrowth is a person who has been on steroids, hormone medication, cortisone, the entire gamut of prescriptions and over-the-counter drugs, especially ulcer medications such as Tagamet and Zantac, and oral contraceptives. As far as I'm concerned, the sugar and junk food diet that most people have is also a drug."

SYMPTOMS

Classical symptoms of a yeast infection are itching, redness, irritation, and a cottage cheese–like curdly white discharge. Symptoms are not always obvious, but a gynecologist can often confirm whether or not a yeast infection exists by looking at a smear under the microscope or creating a culture to see if yeast colonies form.

Clearing up immediate symptoms is relatively simple. Many over-the-counter preparations, including homeopathic remedies, exist for that purpose. The trick, according to Dr. Marjorie Ordene, a holistic gynecologist from Brooklyn, New York, is to treat the overall yeast syndrome, not just the local infection.

"Often the vaginal itching will be the impetus for the person to come to the doctor, but it is not the only problem they have. Unless the whole person is treated, the yeast is bound to recur." Dr. Ordene breaks down symptoms of a yeast syndrome into five categories:

GENERAL SYMPTOMS—Low energy and fatigue, brain fog, depression, headaches, muscle and joint pains, memory loss, extreme sensitivity to chemicals, recurrent urinary infections, light-headedness

DIGESTIVE SYMPTOMS—Gas, bloating, intermittent constipation and diarrhea, indigestion, intestinal cramps

RESPIRATORY SYMPTOMS—Chronic postnasal drip, frequent coughs, sore throats, colds, asthma, allergies

SKIN PROBLEMS—Eczema, itching, rashes, fungal infections

HORMONAL PROBLEMS—Menstrual irregularities, menstrual cramps, premenstrual syndrome, mood swings, problems with the endocrine glands, hypothyroidism, hypoglycemia or diabetes

As noted, the infection is more likely to take hold if a woman has a less than healthy immune system. "If the person who gets a yeast infection has a weak immune system, then the yeast, which comes out in the stool, can creep up. It grows like little tree branches, into the perineum and vaginal area. If the pH is off, it can cause an infection in that area," Dalton says.

CLINICAL EXPERIENCE

Since the intestines serve as a reservoir for much of the yeast, a stool study may reveal an overgrowth. Excess yeast here indicates that yeast is present in other parts of the body, including the vagina, and is causing recurrent yeast infections.

A simple skin test may reveal a yeast allergy as well. Red or itchy skin indicates a problem. Often the results are seen quickly, within ten to fifteen minutes, although sometimes there is a delayed reaction or none at all.

These tests are not always reliable, according to Dr. Crook. "Although we physicians generally like to have a test that can say you do or do not have a particular condition, such as a chest X-ray to see whether your heart is enlarged, there is not presently a single, simple laboratory test that can say whether you do or do not have a yeast-related problem. If a woman has a vaginal infection, a lab study of the secretion may help identify the yeast. Sometimes a culture may. But they are not 100 percent accurate. They may not be more than 50 percent accurate. There are studies done on stools because yeast grows there, but those are not reliable either. The best we can do is to suspect it, and then to note the response of a person to a sugar-free special diet, and oral antiyeast medication, both prescription and nonprescription."

ALTERNATIVE THERAPIES

Yeast-Free Diet

A yeast-free diet is both diagnostic and therapeutic. If a woman feels better when following the diet, this indicates a yeast sensitivity. The diet should be observed for several weeks at a minimum, and may be followed indefinitely. Some people feel much better and choose to eat this way permanently. Foods can be added back gradually, however, to see their effect. If symptoms recur, the reintroduced food should be avoided.

There are two basic principles to follow on a yeast-free diet:

AVOID SWEETS—The relationship between sugar and yeast was seen in a study performed at St. Jude Hospital in Memphis, Tennessee, where mice who were fed sugar had two hundred times greater yeast concentration than mice who were not. Yeast feeds on sugar, causing many symptoms, especially digestive problems such as gas and bloating. Avoiding sugar entails more than just not adding granulated sugar to cereal or tea; it means checking labels and staying away from corn syrup, maltose, artificial sweeteners, fructose, cornstarch, sodas, and lactose, a milk sugar found in dairy products.

AVOID FOODS CONTAINING YEASTS AND MOLDS—These include baked foods such as breads, muffins, cakes, cookies, and other refined carbohydrates, commercial fruit juices, tomato sauce (unless homemade with fresh tomatoes), foods containing vinegar, pickled foods, smoked foods, alcohol, fermented foods, smoked meats, dried fruits, mushrooms (except for shiitake), pistachio nuts, and peanuts. Leftovers may be moldy as well.

What you can eat are healthful foods that do not contain yeasts and molds. Included are whole grains, such as brown rice, millet, amaranth, quinoa, and barley, as well as fresh vegetables. Lots of steamed green vegetables are particularly beneficial because they are abundant in purifying chlorophyll. Also allowed are sea vegetables; whole wheat matzoh; sourdough rye bread; popcorn; tortillas;

tofu; miso; plain yogurt; lean meats; fresh fish; organically fed, free-range poultry; and eggs from free-range chickens. Organic extra-virgin olive oil, when used sparingly, can inhibit yeast overgrowth, according to recent studies. Raw garlic or lightly cooked garlic helps get rid of candida in the intestines.

Supplements

Sometimes diet alone is not enough. After all, yeast has been in the body for years. The following supplements provide additional needed help:

FLORA—The flora found in Lactobacillus acidophilus and bifida bacteria can be taken in powder form or as sugar-free yogurt. The effectiveness of flora was noted in a New York Medical School study of women with recurrent vaginal yeast infections. Those eating sugar-free yogurt had fewer infections than those who did not. Flora repopulate the intestinal tract with good bacteria, which in turn crowd out the yeast. The effects of flora are temporary, so the powder or yogurt should be consumed on a daily basis.

ANTIFUNGAL, ANTIYEAST AGENTS—Over-the-counter preparations, such as citrus seed extract, kyolic garlic, caprylic acid, pau d'arco, and berberine, may be helpful. Sometimes prescription agents such as nystatin are needed. These remedies get rid of excess yeast only. Since they are not absorbed into the blood, they are safe to take, even during pregnancy and while nursing.

HOMEOPATHIC CANDIDA—Helps desensitize the body to yeast.

GARLIC SUPPOSITORIES—Simple insertion of a clove of garlic into the vagina has a powerful healing effect. *The New Our Bodies, Ourselves* suggests that the clove should be peeled but not nicked, and then wrapped in gauze before inserting.

A strong body is better able to rebalance its health. In addition to supplements that target yeast infections specifically, the following nutrients provide overall nutritional support:

MULTIVITAMIN/MINERAL SUPPLEMENT—Formulas containing zinc, magnesium, yeast-free vitamins, trace minerals, and essential fatty acids boost immune function and help prevent recurrent yeast infections.

CHLOROPHYLL—Cleanses the intestines and purifies the blood.

ESSENTIAL FATTY ACIDS—3,000 milligrams of evening primrose, borage, or blackcurrant seed oil daily in three divided doses, or one tablespoon of organic flaxseed oil. (Never cook flaxseed oil, and keep refrigerated.)

VITAMIN C—3,000 to 5,000 milligrams daily in three divided doses helps fight infections.

B-COMPLEX—50 to 100 milligrams with each meal combats stress.

Herbs
The following Asian and Western herbs can help alleviate yeast problems:

DIGESTIVE HARMONY AND HERBASTATIN—Digestive Harmony is a combination of bitter herbs that work together to cleanse the digestive tract and other internal organs of yeast infections. Herbastatin gets rid of yeast caused by phlegm.

YU DAI WAN—This Chinese remedy helps to eliminate creamy discharges.

KU SHEN—Used as a wash to clean the vagina.

BLACK WALNUT TINCTURE—Thirty drops three times daily, added to water before meals.

PAU D'ARCO—This herb has wonderful immune-enhancing and antifungal properties. As a tea, take three to four cups daily.

SUMMA—This is another good herbal tea for helping the immune system.

Also helpful are goldenseal, bearberry, Oregon grape, German chamomile, aloe vera, rosemary, ginger, alfalfa, red clover, and fennel.

Colon Therapy
"My battle with Candida lasted a long time," says colon therapist Tovah Finman-

Nahman. "I tried everything, including a strict diet, antifungals, and vitamin C drips. But I never got it under control until I started doing colonics. Then I saw quick results. The gas and bloating went away, and my chronic fatigue amazingly disappeared. I have seen similar results with a lot of people who come to see me. I can't stress how good colonics are."

What makes colon therapy such an effective treatment? First, it creates a clean internal environment. "We want a good environment so that flora can grow and flourish. That is paramount when we have candida overgrowth," says Finman-Nahman. Second, colonics calm an irritated colon: "Herbs can be added to the water, such as pau d'arco, which has antifungal properties. Yellow dock can also be added to soothe any inflammation. Fennel can be used to dissipate gas and eliminate the bloating that a lot of people with candida tend to get. Aloe vera gel is absolutely wonderful. It is very soothing to an inflamed colon. And of course, it can be taken orally in the form of aloe vera juice.

"In conjunction with colonics, psyllium can be taken orally. This moisturizes impacted fecal material in the congested colon, which further aids cleaning.

"People ask, 'How many colonics should I get?' That depends on the individual. The more the merrier. For a healthy person I recommend at least ten in a series, and then a maintenance program. Sometimes, it can take as long as six months to get candida under control because it is a very hearty bacteria. When yeast is at the point of being candidiasis, it can grow through the colon walls and run rampant. The more we cleanse, the better our chance of getting it under control and regaining health."

Aromatherapy
Tea tree oil is scientifically shown to be antifungal, antiyeast, and antiviral. One tablespoon of the oil added to a pint of water, and used in a douche, helps eliminate yeast infections. Follow this by placing acidophilus tablets or capsules into the vagina to reestablish proper vaginal bacteria.

Lifestyle Factors
Nutritionist Gracia Perlstein notes the following important habits for minimizing the incidence of vaginal infections:

- Wear underpants with a cotton crotch so that air can circulate.

- Avoid pantyhose or any tight-fitting clothing for the same reason.

- Develop good toilet habits of always wiping from front to back. This keeps anal bacteria from entering the vagina.

- Avoid feminine hygiene sprays and powders, which can cause irritation. Douching is not necessary; a healthy vagina is naturally clean.

- Keep stress under control. Take a few deep breaths. Go for a brisk walk in the open air. Do something to alleviate the stress that builds up.

Homeopathy

Since homeopathy treatments are chosen according to symptoms, deciding on a remedy depends on the quality of the discharge and the sensations, according to the late Dr. Ken Korins. Here he offers some of the major remedies for vaginal yeast infections:

PULSATILLA—This remedy is often indicated in vaginitis. The woman has a thick, yellowish-to-green discharge. Sometimes the consistency is milky or creamy. Mentally, she is often moody, gentle, and weepy, and craves sympathy.

SILICA—The main symptom is an itching of the vulva and vagina. It is sensitive to touch. The discharge tends to be thin, and sometimes curdly.

KREOSOTUM—The person has violent symptoms. Discharges are excoriating, burning is profuse, and there is a foul odor, as well as violent itching and a burning and swelling of the labia. Discharge tends to be yellow and may actually have a watery, bloody consistency.

HEPAR SULPH—Symptoms are similar to Silica, but more chronic. The vagina itches, particularly after sexual intercourse, and often has an odor similar to that of old cheese. Both Hepar sulph and Silica can be used to treat sores or cysts, particularly Bartholin's cysts.

KALI BICHROMIUM—Here discharges tend to be thick, green, and sometimes jellylike.

ALUMINA—Discharge is thick and transparent.

NITRIC ACID—Helps when there are sores or ulcers on the vaginal mucosa. The sensation tends to be a sharp, sticking pain. Discharges are brown. Often, there is a stain on underwear that leaves a yellow perimeter.

MERCURIUS—The discharges are excoriating but greenish and bloody. There is a sensation of rawness.

MEDORRHINUM—Discharge is thick and acrid, with a sensation way up in the uterus.

Wellspring for Women Treatment
The holistic program at the Wellspring for Women clinic treats chronic cases of yeast infection. As Carol Dalton points out, the conventional treatment for yeast is to prescribe antifungal medications. "If a woman went to a more traditional medical care facility, that would be the first choice. It would be an antifungal of some sort in either a vaginal or an oral preparation.

"The problem with this approach is that you are not really addressing why this problem develops in the first place; why there is an unhealthy environment that allows this organism to grow. By prescribing these drugs, you are actually adding to the imbalance in the environment. This makes it even more likely that the person is going to pick it up again or that she will develop a yeast infection, because you have killed off her normal bacteria and allowed yeast to overgrow there. Often that starts a cycle of bacteria, then yeast, sometimes even developing into bladder infection because the whole area gets so inflamed."

Dalton notes that she often sees patients who have had chronic infections for a long time. "What we try to do is establish what their general immune system looks like. Then we try to help them systemically to get that into balance.

"We look at their diet, their lifestyle, their stress factors, their supplements, all those things, and try to help them create a healthier, better balance. For example, if the woman was low on protein in her diet and eating a lot of sugar and carbs, then we might recommend a lower-carb, lower-sugar diet so that we are not feeding the yeast.

"If the woman is not doing any kind of supplementation, we would tend to recommend things to raise the immune system and to help balance the flora in the vagina. We might suggest B-complex vitamins, zinc, beta-carotene, vitamin C, all of those things that seem to help the immune system in general."

Dalton also uses natural suppositories to treat the yeast, as well as oral anti-fungal remedies including garlic. This is a traditional treatment. "I've even had patients who were told to tie some dental floss onto a clove of garlic or to thread it through a garlic clove and insert the clove in the vagina. It is very antifungal, so it probably does work.

"There are many ways to treat this, but the basic premise when you have developed a chronic problem should be to look at the whole body."

Describing the difference between acute versus chronic yeast infections, Dalton says, "If somebody gets a onetime infection, then perhaps she has a new partner and is having more sex than usual. In that case I would recommend she get some over-the-counter Monistat cream or use a little antifungal vaginal gel for a few days, to get rid of it. However, if it's an ongoing problem, we try to look more at the whole person and why she is having infections over and over again."

For chronic yeast problems, Dalton looks at the digestive system, because there is likely a yeast imbalance in the digestive system. That means the woman is getting more vaginal contamination than average. "Often you'll see symptoms such as gas, bloating, constipation or diarrhea, and rectal itching."

In chronic cases, it is important to determine what strain of yeast is present. At Wellspring for Women, Dalton says, "We do tests through our local lab or, more often than not, through Great Smokies Lab in North Carolina. The patient gets a kit from the clinic and takes a stool sample, and it's sent to North Carolina to be analyzed. With chronic yeast, the problem is that over time the yeast will mutate into a form that becomes resistant to most, if not all, of the medications typically used to treat yeast. The lab not only cultures but also tests the strain or strains that are found for sensitivities to medications and natural treatments. We have sometimes found yeast that has become resistant to garlic, for example. Though garlic in general is considered a great antifungal, there are some yeast strains that have mutated into a form in which garlic doesn't bother them at all—in fact, they probably thrive on it. And the same is true for resistance to various types of medication.

"So for chronic problems, we not only look a little deeper into the person's situation—into her lifestyle and habits—but we try to identify the exact organism we are dealing with and what that organism is sensitive to, so that we can help the person get rid of it completely."

PATIENT STORY

I had a patient who had a chronic yeast infection for about twelve years. It developed out of chronic bladder infections. She was given so many antibiotics that they ended by killing off the normal bacteria in the gut, which allowed the yeast to overgrow. Eventually that developed into vaginal yeast infections. We worked on it systemically. We tested to find out what organism she had and what it was sensitive to. We looked at her diet and her stress levels, which were high. After medication as well as natural treatments, we thought we'd gotten rid of it.

"Recently she had to be on antibiotics for twelve weeks for an abscessed tooth, so we wanted to check her. We found that she was fine. She had gone three months on antibiotics and there was no sign of yeast at all. We felt that she was really clear of it, since, being on the antibiotics that long, any average woman would have gotten a yeast infection. She was able to avoid it. So that was a very good sign that she was clear.

—*Carol Dalton*

Trichomonas

Trichomonas is another vaginal infection, caused by a one-celled protozoan called *Trichomonas vaginalis*. Trichomonas, says herbalist Amanda McQuade Crawford, "is usually sexually transmitted. It's a parasite, not a virus or a bacterium, and is not to be confused with trichinosis, the infestation of worms that can result from eating uncooked pork."

SYMPTOMS

Trichomonas causes an inflammation of a woman's vaginal lining. The symptoms, says Crawford, are intense vaginal itching, irritation, and discharge. These symptoms are worse than similar symptoms that appear with bacterial vaginitis or yeast infections. The thin vaginal discharge trichomonas produces is yellow or green, and occasionally gray, and has a bubbly or frothy appearance. This discharge produces a burning sensation; a raw feeling; and a characteristic bad, fishy smell. Sexual intercourse is painful.

Trichomonas is a very serious condition, and it is important to know how it is distinct from other vaginal infections. Some general medical symptoms are also present: fever, chills, nausea, and fatigue. It can mimic a bladder infection (cystitis). The organisms that cause trichomonas can sit in the tissues of the vagina or the urethra, or hidden away deep in some of the glands inside the vagina, which makes it difficult to treat with natural remedies. When the infection goes on, you need to consult a licensed health care practitioner.

TREATMENT

In herbal treatment, Crawford indicates, "We try to eliminate the parasite by optimizing natural immune system defenses and work on preventing a recurrence at the same time. This means eliminating risk factors, particularly unsafe sex. The woman's sex partners may need to be tested to see if they require treatment. If they test positive, they need to be tested until they are shown to be negative. It's not enough just to have the symptoms go away. The herbal treatment requires consistency and should be done for at least two months before a retest to see if the parasite has disappeared."

One of the best herbal treatments is cassia bark. Others are myrrh and barberry root. These herbs together are often used to kill off the parasite causing the infection. Tonics promoting long-term immune system health also offer benefits. Two herbs used for this purpose are reishi, a Chinese mushroom, and astragalus root. Astragalus has often been used to boost immunity, especially with long-term infections.

Crawford cautions, "The herbs that are strong enough to kill the organism are ones that taste particularly bad. I say that so that women will know, when they are treating themselves for this, that it is not something like a beverage herbal tea. To take it will require some rigor and some willingness to gulp the things down." You can also take these herbs in capsule form. It can take as long as two months to eliminate the infection.

To make a capsule, combine 4 ounces cassia with 3 ounces barberry root. Add to that 3 ounces reishi mushrooms and 2 ounces astragalus. These herbs can be mixed together and put into capsules at home very easily. It's also very affordable.

If you don't want to take them as powdered herbs in capsules, you can take them in extracts and tinctures. The proportions would be the same, and the dose would be 1 teaspoon in 1 cup of water with meals four times a day for six to eight months.

Alternatively, you can take the herbs separately, although if you do, after three weeks you might encounter a little stomach distress. In that case, dilute them with even more water and be sure to take them with meals so that there is some food in your stomach. This will slow down the speed with which the herbs get into your bloodstream but will not neutralize their effects.

Don't forget that what you eat can also help the body heal. For trichomonas there is no one specific food that will make the difference. Crawford's recommendations are to decrease excess sugar and refined carbohydrates. Eat low-protein, high-quality whole foods with at least four to five servings a day of fresh fruits and vegetables in season. She says you must keep in mind that "We are eating foods that will nourish our whole being, not just the fruits or plants that will kill off parasites, because that won't get to the root of the whole problem."

Dalton also recommends certain supplements. She cites "good research on using fairly high doses of zinc, C, and beta-carotene, which seem to systemically help the body throw off trichomonas."

Crawford uses douches in her treatment. One douche formula is cassia bark combined with equal amounts of licorice root bark to soothe the irritated, raw vaginal lining. Simmer 1 ounce of each on low heat for about fifteen minutes, then strain and use the tea as a douche.

A douche Dalton recommends contains aloe, vinegar, and tea tree oil. This is a drawing solution that helps get rid of the infection.

Crawford warns, "The thing to remember about douching is that it has some short-term benefits but also some long-term drawbacks. It should not be done every day, but only to relieve symptoms. At the same time, you must undergo a long-term treatment, such as taking the capsules, to deal with the root of the problem."

After six or eight weeks on the herbal treatment, get tested to see if the parasite has been eliminated. If it is still present, use the herbal treatment for an additional two weeks.

Crawford also notes that there's a need to counter the effect of the stronger herbal remedies. "If you are going to continue taking fairly strong herbs to kill off a small living organism, it's necessary to take some other herbs to help you counteract the negative side effects of these strong herbs. One of these counteracting herbs would be milk thistle. Take it as a standard extract, or in one of the many proprietary forms that are now in the marketplace. The dose would be 300 or 400 milligrams a day." Milk thistle can help the body develop long-term immunity as well as cope with the other herbs being used to treat the infection.

PATIENT STORY

Trichomonas is generally treated with a drug called Flagyl. In traditional medicine, it's thought that Flagyl or other antiparasitic drugs are the only way to treat this. About twenty years ago I had a patient who had a resistant case of trichomonas. She had been in the university hospital in Denver and they had given her intravenous Flagyl. Still they had not been able to get rid of the trichomonas. We used the douche solution and oral supplements to boost her immune system, and, lo and behold, in about three weeks, the trichomonas was gone and never recurred. So the natural treatments really can work if people are willing to put forward the effort. Obviously, it's easier in many cases to take a pill or two a day than to do all of this regime. However, it helps the body be healthier in general.

—*Carol Dalton*

Bacterial Vaginosis

Bacterial vaginosis (BV) is caused by Gardnerella, a gram-negative bacterium that hates oxygen. An alternative treatment that has been used at women's health clinics across America is to mix 1 cup of distilled or sterilized water and 1 tablespoon of a 3 percent solution of hydrogen peroxide. Douche with this mixture once a day for a week. Then repeat every three days, for an additional two weeks. The hydrogen peroxide and distilled water increase oxygen in the vaginal canal and tissues, which is antagonistic to the Gardnerella. This douche is a noninvasive, effective way to treat the problem. If it doesn't work within a week to ten days, consult a licensed health practitioner for other kinds of help that might be appropriate.

Plants containing phytochemicals with antibacterial/antifungal activity, in order of potency, include:

Coptis chinensis (Chinese goldthread)
Coptis sp. (generic goldthread)
Mangifera indica (mango)
Coptis japonica (huang lia)
Hydrastis canadensis (goldenseal)
Hamamelis virginiana (witch hazel)

Phyllanthus emblica (emblic)

Punica granatum (pomegranate)

Quercus infectoria (aleppo oak)

Berberis vulgaris (barberry)

Phellodendron amurense (huang po)

Argemone mexicana (prickly poppy)

Fragaria sp. (strawberry)

Rheum rhaponticum (rhubarb)

Glycine max (soybean)

Chapter 60

Varicose Veins

Varicose veins, a common condition in women that usually affects the lower extremities, is the result of damaged valves in the veins. Normally, these tiny valves ensure that the blood flowing through the veins will return fully to the heart. But when these valves are injured, and do not open and close properly, some of the blood runs backward in the veins, pools, and finally engorges the vessels. Varicose veins are large, contorted, unsightly, and sometimes even painful.

Causes

Three mechanisms help return blood to the heart, says Dr. Leon Chaitow, a naturopath, osteopath, and acupuncturist from England, in an article on the HealthWorld Online website (www.healthy.net): the action of muscles through which veins run, the pulsation of arteries that run alongside veins, and the movement of the diaphragm during breathing. Thus, he says, poor breathing function and lack of exercise, as well as various mechanical stresses, such as those resulting from occupations that require long periods of standing, will make venous return less efficient. Other factors that can increase the chance of developing varicose veins are inadequate fiber, vitamins C and E, and bioflavonoids in the diet; increased pressure in the pelvis, as from chronic constipation; and use of birth control pills.

Another cause of varicose veins, says Dr. Chaitow, is thrombophlebitis, a condition in which the veins are obstructed due to clot formation or an aggregation of platelets and fibrin, which restricts blood flow, causing inflammation and damage to the veins.

Herbalist David L. Hoffman lists several other reasons why the walls of the veins receive inadequate support, resulting in varicose veins:

OBESITY—A buildup of fatty tissue in the legs results in inadequate support for veins.

GENETIC PREDISPOSITION—In about 40 percent of cases, there seems to be an inherited tendency to varicosity.

AGE—Over time the connective tissue that supports the veins degenerates, and a decrease in exercise worsens the problem.

TIGHT CLOTHING—Tight clothing constricts and weakens tissue.

PREGNANCY—Pregnancy creates intrapelvic pressure, which interferes with venous return.

Symptoms

According to Dr. Chaitow, the earliest symptom is feeling leg fatigue more often than usual. Other standard symptoms are an ache and heavy feeling in the legs, itching in the skin over the veins, and swelling, sometimes of the entire leg. The skin is discolored, and sometimes an eczema develops, with a breakdown of the skin that may lead to ulcers.

Clinical Experience

Standard procedures for treating varicose veins include elevating the legs, wearing elastic stockings, and, in severe cases, surgery.

Many types of support stockings are available, but it is best to buy them at a pharmacy or surgical supply store, where they will be better quality. If you have a severe problem with varicose veins, you might look into custom-made surgical support stockings. In this country, two companies, Jobst and Sigvaris, make them. If you can't afford support stockings, sometimes an Ace bandage will give you the support you need. Wrap a three- or four-inch bandage around the leg where the varicosity is a problem. This may require wrapping your legs from the toes to the groin if the problem is severe.

With early intervention, the following natural remedies have a high rate of effectiveness.

NUTRIENTS AND HERBS

Certain foods and supplements may strengthen the integrity of the vein wall. These include dark-skinned fruits and berries, such as blueberries, cherries, and purple grapes. Vitamin C with bioflavonoids, especially quercetin or bilberry, improves elasticity, so that blood can return more effectively to the heart.

Dr. Chaitow also recommends vitamin E, in a daily dose of 500 to 800 IU, which is thought to help develop other channels of circulation, thus relieving the pressure in the veins. Vitamin E can also be applied directly to leg ulcers. Selenium, which works together with vitamin E, should also be taken daily in a dose of 50 micrograms. Essential fatty acids in the form of 500 milligrams of evening primrose oil and four to six capsules of EPA (eicosapentaenoic acid) a day will help decrease the likelihood of inflammation and lower the viscosity of the blood. Finally, he says, it is essential to consume enough fiber to keep the bowels functioning well so that no straining occurs.

Astringent herbs, such as horse chestnut, witch hazel, gotu kola, and butcher's broom, are good to take, although the first two should not be used when pregnant or lactating. Naturopathic physicians often recommend 1,000 milligrams of butcher's broom, two to three times daily, for pregnant women in their third trimester who are troubled by varicose veins or hemorrhoids.

David Hoffman adds that prickly ash and ginkgo can be used to stimulate circulation; hawthorn, yarrow, horse chestnut to tone the veins; comfrey to soothe irritation and heal wounds. He offers the following lotion, which can be used as necessary to relieve irritation:

- 8 parts distilled witch hazel
- 1 part horse chestnut tincture
- 1 part comfrey tincture
- Rose water, if desired

Another factor to consider is dietary support for the liver. This is because a congested liver backs up venous circulation and places additional pressure on the veins, which can then damage valves. Foods such as beets and artichokes and herbs such as milk thistle and dandelion can improve liver circulation. At the same time, it is important to refrain from substances known to cause liver damage, such as drugs, alcohol, and other harsh chemicals.

EXERCISE

The main way to help relieve varicose veins is to do what you can to keep your blood flow moving, in spite of the fact that the veins are not doing their job properly. Helping the blood flow counteracts some of the problems caused by the damaged valves. Daily exercise is key. It is also important for keeping weight down. Excess weight creates stress on the body. Maintaining one's optimal weight lessens stress on the body, which, in turn, decreases the chance of damaging the valves in the veins. In addition, exercise improves overall circulation in the arteries and veins. Dr. Chaitow suggests exercises that involve contracting the leg muscles, circling the ankles, and upside-down bicycling movements.

Of particular benefit are maneuvers that take pressure off the legs. It is helpful to sit with your feet and legs elevated, waist-level or higher, whenever you can. This allows gravity to help the blood flow back to your heart. Inverted postures in yoga or even just lying on a slant board with the legs elevated for a few minutes a day are beneficial. You can also raise the foot of your bed by six to twelve inches. Medical magnets can be placed over the feet for added healing power. Maneuvers that take weight off the feet are particularly important for people who work in occupations in which they are constantly on their feet.

Another form of exercise to consider is qi gong, which strengthens the veins' ability to pump blood back to the heart.

CHELATION THERAPY

Chelation therapy flushes toxins out of the blood. Many people know that chelation therapy improves arterial integrity, but few realize that it can aid venous circulation as well, thereby helping varicose veins. Chelation therapy also helps to overcome liver congestion and thrombophlebitis, two conditions that put women at risk for varicose veins. (See chapter 1 for a more in-depth discussion of chelation therapy.)

ADDITIONAL SUGGESTIONS

Dr. Tori Hudson, a naturopath in Portland, Oregon, offers the following tips in her column in *Prevention* magazine:

- Eat a high-fiber diet.
- Avoid standing for long periods and lifting heavy objects.
- Use supplements: Every day take 1,000 milligrams of vitamin C, 1,000 milligrams of bioflavonoids, 150 milligrams of pycnogenols, and 400 IU of vitamin E.

Dr. Chaitow adds a few more suggestions:

- Instead of standing still, shift from one leg to the other, or walk gently back and forth.
- Don't cross your legs when you sit.
- Take warm, not hot, baths, and end by splashing cold water on the legs.
- Take regular sitz baths, alternating between hot and cold, but finish with cold; this stimulates circulation.
- Alexander technique and osteopathic manipulation both improve body mechanics and thereby aid circulation.
- Garlic is excellent for thinning the blood; Dr. Chaitow recommends two or three capsules or raw cloves a day.

Research Update

An increasing body of evidence is showing the benefits of natural modalities to overall health and well-being. Following is a sample of recent peer-reviewed scientific studies regarding varicose veins.

According to a 2012 article in *Life Extension Magazine*, studies have indicated that diosmin, derived from the flavonoid herperdin, is a first line treatment for chronic venous disease. A prescription medication in some European countries, the extract is taken orally and has been found to help maintain healthy blood flow as well as vascular tone and elasticity. It is also used for hemorrhoids.

Chapter 61

Vision Problems

Problems of the eye range from minor inconveniences to severe, debilitating conditions. According to the Centers for Disease Control and Prevention (CDC), some eighty million Americans have potentially blinding eye diseases. As the aging population continues to grow, the number of people with cataracts, glaucoma, macular degeneration, diabetic retinopathy, and other serious eye disorders will increase. Scientific evidence indicates that vision problems can be often prevented with early detection and treatment, as well as healthy behaviors and lifestyle choices throughout the lifespan. This comes as no surprise to the natural healing community, but now appears to be acknowledged by mainstream medicine, too. On its website, the CDC tells about the association between age-related eye problems and risk factors such as smoking and ultraviolet light exposure. Furthermore, it says, "Additional modifiable factors that might lend themselves to improved ocular health include a diet rich in antioxidants and maintenance of normal levels of blood sugar, lipids, total cholesterol, body weight, and blood pressure combined with regular exercise."

Common Eye Disorders

Cataract, the primary cause of vision loss in the US, occurs when the lens of the eye becomes cloudy as a result of tissue breakdown and protein clumping. It can affect one or both eyes, and usually develops slowly. According to 2013 data from the CDC, the number of people who have cataracts is expected to surge from 20.5 million in 2013 to more than 30 million by 2020.

Glaucoma is characterized by increased pressure within the eye. It can damage the optic nerve and lead to vision loss and blindness. Glaucoma is associated with

normal aging, as well as injury, infection, blood vessel blockage, and inflammatory disorders. In the early stages, there are usually no symptoms.

Diabetic retinopathy involves progressive damage to the blood vessels of the
retina. It is a common complication of diabetes. Over time, high blood sugar
deprives the light-sensitive tissue at the back of the eye from receiving necessary
nutrients. As with the other conditions, vision loss from diabetic retinopathy can
be prevented if diagnosed early and managed properly.

Nearly two million Americans have macular degeneration, also known as age-
related macular degeneration (AMD), with an additional seven million showing
early signs of the disease. AMD affects the macula, which is the central part of the
retina responsible for central vision. Central vision is needed for seeing fine
details clearly, and is important for daily activities such as reading and driving. The
more common type of the disease, dry AMD, occurs over time as the macula
thins and tiny yellow deposits under the retina, called drusen, form and grow.
Wet AMD, which accounts for 10 to 30 percent of cases, progresses more rapidly
than the dry form. When it occurs, abnormal blood vessels behind the retina
start to grow under the macula, causing leakage of blood and fluid, and subsequent
scarring. In the early stages of wet AMD, straight lines often look wavy.

Myopia, or nearsightedness, affects nearly one out of every three Americans.
It is so common that most people view it as an inevitable part of aging. However,
experiences in children with myopia have shown that it may be associated with
deficiencies and imbalances in nutrients, including selenium, magnesium,
chromium, zinc, calcium, vitamin C, and folic acid.

Vision loss can also be caused by infections, eye injuries, inherited eye diseases, and stroke. Other, less serious eye problems that may cause varying levels
of discomfort include floaters, which are typically normal, small specks that float
across the field of vision; dry eyes, which can cause itching and burning; and eye
strain, caused by overuse.

General Considerations

The National Eye Institute offers the following general guidelines for promoting
healthy vision: schedule regular, comprehensive examinations that include dilation of the eyes (especially important since many diseases often have no warning
signs); know your family's eye health history; maintain a healthy weight; use protective eye wear; rest your eyes as needed; and do not smoke. Dietary recom-

mendations include dark leafy green vegetables such as kale, spinach, and collard greens, and fish such as salmon, tuna, and halibut, which are high in omega-3 fatty acids.

Natural Therapies

According to an article on eye health on the *Life Extension* website (www.lifeextension.com), many lifestyle and nutritional interventions have been found to prevent and reduce the severity of eye problems. These include exercise, controlling blood sugar, diet, and nutritional supplementation.

Whole body exercise can decrease drusen formation associated with macular degeneration. Walking and running have been shown to reduce the risk of cataracts. People with diabetic retinopathy appear less likely to engage in regular movement activities as recommended by the American Diabetes Association.

Research indicates that uncontrolled blood sugar can increase the progression of eye diseases. Foods that have a high glycemic index, such as high fructose corn syrup, potatoes, fruit juices, and dried fruit, should be avoided or limited. Unsweetened dairy products, meat, fish, poultry, nuts, seeds, and other low glycemic foods are preferred.

Other dietary recommendations include increasing overall consumption of fruits and vegetables, with particular focus on phytonutrients as found in kale and collard greens, as well as beans, okra, and plantains. Improved eye health has also been associated with a Mediterranean diet emphasizing whole grains, legumes, olive oil, and fish, in addition to fruits and vegetables.

A number of supplements may help to lower the risk of eye diseases. These include the B-complex vitamins, vitamin A, vitamin C, vitamin E, vitamin D, lipoic acid, and zinc. Omega-3 fatty acids are useful in regulating the formation of blood vessels that can distort vision. Among the phytochemicals, carotenoids such as lutein, zeaxanthin, and meso-zeaxanthin have been shown to reduce the occurrence of macular degeneration and cataract formation, and astaxanthin has been linked to decreased eye strain and fatigue. Other supplements with antioxidant and anti-inflammatory properties include Ginkgo biloba, curcumin, and resveratrol, a phytochemical found in grapes, cranberries, and peanuts. Taurine may help with corneal disease, as it supports the regeneration and removal of worn out tissue. Cineraria is a homeopathic remedy that increases lymph flow around the eyes, thereby removing toxins and improving visual clarity.

Research Update

An increasing body of evidence is showing the benefits of natural modalities to overall health and well-being. Following is a sample of recent peer-reviewed scientific studies regarding vision problems.

A 2013 study published in *Investigative Ophthalmology and Visual Science* found that larger macular drusen were less likely in participants who were physically active seven or more hours per week compared to those who exercised two or fewer hours per week, leading the investigators to conclude that "a physically active, heart-healthy lifestyle prevents the earliest manifestation of AMD." A lower cataract risk was significantly associated with both running and walking in a 2013 study in *Medicine and Science in Sports and Exercise*. Researchers reported in *Epidemiology* (2013) that patients with type 2 diabetes who ate an average of 253 grams of fruit per day had a 50 percent lower risk of incident retinopathy compared with those who had an average of 23 grams per day.

A 2012 study published in *Ophthalmologica* found that daily consumption of black currant anthocyanins was associated with a notable drop in eye pressure in patients with open-angle glaucoma.

III.

ALTERNATIVE HEALTH RESOURCES

Chapter 62

Recipes For Good Health

BREAKFAST

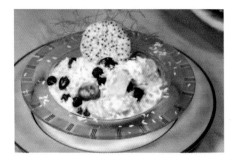

TROPICAL PARADISE RICE CEREAL

2 cups coconut milk
1 cup pitted fresh or frozen
  pomegranate
½ cup chopped pineapple
¼ cup shredded unsweetened coconut
2 cups cooked sweet rice
½ cup chopped macadamia nuts, toasted (see note below)

2 tablespoons almond extract
1 tablespoon vanilla extract

In a medium saucepan, combine the coconut milk, banana, cherries, and pineapple. Cook over medium-low heat for 2 to 3 minutes. Add the remaining ingredients, mix well, and cook an additional 2 to 3 minutes. Serve hot. *Serves 2*

Note: To toast the nuts, use a food dehydrator at 125 degrees overnight. This is for all nuts and seeds.

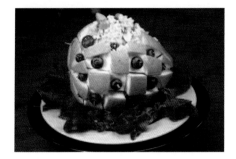

MILLET CRUNCH

6 ounces millet
2 ounces almonds, whole
1 teaspoon blueberry
    concentrate
Pinch of cinnamon

Cook millet in a saucepan in 13 ounces water. When water comes to a boil, lower heat and cook until water is absorbed. Stir occasionally. Add remaining ingredients. Mix well. *Serves 1*

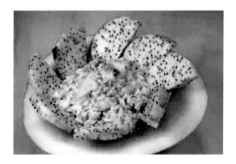

CARIBBEAN POWER BREAKFAST

6 ounces basmati rice, cooked
    (room temperature)
3 ounces mango
1 ounce papaya
1 ounce pineapple
1 tablespoon manuka honey
Pinch of cinnamon

Combine all ingredients. Mix well. *Serves 1*

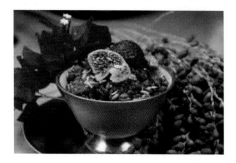

BERRY SUNRISE

6 ounces brown rice, cooked
   (room temperature)
3 ounces blueberries
3 ounces blackberries
3 ounces strawberries, halved
1½ ounces sunflower seeds
1½ ounces figs, chopped
Sprinkle of coconut, shredded and unsweetened

Combine all ingredients. Mix well. *Serves 1*

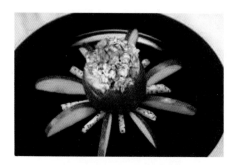

SCOTTISH OATMEAL

6 ounces steel cut Scottish
   oatmeal, cooked (room
   temperature)
2 ounces gooseberries or
   mulberries
1½ ounces dried apricots,
   chopped
2 teaspoons prime grade
   maple syrup
Pinch of cinnamon

Combine all ingredients. Mix well. *Serves 1*

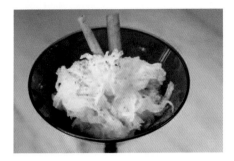

CANADIAN MAPLE SQUASH

6 ounces spaghetti squash
2 tablespoons maple syrup
1½ ounces brewer's yeast
1 tablespoon plant-based
    protein powder
Pinch of cinnamon

Preheat oven to 400 degrees. Cut squash in half, remove the seeds and discard. Place in baking dish cut side down, with 1/3 inch water. Bake for 40 minutes. When cooled, spoon out squash and place in a bowl. Add remaining ingredients and mix well. *Serves 1*

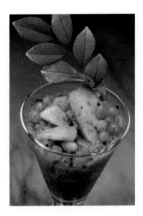

AMISH AMARANTH

6 ounces amaranth, cooked
    (room temperature)
3 ounces peaches, cut into
    bite size pieces
1 tablespoon honey
Pinch of anise
Pinch of allspice

Combine all ingredients and mix well. *Serves 1*

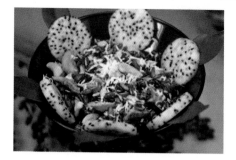

MIXED NUTS WITH RICE

6 ounces brown rice, cooked
   (room temperature)
1½ ounces coconut, shredded
   (unsweetened)
1 ounce cashews, chopped
1 ounce almonds
1 ounce walnuts
2 ounces dried apricots,
   chopped
2 ounces sunflower seed butter

Combine brown rice with coconut, all nuts, sunflower seed butter, and apricots. Puree half the mixture in blender with 2 ounces water until coarsely ground. Add to the rest of the rice. *Serves 1*

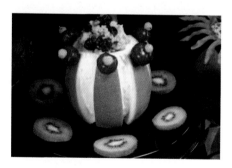

MEDITERRANEAN MILLET

6 ounces millet, cooked
   (room temperature)
2 ounces Thompson raisins
1 tablespoon manuka honey
⅛ teaspoon fennel powder
⅛ tablespoon anise
Pinch of cardamom
Pinch of cinnamon

Combine all ingredients. Mix well. *Serves 1*

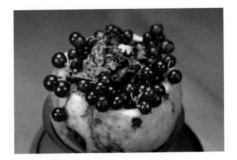

AMARANTH CHERRY DELIGHT

6 ounces amaranth, cooked
(room temperature)
4 ounces frozen cherries
2 ounces pecans, chopped
3 ounces dried peaches,
chopped
Pinch of clove
Pinch of allspice

Combine all ingredients. Mix well. *Serves 1*

SALADS

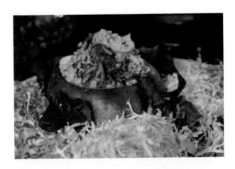

SPICY BASMATI MARINADE

3 ounces basmati rice, cooked (chilled)
2 ounces sunflower sprouts
3 ounces spinach, coarsely chopped
3 ounces marinated artichoke hearts,
chopped to bite-size pieces
2 tablespoons extra virgin olive oil
1 teaspoon coconut oil
2 teaspoons cider vinegar

½ teaspoon salt
½ teaspoon basil
¼ teaspoon curry powder
Pinch of cayenne

Combine all ingredients and mix well. Allow to set in refrigerator overnight for best taste. Serve chilled. *Serves 1*

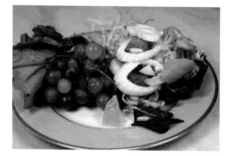

PECAN, WALNUT, AND PINE NUT SALAD

1 cup sliced fennel root
3 cups mixed mesclun greens
½ cup diced fresh peaches
1 diced pear
2 peeled sliced fresh seedless oranges
¼ cup chopped pecans

¼ cup walnuts
¼ cup pine nuts

Combine fennel, mesclun greens, oranges, pear, and peaches in a large salad bowl. Toss with a light, sweet salad dressing, such as orange vinaigrette, and top with walnuts, pecans, and pine nuts. Serve chilled. *Serves 3*

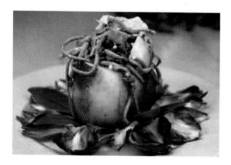

COOL GARDEN NOODLES

3 ounces brown rice, cooked
   (chilled)
3 ounces mung bean noodles,
   cooked (chilled)
3 ounces avocado, chopped into
   bite-size pieces
3 ounces marinated artichoke hearts,
   chopped into bite-size pieces
2 tablespoons coconut oil
2 tablespoons avocado or flax seed oil
1 teaspoon chopped fresh parsley

½ teaspoon minced garlic
½ teaspoon basil
½ teaspoon salt
Pinch of ginger

Combine all ingredients and mix well. *Serves 2*

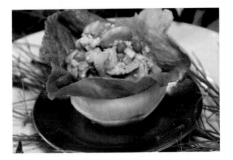

CRUNCHY PENNE SALAD

3 ounces yellow squash, cubed
3 ounces celery, chopped
3 ounces scallions, chopped
3 ounces olive oil
1½ ounces miso

½ teaspoon cumin
Pinch of cayenne
3 ounces black-eyed peas, cooked (chilled)
6 ounces penne brown rice pasta, cooked

Cook pasta until done then blanch under cold water. Combine squash, celery, and scallions in a bowl. Set aside. In a blender, combine oil, miso, and ¼ cup water. Blend until smooth. Add vegetables to miso mixture and blend until coarsely ground. Add cumin and cayenne. Combine with black-eyed peas and rice penne. Mix thoroughly. *Serves 2*

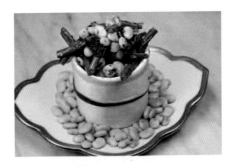

GARBANZO BEAN AND LIMA BEAN SEAWEED SALAD

1 ounce dulse, dry
3 ounces snap beans, cut into
   1-inch pieces
3 ounces garbanzo beans, cooked
   (chilled)
3 ounces lima beans, cooked (chilled)
2 tablespoons olive oil
1 teaspoon dill

1 teaspoon tarragon
½ teaspoon salt
Juice of ½ lemon

Soak and rinse dulse 2 or 3 times in cold water. Steam snap beans for 10 minutes. Mix all ingredients together. Serve chilled. *Serves 2*

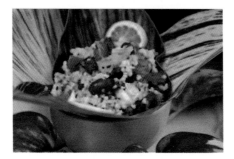

PERSIAN MILLET SALAD

3 ounces garbanzo beans,
   cooked (chilled)
3 ounces millet, cooked (chilled)
3 ounces red and yellow pepper,
   chopped
3 ounces onion, chopped
1 teaspoon tarragon

¼ teaspoon anise
½ teaspoon salt
Pinch of celery seed
2 tablespoons sesame oil

Combine all ingredients and mix well. Serve hot or cold. *Serves 1*

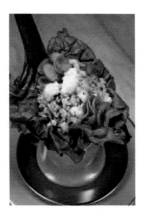

TEX MEX MARINADE

3 ounces cauliflower flowerets,
   in bite-size pieces
3 ounces kidney beans, cooked (chilled)
3 ounces avocado, cut into ½-inch
   cubes
1½ ounces sunflower seeds
2 ounces shallots, chopped
1 ounce shredded coconut
   (unsweetened)

2 tablespoons toasted sesame oil
1 teaspoon tarragon
½ teaspoon basil
1 teaspoon soy sauce
¼ teaspoon salt
2 teaspoons cider vinegar
Pinch of cayenne
Pinch of mild jalapeño

Steam cauliflower for 8 minutes. Combine with the remaining ingredients and mix well. Serve chilled. *Serves 2*

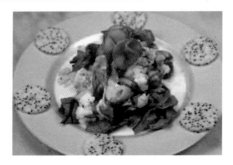

ZESTY PECAN ARUGULA SALAD

3 ounces arugula, coarsely chopped
3 ounces cauliflower flowerets,
　in bite-size pieces
3 ounces avocado, cut into
　bite-size pieces
3 ounces marinated artichoke hearts, cut into bite-size pieces
2 ounces pecans, chopped
1½ ounces shallots, chopped

1½ tablespoons coconut oil
1 teaspoon lemon juice
¼ cup fresh basil
½ teaspoon salt

Combine all ingredients and mix well. *Serves 1*

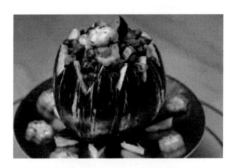

PINTO BEAN SALAD

3 ounces pinto beans, cooked
　(chilled)
3 ounces onion, chopped
3 ounces tomato, chopped
3 ounces green pepper, chopped
1½ ounces walnuts
2 tablespoons toasted sesame oil

½ teaspoon minced garlic
½ teaspoon tarragon
¼ teaspoon basil
1 teaspoon salt

Combine all ingredients. Serve at room temperature. *Serves 2*

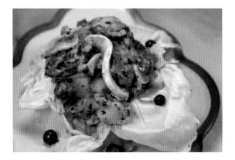

MIDDLE EASTERN POTATO SALAD

1 medium-sized potato	½ teaspoon basil
1½ ounces sesame seeds	½ teaspoon salt
3 ounces scallions, chopped	1½ ounces tahini
3 ounces mushrooms, sliced	2 tablespoons sesame oil
1½ ounces coconut flour	
½ teaspoon cumin	

Preheat oven to 400 degrees. Bake potato for 40 minutes. When cooled, cut into ½-inch cubes. Toast sesame seeds in a skillet, without oil, for 3 minutes over low heat. Set aside. In a separate bowl, combine vegetables with remaining ingredients, except oil, and 2 ounces water. Sauté all ingredients, including potato cubes, with coconut flour for 4 minutes over medium heat. Place in a bowl, and add sesame seeds and salt. Mix well. Serve hot. *Serves 2*

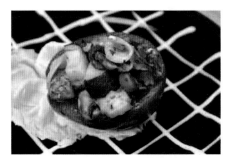

MEDITERRANEAN MUSHROOM AND POTATO SALAD

1 medium-sized potato	¼ teaspoon basil
3 ounces mushrooms, chopped	¼ teaspoon oregano
medium fine	½ teaspoon salt
3 ounces okra, cut into ½-inch pieces	1½ tablespoons olive oil
3 ounces onion, chopped	
3 ounces tomato, chopped	
1½ ounces scallions, chopped	

Preheat oven to 400 degrees. Bake potato for 45 minutes. When cooled, cut into ½-inch cubes. Sauté vegetables, basil, oregano, and salt in olive oil over low heat for about 5 minutes. Combine all ingredients. Mix well. Serve hot. *Serves 2*

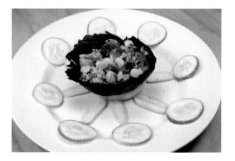

MULTI-SPROUT VITALISM SALAD

3 ounces brussels sprouts
3 ounces cannellini beans, cooked
(chilled)
3 ounces barley, cooked (chilled)
3 ounces mung bean and alfalfa
sprouts
1½ ounces Brazil nuts, chopped

2 tablespoons olive oil
1 teaspoon soy sauce
½ teaspoon chopped parsley
½ teaspoon rosemary
½ teaspoon salt

Steam brussels sprouts for 10 minutes. Combine all ingredients and mix well. Serve cool. *Serves 2*

SOUPS

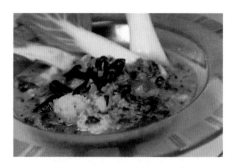

HEART HEALTHY BEAN SOUP

3 ounces kidney beans
6 ounces cauliflower flowerets,
in bite-size pieces
6 ounces watercress, coarsely chopped
1 teaspoon minced onion
3 tablespoons avocado oil

½ teaspoon basil
½ teaspoon salt
Pinch of cayenne

Soak beans overnight in water. In the morning, rinse well and add 4 cups of fresh water. Bring beans to a boil and lower to medium heat. Place the cover on the pot. The beans should cook for about 2 hours. After 1½ hours add remaining ingredients and continue cooking for an additional 30 minutes. Puree half the amount in blender for about 15 seconds and return to the rest of the soup. Mix well. Cook for an additional 10 minutes. *Serves 2*

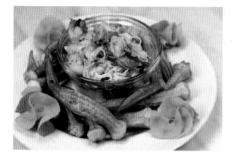

VIETNAMESE RICE NOODLE SOUP

5 tablespoons extra virgin olive oil
½ cup sliced zucchini
½ cup sliced potatoes
½ cup sliced celery
1 cup diced onions
1 cup sliced mushrooms
¼ cup chopped fresh parsley
½ cup broccoli florets

1 teaspoon Himalayan pink sea salt
¼ teaspoon freshly ground black pepper
Pinch of cayenne pepper
¼ cup chopped fresh dill
6 cups water
2 cups uncooked brown rice noodles
4 cloves crushed garlic

In a large saucepan, heat oil over medium heat and sauté vegetables about 10 minutes. Add remaining ingredients, except rice noodles, and let simmer over medium-low heat for 25 to 35 minutes. Add the noodles 10 minutes before finishing. *Serves 2*

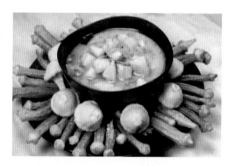

NEW ENGLAND CREAMY POTATO CHOWDER

1 cup peeled, cubed potatoes
¼ cup sliced celery
½ cup diced onions
2 tablespoons olive oil
¼ teaspoon Himalayan pink sea salt
Dash of cayenne

Dash of freshly ground black pepper
1½ cups of water
1 vegetable bouillon cube (morga)
1 to 2 cups rice milk
1 cup fresh peppermint for garnish

In a large saucepan, sauté potatoes, celery, and onions in the oil over medium heat for 10 minutes. Add remaining ingredients and cook, covered, over medium to low heat for 25 to 30 minutes. Garnish with peppermint. *Serves 3*

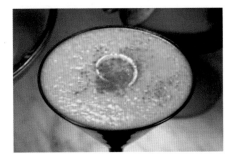

CARIBBEAN SQUASH SOUP

1 medium-sized butternut
  squash
1½ ounces sunflower seeds,
  raw
2 teaspoons maple syrup
½ teaspoon curry
Pinch of cinnamon
3 ounces celery, chopped

Preheat oven to 400 degrees. Cut squash in half. Remove seeds and discard. Place in a baking pan, cut side down, with ½ inch water. Bake for 40 minutes. When cool, remove skin and place squash in a blender along with remaining ingredients, except for celery, and 2 cups of water. Blend until smooth; add the celery. Mix well. Transfer to medium saucepan. Cook over low heat for about 20 minutes or until thoroughly heated. *Serves 1*

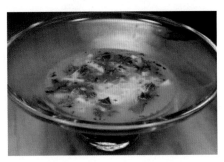

GARY'S NOODLE SOUP

1 cup gluten-free noodles
6 ounces celery chopped
2 ounces sunflower seeds, raw
2 ounces raw pumpkin seeds
2 tablespoons maple syrup

½ teaspoon curry
Pinch of cinnamon

Put vegetables in medium saucepan with 4 cups water. Bring to a boil and add remaining ingredients, except for noodles. Lower to medium heat and continue cooking an additional 10 minutes. Puree half of this mixture in blender for about 15 seconds and then return to saucepan. Add noodles and cook for an additional 10 minutes. *Serves 2*

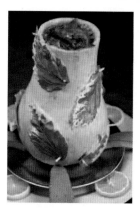

SPICY VEGETABLE SOUP

3 ounces mung beans
3 ounces onions, sliced
2 ounces celery, chopped
2 ounces red cabbage, sliced
Pinch of chili peppers
Pinch of jalapeño peppers
Pinch of cayenne

½ teaspoon salt
½ teaspoon oregano
1 cup fresh basil
6 ounces basmati rice, cooked
1 teaspoon chopped fresh parsley
3 tablespoons coconut oil

Soak beans overnight in water. In the morning, rinse the beans, pour into saucepan and add 4 cups water. Bring beans to a boil and lower to medium heat. Place the cover on the pot. After 1 hour, add the vegetables, oil, and seasonings. Puree half the mixture in the blender for 15 seconds or until coarsely ground. Return to the soup along with the basmati rice. Mix well and cook for an additional 10 minutes. *Yields 4 to 5 cups*

LUNCH AND DINNER ENTREES

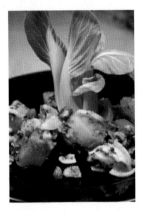

BUTTERNUT SQUASH

3 ounces butternut squash
1½ ounces shallots, chopped fine
2 ounces walnuts
2 tablespoons olive oil
1 teaspoon chopped fresh dill
¼ teaspoon thyme

½ teaspoon basil
½ teaspoon salt
3 ounces avocado, sliced

Preheat oven to 400 degrees. Lightly oil 4 x 8 baking pan with sunflower oil. Cut squash in half, remove seeds and discard. Place squash halves in baking pan, cut side down, with ½ inch water. Bake for 40 minutes. Take squash out of oven, and lower heat to 350 degrees. When cool enough to handle, remove skin from squash and cut squash into 1-inch cubes. Combine the shallots with the squash and transfer to baking pan. In a blender, place walnuts, oil, dill, thyme, basil, and salt. Puree until smooth. Pour over squash and shallots, and bake for 20 minutes. Top with avocado.
Serves 2

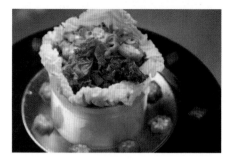

DELTA DELIGHT

3 ounces spinach, chopped
3 ounces okra, sliced
3 ounces red pepper, chopped
3 ounces split peas, cooked
1½ tablespoons toasted sesame oil
½ teaspoon soy sauce
Pinch each of cayenne pepper, Cajun seasoning, and black pepper

½ teaspoon tarragon
½ teaspoon salt
3 ounces brown rice, cooked

Steam spinach, okra, and pepper for 7 minutes or until tender. Puree split peas in the blender along with oil, soy sauce, tarragon, salt, and ¼ cup water until mixture achieves sauce consistency. Pour split peas over vegetables and brown rice and serve warm. *Serves 2*

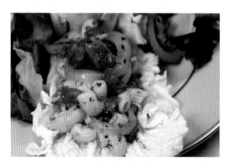

OLIVE RICE PASTA

3 ounces Portobello mushrooms,
    sliced
6 ounces onions, sliced
3 ounces tomato, chopped
½ cup fresh basil
¼ teaspoon oregano

½ teaspoon tarragon
½ cup mixed olives—green, brown, red
½ teaspoon salt
2 tablespoons olive oil
6 ounces rice pasta, cooked

Sauté mushrooms, onions, and tomato with basil, oregano, tarragon, and salt in olive oil for 5 minutes. Combine with rice pasta and toss gently. Serve warm. *Serves 2*

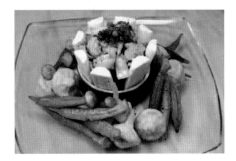

SAVORY FLORENTINE

3 ounces coconut flour
¼ cup minced onions
½ teaspoon thyme
½ teaspoon oregano
½ teaspoon salt
½ teaspoon soy sauce

2 tablespoons coconut oil
3 ounces arugula, coarsely chopped
3 ounces marinated artichoke hearts, chopped into bite-size pieces
3 ounces brown rice, cooked

Combine flour with onion, thyme, oregano, salt, soy sauce, and oil. Mix well. Sauté flour mixture with vegetables and sunflower oil in skillet or wok. Add rice and sauté for 7 minutes. *Serves 2*

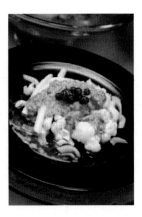

BELOW THE BORDER QUICK MEAL

3 ounces asparagus, cut in
   ½-inch pieces
4 ounces cauliflower flowerets,
   in bite-size pieces
3 ounces celery, chopped
6 ounces kidney beans, cooked
1½ ounces filberts, chopped
   medium fine
2 ounces pine nuts

2 tablespoons olive oil
¾ teaspoon chopped fresh dill
½ teaspoon chili powder
¼ teaspoon basil
¼ teaspoon celery seed
½ teaspoon minced garlic
½ teaspoon salt
1 teaspoon jalapeño peppers

Steam asparagus and cauliflower for approximately 10 minutes. Combine with celery. Set aside. In a blender, place beans, pine nuts, and remaining ingredients. Puree until smooth. Pour this sauce over the asparagus mixture. Serve at room temperature. *Serves 2*

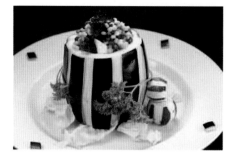

GREEN BARLEY SPLIT

6 ounces split peas, cooked
6 ounces spinach, chopped coarsely
6 ounces barley, cooked
6 ounces asparagus, cut into
   1-inch pieces

3 tablespoons olive oil
½ teaspoon minced garlic
½ teaspoon salt
½ teaspoon black pepper salt
1 teaspoon tarragon

Preheat oven to 375 degrees. Lightly grease a 4 x 8 baking pan with olive oil. Combine all ingredients together. Toss and mix well. Transfer to baking pan and bake for 15 minutes or until thoroughly heated. *Serves 3*

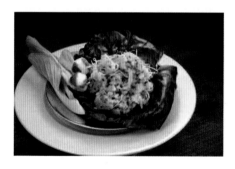

MEDITERRANEAN RICE

3 ounces celery, chopped
2 ounces shallots,
   chopped finely
3 ounces brown rice, cooked
2 tablespoons olive oil
2 teaspoons tarragon
¼ teaspoon dill

¾ teaspoon salt
½ teaspoon soy sauce
3 ounces broccoli sprouts
2 ounces macadamia nuts, chopped
3 ounces cider vinegar

Sauté celery and shallots with brown rice in a skillet with olive oil for 5 minutes. Add herbs, salt, and soy sauce. Transfer to bowl. Add sprouts, macadamias, and cider vinegar. Mix well and serve at room temperature. *Serves 1*

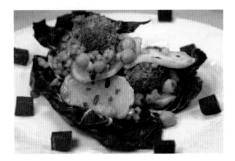

CURRIED PEAS WITH VEGGIES

4 ounces turnips,
   sliced ¼ inch thick
3 ounces broccoli florets,
   in bite-size pieces
4 ounces peas, cooked
4 ounces barley, cooked

2 tablespoons minced fresh chives
2 tablespoons coconut oil
1 teaspoon curry
Juice of 1 lemon

Steam turnips and broccoli for 8 minutes. Combine with remaining ingredients. Mix well. Serve warm. *Serves 2*

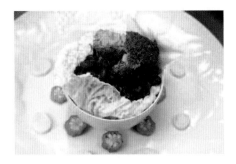

ARGENTINIAN RICE

3 ounces cauliflower florets,
   in bite-size pieces
2 tablespoons fresh chopped parsley
2 tablespoons toasted sesame oil
½ teaspoon soy sauce
¼ teaspoon black pepper
¼ teaspoon anise

¾ teaspoon salt
6 ounces black beans, cooked
4 ounces brown rice, cooked
3 ounces avocado, sliced

Preheat oven to 375 degrees. Lightly grease a 4 x 8 baking pan with toasted sesame oil. Steam cauliflower for about 5 minutes. Combine all ingredients except for the avocado. Mix well. Transfer to baking pan and bake for 15 minutes. Garnish with avocado slices. *Serves 2*

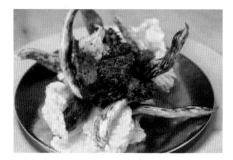

TASTE OF INDIA CASSEROLE

4 ounces coconut flour
4 ounces split peas, cooked
3 tablespoons coconut oil
2 teaspoons curry
1 teaspoon minced garlic
¾ teaspoon salt

¼ teaspoon thyme
3 ounces spinach, coarsely chopped
3 ounces cauliflower,
    cut into bite-size pieces
3 ounces brown rice, cooked
3 ounces avocado, sliced

Preheat oven to 375 degrees. Lightly grease 4 x 8 baking pan with coconut oil. In a blender, combine coconut flour, split peas, oil, curry, garlic, salt, thyme, and ¼ cup water. Separately, combine spinach, cauliflower, and brown rice. Transfer to covered baking pan, add the flour and the beans, and bake for 15 minutes. Place avocado slices on top for garnish. *Serves 2*

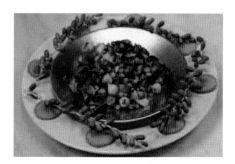

CHICKPEA CASSEROLE

3 ounces chick peas, cooked
3 ounces barley, cooked
3 ounces turnip greens, chopped
3 ounces cashew nuts, chopped
2 tablespoons coconut oil
2 teaspoons chopped fresh mint leaves

1 teaspoon thyme
1 teaspoon curry
¾ teaspoon salt
½ cup fresh basil

Preheat oven to 375 degrees. Lightly grease a 4 x 8 baking pan with coconut oil. Combine all ingredients and mix well. Transfer to baking pan and bake for 15 minutes. *Serves 2*

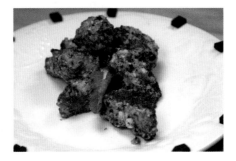

HONEY MUSTARD TEMPEH

3 ounces tempeh, cut into
  ½-inch pieces
3 ounces macadamia nuts, chopped
2 teaspoons fresh chives, minced

2 teaspoons tarragon
½ teaspoon salt
2 tablespoons coconut oil
2 tablespoons honey mustard

Preheat oven to 350 degrees. Lightly grease baking sheet with coconut oil. Sauté tempeh in coconut oil for 3 minutes. Blend macadamia nuts in blender until finely ground. Mix nut meal with chives, tarragon, and salt as well as 1 ounce water. Dip tempeh in this batter and place on baking sheet. Place in oven for 15 minutes. Upon removal from the over baste the mustard upon the tempeh. *Serves 1*

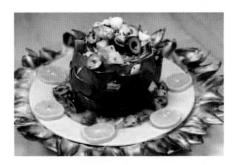

MUSHROOM STUFFED ARTICHOKES

4 artichokes
4 tablespoons orange juice
4 tablespoons plus 1 teaspoon
  lemon juice
2 tablespoons mint
1 cup diced Portobello mushrooms
2 cups water
½ cup chopped avocado
¼ cup chopped fresh tomatoes
¼ cup chopped black pitted olives

1 cup chopped onions
2 tablespoons extra virgin olive oil
1 cup chopped fresh basil
3 tablespoons toasted sesame seeds
2 tablespoons cayenne pepper
½ cup roasted macadamia nuts
1 teaspoon salt
1 sliced lemon (for garnish)

Trim the thorns from the artichoke leaves with a pair of scissors and trim the bottoms so they will stand upright. In a medium saucepan, simmer the artichokes in the water and lemon juice over medium heat for about 50–60 minutes, until the leaves pull out easily. Remove the artichokes from the water and let them cool. Gently pull out the center leaves and scoop out the fuzzy choke with a spoon. Combine the remaining ingredients including the sautéed mushrooms in a small mixing bowl and stir well. Spoon the stuffing mixture into the centers of the artichokes and garnish with lemon slices. *Serves 4*

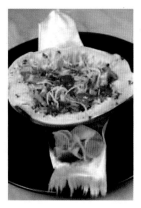

SPAGHETTI SQUASH SPAGHETTI

3 ounces spaghetti squash	2 tablespoons olive oil
6 ounces tomato, chopped	¼ teaspoon basil
3 ounces scallions, chopped	1 teaspoon salt
3 ounces green pepper, chopped	Pinch of black pepper
1½ ounces onion, chopped	Pinch of cayenne

Preheat oven to 400 degrees. Cut squash in half; remove the seeds and discard them. Place the halves in a baking pan cut side down, with ⅓ inch water. Bake for 40 minutes. Sauté the tomato, scallions, green pepper, and onion in the skillet with olive oil for 5 minutes. Add the basil and salt. Remove the spaghetti from the squash and combine with the sautéed mixture. Toss gently. Serve hot. *Serves 1*

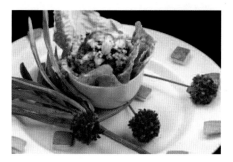

MILLET MAGIC

3 ounces millet, cooked	½ teaspoon salt
3 ounces mushrooms, sliced	¼ teaspoon cumin
3 ounces green pepper, chopped	¼ teaspoon basil
3 ounces onion, chopped	2 ounces coconut flour
1½ ounces pumpkin seeds	Sesame oil
2 tablespoons olive oil	1 cup fresh basil

Preheat oven to 350 degrees. Lightly grease a 4 x 8 baking dish with olive oil. Combine all ingredients together gradually stirring in coconut flour. Transfer to covered baking dish and bake for 20 minutes. *Serves 1*

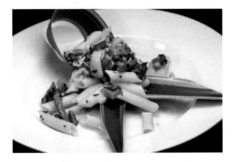

BASIL RICE PASTA

2 cups chopped fresh tomatoes
1 cup sweet peas
1 cup chopped green beans
1 cup chopped yellow onions
4 tablespoons capers
1 cup diced yellow and red
    sweet peppers

2½ cups chopped fresh basil
⅓ teaspoon sliced garlic
¼ cup extra virgin olive oil
4 cups cooked rice pasta
Dash of black pepper
Dash of cayenne
1 teaspoon fennel

In a large saucepan, sauté all the ingredients, except the rice pasta, in the oil for 10 to 15 minutes. Serve hot as a sauce over the cooked spaghetti. *Serves 3 to 4*

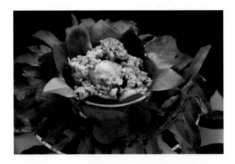

AROMATIC GREEN CASSEROLE

3 ounces snap beans, cut into
    bite-size pieces
3 ounces brussels sprouts, cut into
    bite-size pieces
3 ounces broccoli, cut into
    bite-size pieces
2 ounces walnuts, chopped
2 tablespoons coconut oil
½ teaspoon chopped fresh dill

¼ teaspoon sage
¾ teaspoon sea salt
Juice of 1 lemon
Pinch of cayenne
1 teaspoon tarragon

Steam beans, brussels sprouts, and broccoli for 8 minutes. Combine beans and walnuts with remaining ingredients and ¼ cup water. Transfer to blender and puree until smooth. Pour sauce over vegetables. Serve hot or cold. *Serves 2*

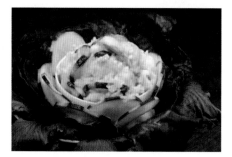

AROMATIC RICE

5 teaspoons peanut oil
¼ cup chopped zucchini
1 cup chopped yellow onions
½ teaspoon chopped shallots
¼ cup chopped unsalted roasted
  peanuts
½ cup roasted macadamia nuts
1 teaspoon fennel

3 cups cooked long grain brown rice
5 artichoke hearts
¼ cup canned water chestnuts
3 teaspoons chopped garlic
4½ teaspoons chopped fresh
  mint for garnish
¾ teaspoon sea salt
2 tablespoons raw honey

Heat the peanut oil in a skillet or wok over high heat until hot but not smoking. Add
the zucchini, onions, and shallots, and sauté over medium heat for 5 minutes. Add
the remaining ingredients one at a time, stirring after each addition, and cook until
hot. Garnish with chopped mint. *Serves 4*

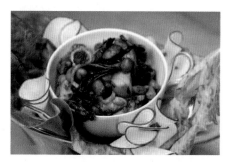

SOUTHERN SOUL DISH

1 cup finely chopped kale,
  steamed 5 minutes
1 cup diced apples
4½ teaspoons apple juice
1 cup sliced mushrooms
½ cup sliced fennel root
1 cup black-eyed peas,
  steamed 15 minutes
½ teaspoon cayenne

1 teaspoon sea salt
1 teaspoon freshly ground black pepper
2 tablespoons extra virgin olive oil
3 tablespoons chopped fresh parsley
3 teaspoons ground cinnamon
1 teaspoon ground nutmeg
½ cup toasted almonds
2 tablespoons maple syrup

In a large saucepan, sauté kale, apples, mushrooms, fennel, salt, pepper, and cayenne
in oil over medium-high heat for 7 minutes. Add the remaining ingredients and cook
an additional 10 minutes. Serve hot. *Serves 3 to 4*

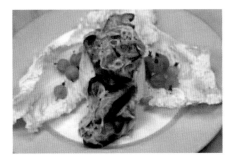

THAI PEANUT RICE NOODLES

1 cup diced yellow onions
½ cup sliced scallions
¼ cup diced celery
7 tablespoons toasted sesame oil
1 cup stemmed and sliced
  shitake mushrooms
1 clove garlic
¼ cup smooth almond butter

3 tablespoons pure maple syrup
1 teaspoon fresh lime juice
½ cup plus tablespoon water
2 drops hot chili oil or Tabasco sauce
Gomasio (sesame salt) to taste
¼ pound cooked rice noodles
1 teaspoon sea salt
Pinch of cayenne

Combine 1 tablespoon oil, garlic, almond butter, maple syrup, cayenne, lime juice, water, and hot chili oil in a blender and mix until smooth, 2 to 3 minutes, and set aside. In a large saucepan, heat the oil over medium heat, then sauté the scallions and mushrooms for 8 to 10 minutes. Remove from the heat and stir in the gomasio and peanut sauce. Toss the rice noodles with the sauce in large bowl until all the noodles are covered. Chill for an hour and a half and serve cold. *Serves 2 to 4*

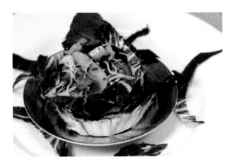

ANGEL HAIR ITALIAN STYLE

1 cup sliced mushrooms
1 cup sliced radicchio
1 cup fresh or frozen peas
1 cup soy parmesan cheese (non-dairy)
4 cups cooked angel hair rice pasta
1 cup fresh basil

1 cup sliced black pitted olives
1 tablespoon sea salt
¾ teaspoon freshly ground black pepper
½ cup rice milk
4 tablespoons capers
1 tablespoon tarragon

In a large saucepan, heat the oil over medium heat and sauté the mushrooms and peas for 6 minutes or until tender. Add the capers, basil, fennel, tarragon, salt, pepper, and milk. Cover and cook for another 2 minutes. Add the radicchio and cook for 1 additional minute. Remove from heat and toss with the cheese and rice pasta. *Serves 3 to 4*

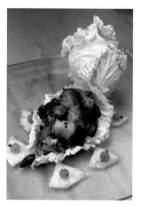

TANTALIZING TEMPEH

2 cups cubed tempeh	2 teaspoons crushed garlic
1 cup cubed pineapple	3 tablespoons tamari
½ cup chopped macadamia nuts	1 cup broccoli florets
1 cup sweet basil leaves	2 tablespoons sliced scallions
¼ cup toasted sesame seeds	2 tablespoons hot sesame oil

In a large saucepan, sauté all the ingredients in the oil over medium heat for 5 to 10 minutes, stirring constantly. Serve with brown rice. *Serves 2*

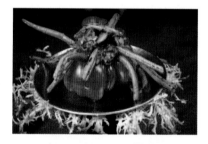

YOUR MOMMA'S STRING BEANS

4 cups string beans, strings removed	2 tablespoons peppercorns
1½ cups chopped or sliced onions	½ teaspoon red pepper
6 cloves garlic, sliced	1 teaspoon dill
5 cups sliced mushrooms	3 cups chopped fresh tomatoes
1 cup chopped fresh basil	¼ cup extra virgin olive oil
3 tablespoons chopped fresh parsley	1 cup grated soy parmesan cheese
1 teaspoon chopped fresh oregano	(non-dairy)
4 tablespoons maple syrup	

In a large saucepan, sauté the string beans, onions, garlic, mushrooms, basil, parsley, oregano, peppercorns, red pepper, maple syrup, and dill in the oil over medium-high heat for 5 to 7 minutes. Add the tomatoes and cook another 15 to 20 minutes. Garnish with the cheese and serve with brown rice. *Serves 3 to 4*

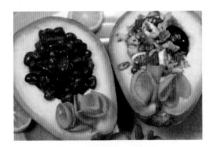

BRAZILIAN RICE

1 cup chopped onions
1 fresh tomato, chopped, or
  ½ cup prepared tomato sauce
1½ teaspoons drained,
  crushed capers
½ cup large pitted black olives
½ cup hearts of palm
1 bay leaf
2 cups cooked basmati rice
2 tablespoons maple syrup

2 tablespoons roasted sunflower seeds
2 tablespoons pumpkin seeds
¼ teaspoon cayenne
¼ teaspoon dried thyme
½ teaspoon freshly ground black pepper
¼ teaspoon chili pepper
4 cloves crushed garlic
1 teaspoon sea salt
4 tablespoons extra virgin olive oil

In a large sauce pan, sauté the onions, tomatoes, capers, olives, and bay leaf in oil over medium heat until the onions are clear. Add the remaining ingredients and sauté another 4 minutes until hot. Serve with black beans. *Serves 4*

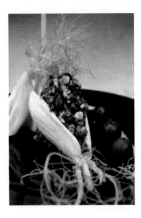

KIDNEY BEAN CURRY

1½ ounces filberts, chopped
2 tablespoons coconut oil
3 tablespoons tarragon
¾ teaspoon basil
¾ tablespoon salt

1 teaspoon curry
3 ounces brown rice, cooked
3 ounces kidney beans, cooked
1½ ounces cashew pieces
1 cup fresh basil

Preheat oven to 375 degrees. Lightly grease 4 x 8 baking dish with coconut oil. Place filberts in blender with ¼ cup water, oil, tarragon, basil, salt, and curry. Blend until mixture achieves sauce consistency. Combine brown rice and beans. Transfer to baking dish. Top with filbert sauce. Sprinkle on cashews. Bake with cover for 15 minutes. *Serves 2*

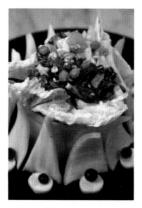

STIR-FRIED KOMBU

1 cup sweet peas	1 cup cubed firm tofu
1 cup diced yellow and red	4 tablespoons tamari
sweet peppers	¼ cup sun-dried tomatoes
2 cups chopped bok choy	1 cup kombu, soaked and drained
2 tablespoons mustard powder	(see below)
5 cloves garlic, crushed	4 tablespoons toasted hot sesame oil

In a large sauce pan, sauté the peas, peppers, bok choy, mustard powder, and garlic in the oil, over medium heat, for 15 minutes. Add the tofu and cook an additional 2 to 3 minutes. Add the tomatoes, tamari, and kombu, mix in lightly and serve with brown rice. *Serves 2*

Note: Kombu leaves will disintegrate if stirred vigorously. Soak for 10 to 20 seconds, drain, and use.

DESSERTS

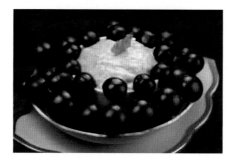

PEACH JULEP PUDDING

6 ounces peaches, sliced	1½ ounces walnuts
3 ounces barley, cooked	1 teaspoon vanilla
8 ounces peach juice	2 teaspoons fresh mint
4 ounces coconut sweetener	1 teaspoon lemon juice

Place all ingredients in blender. Puree until smooth. Transfer to saucepan and set over medium heat for 5 minutes, stirring frequently. Chill for 45 minutes in refrigerator. *Serves 2*

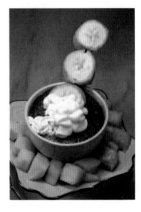

RICE PUDDING

3 ounces mango
3 ounces brown rice, cooked
5 teaspoons carob powder
1½ ounces sunflower seeds

1 ounce date sugar
1 teaspoon vanilla
1½ ounces dates
2 heaping teaspoons egg replacer

Combine all ingredients and puree until smooth. Transfer to saucepan and cook over medium heat for 5 minutes, stirring frequently. Chill in refrigerator for 45 minutes. *Serves 2*

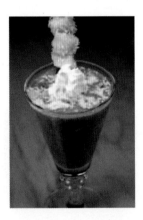

MANGO PUDDING

6 ounces mango
3 ounces brown rice, cooked
1½ ounces coconut, shredded
(unsweetened)

1¼ cups coconut milk
1½ ounces dates
2 heaping teaspoons egg replacer
Pinch of cinnamon

Combine all ingredients in blender and puree until smooth. Transfer to saucepan and cook over medium heat for 5 minutes, stirring frequently. Chill in refrigerator for 45 minutes. *Serves 2*

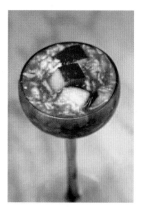

PAPAYA PUDDING

3 ounces papaya
3 ounces oatmeal, cooked
¾ cup apple juice
3 tablespoons honey

2 heaping teaspoons egg replacer
Pinch of cinnamon
3 ounces apples, cut into ½-inch cubes

Combine all ingredients in blender except apples. Puree until smooth. Transfer to saucepan and cook over medium heat for about 5 minutes. Add apples and stir. Chill in refrigerator for 45 minutes or until set. *Serves 2*

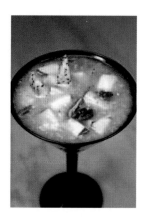

APPLE-PAPAYA PUDDING

6 ounces pineapple
¾ cup papaya juice
3 tablespoons honey
2 tablespoons egg replacer

Pinch of cinnamon
4½ ounces apples, chopped
1½ ounces pecans, chopped
1 ounce macadamia nuts

Combine all ingredients in blender except apples and pecans. Puree until smooth. Transfer to saucepan and cook over medium heat for 5 minutes. Add apples and nuts. Chill 45 minutes in refrigerator. *Serves 2*

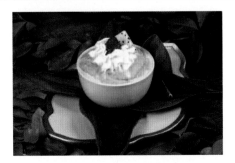

STRAWBERRY KIWI PUDDING

5 ounces strawberries
2 ounces kiwi
3 ounces millet, cooked
½ cup maple syrup
¾ cup coconut milk
2 heaping teaspoons egg replacer

1 teaspoon vanilla
1 teaspoon fresh mint
1 teaspoon lemon juice
Pinch of cinnamon
1½ ounces slivered almonds

Place all ingredients in blender, except almonds. Puree until smooth. Transfer to saucepan and set over medium heat for 5 minutes, stirring constantly. Chill for 45 minutes in the refrigerator. Top with almonds when chilled. *Serves 3*

Chapter 63

Selecting An Alternative Health Practitioner

Alternative health practitioners can help define the weak links in your body's structure and function and then direct you toward optimal personal care. There are many different approaches, but some general guidelines are worth mentioning here.

Your Rights As a Patient

A good alternative medical practitioner will perform at least these three basic types of analysis before prescribing any treatment plan: (a) Take a detailed medical history; (b) perform a physical examination that goes beyond conventional methodologies; and (c) study carefully the results of appropriate laboratory tests taken at the time of the history taking and the physical examination.

In addition, you have the right to expect that the practitioner will include in his or her repertory some or all of the following:

- As many noninvasive diagnostic techniques as possible.
- An awareness of the potential diagnostic value of even very minor signs and symptoms in the prevention of major dysfunction.
- A preference for noninvasive over invasive techniques; for example, substances will be administered orally rather than intravenously (except when a condition calls for the more direct route).
- A recognition of the importance of strengthening the body's

resistive capacities and an interest, wherever possible, in attempting to repair any malfunctioning organ or gland.

■ A tendency, whenever possible, to treat the primary weak link first if more than one has been discovered. (For example, if the stomach is producing insufficient hydrochloric acid, resulting in the malabsorption of calcium, among other substances, the resulting calcium deficiency could lead to osteoarthritis, periodontal disease, or skin problems; by treating the hydrochloric acid insufficiency, the physician would be treating the primary weak link.)

■ An approach that treats the person as a whole person, not just a collection of ailing parts.

■ The demonstrated ability to listen carefully and to skillfully classify any relevant symptoms to arrive at the best possible diagnosis.

■ An orientation toward optimal health and sensitivity to dysfunctions that signal an imbalance in the individual.

■ Familiarity with a combination of approaches to help the person regain balance. (For example, in addition to orthodox treatments, the physician's recommendations may include advice about stress reduction and lifestyle changes to reduce or eliminate causative factors in the environment.)

■ A willingness to refer the individual, when the condition warrants, to other medical practitioners whose specialized knowledge in a given area may be necessary to provide the most valuable restorative program.

■ A demonstrated awareness of the importance of the individual's own attitudes toward health and disease, and a willingness to communicate openly with the individual.

Your Role As a Patient

Your alternative health practitioner should expect you to be an active, committed participant in the process, not a passive, disinterested patient who accepts everything the doctor recommends.

One form of this active participation may be the questions you ask with a view to getting the important information you need to help in your contributions to the healing process. Some examples are:

- What, specifically, is being treated?
- How do you know that that's the problem?
- What are some realistic goals in my situation?
- What is the time frame?
- Does every individual with this condition get exactly the same tests and treatments?
- What are my weak links?
- Are these tests and this treatment relevant to my body and my condition?

The Importance of Commonplace Symptoms

Many people are living with symptoms that, because they are mild and do not constitute a full-blown disease state, are accepted, needlessly, as being an inevitable consequence of getting older. In fact, such people are often told by their conventional physicians, "Nothing is wrong with you. Everything is normal." And yet, the symptoms may be early warnings that something is out of balance. Gas in the lower bowel (flatulence), belching, heaviness in the stomach, heartburn, and bloating, for example, may all be indicators of a malfunctioning digestive system, depending on their frequency and severity. These conditions are not normal in a healthy state, and they are often correctable.

Similarly, many of the symptoms that accompany delayed allergic reactions (the masked, cyclical allergies) are widely accepted as normal, and therefore to be tolerated for no better reason than "that's the way it is." The failure to recognize a connection between these symptoms and allergies may be due to the fact that they do not appear for upward of thirty hours after the ingestion of the offending food or chemical substance. Typical symptoms are headache, irritability, anxiety, sudden changes of mood, and excessive fatigue, as well as unexplained body aches and pains. These symptoms may not be severe enough to be labeled disease states, so the underlying cause is repeatedly overlooked or denied by traditional practitioners. Even when the disorders are recognized, their true significance may still be missed by those who try to reverse the symptoms without addressing the underlying causes for their appearance.

Thus frequent colds, recurring infections, and fatigue are all part of the warning mechanisms used by the body to signal a malfunctioning immune system. But they are rarely recognized as such. The phenomenal sales of cold remedies, for example, reflect how little attention is paid to strengthening the immune system—an approach that would far more effectively reduce the incidence of these and other disorders.

Types of Therapies

It has never been my policy to make specific recommendations, to suggest to a person that a specific practitioner is the best doctor to see. The quality of a doctor's health care may depend on both the physician and the patient, as well as on their mutual compatibility. This is not something I, or anyone else, can predict in advance. But I still feel that people should be given some direction. So, what I have done here is supplied a directional guide. Below are descriptions of the therapies described in this book. Where applicable, I have listed organizations to contact for referrals or more information.

ACUPRESSURE

Acupressure, also known as shiatsu, is based on the principle that a vital energy, called qi (chi), flows through the body. The primary cause of pain is an imbalance in this energy. The goal of the healer is to balance the client's energy so that pain and discomfort do not manifest or, if they do appear, will be relieved.

The practitioner concentrates on certain pressure points that have metaphoric names that tell us something of what they do or how they are to be worked with. He or she uses thumbs, fingers, palms, forearms, elbows, and even knees to apply pressure to specified points in the body to modulate the flow of energy. During a treatment, the client lies on the floor on a comfortable padded surface, such as a futon, fully clothed or undressed to her level of comfort. What the client feels is pressure, which can be gentle or deeper at the places where the practitioner is working. As the pressure continues, the patient will generally feel relaxed and energized at the same time.

Acupressure is good for treating a variety of different pains. It is especially beneficial in combating chronic pain in the back, neck, or shoulders, but it has also proved effective in treating whiplash, herniated disk, and nerve problems, such as Bell's palsy.

CONTACT:

AMERICAN ORGANIZATION FOR BODYWORK THERAPIES OF ASIA
(856) 809-2953
www.aobta.org

ACUPUNCTURE

Acupuncture sees pain as derived from blocked energy or qi (chi). In treating this blockage, the practitioner has to determine whether it stems from an overabundance or a deficiency in energy, so the treatment can be adjusted depending on whether it is necessary to strengthen or decrease qi. To accomplish this, the acupuncturist will work to open blocked energy pathways, so that healing energy can go directly to the point in the body where it is needed, thereby stimulating the body's natural healing capacities.

The acupuncturist first records the patient's medical history in the manner of a conventional doctor. Then, with the patient lying down or seated, depending on the area to be treated, fine-gauge, stainless steel needles are inserted into significant points and meridians (channels through which qi flows) to exert different physiological effects on the body and induce both relaxation and energization. The patient will remain in this position from twenty to thirty minutes, though an appointment with an acupuncturist may last up to an hour, since part of the time will be spent consulting about the employment of other traditional and herbal treatments that might be recommended. Bodywork and massage might also be included in the session.

According to Abigail Rist-Podrecca, a registered nurse, acupuncture works by "dilating the blood vessels, so that the vessels can open. You get more circulation, more of the nutrients, more oxygen flowing through the meridians."

Practitioners attend three- to four-year postgraduate-type programs. Schools are accredited for master's degree programs through the National Accreditation Commission of Schools and Colleges of Acupuncture and Oriental Medicine. A certification examination is offered through the National Certification Commission for Acupuncture and Oriental Medicine. A minimum of 1,300 hours of training is required to sit for this exam. Medical doctors and dentists rarely require specialized training to perform acupuncture, although training is available through the American Academy of Medical Acupuncturists.

CONTACT:

AMERICAN ACADEMY OF MEDICAL ACUPUNCTURE
(310) 379-8261
www.medicalacupuncture.org

AMERICAN ASSOCIATION OF ACUPUNCTURE AND ORIENTAL MED-
ICINE
(866) 455-7999
www.aaaomonline.org

NATIONAL CERTIFICATION COMMISSION FOR ACUPUNCTURE AND
ORIENTAL MEDICINE
(904) 598-1005
www.nccaom.org

ALEXANDER TECHNIQUE

Alexander technique is based on the concept that all of us know how to move comfortably as children but lose that natural flexibility over time. The teacher acts to help the student recapture this freedom and lightness of movement. Practitioners see themselves as teachers, and their sessions not as therapy but as teaching.

Each session is an experiential process in which the teacher guides the student with hands-on training to help her learn a new way of moving, by means of the teacher's hands stimulating the student's nervous system.

This technique can help mothers, for example, learn how to bend over and lift children in a new way that avoids stress on the back.

There are ten affiliated societies for teachers of Alexander technique worldwide. Teacher certification requires 1,600 practical hours over a three-year period.

CONTACT:

AMERICAN SOCIETY FOR THE ALEXANDER TECHNIQUE
(800) 473-0620
www.alexandertech.org

APPLIED KINESIOLOGY

This discipline is related to Chinese acupuncture. Practitioners use it to determine which foods and herbs are best assimilated by the individual, in order to develop a healing diet and supplementation program that is finely calibrated to the person's own biology.

The patient extends her arm at shoulder level while holding a food or supplement in the other hand, and the practitioner pushes down on the extended arm. If the substance is appropriate for her, the arm will be strong and harder to force down. If the substance is not good for her, the arm will be weak. This is because the body can feel the value of the substance. Using various techniques, kinesiologists can study these reactions more precisely to determine proper individual diet.

CONTACT:

INTERNATIONAL COLLEGE OF APPLIED KINESIOLOGY
(913) 384-5336
www.icakusa.com

AROMATHERAPY

Aromatherapy depends on the therapeutic powers of essential oils. These oils are commonly used in skin and body care products in the United States, but their medicinal properties have long been accepted in other countries, particularly France, where, in many instances, their antimicrobial properties make them acceptable replacements for drug therapy. Pure essential oils can be used to cure cold and canker sores, calm the emotions, diminish joint swelling, clear the nasal passages and lungs, balance hormones, and for many other applications.

CONTACT:

NATIONAL ASSOCIATION FOR HOLISTIC AROMATHERAPY
(919) 894-0298
www.naha.org

AYURVEDA

Ayurveda means "the science of life." It is a system of medicine widely used in India for the past 4,000 years. Ayurveda believes that balance is the key to perfect health. It basically determines which of three body-mind types a person belongs to and, based on that type, helps people choose the type of foods he or she should eat as well as the best type of exercise. For more information, read *Perfect Health and Ageless Body, Timeless Mind* by Deepak Chopra.

CONTACT:

THE AYURVEDIC INSTITUTE
(505) 291-9698
www.ayurveda.com

BACH FLOWER REMEDIES

The Bach flower remedies were developed by Dr. Edward Bach during the 1930s. They consist of thirty-eight plant extracts that are used to treat physical and emotional problems. The extracts used in each case are selected according to the individual patient's personality. For instance, for a person who is critical and intolerant of others, the suggested remedy derives from the beech tree. For some with an unhealthy fear of the unknown, a remedy derived from the aspen would be prescribed. Bach flower remedies are said to have positive effects on the psychological and emotional stresses that underlie many illnesses.

CONTACT:

FLOWER ESSENCE SOCIETY
(800) 736-9222
www.flowersociety.org

BACH CENTRE
www.bachcentre.com

BACH FLOWER EDUCATION
(800) 928-1270
www.bachflowereducation.com

BIOFEEDBACK

Biofeedback is a technique that teaches a person to consciously regulate normally involuntary bodily processes, such as heartbeats, brain waves, blood pressure, and muscle tension. The bodily process, such as heart rate, may be monitored by electronic equipment or by natural observation, such as holding a finger against an artery. With practice, the patient learns to slow down the heart rate, relax tension, and so on. Biofeedback is helpful for conditions such as migraine, tension headache, digestive upset, and other disorders that are aggravated by stress.

Practitioner certification is recommended but not required. Practitioners are certified through the Biofeedback Certification Institute of America.

CONTACT:

ASSOCIATION FOR APPLIED PSYCHOPHYSIOLOGY AND BIOFEEDBACK
(800) 477-8892
www.aapb.org

BIOFEEDBACK CERTIFICATION INTERNATIONAL ALLIANCE
(720) 502-5829
www.bcia.org

BODY ROLLING

Body rolling, a form of bodywork developed by Yamuna Zake, uses a six- to ten-inch ball in a series of routines designed to elongate muscles and increase blood flow in all parts of the body. As the body weight presses into the ball, the ball applies pressure onto bone and creates traction that allows the entire length of a muscle to release. Body rolling is useful for relieving pain and tension in many parts of the body.

YAMUNA BODY ROLLING
(212) 367-9570
www.yamunabodyrolling.com

CHELATION THERAPY

Chelation therapy flushes toxins out of the blood. A synthetic amino acid, EDTA, is administered to the patient through an intravenous drip. The EDTA moves through the blood vessels and attaches itself to heavy metals in the blood such as mercury and lead, holding on to these substances until they are washed out of the body in the urine. Chelation therapy is being used increasingly to treat heart disease as well as other illnesses. Protocols for the intravenous administration of EDTA are set by the American College for the Advancement of Medicine (ACAM) and require a prior medical examination. Certification is provided to MDs and DOs who satisfy requirements from the American Board of Clinical Metal Toxicology.

CONTACT:

AMERICAN COLLEGE FOR ADVANCEMENT IN MEDICINE
(800) 532-3688
www.acamnet.org

AMERICAN BOARD OF CLINICAL METAL TOXICOLOGY
(419) 358-0273
www.abcmt.org

CHIROPRACTIC

Chiropractic treatment involves the manual manipulation of vertebrae that have become misaligned, exerting pressure on nerves and blocking the flow of energy to various organs. The manipulation is called an adjustment. It involves the chiropractor's gentle and painless application of direct pressure to the spine and joints. The chiropractor may squeeze or twist the torso, pull or twist the limbs, or wrench the head or back. In this manner she or he is readjusting the spinal column to restore the normal relationship of one vertebra to another. This eliminates the body's energy blocks.

Chiropractic is effective in dealing with pain and as a preventive measure because it relieves nerve pressure as the spine is properly adjusted.

While chiropractic is still far from being accepted as a part of standard health care, it attracts more patients now than ever before and is more accepted than ever before by the mainstream medical community. There are now about twenty chiropractic colleges nationwide, and chiropractors can get licensed in all fifty states. Some liberal arts colleges offer undergraduate degrees in chiropractic, and some facilities at member hospitals of the American Hospital Association have been opened to chiropractors.

CONTACT:

AMERICAN CHIROPRACTIC ASSOCIATION
(703) 276-8800
www.acatoday.com

INTERNATIONAL CHIROPRACTORS ASSOCIATION
(800) 423-4690
www.chiropractic.org

COLON THERAPY

Colon cleansing refers to washing out the colon in order to remove toxic buildups. First the colon is irrigated with warm water, washing out encrustations and old fecal matter. Next, healing substances to reduce inflammation and strengthen the colon wall are infused.

CONTACT:

AMERICAN ASSOCIATION OF NATUROPATHIC PHYSICIANS
(866) 538-2267
www.naturopathic.org

INTERNATIONAL ASSOCIATION FOR COLON HYDROTHERAPY
(210) 366-2888
www.i-act.org

CRANIOSACRAL THERAPY

The sacral region is at the bottom of the spine. Between that region and the head there should be maintained a balanced relation for the health of the organism. If a restriction is experienced at that point, pain will be felt and other problems may arise.

In craniosacral therapy, the practitioner places her or his hands on the patient's body in such a way as to bring the cranium and sacrum back into alignment and to reestablish a natural rhythm between them. Treatment usually centers on the head or lower back, although it may be done on many different parts of the body.

CONTACT:

BIODYNAMIC CRANIOSACRAL THERAPY ASSOCIATION OF NORTH
AMERICA
(734) 904-0546
www.craniosacraltherapy.org

INTERNATIONAL ASSOCIATION OF HEALTH CARE PRACTITIONERS
(800) 311-9204
www.iahp.com

DETOXIFICATION THERAPY

A person whose health is compromised, or on a diet that is too high in fats, processed proteins, and refined foods, has a reduced capacity to rid the body of toxins. When this happens, the toxins accumulate.

Frances Taylor, coauthor of *The Whole Way to Natural Detoxification*, explains: "As we journey through life the way most people do, we become overloaded with the toxins that absorb in the body. Unless we do something to get rid of these things, our bodies become overloaded and our health suffers. We develop symptoms such as headaches, digestive problems, sluggishness, after-meals fatigue. Many health benefits can be obtained by simply detoxifying the body."

Among the methods of detoxification are diet, nutritional supplementation, chelation therapy, colon cleansing, detox baths, exercise, deep breathing, and bodywork.

CONTACT:

AMERICAN ASSOCIATION OF NATUROPATHIC PHYSICIANS
(866) 538-2267
www.naturopathic.org

AMERICAN COLLEGE FOR ADVANCEMENT IN MEDICINE
(800) 532-3688
www.acam.org

ENZYME THERAPY

Enzyme therapy uses enzymes to cure illness and enhance life. South American

Indians used papaya as a healing agent, and medieval Europeans used the milky juice of plants of the spurge family for medical reasons. Today, many practitioners advocate enzyme supplementation to enable vitamins and other supplements, as well as food, to be properly absorbed.

There are many different types of enzyme therapy. One example is that which relies on the Wolfe and Benitez formulas, which combine animal and vegetable enzymes. The preparations are said to be powerful weapons against bacteria and other invasive microorganisms. Many naturopaths and chiropractors use enzyme therapy.

CONTACT:

LOOMIS INSTITUTE OF ENZYME NUTRITION
(800) 662-2630
www.loomisinstitute.com

ENZYME TECHNICAL ASSOCIATION
(202) 739-5612
www.enzymeassociation.org

FELDENKRAIS

Feldenkrais is a practice that helps eliminate poor movement habits and relieve chronic tensions. It uses very gentle movements that the student does herself, guided by the instructor, while lying on the floor. Alternatively the student lies on a massage table and the teacher uses a hands-on approach, taking the student through gentle movements to enable the student to let go of a chronic holding pattern.

The goal is to learn to differentiate between parts of the body that are relaxed and parts that are still tense. Thus the nervous system learns a new way of functioning.

CONTACT:

FELDENKRAIS METHOD OF SOMATIC EDUCATION
(781) 876-8935
www.feldenkrais.com

GUIDED IMAGERY

Guided imagery can be practiced either by an individual with a therapist or in a group setting. In the individual setting, the practitioner helps the client elicit her own mental images, which she then interacts with, perhaps in dialogue. For example, if the client is ill, she may call up images of the distressed part of her body and encourage it to heal through an imagistic interaction.

In a group, a facilitator helps the participants concentrate on building certain images whose healing power they can tap into. In this setting, the participant has the added benefit of being able to discuss the process with another participant afterward so as to further affirm and enrich the healing process.

CONTACT:

ACADEMY FOR GUIDED IMAGERY
(424) 242-6369
www.acadgi.com

ACADEMY OF INTEGRATIVE HEALTH AND MEDICINE
(218) 525-5651
www.aihm.org

AMERICAN HOLISTIC NURSES ASSOCIATION
(800) 278-2462
www.ahna.org

HELLERWORK

Hellerwork is a bodywork technique derived from Rolfing (see below). Both modalities work to improve body structure with deep tissue work, but Hellerwork, unlike Rolfing, is not painful. The practice has three components. In the first, hands-on part, the practitioner finds a misalignment in the body and works with the client to release it.

The second part is movement education. The practitioner analyzes the patient's posture and movements, then offers more relaxed and stressless ways to move. The third component is body-mind dialogue, whose purpose is to identify emotional patterns that underlie dysfunctional movement patterns.

CONTACT:

HELLERWORK INTERNATIONAL
(714) 873-6131
www.hellerwork.com

HERBAL MEDICINE

American interest in herbal medicine has exploded in recent years. Not long ago, we had to seek out an herbalist or visit a health food store to obtain herbal formulas. Today supplements are being manufactured by mainstream drug and vitamin companies, and can be found on store shelves everywhere. The National Institutes of Health has even established an office to maintain a database and fund research into herbals. It may seem as if herbal medicine is a new field. In actuality, herbs have been used for healing for as far back as we can trace the existence of humans.

Herbs can play a vital role in our day-to-day lives by stimulating our immune systems. Many people find that their health seems to be sapped by recurring or chronic colds and viruses. Synthetic drugs, far from being a solution, seem merely to encourage new, more resistant strains of bacteria and viruses. People with more serious immune problems, such as AIDS and cancer, can help their systems to fight back as much as possible by using herbs to stimulate a healthy immune system.

In addition to fresh herbs and dried herbs, there are several other forms in which herbal medicines can be taken. Infusions and decoctions, two of the simpler forms, are both made with boiling water. Tinctures are made by macerating herbs in a mixture of water and alcohol for at least two weeks. Ointments, which are useful for treating some skin conditions, can be made with herbs and oils.

CONTACT:

AMERICAN HERBALISTS GUILD
(617) 520-4372
www.americanherbalistsguild.com

HERB RESEARCH FOUNDATION
(303) 449-2265
www.herbs.org

AMERICAN ASSOCIATION OF NATUROPATHIC PHYSICIANS
(866) 538-2267
www.naturopathic.org

HOMEOPATHY

Homeopathy is based on the Law of Similars, the principle that what causes illness can also cure it. If a person has a head cold, you would give the person a substance that would cause cold symptoms in a healthy person, but in a sick person it helps to cure them. Homeopathy is limited in scope at this time in the United States, although 100 years ago it was the prevailing form of medicine—until allopathic medicine, and the American Medical Association in particular, launched an intensive drive against it, which culminated in its being virtually banned in this country.

Recently, there has been a renewed interest in homeopathy, and growing numbers of physicians are using its principles. Homeopathy is particularly effective in the treatment of fevers, bacterial infections, toxicity, and the cumulative effects of alcohol, drugs, tobacco, caffeine, or sugar. It is not recommended for cancer, AIDS, or heart disease.

CONTACT:

HOMEOPATHIC ACADEMY OF NATUROPATHIC PHYSICIANS
(541) 708-1827
www.hanp.net

NATIONAL CENTER FOR HOMEOPATHY
(703) 506-7667
www.homepathic.org

COUNCIL FOR HOMEOPATHIC CERTIFICATION
(866) 242-3399
www.homeopathicdirectory.com

HYDROTHERAPY

Hydrotherapy is a traditional naturopathic method that uses hot and/or cold water to treat a range of ailments, including urinary tract inflammations, fibrocystic breast disease, migraine headaches, and infertility. For urinary tract inflammations, for example, sitz baths or hot compresses can be used to stimulate blood circulation and remove toxins from the pelvic area. For migraines, there are many inventive forms of hydrotherapy that involve applying cold to the head and heat to the feet.

CONTACT:

AMERICAN ASSOCIATION OF NATUROPATHIC PHYSICIANS
(866) 538-2267
www.naturopathic.org

MASSAGE THERAPY

Massage therapy is used to treat a variety of ailments, including muscle spasm and pain, soreness, swelling and inflammation, temporomandibular joint syndrome, whiplash, headaches, and stress. It helps to release tension and enhance relaxation. It can help in detoxification. Some states require massage therapists to be licensed, others do not. Many massage therapists perform a variety of bodywork techniques.

CONTACT:

AMERICAN MASSAGE THERAPY ASSOCIATION
(877) 905-0577
www.amtamassage.org

MIDWIFERY

Midwives help women give birth, providing care and advice during pregnancy and after a baby is born. They may also provide general gynecological care. Midwives work in homes, clinics, birthing centers, and hospitals. Midwifery views pregnancy as a natural, normal, and individual process in which medical intervention should be as minimal as possible. Most midwives only accept women who are likely to have a normal delivery and are not considered at high risk for complications.

Certified nurse-midwives (CNMs) are registered nurses who have been trained in midwifery and certified by the American College of Nurse-Midwives. Some states require nurse-midwives to have a special license. Other states allow them to practice under their nursing license. Most CNMs have back-up doctors at hospitals.

Lay midwives have no formal training in midwifery. A few states license lay midwives.

CONTACT:

AMERICAN COLLEGE OF NURSE-MIDWIVES
(240) 485-1800
www.acnm.org

NATURAL HYGIENE

Natural hygiene is the practice of creating optimal conditions for the body and its constituent cells, tissues, and organs to pursue and sustain health. This means environmental purity of air, food, and water; a balanced primordial diet based on natural foods; and stress reduction and management. It precludes the use of most drugs, since they are antithetical to a modality that perceives illness to be due to inappropriate nutrition and toxic accumulations (drugs are usually toxic substances). Finally, it means a symbiotic relationship of all humankind and harmony with God and nature.

CONTACT:

INTERNATIONAL NATURAL HYGIENE SOCIETY
www.naturalhygienesociety.org

AMERICAN ASSOCIATION OF NATUROPATHIC PHYSICIANS
(866) 538-2267
www.naturopathic.org

NATUROPATHY

Naturopathic physicians can treat most conditions. They are not, however, allowed to perform major surgery (although they can perform minor surgery). Their very extensive background is centered in the botanical sciences, including the use of herbs and tinctures with a wide variety of natural immune-stimulating properties. Becoming a doctor of naturopathic medicine requires four years of graduate-level study in the medical sciences. The accrediting agency is the Council on Naturopathic Medical Education (CNME).

The naturopath practices a natural form of health care whose traditions precede the advent of modern medicine. In this the naturopath resembles the traditional Tibetan physician, who must be able to identify nearly one thousand different healing herbs, mineral sources, and animal sources. The naturopath has years of extensive study in the healing potential of such substances. He or she is also able to understand muscular and skeletal bodily adjustment. Naturopaths use a much broader basis for diagnosis than do conventional allopathic physicians.

CONTACT:

AMERICAN ASSOCIATION OF NATUROPATHIC PHYSICIANS
(866) 538-2267
www.naturopathic.org

AMERICAN NATUROPATHIC MEDICAL ASSOCIATION
(888) 202-4440
www.anma.com

ORTHOMOLECULAR MEDICINE

Orthomolecular medicine is an alternative approach to mental and physical health whose goal is to identify and treat the root cause of disease. The objective is to balance and rebuild the whole body, not merely to mask or suppress symptoms. To do this, orthomolecular physicians try to establish equilibrium among the essential nutrients that may be lacking, present in excess, or are being poorly absorbed. Orthomolecular physicians are conventionally trained medical doctors who feel that such an imbalance is often responsible for psychiatric as well as physical disorders.

The physician looks at diet, glandular function, glucose metabolism, and a host of other biochemical factors that may play a role in the patient's mental health. Imbalances in the body are corrected through judicious use of vitamins, minerals, amino acids, and other naturally occurring nutrients. Orthomolecular physicians frequently use a very high-dose vitamin regimen.

CONTACT:

INTERNATIONAL SOCIETY FOR ORTHOMOLECULAR MEDICINE
(416) 733-2117
www.orthomed.org

ORTHOMOLECULAR DEVELOPMENT

(316) 682-3100

www.orthomolecular.org

POLARITY THERAPY

Polarity therapy is based on the belief that any stagnation or stopping of the natural flow of energy in the human body is the underlying cause of disease. The naturally occurring positive and negative energy fields of the body are in a polarity relationship with each other. However, when the energy is blocked, it turns neutral, and the surrounding tissues stagnate and become painful.

Practitioners use light forms of touch, gentle manipulation, and techniques such as rocking to restore the flow of energy, relieving stress and pain and encouraging healing.

Polarity therapy is particularly useful for depression, anxiety, fatigue, headaches, fibromyalgia, and other conditions involving emotional blockages. Standards of practice and a code of ethics are established by the American Polarity Therapy Association.

CONTACT:

AMERICAN POLARITY THERAPY ASSOCIATION

(336) 574-1121

www.polaritytherapy.org

QI GONG

The Chinese phrase *qi gong* means "air" (considered the vital essence) and "work." This traditional Asian practice utilizes aerobic exercise, meditation, relaxation techniques, and isometrics to control the vital energy of the body in the most efficient way. Like many Chinese practices, it emphasizes the unity of mind, spirit, and world.

The central practice is a combination of breathing, movement, and shallow meditation, in which the person is aware of what is going on but in a tranquil state in which positive images flow quietly through a relaxed mind. Once the person is in this state, the flow of the *qi* through the body is stimulated. This unobstructed flow will heal sickness or increase an existing sense of wellness.

CONTACT:

QI GONG ASSOCIATION OF AMERICA
(888) 9-QIGONG
www.qi.org

AMERICAN ASSOCIATION OF ACUPUNCTURE AND ORIENTAL MEDICINE
(866) 455-7999
www.aaaomonline.org

REFLEXOLOGY

Reflexology is based on the principle that people have reflex areas in their feet that correspond to every part of the body. The locations of the reflex points on the foot correspond to the way the organs and glands are distributed within the body. Massaging these specific areas on the feet thus helps to improve the functioning of particular organs and glands.

For example, the toes reflect the head area, the ball of the foot represents the chest area, and so on. The practitioner presses his or her fingers into the foot, using a variety of techniques, to massage and relax ill or stressed parts of the body.

CONTACT:

REFLEXOLOGY ASSOCIATION OF AMERICA
(980) 234-0159
www.reflexology-usa.org

INTERNATIONAL COUNCIL OF REFLEXOLOGISTS
www.icr-reflexology.org

REIKI

Reiki is a type of massage therapy or bodywork in which pressure-point techniques are used to move energy through the body in order to create balance and harmony. The practice, Japanese in origin, teaches the student to attain an attunement with the universal energy.

Whereas many Asian techniques involve learning a discipline to guide the flow of energy, in Reiki the student attains attunement from a Reiki Master, who transmits it during a ritual process. This single attunement can never be lost, although with further attunements one can move to a higher spiritual level. There are schools of Reiki with three levels or "degrees" of proficiency.

CONTACT:

INTERNATIONAL ASSOCIATION OF REIKI PROFESSIONALS
www.iarp.org

ROLFING

According to practitioners of Rolfing, pain is caused by chronic shortenings in the tissue. Correction of the pain can be accomplished by soft-tissue manipulation. This manipulation creates order in the body so that the client stands tall and free of restriction.

Rolfing is generally performed in a series of ten sessions, designed to address all the shortenings in the structure systematically. Each session works in a different area. The basic goal of Rolfing is not pain relief per se; still it has been found useful for TMJ, frozen shoulder, carpal tunnel syndrome, tennis elbow, chronic hip problems, sciatica, cervical neuropathies, and knee, foot, and ankle problems.

The Rolf Institute of Structural Integration certifies Rolfers.

CONTACT:

ROLF INSTITUTE OF STRUCTURAL INTEGRATION
(303) 449-5903
www.rolf.org

THERAPEUTIC TOUCH

Therapeutic Touch represents a reinvigoration of the old process of the laying on of hands, whereby the subtle touch of a healer on the patient's body will infuse her with positive energy. This therapy was originally developed by nurses and emphasizes the nurturing aspect of the practitioner.

A key ingredient of the practice is compassion for the patient being touched. Unlike most of the therapies reviewed here, this technique requires minimal training, which is why it is widely practiced by both professional medical practitioners and laypeople.

The Therapeutic Touch International Association is responsible for guidelines and curricula for teaching practitioners. There is no certification program.

Therapeutic Touch can be practiced by nurses after a twelve-hour or minimum six-hour program.

CONTACT:

THERAPEUTIC TOUCH INTERNATIONAL ASSOCIATION
(518) 325-1185
www.therapeutic-touch.org

TRADITIONAL CHINESE MEDICINE

Traditional Chinese medicine is based on ancient Taoist philosophy, which treats the whole person. The philosophy is that body and mind are one; there is no separation between the two. When qi, or universal energy, flows freely through the meridians, a person is healthy, but when qi is blocked or disrupted, the person develops pain or illness.

Practitioners begin by examining the patient to identify patterns of disharmony. They then prescribe herbal remedies based on these patterns.

CONTACT:

AMERICAN ASSOCIATION OF ACUPUNCTURE AND ORIENTAL MEDICINE
(866) 455-7999
www.aaaomonline.org

TRAGER TECHNIQUE

According to the theory behind Trager technique, pain is caused when someone frequently tightens her muscles in movement and posture. To correct this, the practitioner uses gentle motions to increase the patient's pleasure in the quality of her tissues and decrease the restriction and sense of holding. Gentleness is important, so that no message is sent to the body telling it that pain is on the way or that causes the patient to tighten up.

The movement reaches into the central nervous system to convey the sensations of pleasure, lengthening, softening, and opening to the tissues and joints. This practice is used to relieve lower back, neck, and upper back pain; sciatica; migraines; TMJ disorders; carpal tunnel syndrome and other repetitive stress disorders.

The Trager Institute offers information, training, and certification in the Trager approach.

CONTACT:

UNITED STATES TRAGER
ASSOCIATION
(440) 834-0308
www.tragerus.org

TRAGER INTERNATIONAL
www.trager.com

YOGA

Yoga is a system of mental and physical exercise. It combines physical postures, breathing exercises, and meditation. Studies have shown that yoga can help improve overall health and prevent and/or manage many conditions and diseases. Among other things, it has been proven to reduce stress, improve metabolism, enhance blood flow, aid digestion, and manage menstrual problems. Various forms of yoga have become popular in the United States and Europe.

CONTACT:

iNTERNATIONAL ASSOCIATION OF YOGA THERAPISTS
(928) 541-0004
www.iayt.org

Chapter 64

Resource Guide

Below you will find contact information for many of the alternative health practitioners whose work and/or wisdom are profiled in this book. A number of them were interviewed by me for my syndicated radio show, *The Gary Null Show*, on the Progressive Radio Network. Please note that this material is provided for informational purposes only, and should not be viewed as individual recommendations or endorsements.

DR. LAURIE AESOPH
717 S. Duluth Avenue
Sioux Falls, SD 57104
(605) 339-9080
aesoph@worldnet.att.net

DR. LISE ALSCHULER
7331 East Osborn Drive, Suite 330
Scottsdale, AZ 85251
(480) 990-1111
www.lisealschulernd.com

NINA ANDERSON
PO Box 36
East Canaan, CT 06024
(860) 824-5301

DR. RICHARD ASH
Ash Center for Complementary Medicine
800A 5th Avenue
New York, NY 10021
(212) 758-3200
www.ashcenter.com

DR. NEAL BARNARD
5100 Wisconsin Avenue, N.W., Suite 400
Washington, DC 20016
(202) 686-2210
www.pcrm.org

DR. ZUZANA BIC
University of California, Irvine
Irvine, CA 92697
faculty.sites.uci.edu/zbic/

JEANETTE BREEN
Baldwin Midwifery Service
660 Merrick Road
Baldwin, NY 11510
(516) 223-1251
www.jeanettebreen.com

DR. PETER BREGGIN
101 East State Street
Ithaca, NY 14850
(607) 272-5328
www.breggin.com

DR. JENNIFER BRETT
The Acupuncture Institute
University of Bridgeport
126 Park Avenue
Bridgeport, CT 06604
(203) 576-4122
jbrett@bridgeport.edu

DR. ART BROWNSTEIN
932 Ward Avenue
Honolulu, HI 96814
(808) 535-5556
www.docbrownstein.com

STEPHEN HARROD BUHNER
Foundation for Gaian Studies
Silver City, NM 88061
(575) 538-5498
www.gaianstudies.org

SUSAN BUCCI
86 Coppersmith Road
Levittown, NY 11756
(516) 731-4648

DR. CHRISTOPHER CALAPAI
1900 Hempstead Turnpike
East Meadow, NY 11554
(516) 794-0404
www.drcalapai.net

DR. HYLA CASS
1608 Michael Lane
Pacific Palisades, CA 90272
(866) 778-2646
www.cassmd.com

DR. ROBERT CATHCART (deceased)
www.orthomolecular.org

ROBERTA CERTNER
677 West End Avenue
New York, NY 10025
(212) 865-7505

DR. DAWSON CHURCH
3340 Fulton Road, #442
Fulton, CA 95439
(707) 525 9292
www.dawsonchurch.com

DR. JANE CICCHETTI
12 Elk Mountain Road
Asheville, NC 28804
www.janecicchetti.com

DR. ANTHONY CICHOKE
PO Box 25408
Portland, OR 97298
(503) 654-3225

DR. GABRIEL COUSENS
Tree of Life Center US
686 Harshaw Road
Patagonia, AZ 85624
(866) 394-2520
www.treeoflifecenterus.com

DR. WILLIAM CROOK (deceased)
www.yeastconnection.com

DR. MARTIN DAYTON
18600 Collins Avenue
Sunny Isles Beach, FL 33160
(305) 931-8484
www.daytondandesmedical.com

DR. CHRISTINE DOHERTY
354 Nashua Street
Milford, NH 03055
(603) 672-3600
www.pointnatural.com

DR. CALDWELL ESSELSTYN
Cleveland Clinic Wellness
Institute
1950 Richmond Road
Lyndhurst, OH 44124
(216) 448-8556
www.dresselstyn.com

TOVAH FINMAN-NAHMAN
Lifeline Hygienics
150 Theodore Fremd Avenue
Rye, NY 10580
(914) 921-5433
www.lifelinehygienics.com

DAVID FROME
Frome Center for Physical Therapy
241 West 37th Street
New York, NY 10018
(973) 509-8464
www.fromept.com

DR. HERBERT GOLDFARB
170 William Street
New York, NY 10038
(973) 699-1904
www.nohysterectomy.com

DR. PAT GORMAN
5 East 17th Street
New York, NY 10003
(212) 620-0506

DR. SARA GOTTFRIED
Gottfried Institute
2625 Alcatraz Avenue, Suite 369
Berkeley, CA 94705
www.saragottfriedmd.com

DR. JANE GUILTINAN
Bastyr Center for Natural Health
3670 Stone Way N.
Seattle, WA 98103
(206) 834-4100
www.bastyrcenter.org

MICHAEL GURIAN
(509) 624-0623
www.michaelgurian.com

DR. ELSON HAAS
25 Mitchell Boulevard
San Rafael, CA 94903
(415) 472-2343
www.hasshealthonline.com

LETHA HADADY
New York, NY
www.asianhealthsecrets.com

DR. JESSE HANLEY
22917 Pacific Coast Highway
Malibu, CA 90265
(310) 457-5806
www.jessehanleymd.com

DR. TORI HUDSON
www.drtorihudson.com

DR. VICKI HUFNAGEL
www.drhufnagel.com

DR. HAL A. HUGGINS (deceased)
www.hugginsappliedhealing.com

DR. MICHAEL JANSON
411 Waverly Oaks Road
Waltham, MA 02452
(386) 409-7747
or
225 N. Causeway
New Smyrna Beach, FL 32169
www.drjanson.com

KIM JESSOR
114 Fulton Street
New York, NY 10038
(718) 398-9421

DR. DAVID KAUFMAN
210 Central Park South
New York, NY 10019
(212) 969-9540

DR. RAPHAEL KELLMAN
150 East 55th Street
New York, NY 10022
(212) 717-1118
www.raphaelkellmanmd.com

JANE KOSMINSKY
41 West 72nd Street
New York, NY 10023
(212) 724-9755
www.balanceofwellbeing.com

SUSAN LACINA
1111 Amsterdam Avenue
New York, NY 10025
(212) 523-4472

DR. STEPHEN LANGER
3031 Telegraph Avenue
Berkeley, CA 94705
(510) 548-7384

DR. MICHAEL LESSER
2340 Parker Street
Berkeley, CA 94704
(510) 845-0700

SUSAN LEVIN
Director, Nutrition Education
Physicians Committee for Responsible
Medicine
5100 Wisconsin Avenue, N.W.
Washington, DC 20016
(202) 686-2210
www.pcrm.org

DR. WARREN LEVIN
www.warrenmlevinmd.net

DR. RANDINE LEWIS
11359 Main Street
Roscoe, IL 61073
www.thefertilesoul.com

DR. ELIZABETH LIPSKI
8556 Light Moon Way
Laurel, MD 20723
(828) 423-0670
(828) 645-7224
www.lizlipski.com

DR. GENNARO LOCURCIO
112 Lexington Avenue
New York, NY 10016
(212) 696-2680

DR. JAY LOMBARD
1730 South Federal Highway
Delray Beach, FL 33483
(561) 654-1300
www.drjaylombard.com

SUSANA LOMBARDI
We Care Spa
18000 Long Canyon Road
Desert Hot Springs, CA 92241
(800) 888-2523
www.wecarespa.com

DR. NANCY LONSDORF
1100 N. 4th Street, Suite 105
Fairfield, IA 52556
(641) 469-3174
www.drlonsdorf.com

DR. SARALYN MARK
SolaMed Solutions
Washington, DC
(202) 230-4101
www.solamedsolutions.com

DR. JOHN MCDOUGALL
PO Box 14039
Santa Rosa, CA 95402
(800) 941-7111
www.drmcdougall.com

DR. LANCE MORRIS
1601 North Tucson Boulevard
Tucson, AZ 85716
(520) 322-8122

DR. CHRISTIANE NORTHRUP
PO Box 199
Yarmouth, ME 04096
www.drnorthrup.com

DR. LINDA OJEDA
PO Box 2914
Alameda, CA 94501
(800) 266-5592

DR. MARY E. OLSEN
11 Renwick Avenue
Huntington, NY 11743
(631) 421-1248

SHARON OLSON
20-61 32nd Street
Astoria, NY 11105
(718) 726-3817

DR. MARJORIE ORDENE
2515 Avenue M
Brooklyn, NY 11210
(718) 258-7882
www.marjorieordene.com

DR. DEAN ORNISH
www.deanornish.com

DR. SANGEETA PATI
954 Lake Baldwin Lane
Orlando, FL 32814
(407) 478-9797
www.sajune.com

DOLORES PERRI
140 West End Avenue
New York, NY 10023
www.doloresperri.com

DR. JOHN PITTMAN
Carolina Center for Integrative Medicine
4505 Fair Meadow Lane
Raleigh, NC 27607
(919) 571-4391
www.carolinacenter.com

DR. JOSEPH PIZZORNO
www.drpizzorno.com

DR. MITCHELL PROFFMAN
144-02 69th Avenue
Flushing, NY 11367
(718) 268-9080
www.chirohands.com

DR. STEPHANIE ODINOV PUKIT
20 West 20th Street, Suite 1002
New York, NY 10011
(212) 206-8100

DR. DORIS RAPP
(800) 787-8780
www.drrapp.com

**DR. JUDYTH REICHENBERG-
ULLMAN**
123 4th Avenue
Edmonds, WA 98020
(425) 774-5599
www.healthyhomepathy.com

DR. SUSANNA REID
1661 High Street
Eugene, OR 97401
(541) 683-7000

DR. UZZI REISS
Beverly Hills Anti-Aging
Center
414 Camden Drive
Beverly Hills, CA 90210
(310) 247-1300
www.uzzireissmd.com

ABIGAIL RIST-PODRECCA
44 East 32nd Street
New York, NY 10016
(212) 685-2848

DR. HOWARD ROBINS
200 West 57th Street
New York, NY 10019
(212) 581-0101

DR. MARWAN SABBAGH
10515 W. Santa Fe Drive
Sun City, AZ 85351
www.bannerhealth.com

DR. RAY SAHELIAN
www.raysahelian.com

DR. MICHAEL SCHACHTER
Schachter Center for Complementary
Medicine
Suffern, NY 10901
(845) 368-4700
www.mbschachter.com

DR. SHERRILL SELLMAN
www.whatwomenmustknow.com

DR. MARCEY SHAPIRO
1152-A Solano Avenue
Albany, CA 94706
(510) 525-2200
www.marceyshapiromd.com

DR. SUSAN SILBERSTEIN
130 Almshouse Road
Richboro, PA 18954
(888) 551-2223
www.beatcancer.org

DR. CHARLES SIMONE
123 Franklin Corner Road
Lawrenceville, NJ 08648
(609) 896-2646
www.drsimone.com

DR. CARL SIMONTON (deceased)
www.simontoncenter.com

DR. PRISCILLA SLAGLE
24 Scarborough Way
Rancho Mirage, CA 92270
(760) 322-7797
www.thewayup.com

DR. DAVID STEENBLOCK
187 Avenida La Pata
San Clemente, CA 92673
(949) 367-8870
www.davidsteenblock.com

**DR. JANICE STEFANACCI
STEWARD**
9 Berkshire Heights Road
Great Barrington, MA 01230
(413) 644-9827
www.fruitionservices.com

DR. WALT STOLL (deceased)
www.askwaltstollmd.com

SARAH SUATONI
www.sarahsuatoni.com

DR. CYNTHIA THAIK
2701 W. Alameda Avenue
Burbank, CA 91505
(818) 842-1410
www.drcynthia.com

DR. JASON THEODOSAKIS
6890 E. Sunrise Drive
Tucson, AZ 85750
www.drtheo.com

ROGER TOLLE
www.rogertolle.net

STEPHANIE TOURLES
Oreland, ME
www.stephanietourles.com

DANA ULLMAN
2124 Kittredge Street
Berkeley, CA 94704
(510) 649-0294
www.homeopathic.com

DR. ROBERT ULLMAN
123 4th Avenue
Edmonds, WA 98020
(425) 774-5599
www.healthyhomepathy.com

DR. ELIZABETH VLIET
2200 River Road
Tucson, AZ 85718
(520) 797-9131
www.herplace.com

NILSA VERGARA
7609 34th Avenue
Jackson Heights, NY 11372
(718) 651-2260

DR. MICHAEL WALD
55 Crow Hill Road
Mount Kisco, NY 10549
(914) 552-1442
www.blooddetective.com

DR. LYNNE WALKER
29399 Agoura Road
Agoura Hills, CA 91301
(818) 584-0058
www.alternativepharmacy.com

DR. ALLAN WARSHOWSKY
150 Purchase Street
Rye, NY 10580
(914) 967-1630
www.doctorallan.com

DR. JULIAN WHITAKER
www.drwhitaker.com

DR. JONATHAN WRIGHT
6839 Fort Dent Way
Tukwila, WA 98188
www.tahomaclinic.com

DR. JOSE YARYURA-TOBIAS
935 Northern Boulevard
Great Neck, NY 10021
(516) 487-7116
www.behavioralinstitute.com

DR. JANET ZAND
(800) NEO-4040
www.neogenis.com

DR. VICTOR ZEINES
57 West 57th Street #1008
New York, NY 10019
(212) 813-9461
www.natdent.com

TINA CHUNNA ZHANG
Wu Tang Physical Culture Association
217 Centre Street
New York, NY 10013
(347) 558-5674
www.qigongforwomen.com

Chapter 65

References and Resources

CHAPTER 1: DIET AND NUTRITION

Singh GM, et al. Estimated Global, Regional, and National Disease Burdens Related to Sugar-Sweetened Beverage Consumption in 2010. *Circulation*. Published online ahead of print 06-29-15. doi:10.1161/CIRCULATIONAHA.114.010636.

CHAPTER 6: NATURAL MEDICINE CABINET

Gray S, et al. Cumulative Use of Strong Anticholinergics and Incident Dementia: A Prospective Cohort Study. *JAMA Int Med*. 2015;175(3):401-407. doi:10.1001/jamainternmed.2014.7663.

Meletis ND, Wilkes K. Seasonal Allergies and Asthma: Removing Total Burden for Powerful Symptom Relief and Whole Body Wellness. *Townsend Letter*, May 2014. Web. Accessed July 15, 2015.

CHAPTER 10: SKIN CARE

Chalopin M, et al. Estrogen Receptor Alpha as a Key Target of Red Wine Polyphenols Action on the Endothelium. *PLoS One*. 2010 Jan 1;5(1):e8554.

Cho S, et al. Dietary Aloe Vera Supplementation Improves Facial Wrinkles and Elasticity and It Increases the Type I Procollagen Gene Expression in Human Skin *In Vivo*. *Ann Dermatol*. 2009;21(1):6-11. doi:10.5021/ad.2009.21.1.6.

Goldfaden D. Revitalize Aging Skin With Topical Vitamin C, *Life Extension Magazine*, May 2009. Web. Accessed July 15, 2015.

Goldfaden R, Goldfaden, D. Topical Resveratrol Combats Skin Aging, *Life Extension Magazine*, November 2011. Web. Accessed July 15, 2015.

Look Younger With This Anti-Aging Plant, *Institute for Natural Healing*, December 2012. Web. Accessed July 15, 2015.

Optimal Skin Protection With Vitamin D, *Life Extension Magazine*, June 2010. Web. Accessed July 15, 2015.

Potapovich AI, et al. Plant Polyphenols Differentially Modulate Inflammatory Responses of Human Keratinocytes By Interfering With Activation of Transcription Factors Nfkb and Ahr And EGFR-ERK Pathway. *Toxicol Applied Pharmacol*. 2011 Jul 12.

Surjushe A, et al. Aloe Vera: A Short Review. *Indian J Dermatol*. 2008;53(4):163-166. doi:10.4103/0019-5154.44785.

Tabassum N, Hamdani M. Plants Used to Treat Skin Diseases. *Pharmacogn Rev*. 2014 Jan-Jun;8(15):52–60.

CHAPTER 12: HAIR CARE

Norek D. Vitamins and Herbs for Strong, Healthy Hair. *Naturalnews.com*, January 23, 2012. Web. Accessed July 23, 2015.

CHAPTER 14: AGING

Chowanadisai W, et al. Pyrroloquinoline Quinone Stimulates Mitochondrial Biogenesis Through Camp Response Element-Binding Protein Phosphorylation and Increased PGC-1alpha Expression. *J Biol Chem*. 2010 Jan 1;285(1):142-152.

Downey M. Powerful Protection Against Cellular Aging, *Life Extension Magazine*, 2012. Web. Accessed July 15, 2015.

Klatz R, Goldman R. The Harmony Between Naturopathic Medicine and Anti-Aging Medicine. *Townsend Letter*, February/March 2015. Web. Accessed July 15, 2015.

Misra HS, et al. Pyrroloquinoline-Quinone and Its Versatile Roles in Biological Processes. *J Bioscience*. 2012 Jun;37(2):313-325.

Mitchell T. Vitamin K: Stunning New Research Shows that Vitamin K May Be One of the Most Extraordinary Anti-aging Vitamins Ever Discovered. *Life Extension Magazine*, Feb. 2000. Web. Accessed July 15, 2015.

Rahway, S. The Youth Restoring Benefits of NAD+, *Life Extension Magazine*, November 2014. Web. Accessed July 15, 2015.

CHAPTER 17: ADDICTION

Darvishzadeh-Mahani F, et al. Ginger (Zingiber officinale Roscoe) Prevents the Development of Morphine Analgesic Tolerance and Physical Dependence in Rats. *J Ethnopharmacol*. 2012 Jun 14;141(3):901-907. doi: 10.1016/j.jep.2012.03.030. Epub 2012 Mar 26.

Joslin, M. Novel Methods to Cure Drug Addiction. *Life Extension Magazine*, October 2011. Web. Accessed July 15, 2015.

Lee B, et al. Acupuncture Stimulation Attenuates Impaired Emotional-Like Behaviors and Activation of the Noradrenergic System during Protracted Abstinence following Chronic Morphine Exposure in Rats. *Evid Based Complementary Altern Med.* 2014. http://dx.doi.org/10.1155/ 2014/216503.

Shivani R, et al. The Effect of a Yoga Intervention on Alcohol and Drug Abuse Risk in Veteran and Civilian Women with Posttraumatic Stress Disorder. *J Altern Complement Med.* 2014 Oct;20(10): 750-756. doi:10.1089/acm.2014.0014.

CHAPTER 18: ADRENAL FATIGUE

Olsson EM, et al. A Randomised, Double-Blind, Placebo-Controlled, Parallel-Group Study of the Standardised Extract Shr-5 of the Roots of Rhodiola Rosea in the Treatment of Subjects With Stress-Related Fatigue. *Planta Med.* 2009 Feb;75(2):105-12. doi: 10.1055/s-0028-1088346. Epub 2008 Nov 18.

CHAPTER 19: ALZHEIMER'S DISEASE

Ahmed A, et al. Cannabinoids in Late-Onset Alzheimer's Disease, *Clin Pharmacol Ther.* 2015 Jun;97(6):597-606. Epub 2015 Apr 17.

Nishteswar K, et al. Role of Indigenous Herbs in the Management of Alzheimer's Disease. *Ancient Sci Life.* 2014;34:3-7.

Sang Z, et al. Design, Synthesis and Evaluation of Scutellarein-O-Alkylamines as Multifunctional Agents for the Treatment of Alzheimer's Disease. *Eur J Med Chem.* 2015 Apr 13;94:348-366. Epub 2015 Mar 4.

CHAPTER 20: ANEMIA

Ahmed F, et al. Long-Term Intermittent Multiple Micronutrient Supplementation Enhances Hemoglobin and Micronutrient Status More Than Iron + Folic Acid Supplementation in Bangladeshi Rural Adolescent Girls With Nutritional Anemia. *J Nutr.* 2010 Oct.;140(10):1879-1886.

Deniau AL, et al. Multiple Beneficial Health Effects of Natural Alkylglycerols From Shark Liver Oil. *Mar Drugs* 2010;8(7):2175-2184.

Haider BA, et al. Effect of Multiple Micronutrient Supplementation During Pregnancy on Maternal and Birth Outcomes. *BMC Public Health* 2011;11 Suppl 3:S19.

Kelly A, et al. Safety and Efficacy of High-dose Daily Vitamin D3 Supplementation in Children and Young Adults With Sickle Cell Disease, *J Ped Hematol Oncol.* 2015;37(5) e308.

Low Vitamin D Levels Raise Anemia Risk in Children, Hopkins-Led Study Shows, John's Hopkins Children's Center Press Release, Oct. 2013. Web. Accessed July 15, 2015.

Sim JJ, et al. Vitamin D Deficiency and Anemia: A Cross-Sectional Study. *Ann Hematol.* 2010 May;89(5):447-452.

CHAPTER 21: ANXIETY

Abdali K, et al. HR. Effect of St John's Wort on Severity, Frequency, and Duration of Hot Flashes in Premenopausal, Perimenopausal and Postmenopausal Women: A Randomized, Double-Blind, Placebo-Controlled Study. *Menopause.* 2010 Mar;17(2):326-331.

Hood SD, et al. Effects of Acute Tryptophan Depletion in Serotonin Reuptake Inhibitor-Remitted Patients With Generalized Anxiety Disorder. *Psychopharmacol.* (Berl). 2010 Feb;208(2):223-232.

Lipovac M, et al. Improvement of Postmenopausal Depressive and Anxiety Symptoms After Treatment with Isoflavones Derived from Red Clover Extracts. *Maturitas.* 2010 Mar;65(3):258-261.

Sartori SB, et al. Magnesium Deficiency Induces Anxiety and HPA Axis Dysregulation: Modulation by Therapeutic Drug Treatment. *Neuropharmacol.* 2012 ;62(1):304-312.

CHAPTER 22: ARTHRITIS

Tao R, et al. Pyrroloquinoline Quinone Slows Down the Progression of Osteoarthritis by Inhibiting Nitric Oxide Production and Metalloproteinase Synthesis. *Inflammation* 2015 Aug;38(4):1546-1555.

O'Dell J, et al. Therapies for Active Rheumatoid Arthritis after Methotrexate Failure. *N Engl J Med* 2013; 369:307-318.

Preston W. Rebuild Aging Joints, *Life Extension Magazine*, 2011. Web. Accessed July 15, 2015.

Qi, Q. Lv et al. Comparison of Tripterygium Wilfordii Hook F With Methotrexate in the Treatment of Active Rheumatoid Arthritis (TRIFRA): A Randomised, Controlled Clinical Trial. *Ann Rheum Dis.* 2015;74:1078-1086.

CHAPTER 23: BIRTH CONTROL

Pallone SR, Bergus GR. Fertility Awareness-Based Methods: Another Option for Family Planning. *J Am Board Fam Med.* 2009 Mar-Apr;22(2): 147-157.

CHAPTER 24: BREAST CANCER AND OTHER BREAST DISEASES

Alipour S, et al. Benefits and Harms of Phytoestrogen Consumption in Breast Cancer Survivors. *Asian Pac J Cancer Prev*. 2015;16(8):3091-3396.

Aragón F. Modification in the Diet Can Induce Beneficial Effects Against Breast Cancer. *World J Clin Oncol*. 2014 Aug. 10;5(3):455-464.

Bilal I, et al. Phytoestrogens and Prevention of Breast Cancer: The Contentious Debate. *World J Clin Oncol*. 2014 Oct 10;5(4):705-712.

Brownstein D. Statins More Than Double Breast Cancer Risk. Dr. Brownstein's Blog. March 25, 2014. Web. Accessed July 2015.

Elgazar AF, et al. Anti-Hyperglycemic Effect of Saffron Extract in Alloxan-Induced Diabetic Rats. *Eur J Biol Sci*. 2013;5(1):14-22.

Fritz H, et al. Soy, Red Clover, and Isoflavones and Breast Cancer: A Systematic Review. Shioda T, ed. *PLoS One*. 2013;8(11):e81968.

Gutheil WG, et al.: An Agent Derived from Saffron for Prevention and Therapy for Cancer. *Curr Pharm Biotechnol*. 2012 Jan;13(1):173-179.

Holtz, M. Novel Citrus Extract Blocks Deadly Cancer Cell Signaling, *Life Extension Magazine*, July 2011. Web. Accessed July 15, 2015.

How Curcumin Protects Against Cancer, *Life Extension Magazine*, 2011. Web. Accessed July 15, 2015.

Kim SH, et al. Proposed Cytotoxic Mechanisms of the Saffron Carotenoids Crocin and Crocetin on Cancer Cell Lines. *Biochem Cell Biol*. 2014 Apr;92(2):105-111.

Luoma ML, et al. Experiences of Breast Cancer Survivors Participating in a Tailored Exercise Intervention: A Qualitative Study. *Anticancer Res*. 2014 Mar;34(3):1193-1199.

MacDonald B. Improving Breast Cancer Survivorship with Lifestyle Changes. *Townsend Letter*, August/September 2014. Web. Accessed July 15, 2015.

Provos J. Anticancer Properties of Saffron, *Life Extension Magazine*, March 2015. Web. Accessed July 15, 2015.

Teegarden D, et al. Redefining the Impact of Nutrition on Breast Cancer Incidence: Is Epigenetics Involved? *Nutr Research Rev*. 2012;25(1):68-95.

Woo, HD, et al. Differential Influence of Dietary Soy Intake on the Risk of Breast Cancer Recurrence Related to HER2 Status. *Nutr Cancer* 2012;64(2)198-205.

CHAPTER 25: CERVICAL DYSPLASIA, FIBROIDS, AND REPRODUCTIVE SYSTEM CANCERS

Merritt M, et al. Investigation of Dietary Factors and Endometrial Cancer Risk Using a Nutrient-wide Association Study Approach in the EPIC and Nurses' Health Study (NHS) and NHSII. *Cancer Epidemiol Biomarkers Prev*. 2015 Feb. 24;466-471; doi:10.1158/1055-9965. EPI-14-0970.

Piyathilake CJ, et al. Folate and Vitamin B_{12} May Play a Critical Role in Lowering the HPV 16 Methylation–Associated Risk of Developing Higher Grades of CIN. *Cancer Prev Res*. 2014 Nov. 7;1128-1137. doi: 10.1158/1940-6207.

Roshdy E. Treatment of Symptomatic Uterine Fibroids With Green Tea Extract: A Pilot Randomized Controlled Clinical Study. *Int J Womens Health* 2013;5:477–486. Published online 2013 Aug 7. doi: 10.2147/IJWH.S41021.

Zhang D. Antiproliferative and Proapoptotic Effects of Epigallocatechin Gallate on Human Leiomyoma Cells. *Fertil Steril*. 2010 Oct;94(5):1887-1893. doi:10.1016/ j.fertnstert.2009. 08.065. Epub 2009 Oct 12.

CHAPTER 26: CHRONIC FATIGUE SYNDROME

Belcaro G, et al. Improved Management of Primary Chronic Fatigue Syndrome With the Supplement French Oak Wood Extract (Robuvit®): A Pilot, Registry Evaluation. *Panminerva Med*. 2014 Mar;56(1):63-72.

Brewer JH, et al. Detection of Mycotoxins in Patients with Chronic Fatigue Syndrome. *Toxins* 2013;5(4):605–617. doi:10.3390/toxins5040605.

Coenzyme Q10 Levels Reduced in Chronic Fatigue Syndrome. *Life Extension Update*, February 2010. Web. Accessed July 15, 2015.

Franco M. New Option for Chronic Fatigue Syndrome. *Life Extension Magazine*, December 2014. Web. Accessed July 15, 2015.

Leong PK, et al. Yang/Qi Invigoration: An Herbal Therapy for Chronic Fatigue Syndrome with Yang Deficiency? *Evid. Based Complementary Altern Med*. 2015;945901. doi:10.1155/2015/945901.

CHAPTER 27: DEPRESSION

Lewis JE, et al. The Effect of Methylated Vitamin B Complex on Depressive and Anxiety Symptoms and Quality of Life in Adults with Depression. *ISRN Psychiatry*. 2013; 621453.

Naqvi SH, et al. Predictors of Depression in Women With Polycystic Ovary Syndrome. *Arch Womens Ment Health*. 2015 Feb;18(1):95-101. doi: 10.1007/s00737-014-0458-z.

Prousky JE. The Manifestations and Triggers of Mental Breakdown, and its Effective Treatment by Increasing Stress Resilience With Psychosocial Strategies, Therapeutic Lifestyle Changes, and Orthomolecular Interventions. *Townsend Letter*. February/ March 2015. Web. Accessed July 15, 2015.

Stough C, et al. The Effect of 90 Day Administration of a High Dose Vitamin B-Complex on Work Stress. *Hum Psychopharmacol*. 2011;26:470–476.

CHAPTER 28: DEMENTIA

Chen LP, et al. Clinical Research on Comprehensive Treatment of Senile Vascular Dementia. *J Tradit Chin Med*. 2011;31(3):178-181.

Jesky R, Hailong C. Are Herbal Compounds the Next Frontier for Alleviating Learning and Memory Impairments? An Integrative Look at Memory, Dementia and the Promising Therapeutics of Traditional Chinese Medicines. [Review]. *Phytother Res*. 2011;25(8):1105-1118. doi: 10.1002/ptr.3388.

Perry E, Howes MJ. Medicinal Plants and Dementia Therapy: Herbal Hopes for Brain Aging? *CNS Neurosci Ther*. 2011 Dec;17(6):683-698. Doi: 10.1111/J.1755-5949.2010.00202.X. Epub 2010 Oct 18.

Samaras N, et al. Dementia Prevention: Potential Treatments and How to Target High Risk Patients. *Rev Med Suisse*. 2013; 9(387):1116-1119.

Wang BS, et al. Effectiveness of Standardized Ginkgo Biloba Extract on Cognitive Symptoms of Dementia With a Six-Month Treatment: A Bivariate Random Effect Meta-Analysis. *Pharmacopsych*. 2010;43(3):86-91.

CHAPTER 29: DIABETES

Morstein M. The Role of Nutritional and Botanical Agents in the Management of Type 2 Diabetes Mellitus. *Townsend Letter*, April 2014. Web. Accessed July 15, 2015.

Neelakantan N. Effect of Fenugreek (Trigonella Foenum-Graecum L.) Intake on Glycemia: A Meta-Analysis of Clinical Trials. *Nutr. J*. 2014;13:7. doi:10.1186/1475-2891-13-7.

Kelleher S, et al. Zinc in Specialized Secretory Tissues: Roles in the Pancreas, Prostate, and Mammary Gland. *Adv Nutr*. 2011;(2):101-111. doi: 10.3945/an.110.000232.

Rungseesantivanon S, et al.. Curcumin Supplementation Could Improve Diabetes-Induced Endothelial Dysfunction Associated With Decreased Vascular Superoxide Production and PKC Inhibition. *BMC Complement Altern Med*. 2010;10:57.

Szkudelski T, Szkudelska K. Anti-Diabetic Effects of Resveratrol. *Ann N Y Acad Sci*. 2011 Jan;1215:34-39. doi:10.1111/j.1749-6632.2010.05844.x.

Takikawa M, et al. Dietary Anthocyanin-Rich Bilberry Extract Ameliorates Hyperglycemia and Insulin Sensitivity Via Activation of AMP-Activated Protein Kinase in Diabetic Mice. *J Nutr*. March 2010;140(3)527–533.

CHAPTER 30: DIGESTIVE DISORDERS

Dinleyici EC, et al.. Effectiveness and Safety of Saccharomyces Boulardii for Acute Infectious Diarrhea. *Exp Opin Biol Ther*. 2012 April;(12)4:395-410. doi:10.1517/14712598.2012.664129.

Fahey JW, et al. Protection of Humans by Plant Glucosinolates: Efficiency of Conversion of Glucosinolates to Isothiocyanates by the Gastrointestinal Microflora. *Cancer Prev Res*. 2012 April(5):603-611. Published OnlineFirst February 7, 2012. doi:10.1158/1940-6207.CAPR-11-0538.

Ishikawa H. Beneficial Effects of Probiotic Bifidobacterium and Galacto-Oligosaccharide in Patients With Ulcerative Colitis: A Randomized Controlled Study. *Digestion*. 2011;84(2):128-133. doi: 10.1159/000322977. Epub 2011 Apr 28.

Parekh, PJ. The Influence of the Gut Microbiome on Obesity, Metabolic Syndrome and Gastrointestinal Disease. *Clin Trans Gastroenterol*. (2015) 6, e91. doi:10.1038/ctg.2015.16. Published online June 18, 2015.

Saez-Lara MJ, et al. The Role of Probiotic Lactic Acid Bacteria and Bifidobacteria in the Prevention and Treatment of Inflammatory Bowel Disease and Other Related Diseases: A Systematic Review of Randomized Human Clinical Trials. *BioMed Res Intern*. 2015;2015:505878. doi:10.1155/2015/505878.

Stokel K. Block Acid Reflux to Prevent Esophageal Problems. *Life Extension Magazine*, November 2013. Web. Accessed July 15, 2015.

Triantafillidis JK, et al. The Role of Enteral Nutrition in Patients with Inflammatory Bowel Disease: Current Aspects. *BioMed Res Intern*. 2015;2015:197167. doi:10.1155/2015/197167.

CHAPTER 31: EATING DISORDERS

Carei TR, et al. Randomized Controlled Clinical Trial of Yoga in the Treatment of Eating Disorders. *J Adolesc Health.* 2010 Apr;46(4):346-351.

Ozier AD, Henry BW. Position of the American Dietetic Association: Nutrition Intervention in the Treatment of Eating Disorders. *J Am Diet Assoc.* 2011 Aug;111(8):1236-1241.

Setnick J. Micronutrient Deficiencies and Supplementation in Anorexia and Bulimia Nervosa: A Review of Literature. *Nutr Clin Pract.* 2010 Apr;25(2):137-142.

Vancampfort D, et al. A Systematic Review of Physical Therapy Interventions for Patients With Anorexia and Bulemia Nervosa. *Disabil Rehabil.* 2014; 36(8):628-634.

CHAPTER 32: ENDOMETRIOSIS

Kong S, et al. The Complementary and Alternative Medicine for Endometriosis: A Review of Utilization and Mechanism. *Evid-Based Complementary Altern Med*, 2014:146383. doi:10.1155/2014/146383.

Rudzitis-Auth J, et al. Resveratrol is a Potent Inhibitor of Vascularization and Cell Proliferation in Experimental Endometriosis. *Human Reprod.* 2013;28(5):1339–1347.

Wang CC, et al. Prodrug of Green Tea Epigallocatechin-3-Gallate (Pro-EGCG) as a Potent Anti-Angiogenesis Agent for Endometriosis in Mice. *Angiogen.* 2013;16(1):59–69.

Xiang DF, et al., Effect of Abdominal Acupuncture on Pain of Pelvic Cavity in Patients With Endometriosis. *Chin Acupun Moxibust.* 2011;31(2):113–116.

Zhang Z, et al. Therapeutic Potential of Wenshen Xiaozheng Tang, A Traditional Chinese Medicine Prescription, For Treating Endometriosis. *Reprod Sci.* 2013;20(10):1215–1223.

CHAPTER 33: ENVIRONMENTAL ILLNESS

Forsgren S, et al. Mold and Mycotoxins: Often Overlooked Factors in Chronic Lyme Disease. *Townsend Letter*, July 2014. Web. Accessed July 15, 2015.

Peterson BS, et al. Effects of Prenatal Exposure to Air Pollutants (Polycyclic Aromatic Hydrocarbons) on the Development of Brain White Matter, Cognition, and Behavior in Later Childhood. *JAMA Psychiatry.* 2015;72(6):531-540.

CHAPTER 34: FIBROMYALGIA

Arranz LI, et al. Fibromyalgia and Nutrition, What Do We Know? *Rheumatol Int.* 2010 Sep;30(11):1417-1427.

Bagis S, et al. Is Magnesium Citrate Treatment Effective on Pain, Clinical Parameters and Functional Status in Patients With Fibromyalgia? *Rheumatol Int.* 2013 Jan;33(1):167-172.

Cordero MD, et al. Oxidative Stress Correlates with Headache Symptoms in Fibromyalgia: Coenzyme Q10 Effect on Clinical Improvement. *PLoS One.* 2012;7(4): e35677. doi:10.1371/journal.pone.0035677.

Curtis K, et al. An Eight-Week Yoga Intervention is Associated With Improvements in Pain, Psychological Functioning and Mindfulness, and Changes in Cortisol Levels in Women With Fibromyalgia. *J Pain Research.* 4:189–201. Epub July 2011.

Jones KD, et al. A Randomized Controlled Trial of 8-Form Tai Chi Improves Symptoms and Functional Mobility in Fibromyalgia Patients. *Clin Rheum.* 2012;31(8):1205–1214.

Klatz RK, Goldman R. An Anti-Aging Approach to Fibromyalgia. *Townsend Letter,* December 2011. Web. Accessed July 15, 2015.

Onieva-Zafra MD, et al. Effect of Music as Nursing Intervention for People Diagnosed With Fibromyalgia. *Pain Manag Nurs.* Published online: 29 Nov 2010.

van Middendorp H, et al. The Effects of Anger and Sadness on Clinical Pain Reports and Experimentally-Induced Pain Thresholds in Women With and Without Fibromyalgia. *Arthritis Care Res.* 2010 Oct;62(10).

Wang C, et al. A Randomized Trial of Tai Chi for Fibromyalgia. *N Engl J Med.* 2010 Aug;363:743–754.

CHAPTER 36: HEART DISEASE

Ahmadi N,et al. Aged Garlic Extract With Supplement is Associated With Increase in Brown Adipose, Decrease in White Adipose Tissue and Predict Lack of Progression in Coronary Atherosclerosis. *Int J Cardio.* 2013 Mar 1. Published online: Mar 4, 2013.

Bernstein AM, et al. Major Dietary Protein Sources and Risk of Coronary Heart Disease in Women. *Circulation,* 2010 Aug;122(9):873-883. Epub 2010 Aug. 16.

Chiuve SE, et al. Plasma and Dietary Magnesium and Risk of Sudden Cardiac Death in Women. *Am J Clin Nutr.* 2011 Feb;93(2):253-260. doi: 10.3945/ajcn.110.002253. Epub 2010 Nov 24.

Healy GN, et al. Sedentary Time and Cardio-Metabolic Biomarkers in US Adults: NHANES 2003–06. *Eur Heart J.* 2011 Jan. doi:10.1093/eurheartj/ehq451.

Klatz R, Goldman R. Women Take Heart: An Anti-Aging Approach to Heart Disease. *Townsend Letter,* April 2011, Web. Accessed July 15, 2015.

Rautiainen S, et al. Multivitamin Use and the Risk of Myocardial Infarction: A Population-Based Cohort of Swedish Women. *Am J Clin Nutr.* 2010 Nov;92(5):1251-1256. doi: 10.3945/ajcn.2010.29371. Epub 2010 Sep 22.

Uryash A, et al. Non-Invasive Technology That Improves Cardiac Function after Experimental Myocardial Infarction: Whole Body Periodic Acceleration (pGz). *PLoS One.* 2015 Mar 25;10(3):e0121069. doi: 10.1371/journal.pone.0121069.

CHAPTER 37: HERPES

Antoine TW, et al. Prophylactic, Therapeutic and Neutralizing Effects of Zinc Oxide Tetrapod Structures Against Herpes Simplex Virus Type-2 Infection. *Antiviral Res.* 2012; 96: 363-375.

Bertol JW, et al. Antiherpes Activity of Glucoevatromonoside, A Cardenolide Isolated From a Brazilian Cultivar of Digitalis Lanata. *Antiviral Res.* 2011 Oct;92(1):73-80. doi: 10.1016/j.antiviral.2011.06.015.

Health Concerns: Herpes and Shingles. *Life Extension* website. Accessed July 20, 2015.

Nolkemper S, et al. Mechanism of Herpes Simplex Virus Type 2 Suppression by Propolis Extracts. *Phytomed.* 2010;17:132-138.

Stahl W, Helmut S. B-Carotene and Other Carotenoids in Protection From Sunlight. *Am J Clin Nutr.,* 2012; 96(suppl):1179S-84S.

CHAPTER 38, HIV/AIDS

Health Concerns; HIV/AIDS, *Life Extension.* Web. Accessed July 15, 2015.

Helfer M, et al. The Root Extract of the Medicinal Plant Pelargonium sidoides Is a Potent HIV-1 Attachment Inhibitor. *PLoS One.* 2014 Jan(9):1. e87487. doi:10.1371/journal.pone. 0087487.

Miller TL, et al. The Effect of a Structured Exercise Program on Nutrition and Fitness Outcomes in Human Immunodeficiency Virus-Infected Children. *AIDS Res Hum Retroviruses.* 2010 Mar;26(3):313-319. doi: 10.1089/aid.2009.0198.

Peters BS, et al. The Effect of a 12-Week Course of Omega-3 Polyunsaturated Fatty Acids on Lipid Parameters in Hypertriglyceridemic Adult HIV-Infected Patients Undergoing HAART: A Randomized, Placebo-Controlled Pilot Trial. *Clin Ther.* 2012 Jan;34(1):67-76. doi: 10.1016/j.clinthera.2011.12.001. Epub 2011 Dec 31.

Veljkovic M, et al. Aerobic Exercise Training As a Potential Source of Natural Antibodies Protective Against Human Immunodeficiency Virus-1. *Scand J Med Sci Sports.* 2010;(20)3:469-474. doi: 10.1111/j.1600-0838.2009.00962.x

CHAPTER 40: INFERTILITY

Brogan K. Is Wheat Making You Wait for Babies? The Gluten Infertility Link. *GreenMedInfo.* December 15, 2013. Web. Accessed July 20, 2015.

Chavaroo JE, et al. Use of Multivitamins, Intake of B Vitamins and Risk of Ovulatory Infertility. *Fertil Steril.* 2008 Mar;89(3):668–676.

Choi JM, et al. Increased Prevalence of Celiac Disease in Patients with Unexplained Infertility in the United States: A Prospective Study. *J Reprod Med.* 2011;56(5-6):199-203.

Rice AD, et al. Ten-year Retrospective Study on the Efficacy of a Manual Physical Therapy to Treat Female Infertility. *Altern Ther Health Med.* 2015 Feb 17. pii: at5233. [Epub ahead of print]

CHAPTER 41: LUPUS

Jordan N, et al. Progress with the Use of Monoclonal Antibodies for the Treatment of Systemic Lupus Erythematosus. *Immunother.* 2015 Mar;7(3):255-270. doi: 10.2217/imt.14.118.

Kuhn A., et al., Photoprotective Effects of a Broad-Spectrum Sunscreen in Ultraviolet-Induced Cutaneous Lupus Erythematosus: A Randomized, Vehicle-Controlled, Double-Blind Study. *J Amer Acad Derm.* 2011;64(1):37-48.

Kurien BT, et al. Heat-Solubilized Curry Spice Curcumin Inhibits Antibody-Antigen Interaction in In Vitro Studies: A Possible Therapy to Alleviate Autoimmune Disorders. *Molec Nutr Food Research* 2010;54(8):1202-1209.

Lupus: Systemic Lupus Erythematosus (SLE). Life Extension website. Accessed July 20, 2015.

Muangchan C, et al. Treatment Algorithms in Systemic Lupus Erythematosus. *Arthritis Care Res* (Hoboken). 2015 Mar 16. doi: 10.1002/acr.22589. [Epub ahead of print]

Paintoni S, et al. Phenotype Modifications of T-Cells and Their Shift Toward a Th2 Response in Patients With Systemic Lupus Erythematosus Supplemented With Different Monthly Regimens of Vitamin D. *Lupus.* 2015 Apr;24(4-5):490-498. doi: 10.1177/0961203314559090.

Terrier B, et al. Restoration of Regulatory and Effector T Cell Balance and B Cell Homeostasis in Systemic Lupus Erythematosus Patients Through Vitamin D Supplementation. *Arthritis Res Ther.* 2012 Oct 12;14(5):R221.

Xu JJ, et al. Vitamin D Analog EB1089 Could Repair the Defective Bone Marrow-Derived Mesenchymal Stromal Cells in Patients With Systemic Lupus Erythematosus. *Int J Clin Exp Med.* 2015;8(1):916-921.

CHAPTER 43: MENOPAUSE

Erkkola R, et al. A Randomized, Double-Blind, Placebo-Controlled, Cross-Over Pilot Study on the Use of a Standardized Hop Extract to Alleviate Menopausal Discomforts. *Phytomed.* 2010 May;17(6):389-396.

Hagner-Derengowska M, et al. Effects of Nordic Walking and Pilates Exercise Programs on Blood Glucose and Lipid Profile in Overweight and Obese Postmenopausal Women in an Experimental, Nonrandomized, Open-label, Prospective Controlled Trial. *Menopause.* 2015 Mar 23. [Epub ahead of print]

Manson JE, et al. Menopausal Hormone Therapy and Health Outcomes During the Intervention and Extended Poststopping Phases of the Women's Health Initiative Randomized Trials. *JAMA.* 2013 Oct 2;310(13):1353-1368.

Nadil A. Safely Manage Menopausal Symptoms. *Life Extension Magazine*, August 2014. Web. Accessed July 20, 2015.

Nahidi F, et al Effects of Licorice on Relief and Recurrence of Menopausal Hot Flashes. *Iran J Pharm Res.* 2012 Spring;11(2):541-548.

CHAPTER 44: MENSTRUAL CRAMPS AND IRREGULAR MENSTRUATION

Chao MT, et al. An Innovative Acupuncture Treatment for Primary Dysmenorrhea: A Randomized, Crossover Pilot Study. *Altern Ther Health Med.* 2014 Jan-Feb;20(1):49-56.

Daily JW, et al. Efficacy of Ginger for Alleviating the Symptoms of Primary Dysmenorrhea: A Systematic Review and Meta-analysis of Randomized Clinical Trials. *Pain Med.* 2015 Jul 14. doi: 10.1111/pme.12853. [Epub ahead of print]

CHAPTER 45: MIGRAINES

Gaul C, et al. Improvement of Migraine Symptoms With a Proprietary Supplement Containing Riboflavin, Magnesium and Q10: A Randomized, Placebo-Controlled, Double-Blind, Multicenter Trial. *J Headache Pain.* 2015 Dec;16:516. Doi: 10.1186/S10194-015-0516-6. Epub 2015 Apr 3.

Jackson JL, Kuriyama A, Hayashino Y. Botulinum toxin A for prophylactic treatment of migraine and tension headaches in adults: a meta-analysis. *JAMA.* 2012;307(16):1736-1745

Shaik MM, Gan SH. Vitamin Supplementation as Possible Prophylactic Treatment Against Migraine With Aura and Menstrual Migraine. *Biomed Res Int.* 2015;2015:469529. Doi: 10.1155/2015/469529. Epub 2015 Feb 28.

Wells RE, et al. Complementary and Alternative Medicine Use Among Adults with Migraines/ Severe Headaches. *Headache*. 2011;51(7):1087-1097. doi:10.1111/j.1526-4610.2011.01917.x.

CHAPTER 46: MULTIPLE SCLEROSIS

Fonseca-Kelly Z, et al. Resveratrol Neuroprotection in a Chronic Mouse Model of Multiple Sclerosis. *Front Neurol*. 2012;3:84. Epub 2012 May 24.

Herges K, et al. Neuroprotective Effect of Combination Therapy of Glatiramer Acetate and Epigallocatechin-3-Gallate in Neuroinflammation. *PLoS One*. 2011;6(10):e25456. Epub 2011 Oct 13.

Kozela E, et al. Cannabidiol Inhibits Pathogenic T Cells, Decreases Spinal Microglial Activation and Ameliorates Multiple Sclerosis-Like Disease in C57BL/6 Mice. *Br J Pharmacol*. 2011 Mar 30. Epub 2011 Mar 30.

Marchese, M. Multiple Sclerosis: Environmental Factors and Treatments – Part 2. *Townsend Letter*, December 2012. Web. Accessed July 20, 2015.

Shindler KS, et al. Oral Resveratrol Reduces Neuronal Damage in a Model of Multiple Sclerosis. *J Neuroophthalmol*. 2010;30(4):328–339.

Yadav V, et al. Complementary and Alternative Medicine for the Treatment of Multiple Sclerosis. *Expert Rev Clin Immunol*. 2010; 6(3):381–395.

CHAPTER 48: OBSESSIVE-COMPULSIVE DISORDER

Kisely S, et al. Deep Brain Stimulation for Obsessive Compulsive Disorder: A Systematic Review and Meta-Analysis. *Psych Med*. 2014; 44(16):3533-3542.

Rector NA, et al. A Pilot Test of the Additive Benefits of Physical Exercise to CBT for OCD. *Cogn Behav Ther*. 2015 Jun;44(4):328-340. doi: 10.1080/16506073.2015.1016448. Epub 2015 Mar 4.

Valizadeh M, Valizadeh N. Obsessive Compulsive Disorder as Early Manifestation of B_{12} Deficiency. *Indian J Psychol Med*. 2011 Jul;33(2):203-204.

CHAPTER 49: OSTEOPOROSIS

Bolland MJ, et al. Effect of Calcium Supplements on Risk of Myocardial Infarction and Cardiovascular Events: Meta-Analysis. *BMJ*. 2010;341:c3691.

Gaby A. Do Calcium Supplements Cause Cardiovascular Disease? *Townsend Letter*, January 2011. Web. Accessed July 20, 2015.

Hooshman S, et al. Comparative Effects of Dried Plum and Dried Apple on Bone in Post-menopausal Women. *Br J Nutr.* 2011 Sep;106(6):923-930. doi: 10.1017/S000711451100119X. Epub 2011 May 31.

CHAPTER 50: PARKINSON'S DISEASE

Butt MS , Sultan MT. Coffee and Its Consumption: Benefits and Risks. *Crit Rev Food Sci Nutr.* 2011 Apr;51(4):363-373.

Cassani E, et al. Use of Probiotics for the Treatment of Constipation in Parkinson's Disease Patients. Minerva Gastroenterol Dietol. 2011 Jun;57(2):117-121.

Dobkin RD, et al. Cognitive-Behavioral Therapy for Depression in Parkinson's Disease: A Randomized, Controlled Trial. *Am J Psychiatry.* 2011 Jun 15. [Epub ahead of print]

Gao, X. Habitual Intake of Dietary Flavonoids and Risk of Parkinson Disease. *Neurology.* 2012 Apr 10;78(15):1138-1145.

Lau YS, et al. Neuroprotective Effects and Mechanisms of Exercise in a Chronic Mouse Model of Parkinson's Disease With Moderate Neurodegeneration. *Eur J Neurosci.* 2011 Apr;33(7):1264-1274. doi: 10.1111/j.1460-9568.2011.07626.x. Epub 2011 Mar 7.

Li F, et al. Tai chi and Postural Stability in Patients with Parkinson's Disease. *New Engl J Med.* 2012;366:511–519.

Lieu CA, et al. A Water Extract of Mucuna Pruriens Provides Long-Term Amelioration of Parkinsonism With Reduced Risk for Dyskinesias. *Parkinsonism Relat Disord.* 2010 Aug;16(7):458-465. Epub 2010 May 31.

Parkinson's Disease, Life Extension website. Accessed July 20, 2015.

CHAPTER 52: PREMENSTRUAL SYNDROME (PMS)

Abdollahifard S, et al. The Effects of Vitamin B_1 on Ameliorating the Premenstrual Syndrome Symptoms. *Glob J Health Sci.* 2014 Jul 29;6(6):144-153. doi: 10.5539/gjhs.v6n6p144.

Canning S, et al. The Efficacy of Hypericum Perforatum (St John's Wort) for the Treatment of Premenstrual Syndrome: A Randomized, Double-Blind, Placebo-Controlled Trial. *CNS Drugs.* 2010 Mar;24(3):207-225.

Edilberto A, et al. Essential Fatty Acids for Premenstrual Syndrome and Their Effect on Pro-lactin and Total Cholesterol Levels: A Randomized, Double Blind, Placebo-Controlled Study. *Reprod Health.* 2011 Jan 17:8:2.

Ibrahim RM, et al. Effect of Vitex Agnus Custus (VAC) On Premenstrual Syndromes Among Nursing Students. *J Amer Sci.* 2012;8(4):144-153.

Jang SH, et al. Effects and Treatment Methods of Acupuncture and Herbal Medicine for Premenstrual Syndrome/Premenstrual Dysphoric Disorder: Systematic Review. *BMC Comp Altern Med.* 2014;14:11.

Nevatte T, et al. ISPMD Consensus on the Management of Premenstrual Disorders. *Arch Women's Mental Health.* 2013 Aug;16(4):279-291.

Sohrabi N, et al. Evaluation of the Effect of Omega-3 Fatty Acids in the Treatment of Premenstrual Syndrome: "A Pilot Trial." *Compl Ther Med.* 2013 June;21(3):141-146.

van Die MD, et al. Vitex Agnus-Castus Extracts for Female Reproductive Disorders: A Systematic Review of Clinical Trials. *Planta Medica.* 2013 May;79(7):562-575.

CHAPTER 53: SEXUAL DYSFUNCTION

Chiou YL, Lin CY. The Extract of Cordyceps Sinensis Inhibited Airway Inflammation by Blocking NF- b Activity. *Inflammation.* 2012 Jun;35(3):985-993.

Downey M. The Truth About Male and Female Sexual Dysfunction. *Life Extension Magazine*, October 2013. Web. Accessed July 20, 2015.

Kashani L, et al. Saffron for Treatment of Fluoxetine-Induced Sexual Dysfunction in Women: Randomized Double-Blind Placebo-Controlled Study. *Hum Psychopharmacol.* 2013 Jan;28(1):54-60.

Simon JA. Identifying and Treating Sexual Dysfunction in Postmenopausal Women: The Role of Estrogen. *J Womens Health* (Larchmt). 2011 Oct;20(10):1453-1465.

CHAPTER 54: SEXUALLY TRANSMITTED DISEASES

Blitshteyn, S. Postural Tachycardia Syndrome Following Human Papillomavirus Vaccination. *Eur J Neurol.* 2014 Jan;21(1):135-9. doi: 10.1111/ene.12272. Epub 2013 Sep 16.PMID: 24102827

Kim JH, et al. A Pilot Study to Investigate the Treatment of Cervical Human Papillomavirus Infection With Zinc-Citrate Compound (CIZAR). *Gyn Onc.* 2011;122:303–306.

McGovern C. HPV Vaccine Linked to Nervous System Disorder and Autoimmunity. Greenmedinfo.com, April 24, 2014. Web. Accessed July 20, 2015.

Tomljenovic L, et al. Human Papillomavirus (HPV) Vaccine Policy and Evidence-Based Medicine: Are They at Odds? *Ann Med.* 2013 Mar;45(2):182-193. doi: 10.3109/07853890. 2011.645353. Epub 2011 Dec 22.

Tomljenovic L et al. Postural Orthostatic Tachycardia With Chronic Fatigue After HPV Vaccination as Part of the "Autoimmune/Auto-inflammatory Syndrome Induced by Adjuvants." *J Invest Med High Impact Case Rep* 2014;2(1). doi: 10.1177/2324709614527812

REFERENCES FOR "CAUTION ABOUT THE VACCINES"

Herskovits B, Brand of the Year, February 1, 2007, *Pharmaceutical Executive Magazine*, http://pharamexec.findpharma.com/pharmexec/Articles/Brand-of-the-Year/ArticleStandard/Article/detal/401664, accessed December 26, 2011.

Zimm A and Blum J, Merck Promotes Cervical Cancer Shot by Publicizing Viral Cause, Bloomberg, May 26, 2006, http://www.bloomberg.com/apps/news?pid=2107001&sid =amVj.y3Eynz8, accessed December 27, 2011.

Pettypiece S and Zimm A, Merck Stops Campaign to Mandate Gardasil Vaccine Use, Bloomberg, February 20, 2007, http://www.bloomberg.com/apps/news?pid= 2107001&sid=atbGQuDYx7_c. accessed December 30, 2011.

Bevington C, Researcher, Diane Harper, Blasts Gardasil HPV Marketing, *Off The Radar*, http://offtheradar.co.nz/vaccines/53-researcher-diane-harper-blasts-gardasil-hpv-marketing.html, accessed September 15, 2011.

Siers-Poisson J, The Politics and PR of Cervical Cancer, Part III: Women in Government, Merck's Trojan Horse, *PR Watch*, July 18, 2007,http://prwatch.org/node/6232, accessed 12/27/11.

Levatin J, Why Do Doctors Push Vaccines? Tenpenny Integrative Health Center, December 24, 2011, http://tenpennyimc.com/category/vaccines/, accessed January 3, 2011.

Tomljenovic L and Shaw CA, Human Papillomavirus (HPV) Vaccine Policy and Evidence-Based Medicine: Are They at Odds? *Annals of Medicine*, December 22, 2011; http://informa-healthcare.com/doi/abs/10.3109/07853890.2011.645353, accessed December 23, 2011.

Interview with Tracy Wolf, January 3, 2012.

Interview with William Ronan, January 5, 2012.

Interview with Meryl Nass, January 5, 2012.

Cervical Cancer, American Cancer Society, Cancer.org/cancer/cervical cancer/detailed guide, http://www.cancer.org/Cancer/CervicalCancer/DetailedGuide/index, accessed October 15, 2011.

Rothman SM and Rothman DJ, Marketing HPV Vaccine: Implications for Adolescent Health and Medical Professionalism, *JAMA* 2009, 302(7); 781-786.

Tomljenovic L and Shaw CA, Human Papillomavirus (HPV) Vaccine Policy and Evidence-Based Medicine: Are They at Odds? *Annals of Medicine*, December 22, 2011; http://informa-healthcare.com/doi/abs/10.3109/07853890.2011.645353, accessed December 23, 2011.

Lenzer J, Should Boys be Given the HPV Vaccine? The Science is Weaker than the Marketing, *Discover Magazine*, November 14, 2011.

Tomljenovic L and Shaw CA, Human Papillomavirus (HPV) Vaccine Policy and Evidence-Based Medicine: Are They at Odds? *Annals of Medicine*, December 22, 2011; http://informa-healthcare.com/doi/abs/10.3109/07853890.2011.645353, accessed December 23, 2011.

Erickson N, Dr. Sin Hang Lee: A case study in ethics don't pay, Sane Vax Inc, http://sanevax.org/dr-sin-hang-lee-a-case-study-in-ethics-don%E2%80%99t-pay/, accessed October 15, 2011.

Human Papillomaviruses and Cancer, National Cancer Institute, September 7, 2011,http://www.cancer.gov/cancertopics/factsheet/Risk/HPV/print, accessed January 3, 2012.

Haug CJ, Human Papillomavirus Vaccination—Reasons for Caution, *New England Journal of Medicine*, August 21, 2008, 359; 861-862.

Examining the FDA's HPV Vaccine Records, *Judicial Watch Special Report*, June 30, 2008,http://www.judicialwatch.org/documents/2008/JWReportFDAhpvVaccineRecords.pdf, accessed September 16, 2011.

VAERS—Vaccine Adverse Event Reporting System. http://vaers.hhs.gov/index, accessed October 14, 2011.

Gardasil May Be Causing the Cancer It Pretends to Prevent." *Gaia Health*. N.p., 28 June 2012. Web. 22 Mar. 2013. http://gaia-health.com/gaia-blog/2012-06-28/gardasil-may-be-causing-the-cancer-it-pretends-to-prevent/

Rubin S, Blog Entry for October 2011, National Vaccine Information Center, posted December 29, 2011, http://medalerts.org/analysis/archives/394, accessed December 30, 2011.

Shilhavy, Brian. Merck Now Bribing College Girls to Complete Gardasil Vaccine, *Health Impact News*. http://healthimpactnews.com/2013/merck-now-bribing-college-girls-to-complete-gardasil-vaccine/N.p., 28 Feb. 2013. Web. 25 Mar. 2013. .

Siers-Poisson J, The Politics and PR of Cervical Cancer, Part One: Setting the Stage, *PR Watch*, http://prwatch.org/node/6186, accessed December 27, 2011.

Englund C, India has suspended the use of HPV Gardasil vaccines due to deaths, *American Chronicle*, April 11, 2010,http://www.americanchronicle.com/articles/view/150425, accessed December 27, 2011.

England C, France Says "No" as They Ban Gardasil Ads, Sane Vax, Inc., January 11, 2011, http://offtheradar.co.nz/vaccines/224-france-says-qnoq-as-they-ban-gardasil-ads.htm, accessed December 28, 2011.

Siegrist C et al, Human Papilloma Virus Immunization in Adolescent and Young Adults: A Cohort Study to Illustrate What Events Might be Mistaken for Adverse Reactions, *Pediatric Infect Dis J*. 2007 Nov;26(11):979-84.

Grant B, Merck Published Fake Journal, *The Scientist*, 30th April 2009,http://classic.the-scientist.com/blog/display/55671/, accessed December 15, 2011

CHAPTER 55: STROKE

Cassidy A, et al. Dietary Flavonoids and Risk of Stroke in Women. *Stroke*. Published online before print February 23, 2012. doi: 10.1161/STROKEAHA.111.637835

Kastorini CM, et al. Adherence to the Mediterranean Diet in Relation to Ischemic Stroke Nonfatal Events in Nonhypercholesterolemic and Hypercholesterolemic Participants: Results of a Case/Case-Control Study. *Angiology*. 2012 Oct;63(7):509-515. doi: 10.1177/0003319711427392. Epub 2011 Dec 5.

Oskouei DS, et al. The Effect of Ginkgo biloba on Functional Outcome of Patients with Acute Ischemic Stroke: A Double-blind, Placebo-controlled, Randomized Clinical Trial. *J Stroke Cerebrovasc Dis*. Published Online: July 22, 2013. doi: http://dx.doi.org/ 10.1016/j.jstroke-cerebrovasdis.2013.06.010

Oude Griep LM, et al. Colors of Fruit and Vegetables and 10-Year Incidence of Stroke. *Stroke*. 2011;42:3190-3195. Published online before print September 15, 2011. doi: 10.1161/STROKEAHA.110.611152

Samieri C, et al. Olive Oil Consumption, Plasma Oleic Acid, and Stroke Incidence: The Three-City Study. *Neurology*. Published online before print June 15, 2011. doi: 10.1212/WNL.0b013e318220abeb.

CHAPTER 56: THYROID DISEASE

Kvacheniuk AN, Kvacheniuk EL. The Use of Phytotherapy for Treatment of Thyroid Diseases. *Lik Sprava*. 2012 Apr-Jun;(3-4):99-104.

CHAPTER 57: URINARY INCONTINENCE

Huang AJ, et al. A Group-Based Yoga Therapy Intervention for Urinary Incontinence in Women: A Pilot Randomized Trial. *Female Pelvic Med Reconstr Surg.* 2014 May-Jun;20(3):147-154.

CHAPTER 58: URINARY TRACT INFECTIONS AND INFLAMMATIONS

Altarac S, Papes D. Use of D-Mannose in Prophylaxis of Recurrent Urinary Tract Infections (UTIs) in Women. *BJU Int.* 2014;113:9-10.

de Llano DG, et al. Anti-Adhesive Activity of Cranberry Phenolic Compounds and Their Microbial-Derived Metabolites against Uropathogenic Escherichia coli in Bladder Epithelial Cell Cultures. *Int J Mol Sci.* 2015 May 27;16(6):12119-12130. doi: 10.3390/ijms160612119.

Gaby A. Editorial, Dr. Wright Does It Again: D-Mannose for UTI Prophylaxis Validated in a Clinical Trial. *Townsend Letter*, May 2014. Web. Accessed July 20, 2015.

Jepson RG, et al. Cranberries for Preventing Urinary Tract Infections. Cochrane Database Syst Rev. 2012 Oct 17;10:CD001321. doi: 10.1002/14651858.CD001321.pub5.

Kranj ec B, et al. D-Mannose Powder for Prophylaxis of Recurrent Urinary Tract Infections in Women: A Randomized Clinical Trial. *World J Urol.* 2014;Feb;32(1):79-84. doi: 10.1007/s00345-013-1091-6. Epub 2013 Apr 30.

CHAPTER 60: VARICOSE VEINS

Clachar S. Reducing Dangerous Varicose Veins with Phlebotonics, *Life Extension Magazine*, May 2012. Web. Accessed July 20, 2015.

CHAPTER 61: VISION PROBLEMS

Eye Health. Life Extension website. Accessed July 29, 2015.

Munch IC, et al. Precursors of Age-Related Macular Degeneration: Associations With Physical Activity, Obesity, and Serum Lipids in the Inter99 Eye Study. *Invest Ophthalmol Vis Sci.* 2013;54:3932-3940.

Ohguro H, et al. Two-Year Randomized, Placebo-Controlled Study of Black Currant Anthocyanins on Visual Field in Glaucoma. *Ophthalmologica.* 2012;228:26-35.

Tanaka S, et al. Fruit Intake and Incident Diabetic Neuropathy With Type 2 Diabetes. *Epidemiol.* 2013 Mar;24:204-211.

Williams PT. Walking and Running are Associated With Similar Reductions in Cataract Risk. *Med Sci Sport Exercise.* 2013 Jun;45:1089-1096.

Chapter 66

Testimonials

A BETTER ATHLETE

RICH V.

I came into a support group with long-term negative habits. I eliminated alcohol and cigarettes from my life years ago, but I did eat flesh foods. I indulged in negative emotions, and I dwelled on the worst of a given situation while ignoring any positives. My home was full of objects that I considered to be junk. My self-esteem and energy were low, and there were signs of aging on my skin. I have made progress through vegan living, support group lectures, and detoxification. I detoxed my body and mind; this improved my skin tone. I will not be in the company of negative, complaining people. I post affirmations on my mirror and in my car. They are very beneficial. The supplements have given me new health and vitality. I lost weight and now run 8 miles, not the 5 miles I used to. My sense of smell is improving. New hair grows in with fewer grays. I no longer feel a slump in energy at 3 p.m. each day. My self-esteem is blossoming, and I sing and perform again. My home is uncluttered, and my future priorities are on my agenda.

ACID REFLUX

HOZANA B.

Before: I was slightly overweight and had acute heartburn, acid reflux, and stress and anger toward my teenage son. I am a massage therapist, and I wanted to change my life and learn proper nutrition, so I joined Gary's support group.
Now: I've lost 8 lbs and now have the body I've always wanted. I take organic, vegetarian juices. I no longer have acid reflux. My mind is clearer. I have a successful

relationship with my son, and I handle coworkers without anger. I exercise by powerwalking and my body is alive and energetic. I've uncluttered my mind and my home. Now, I am more open and accepting, less critical, more optimistic and helpful to people.

DOUG

No more heartburn

I was scheduled for gallbladder surgery to relieve chronic heartburn. My pre-operation EKG was abnormal, and I had a quadruple bypass. I decided to change everything and started adopting Gary Null's protocol. I lost weight, have no more heartburn, and enjoy a good sense of health. I am on a strictly vegan protocol.

ADRENAL WEAKNESS

ELEANOR H.

Before the support group, I had physical disorders. My adrenal and thyroid functions were low, leaving me exhausted, stressed, cold, and tired. I did not have energy to exercise. The protocol reversed these problems. I have not had a sinus infection in ages. My hypoglycemia is practically gone. I wake up early without stress, feeling happy and alert. I no longer use prescription medications. My body will heal itself.

AGING WELL

GLORIA, 78 years old

I came into a support group with several physical ailments. I was somewhat overweight. My hair was graying. I had macular degeneration, hypoglycemia, periodontal disease, varicose veins in my legs, and a spinal curvature that, I was told, could become degenerative. I joined a support group. I shed 10 lbs and am filled with renewed self-confidence. My sparse hair is fuller and growing back in a dark color. There is an improvement in the macular degeneration problem I feared would be permanent. I do not have hypoglycemia or periodontal disease. The leg varicosity decreased, and my spinal curvature feels less acute. My amalgam fillings were removed. I returned to school for a degree, and best of all, my family is proud of these reversals. They prepare my special protocol foods when I visit, and they respect my choices.

WILMA & MYRON, 75 years old each

We were not happy with the symptoms of getting old. We both had memory difficulties. I did not like to be a homebody, and I wanted this part of our lives to be active. There is so much to experience and learn. We joined a support group and feel we have reversed aging. We follow the protocol and noticed we have increased brain power. It is sad watching our friends fail physically. They are closed to detoxification and diet changes. We are the only couple in our group not taking medications. I study piano and am writing a book. This is a wonderful time of life.

FRAN, 67 years old

I joined a health support group and followed Gary Null's protocol when obvious and unpleasant signs of aging became too uncomfortable. My skin was sagging and moles grew on it. There were dark age spots on my body. Energy decreased. My LDL and HSL elevated. My hair changed color and I felt my mental function was slowing. The group was a total lifestyle enhancement. The people were optimistic. I influenced them. They influenced me. Today my skin is tight and great; I am more youthful in looks and attitude. The moles fell off. Age spots are gone. My new hair growth is dark brown. LDL and HDL went to zero risk. I have energy galore and my mental function improved from the protocol. I feel absolutely wonderful.

GLORIA, 73 years old

I was hypoglycemic. I used dairy and wheat, and ate flesh foods. My concentration and mental clarity were poor. My energy was low and I suffered from many upper respiratory infections. I joined the year-and-a-half support group because I was a college senior and required extra energy to complete my degree. Today things are quite different. I lost eight pounds and am now size 4 or 6. I feel energetic and do not experience frequent upper respiratory infections. My physician confirmed I do not need stronger glasses. My skin has fewer wrinkles and appears to be brighter. My hair is thicker. I use juices throughout the day without a desire for meals. I learned to honor myself and develop solutions for daily problems by keeping a positive outlook. I am an active walker. I convinced my daughter to use an alternative physician for my granddaughter who was diagnosed psychotic. The child returned to school within two weeks.

RUTH, 75 years old

I have always been a busy person with an active career but I was plagued with frequent illnesses, especially upper respiratory infections. I participated in a health support group two years ago. Before that my diet was quite unhealthy. I ate flesh foods, dairy, sugar, desserts, confections, and breads without regard for health or weight gain. I did not exercise. It was time to correct this imbalance of career and family versus frequent illnesses. I wanted my energy back and decided to improve my life. The initial phase of the detox was interesting. Eliminating "comfort" foods was difficult but so were my options. I stayed with the program. It was uncomfortable at times in restaurants. My friends devoured their toxic food while commenting on my fish and vegetable plate. My hair and skin greatly improved. I have no more upper respiratory infections. Today I am a person holding the tools for healthy aging. My eating companions are rapidly getting old. I work several days a week. I use a stationary bike and lift weights. It's wonderful to hear this positive feedback. My grandson is proud of his attractive, vital grandmother. I am proud of myself.

HELEN, 60 years old

I've been listening to Gary for 25 years. I use Gary's website and read his books. I follow the protocol. I decided I could use a boost of health and joined the retreat group. The impact was tremendous. I was able to understand myself, the relationships in my life, and my fears better. I began power walking, doing yoga exercises, and establishing new social contacts. The eye health lecture was informative. This was a new space for me. The chiropractic treatments were healing. I never felt uncomfortable about my body size. I made new friends, all of them enlightened.

DOROTHEA M., 67 years old

A new beginning at 67 years of age. I am so grateful to you for showing me how to improve life for myself and others. You opened my life to the joy of exploration for myself and others. I now realize there is a world of joy to learn about as I follow my bliss. Thank you for leading me to a healthy body, mind, and spirit.

FLORENCE H.

I wanted to live a healthy life but could not keep on track. I lacked motivation and discipline. I developed both of these skills when I entered a support group. I learned to exercise three times a week, and I began to enjoy and make this my personal routine. I lost weight and feel energetic. I follow the protocol with enjoyment. I foresee a healthier and more vital future.

DAVID Y.

The anti-aging program gave me a pathway toward life expansion. I am happy to be away from the typical American diet. The support group taught me strategies for coping when I am perceived to be different. My body is cleaner. I understand that there are other paths on the road of life.

MARY ANN C.

I began to display the signs of aging. My weight went up with my fatigue, my hair was weaker, and my skin was wrinkling. I was pessimistic about losing my looks. I was in pain because of herniated disks in my neck. I noticed my muscle tone was not as it was just a few years ago. I was determined to turn these conditions around and joined a support group after I heard group members speak about their positive experiences. The group experience was exciting. The group participants were wonderful, optimistic, and helpful to me and each other. We were a family. I lost 20 lbs and have fewer wrinkles today. My hair is healthier. I have less pain in my neck, and with exercise, my muscle tone improved. I do not get colds or flu, and I feel stronger, calmer, and more positive. It's a miracle, but not really. It's cleaning out, building up, and keeping to the protocol.

MARCIA, 77 years old

I was sad about entering old age. I could not recognize myself, with my overweight problem and white, thin hair that was falling out. The hair under my arms and my pubic hair fell out after menopause. I lacked energy and had no sensual emotions. The Gary Null protocol has changed all that and changed my emotional attitude. Just seeing my hair growing back thick and in its original color returned my femininity. My body hair has grown back, too. My libido returned as it was in my early 40s. My energy is phenomenal, and I sleep only four to five hours a night. This is a clean, healthy, youth-preserving program, and it gave me back my life and womanhood.

ALSTON D., 90 years old and self-sufficient
Before

I retired from the Merchant Marines at age 65. I have always been very active and considered myself to be healthy, but considered my future health. I heard Gary Null on the radio and began to read books on health and nutrition.

Now

I follow a vegetarian diet, and I juice. I use a rebounder every morning. I get on the train and travel to Manhattan to buy supplements. I do not see many people my age these days. Most of them have caretakers and are dependent. I am totally self-sufficient; I care for my home and shop, wash my clothes, and even take my curtains down to wash and replace them alone. I do not need anyone to take care of me. I can accomplish my tasks alone. I believe my diet and nutritional supplements are responsible for maintaining my health.

BRIAN C.

I listened to support group members on the radio and decided I would change my life and my body. I had many symptoms of early aging: graying hair, eye-color change, nails growing slowly, scars not healing, hypertension, pock marks on my face, eczema, tension after years in the corporate world. My personal relationships were not going well. I followed the detox protocol, attending meetings, to cleanse my body physically and emotionally, and the results are wonderful. My blood pressure is normal, my skin condition is gone, my hair is growing in blond (my childhood color), and my hairline is reversing. My eyes are returning to their blue color. My nails grow quickly, and the wound scars have disappeared. I left the corporate world, and I find my relationships and attitudes are happier.

ALLERGIES

PETER

As a child my food sensitivities were treated with antibiotics and medications to no avail. I was weak in every aspect of my being, and pale with dark circles under my eyes. Within two weeks on Gary Null's allergy protocol, I felt remarkably better. Nine months later, I find I can tolerate most all foods. My thinking is clear, and my moodiness, depression, lethargy, and poor complexion have reversed. I feel vital, healthy, and alive. I anticipate studying Oriental Medicine, and I continue research on internal energy.

KURT H.

Before

I was fairly healthy. I had seasonal allergies and took Celdane and Claritin. I had digestive problems: food would often get trapped in my esophagus. I drank a lot of caffeine. Then I listened to Gary's radio program. I decided to become vegetarian. I took supplements. I increased my exercising. I went into Gary's one-and-a-half-year detox program (with the wellness support group).

Now

I sleep less. My digestive problem went away. I do not get colds anymore. I have eliminated caffeine and alcohol.

ALAN S.

If anyone was ready to rearrange his life, it was me. I was under heavy stress and felt totally fatigued by midday. I developed allergies. Life was about hurry hurry-hurry and making money. I did not want to continue at this pace. I entered a support group and embarked on a life-enhancing program. The protocol addresses the physical, spiritual, and emotional self. It is life-enhancing. My body feels lighter and cleaner. I have energy all day. I handle stressful situations without internalizing. I discovered that I do not need as many "things" for happiness. Although I make less money, I gain a great deal more on another level. I am exploring life confident. If failures come, they are not major complications. I read *Who Are You, Really?* and discovered I am a dynamic assertive and should not work with others. I am now creating a business venture.

JOANNE, 64 years old

I was diagnosed with chronic fatigue syndrome. I was always exhausted and had many allergies. I did not follow any food plan and was a coffee drinker. I listened to Gary Null on the radio and read *Who Are You, Really?* When an allergy support group opened up, I joined. At that time I took time away from work to recover. I have had excellent results following Gary's protocol. I need less sleep, and am alert and aware of nutrition. I no longer drink coffee. My allergies are practically neither nonexistent nor are signs of chronic fatigue present. Writing forgiveness letters relieved the weight of anger I held and I detached from a painful past. I live in the present. Uncluttering was unpleasant but helped me think clearly. I am actualizing my sense of community responsibility. I now give "professionalism and quality of life" seminars. My husband is supportive of my new lifestyle.

ALZHEIMER'S DISEASE

EGBERT

I was overjoyed to come into a Reversing the Aging support group. My memory was getting worse; I left my car keys in the trunk lock, and my car was stolen. I was not organic, but had been juicing and using supplements for a year before beginning the protocol. Once I used organic produce and juice, I began to feel stronger. I did not get sore throats since I began taking vitamin C at night. I decided to work less. A short time later, I dated a man for the first time since my divorce eight years earlier. I felt happy and prayed for the return of my car. A short time later, I spotted it while taking a long walk on an alternative trail. This increased my spiritual belief. I am building a cohesive relationship between my boyfriend, son, and myself. I sleep better, exercise, and work on an eating plan to prevent overeating.

APPEARANCE

FRAN M., 65 years old

Before

Moles on skin—skin beginning to sag. Dark age spots on body. Decreased energy. LDL. Hair color changing. Mental function slowing.

Now

Skin tighter. More youthful in looks and attitude. Moles fell off. Age spots gone. New hair growth dark brown. LDL normalized. Energetic. Mental function improved.

BILL

I am no longer sluggish and feel stronger both mentally and physically. I sleep less. My face is more colorful, much less pale. I lost 10 pounds and have better tone in my muscles. People comment on how much my appearance has improved.

ARTHRITIS

JOHN

I developed psoriatic arthritis 30 years ago. I underwent surgery to fuse my right wrist. My knees and neck were deteriorating, so I used heavy medications and over-the-counter analgesics. My blood pressure became elevated and I was advised to change careers. My daughter motivated me to join a health support group. Today, I am vegan and eat no sugar or wheat. After I began the protocol and juicing, I became pain-free in four weeks. I take no more medications, and all swelling subsided. My doctor commented that the condition of my knee joints is the best he has observed, and my blood pressure is normal. I am able to take long walks. I have reclaimed my life. Neighbors who have observed my improvement now follow the protocol. One couple, a diabetic and his wife who has multiple sclerosis, report physical improvements. By following the protocol, my cousin lost 10 lbs in two weeks and no longer has heartburn.

PATRICK

My recall and memory is sharp. My skin is clear. I have less nasal mucus, an improved resting heart rate. My tonsil size decreased. No longer do I have dark circles under my eyes and pain from peripheral neuropathy in both legs has diminished as has arthritic pain. I have not been ill since I started the program.

MARIA Q.

I had fatigue and edema. I could not tolerate heat and had migraine headaches, arthritis, and an irregular heartbeat. I lost 15 pounds, and now my energy is very high and so is my optimism.

ELOISE H.

My arthritis and knee stiffness subsided. Inflammation and swelling subsided. My blood pressure is significantly lower. Cholesterol levels are reduced to 159. I lost six pounds, and all my pants fit me. I sleep better and enjoy abundant energy and a sense of well-being.

ALLEN C.

Since I began Gary's protocol, I lost 10 pounds. My arthritis is greatly alleviated, particularly in my knees. I see a considerable improvement in my chronic fatigue condition. I have good energy and require less sleep. My blood pressure dropped, and I now have a positive outlook on life.

HYACINTH

My cholesterol was high. I had dizzy spells. Arthritic fingers, skin and hair showed signs of early aging. My skin is firmer and young looking; the cholesterol level has dropped. My hair is growing back; my nails are firm and pink. The arthritis in my fingers diminished, and I do not have dizzy spells. I think clearly, and I am alert.

CAROL J

Before

Overweight. Low energy. Beginning to get wrinkled skin. Arthritis. Would get involved in negative situations. Liked to eat until very full.

Now

Lost 60 pounds. More stamina. Skin less wrinkled. Arthritis gone. Will not acknowledge negative people or situations. Positive outlook. Do not overreact anymore.

BEATRICE

My arthritis often prevented me from walking. My hair was thinning, and I had a fungal infection on my right heel. I barely had enough energy to get through my daily tasks. I noticed ridges on my fingernails. When I compare myself now to what I was one-and-a-half-years ago, I see a woman without fear and doubt, with hope and optimism, constructing a new life. I have more inspiring dreams than I did in the past, even though my path, at the moment, is not truly constructive. My hair is growing in healthier, the nail ridges have lessened, and I do not have arthritic pain. The heel fungus disappeared. My energy level is high. The homework questions gave me the opportunity to deal with issues directly. Just thinking of an answer redirected my life. My future is a good place. No one can push my buttons anymore.

CAROL J.

I listened to *Natural Living* before entering a support group. I had been to Paradise Gardens [where Gary Null hosts retreats in Naples, Florida] twice, but was not totally vegetarian. Being overweight most of my life caused painful arthritis. My turning point came attending Florida retreats and joining a support group. I quickly adapted to the new lifestyle but hardly exercised. It was when I began yoga lessons that power walking tempted me. It caused joint pain until arthritic symptoms subsided. My energy increased when wheat and dairy were eliminated, and juicing increased. At this point, I became a serious power walker. I lost 15 pounds the first month on the protocol and felt terrific.

Doing support group homework kept me committed to future goals. I moved to a new home, which is uncluttered, and was satisfied to disassociate with the people I felt were obnoxious. I lost 75 pounds. I now belong to a rowing team and race walk with the Gary Null Running and Walking Club.

FELICIA P.

Before

Arthritis. Joint pain. Overweight. Anxious. Depressed. Stressed because son using drugs. Fatigue.

Now

No longer have arthritis or joint pain. Increased energy. Sleep less. Look great. Lost 20 lbs. No longer anxious and depressed. Finding connection to self. Uncluttering. Detaching from son.

TARA

My arthritis has improved and my joints are less painful. Shingles and genital herpes are gone. My allergies have improved and my periods are more regular. I have very little lower back pain and I am not constipated.

KARINA

I was quite ill before I learned how to detoxify. My skin condition was unsightly, my gums bled, and I had neuropathy in my hands and knees, pain from arthritis and kidney disease. Floaters and retinopathy caused slight problems. Tests showed abnormal thyroid levels, and my blood pressure and cholesterol were high. Today, after completing the support group, following Gary's directions, and carefully going with it day by day, I no longer have bad skin. My teeth and gums are fine. I no longer have pain from neuropathy or arthritis. Tests determined that my kidney disease is reduced. My eye problems have disappeared, My thyroid tests read normal, as do my blood pressure and cholesterol blood tests. I have a normal life, and I am thankful for the experience, education and caring I received.

BELL'S PALSY REVERSED

DOLLY F.

Low energy corrected

Before

Although we considered ourselves nutritionally aware and healthy for seniors, my husband and I felt something was missing. We knew our lives and health could improve, but we found no satisfaction in traditional guidelines. We did not want our vitality to diminish as we aged. After listening to Gary Null on the radio, we decided to join one of the first Reversing the Aging Support Groups.

Now

It was easy following the protocol cold turkey. We had vitamin drips. We eliminated all meat, dairy, and chicken from our diet. We are now organic and vegetarian, and we use air, water, and shower filters. We have magnetic appliances. Our amalgam fillings were removed, and we make our home healthier by removing our shoes at the door. When a neurologist confirmed I had Bell's palsy, I had a consult with Gary. We meditate, practice yoga, and run. Our physician daughter now runs. I am a nurse teacher and busier than ever. We feel great juicing and using green, red, and protein powders. My Bell's palsy symptoms subsided within 10 days on the protocol. Our energy is strong, and our bodies feel vital and healthy from the juices and healthy food. We use alternative physicians for diagnosis and treatment if problems occur. This program was very successful for us.

BLADDER—INFECTIONS & BLADDER CONTROL

MILDRED L.

I entered a support group to rid my body of an acute bladder infection that had taken over my life. I sought a natural approach. I did not have good energy and required long hours of sleep each night. I was overly sensitive and easily hurt. I did not stand up for myself. My family was critical of me. This continued during my marriage. I do not have a bladder infection today and can go to museums, on automobile trips, anywhere I wish without running to a bathroom. I learned to appreciate myself and burst into song without realizing it. Finally, I told my family and my husband, "Enough." I will not tolerate their nonsense. Not only did I reverse the emotional and physical conditions in my life, but my husband takes care not to hurt my feelings. I speak my mind and challenge people. Uncluttering opened valuable space in my home and life.

BLEEDING ULCERS

SUSIE

The night my son brought me to the emergency room, I was told I would not have awakened the next day. I had three bleeding ulcers, and I felt angry at my illness. The anemia caused me extreme fatigue, and the daily weight loss I experienced was somewhat of a joke to me. I just did not take it seriously. I was told I might lose 30 percent of my stomach if the condition persisted. I was sent home with medications. Being a vegetarian and researching medical conditions, I used only one medication for my thyroid. I was very stressed without an out. My children suggested I listen to *Natural Living*. The first day I tuned in, Gary mentioned aloe and cabbage juice for ulcers. I bought a juicer and aloe, and I drank the combination. All medication was discarded that day.

Eventually, I joined a support group. Aloe, cabbage juice, and sometimes sauerkraut soothed my problem, but it was the green juices and elimination of dairy, wheat, and other products that really built me up. I am totally organic, vegan, and healthy. My endoscopy revealed no ulcers. I think that is remarkable. I lost 15 lbs on the protocol, and my body began to reshape. At this point, never straying from the program, I have reversed the aging and am emotionally stronger. I made peace with myself and the past by journal writing and power walking, and I enjoy a happy family life with my children and animals. The many support group participants I meet are wonderful, happy, and free people. I am one of them.

BLOOD PRESSURE / HIGH CHOLESTEROL

MICHAEL

I was diagnosed with high blood sugar several years ago. On medication my pressure was 140/80. After being here for two days, experiencing the yoga, the exercise class, the delicious food prepared by chefs, by Wednesday I checked my blood pressure and it was 128/80 without medication. So I'm really glad that I was able to come here and have this life-transforming experience. And I want to recommend this to anyone who wants to get healthy and live a good lifestyle.

STANLEY

I feel like I did 10 years ago. I have reduced blood pressure. I have a better ability to concentrate. I have increased physical strength. I have increased stamina, and I have an increased interest in sex.

JOHN B.

My blood pressure was elevated. It was difficult getting out of bed in the morning. My energy was low, and I felt tired upon awakening. My tongue was coated, and I was slightly overweight. I followed the protocol without question. My blood pressure is lower, I feel great in the morning, my tongue is not coated, and I lost about 8 pounds without dieting. I see improvement in my hair and skin, and acknowledge the protocol to be life restoring.

TOBY

My blood pressure stabilized. I was hospitalized for a diagnosis of appendicitis. I stopped medication and began drinking green juices and taking supplements. A CAT scan two weeks later ruled out appendicitis. I lost 15 pounds. I am less fearful of trying new things and more willing to work toward creating future projects.

NELLY P.

I was slightly overweight. My blood pressure and cholesterol were elevated. I had large fibroids and was given a possible cancer warning by my physician. Excess stress caused chest pain diagnosed as possible angina. Business tension caused worry as I tackled difficult tasks to fulfill my mission helping people in Peru. My husband and I adopted two children but tension affected my family. Then I watched Gary on PBS. I joined a support group and lost 15 pounds. My cholesterol and blood pressure normalized. My family is now vegan. Medical examinations confirmed that I no longer have fibroids. I learned power walking at Paradise Gardens, and I am energetic and patient at home with my children, less of a perfectionist, and I handle stress with humor. I work out in a gym. Friends admire my lovely skin. Life is fulfilling and easier.

GARY L.

My blood pressure improved significantly. My triglycerides dropped to the normal range. I raised my good cholesterol and lowered the bad cholesterol. My homocysteine levels are better than before. I am less depressed and have a more positive outlook on life, with more energy. I also lost 15 lbs so far.

ROSE

My blood pressure shot up. That was just one of the frightening aspects of aging that hit me. I was tired during the day and wanted my vitality back. The best way was to go into a Gary Null Health Support Group. The body is remarkable. In a short amount of time my blood pressure normalized. I feel much more energetic as well.

BOB, 80 years old

I seem to be one of those people who had to get sick before seeking a healthier lifestyle. Before I heard of Gary Null's support groups I suffered headaches, allergies, and several colds and flus a year. Cholesterol and blood pressure were elevated. I ate junk food, pretending everything would work out. Personality-wise I was tense and often irritable. Something had to change; I wanted that thing to be me. I followed the protocol carefully. After a week my energy returned, I slept less, my headaches were gone, and blood pressure and cholesterol levels dropped. I am calmer and more patient, far less irritable. My wife of forty years was a great support. We both benefited with my new health and are thankful we participated in this life-changing process.

MARILYN

Cholesterol dropped from 300 to 215. I have experienced more loving feelings toward my husband, and less anger about taking care of him. I am more understanding and less fearful regarding the future.

DIDI

1 increased my body fat to a healthier level and enjoy sex again. My cholesterol dropped 50 points and HDL went up. No longer crave sweets.

RUDY

Chronic pains in my penis finally dissipated. I think this pain was related to the toxic state I was in prior to the program. My waistline has been greatly reduced, and my muscle mass has increased. I actually began having a thirtyish body instead of a 47-year old body. I have more energy, and my premature gray hair is more natural and brown. I had a fungus on my toes for years, which is beginning to clear up. My joints are moving more freely, my skin is smoother, and I have lessened my propensity for worry and reduced the fear level. I feel more self-assured and confident. This program has helped me become more centered, and enhanced my belief that this [form of natural] happiness is so important. This class is also beginning to restore my belief in spirituality.

NELLI

My blood pressure was 140/90, and cholesterol read 268. I had large fibroids and was warned about cancer. Excess stress created chest pains and angina. I lost 15 pounds. My cholesterol is now 198 and blood pressure is 120/80. My last medical exam was excellent, no trace of fibroids.

I power walk and feel energetic. People compliment my healthy skin. I handle stress with humor and do not react to other people's indifference. All and all, life is healthier.

RONA

I joined the Reversing Aging Group, because I was unfit. I had extremely high blood pressure, and I suffered from occasional swelling of the soles of the feet, which had been diagnosed as an unspecified allergic reaction. Every afternoon I became tired, and I had chest pain. Now, my skin tone has improved, I have stronger nails, my blood pressure is lower, my stamina and fitness level have improved, and I don't have chest pain anymore. The allergic reaction has not occurred since I joined the support group. I am no longer tired in the afternoon. My behavior has also changed. Before I joined the group, I was very angry and stressed, tended to fight fire with fire, and was very confrontational. Now I am a much happier person. This has been noted by numerous colleagues. I no longer allow people to push my buttons. I have a more positive outlook, and I am proactive in attaining career objectives.

GLEN C.

I wanted an improved future without illness. My cholesterol was high and I had great pain from herniated discs, which prevented exercise. I was a compulsive eater and chose an unhealthy diet. I snored and simply did not care for myself. When Gary Null talked about a support group on his radio show, I did not hold back and joined in 2000. I was a student again. The entire time was amazing to me. I learned why my body had problems and what I can do to reverse them. I understood the impact of mediation and forgiveness. I lost 18 pounds and am pain free. I exercise three times a week, practice martial arts, and do not snore. I recover quickly from illness, and feel happy and alert.

IRENE, 66 years old

I lived in a very large home surrounded by years and years of lovely but nonessential objects. It was difficult keeping up with chores. My husband and I lived alone because our children are adults. I was overweight. I had high blood pressure, cardiac arrhythmia, high cholesterol, weak nails, and low energy. I felt this huge, cluttered space around me. I thought that it would be difficult changing my life. I grew accustomed to the way things were but I wanted to be free of physical disabilities and I wanted to feel healthy. I joined a support group and lost thirty pounds. Changes came week by week. My blood pressure normalized. My cholesterol lowered. Energy began to move me mentally and physically. Eventually my arrhythmia ceased. We sold our large home and gave our family the unessential, nostalgic items. We now live in a four-room home. We are much happier and I feel wonderful. I let go of objects and let our future in.

CHARLES, 69 years old

My journey toward improving my health began when I attended a Gary Null seminar. I worked in construction as an ironworker and had several accidents. During my younger years I held several jobs at a time and developed hypertension. It was time to rebuild my physical system. I considered my energy to be adequate for an aging man. I gradually investigated organic foods and vegetarian replacements for flesh foods. My health is maintained with supplements, lifting weights, gardening, and drinking power shakes with red and green powders. I still work in building and construction and just built a playhouse for my grandchildren. Listening to health programs on the radio gave me some information; however, following today's healthier lifestyle and taking proper products supplies me with more energy than I have ever had. I bounce back easily from exhaustion. Except for a constant knee condition, I do not feel the consequences of falling off buildings. I do not have hypertension anymore. My family does not follow or cooperate with my food preparation. I prepare my meals separately and enjoy them. Hopefully, one day my grandchildren will open to this healthy concept. I feel younger than my sixty-nine years and look forward to a happy future.

LILLIAN R.

I have had remarkable results since going on Gary Null's detoxification protocol. My energy level is greatly increased. My blood pressure dropped to a stable, measurable reading. I am no longer constipated. I am totally motivated to heal myself, body and mind, and to bring joy into my life.

MICHAEL C.

The results of my following Gary's protocol are phenomenal. I lost 23 lbs and trimmed over 5 inches from my waist. I eliminated two blood pressure medications. I sleep at least an hour less, and I experience a strong feeling of well-being. My rate of hair loss decreased. I have strength and energy. My joint aches and back pains disappeared. I breathe easier, and my sinuses have cleared up.

JESSIE, 86 years old

I am an eighty-six-year-old woman. My blood pressure was high. My energy was very low. I felt old. My hands were full of age spots. I felt quite discouraged. I joined a Gary Null support group. Once I felt the impact of group interaction I began to feel optimistic about my future. I keep to Gary's protocol. My emotional and physical changes are wonderful. I feel younger and free. I eat organically; I juice and exercise multiple times a week. My blood pressure has lowered and energy has increased. The age spots are lighter. My physical improvements created emotional improvements. I am grateful for this second chance.

RUTH K.

To date, I can happily report wonderful changes on Gary's protocol. I lost 18 lbs, and my blood pressure returned to normal. My energy level increased, and I am not sluggish after meals. Feeling and thinking in a positive mode has increased my self-esteem; I feel good about myself. I did not regain weight, because I am determined to continue the program.

BOB

I had many allergies and frequent upper-respiratory infections. My life was unmanageable, and my stress was overwhelming. My blood pressure and cholesterol were elevated. I heard about Gary Null's support groups and detoxification. I needed to change and decided to enter a group as soon as one was formed. That was the beginning of the best part of my life. My energy built, my headaches stopped, and my cholesterol and blood pressure lowered. I have a new body from exercising, using weights, doing qi gong, and deep breathing. I feel calm, more patient, and less irritable. I love my food and progressive life.

ALICE

I was concerned about my health. My blood pressure and cholesterol were elevated. I had a stressful life due to being mentally fatigued and could not control these feelings. I suffered an acid reflux condition that I assumed was caused by my job. My body was falling apart. I detoxed and carefully followed Gary's protocol. I felt stronger each week and released stress each day. My blood pressure is now normal, my digestion is improved, and I lost fifteen pounds. I do aerobics at home in the morning, yoga during evening hours, bike, walk, and run. My uncluttered environment and journal writing give me a new constructive outlet.

ROSALIND

My blood pressure shot up. That was just one of the frightening aspects of aging that hit me. I was tired during the day and wanted my vitality back. The best way was to go into a Gary Null group. He always used the term "reversing the aging." They were golden words to a fatigued woman. I joined the study. The body is remarkable. Mine immediately responded to the green juices. I eliminated dairy, flesh foods, wheat, and everything Gary and Luanne suggested. In a short amount of time, my blood pressure normalized. I felt more energetic, and after a while, I realized I was younger than my contemporaries. I now exercise five times a week. I was held back by an automobile accident and had to eat hospital food for a while. I recovered quickly, thanks to my healthy immune system. I came home and immediately went back on the protocol.
There is no other choice, and I love it.

PAUL P.

I wanted to feel healthy. Medications did not do the trick, they could not make me healthy, only relieve discomfort for a short period of time. I had high blood pressure and frequent muscle pulls. If a health support group worked for so many other people, I decided to give it a try. The dietary changes created physical improvements in three days. I follow the protocol and writing exercises. I listen to the lectures, and then one day I am told my blood pressure medication is cut in half. I no longer have muscle pulls. The spiritual aspect of our teachings had an impact, and I decided to slow my pace and unclutter my home. It made me feel free. I now consider myself as important as my clients, and I am beginning to understand myself.

NELLIE

My blood pressure was 140/90, and cholesterol read 268. I had large fibroids and was warned about cancer. Excess stress created chest pains and angina. I lost 15 pounds. My cholesterol is now 198 and blood pressure is 120/80. My last medical exam was excellent, no trace of fibroids. I power walk and feel energetic. People compliment my healthy skin. I handle stress with humor and do not react to other people's indifference. All and all, life is healthier.

OLIVER

My cholesterol and blood pressure were elevated. I felt pain in my chest, knees, and ankles in addition to gastric distress. I weighed 238 pounds and was unhappy with brown age spots on my skin. Astigmatism caused discomfort. An Internet acquaintance suggested that I listen to Gary Null to motivate direction. I began psychotherapy. The protocol was successful. I lost 50 pounds in five months and was inspired to continue. My blood pressure and cholesterol lowered. I now exercise one to two hours daily and meditate. Juicing and using supplements improved my endurance. Life is positive without pains. Age spots faded, my astigmatism improved, and my skin texture, nails, and hair are healthy. I learned to let go, not get involved in details or hang on. Today I am involved in research, I live a vegan lifestyle, I am organic, and I put health first for my family and the planet.

JOSEPH I., 63 years old

I read Gary Null's books and listened to *Natural Living* for many years with good results. I have hepatitis, high blood pressure, diabetes, and damaged nerves, and I recently had a bout of Bell's palsy. I also have three bulging disks on my spine. With all of these problems, I sought relief and healing. I decided to follow the protocol. The people that stick to it had good results. Today, I juice, I no longer use eyeglasses during the day, and I am delighted that my blood pressure and diabetes are controlled and that the Bell's palsy did not return for two years. I discontinued weight lifting when my back was injured 10 years ago. I recently resumed lifting weights. I have a lot of energy, and the skin on my face is strong and my nails are healthy and pink. As a senior on a fixed income, I cannot afford a nutritionist. However, I study nutrition with Gary's shows and books. Thank you.

LUIS

At the time I joined a support group, I weighed 155 pounds. My blood pressure was high, and so was my cholesterol. I was not sharp anymore. My memory was not as good as it once was. My hair was growing in thinner, and I felt tired. I listened to Gary Null on the radio and read his books, but when a new support group began, I joined immediately. I was enthusiastic and optimistic immediately. I stayed after class to pass my good feelings on to the group members. I knew I could improve my health and help them improve theirs. Today, I weigh 145 pounds. I am totally organic, juice, use pure water, and have great energy. My hair and eyebrows are thicker. My blood pressure and cholesterol tests are normal. My memory improved, my skin looks great, and I can read without glasses. I eat my last meal before 6 p.m. This experience gave me a new lease on life.

ANDRE D.

Before

High weight. Low muscle mass. High blood pressure. Cholesterol not in normal range. Worked in law firm and was unhappy there. Cynical.

Now

Lost 25 pounds. Gained 7 pounds of muscle. Blood pressure normal. Cholesterol normal. Left his job. No longer cynical. Feels complete and alive. Uncluttered. Sees others as equals. Positive attitude. Is now a personal trainer.

GLENROY A., 68 years old

Before

I was diabetic, developed cellulitis while serving in the military, and had severe knee and lower back disk pain. I could not climb stairs, and I used crutches, a cane. For two months, I was paralyzed and in a wheelchair. My blood pressure and cholesterol were elevated. I ate the typical American diet: flesh foods, wheat, and dairy. Underneath it all, I wanted to be healthy.

Now

My legs are no longer swollen from cellulitis. My backache has subsided. My circulation is normal. I can easily walk up the three flights of steps to my apartment. I buy organic food and follow the protocol: eat fish and use green and red powders and supplementation. My life is active. I am retired and work on a veteran's council. It is wonderful to babysit my granddaughter, feeling lighter and energetic. All my past symptoms are gone. The homework we did in the support group caused me to focus on myself. I learned to be tolerant, less pushy, and more humble. This teaching enhanced my body and my life.

ALICE

Before

I was concerned about my health. My blood pressure and cholesterol were elevated. I had a stressful life and could not control these feelings. I disliked my varicose veins. I suffered with an acid reflux condition that I assumed was caused by my job. My body was falling apart.

Now

I detoxed and carefully followed Gary's protocol. I felt stronger each week and released stress each day. My blood pressure is normal today. My digestion improved, and I have no more acid reflux. I lost 15 lbs. My blood tests are good, and my figure is leaner. I am shapelier. I feel cleaner. I do aerobics at home in the morning, yoga during the evening hours, and bike, walk, and run. My uncluttered environment and journal writing give me a new constructive outlook. I use green juices and green and red powders with supplements. My water is pure. I am organic. I am goal-oriented.

CLARA

I had four children and felt old and unhealthy. I wore size 20. My blood pressure was elevated. I lived a fast and stressful life on an organic farm the city wants to confiscate for open land. I wanted to join a support group for a while, but this time I followed my determination. The support group was a class in biology, nutrition, and human potential. I learned quickly. Today, I wear size 13. We are an organic family and use the green and red powders. Sugar and dairy are out. My daughter had one asthma attack that was not repeated after we eliminated sugar and dairy. I am focused and energetic, and I look forward to my exercises, which I do four to six times a week.

CONNIE

I am 65 years old and thought fatigue, arthritis, high blood pressure, high cholesterol, cataracts, osteoporosis, and overweight were part of aging. My hair and nails were weaker, and I was sensitive to the opinions of others. I decided to go with Gary's research and knowledge. I wanted to be well and happy. I no longer am tired and sluggish. I have no more aches and pains. I lost 20 lbs and look younger. My hair and nails grow in strong, and most of all, I am indifferent to the opinions and criticisms of other people. Look what I did! Bravo for me.

DAMON

I felt frustrated, and I could not muster up energy. I overslept, my hair was graying, my sinus infections drove me mad, and my cholesterol and blood pressure were elevated. This was not me; I had to find a method of true reversal. I went on Gary's protocol carefully. It was easy. I enjoyed new foods. I learned to understand my body mechanisms. My elevated blood levels are normal now. My sinus problems are gone. I sleep less and awake with energy. My hair texture has improved, and I have less graying. I am determined to achieve and to have relationships with my family.

HENRY O.

My life was unmanageable, and my stress was overwhelming. I had many allergies and frequent upper respiratory infections. My blood pressure and cholesterol were elevated. I heard about Gary Null's support groups and detoxification. I needed to change, and I decided to enter a group as soon as one was formed. That was the beginning of the best part of my life. How could green juices clean toxins from one's body? Well, that's exactly what happened with good results. My energy built, my headaches stopped, and my cholesterol and blood pressure lowered. I have a new body since exercising, using weights, and doing qi gong and deep breathing. I feel calm, more patient, and less irritable. I love my food and progressive life.

GLEN

I was overwhelmed by possessions. My home was very large and cluttered. It became too much for my husband and me. My weight, cholesterol, and blood pressure went up. I developed cardiac arrhythmia and lost energy. My nails became weak. We were lost in indecision. Joining a support group gave us the tools to create a new life and future. Detoxing returned my body to health. I lost 30 lbs, which normalized my cholesterol and blood pressure. I am no longer a cardiac patient. My nails are growing in strong. We are energetic, and most of all, we sold our large home, dividing the unessential items among our family, and now live in a four-room house and love it.

BOWEL REGULARITY

JAN S.

Since I started the program, my bowel movements have improved and become more regular. I am more focused, and my anxiety and depression have lessened. My eyesight has improved. I have more energy and sleep better. I lost some weight and feel much better.

BRAIN TRAUMA

YVONNE

Brain surgery left me with numb fingers and cold extremities. I had flu-like symptoms, a constant "frog" in my throat, fatigue the morning, tinnitus, dizziness, constipation, and a general lack of motivation that interfered with my work performance. I was angry and soon went on disability. The first time Gary Null spoke about support groups on his show, I listened but did nothing. At that stage I could not really help myself. Feeling totally locked in I pulled up some inner courage and went to the first meeting. Then, I began the protocol. In a short amount of time, it was evident the protocol was working. I began to feel better; the pains and other symptoms lessened. As I continued and listened to the lectures which were quite penetrating and motivating, I noticed all the symptoms I once had were gone. Today I am a functioning, healthy woman.

FRANK E.

In February 1997, I had brain surgery due to a tuberculum sellae meningioma that was wrapped around my pituitary gland and destroyed my optic nerve. I was diagnosed with hypothyroidism. My craniotomy surgery lasted twenty hours. I was in intensive care three days. I was weak and could not walk or even brush my teeth. I joined a support group eight months after surgery and began the protocol. I came into the Gary Null Running and Walking Club two months later and soon discontinued steroids, seizure pills, Synthroid, laxatives, and antacids. I no longer discuss my illness, but speak of my health. I am naturally positive in thought, behavior, and speech. My physician does not understand my physical, emotional, and mental recovery in so short a time. I feel great and push forward without an attitude of handicap.

MICHAEL

[In the past] seizures began with Alzheimer-like symptoms. Abnormally severe edema in my legs incapacitated me. I was in a coma for 60 days. Nursing home care was considered. My health took an upward turn on the Gary Null protocol. Today I no longer need a compressor for leg edema. My leg size decreased 30 percent. I sleep less and lost 23 pounds. I exercise with hand weights. My blood pressure is lower. My brain speed seems to be faster.

BY-PASS RECOVERY

LOU, 76 years old

I had an unsuccessful quadruple bypass and five years later I was told that I had one month to live without another operation. Now, without the bypass, I underwent chelation therapy, vitamin C drips, and lifestyle changes that have all made a drastic improvement in my quality of life. I am very active now, walking five miles a day. I also dance two to three hours a day. And best of all I have no chest pains.

CANCER

JOHN E.

Cancer stopped. Basal cell and colon cancer reversed. Hepatitis halted. Normalized blood triglycerides, HDL, and LDL. Blood pressure 180/128 to 117/63.

Improvements: Stopped basal cell cancer, lost 15 lbs, reversed colon cancer, halted hepatitis C, normalized blood triglycerides (HDL and LDL), blood pressure significantly dropped.

Mental Changes: Memory has improved greatly.

Breast Cancer

JOYCE

I have just finished a two-week stay at Gary's retreat. It has totally turned my life around. It's been the most incredible experience of my life for a lot of reasons. I came down here as a stage four cancer patient ready to go into hospice and I'm walking out of here, literally walking, without a cane, without anything to help me and feeling better than I've felt in a year—three years. I'm so grateful, so incredibly grateful that I've had this time to re-evaluate a lot of things in my life.

I literally was unable to walk without some type of aid when I came here and within three days I put the cane down and I was walking—and sort of power walking—nothing like what they do down here but I was doing it the best way that I could. So I cannot say enough. I don't even expect people to believe what I am saying because it seems so phenomenal that I would have a breast tumor that would go down almost two-thirds while I'm here because of the attention, because of the energy, because of everything here. I go home a different person. Literally, I go home a different person. I sort of came here against my better judgment, not believing that anything could really make that much of a difference. Knowing that if I had two months left to live that at least maybe Gary Null could help me make the best of those two months. And I go back, fully charged and ready to go to work and continue where I left off three years ago. I was a registered nurse for forty years. I was a certified chemotherapy nurse and worked a lot in heart, lung, liver, kidney transplants. But my belief in chemotherapy was that all my patients that had chemotherapy were dead and I was not going to take it so I wanted the natural route. I had three breast tumors initially three years ago that metastasized into bone cancer, liver cancer, and spinal cancer and at this point, I don't feel like there is any pain there that I was having. I was having excruciating bone pain for which I was taking narcotics—and now that is gone. So I am blessed to have been given this opportunity and for every person that has made this happen. I only wish I could make this happen for other people so they can benefit from this also.

JEAN K.
Cancer gone
Arthritis diminished
Before
I am a lung cancer survivor. I had radiation, chemotherapy, and several body scans, which left me anemic. I also developed osteoarthritis, which incapacitated me. Walking was difficult, and I needed help to board a bus. I used pain medication. My blood pressure was slightly elevated. Although I considered myself to be nutritionally aware, I used dairy. My energy was quite low after cancer treatment. I joined a support group to rebuild my immune system. I wanted to be healthy.
Now
The arthritis has diminished. I no longer require medication. I take walks and prac-

tice yoga. I am totally vegan, drink juices, and follow Gary's protocol totally. The group homework assignments expanded my self-awareness and created new insights. I am delighted with the results of each new blood test. I am cancer-free and optimistic. My work, in the wardrobe department of a theatrical company, is enjoyable, and I look forward to a good season with the crew again.

Stage 3–4 Cancer

LARRY P.

I use the cancer protocol for a testicular tumor. I follow it carefully, and I find I have more energy and feel alive and relaxed. In addition, the skin around my eyes was dry but is now supple, with fewer wrinkles. I am more spiritual and express myself. I focus on weight by simply eating naturally. I do not interact with negative people. I enjoy my job.

KIM

I was a smoker. I worked hard, and I internalized negative issues and work problems. I developed cancer. I followed Gary Null's protocol and used Dr. Revici's methods. I do not smoke today, nor do I internalize negative thoughts. I meditate, exercise, use a rebounder, and feel happier and more peaceful. I work less and take quality time for myself.

ETTAS B.

Before

She had a hysterectomy for uterine cancer, but the cancer returned. She went through chemotherapy and radiation. She had arthritis, psoriasis, and low energy, and she was overweight and unhappy at work.

Now

Her cancer seems to be in full remission. She lost 26 lbs. Her psoriasis is gone. Her hair and skin are healthy, her arthritis is gone, and her immune system is strong. It was through class assignments and other workbook activities that she learned she was hard on herself and came to experience the positive relief of forgiveness of self and others. Etta left her toxic job. She meditates twice daily, exercises, practices yoga, and lifts weights.

Prostate Cancer

EUGENE N.

I was diagnosed with a small melanoma in my right eye. I am legally blind in my left eye. The cancer has not grown for eight months. Migraine headaches virtually disappeared. I lost 35 pounds and my back has improved. Other minor conditions have also improved.

CARDIAC HEALTH

JAMES

I procrastinated myself into a severe cardiac condition. After my angioplasty, I took blood pressure medication and joined Gary's walking club. I was amazed that the walkers and runners, some of whom overcame serious illnesses, were fit and healthy. They made major lifestyle changes. I looked at my life, working 7 a.m. to 9 p.m. without exercise. I was a coffee addict and felt stuck. A change was in order. I joined a group. If you're going with the protocol, go with it all the way . . . and I did. Organic, juicing, powders, vegan, and life changes. We were a great team, the support group people and I. We are different people today. That's what knowledge does. I am aware of labeling and chemicals. I no longer crave caffeine for energy. I ran in two marathons, and I confronted my procrastination. I believe in the power of actualization: "Speak the words, live by the words."

CHRONIC FATIGUE

IRIS

Chronic fatigue and gastro-intestinal problems are less active, and I no longer require naps.

COMPULSIVE EATING

FATIMAH

I was a sugar addict and ate two pounds of it per day, creating a sick, uncomfortable body. I overate using junk food. My energy was low, my skin was bad, and my blood pressure and cholesterol were high. This inability to control myself stressed me. As I listened to Gary, I thought about freeing myself from these habits. I joined a support group. It is wonderful to be free of compulsive eating. I lost 50 pounds. I do not crave sugar. My cholesterol and blood pressure are lower, and I have real, vital energy. Problem solving comes easily, my marriage is happier, and I meditate. The foods I eat are healthy and so is my outlook.

DEPRESSION

MARINA

I had several problems and wanted a solution. The medical community did not have that solution. I was overweight, and that sapped my energy. After menopause, my hair and nails became weak, and I felt very depressed. I was given Prozac for post-menopause syndrome. I was still depressed. Wasn't there any place to go for help for people like me? Finally, I heard about a health support group, and without knowing exactly what it was, I signed up. I joined the group, and it was so interesting, and it was an intelligent class that respected the people attending. I learned how diet affects mood and the body. I followed the protocol and lost weight. I kept it off. I have lots of energy, and my hair and nails are coming back to their premenopausal thickness. I stopped Prozac when I began the protocol, and I feel great. I sleep well, and I have no more depression.

ATHENA, 60 years old

I had premenstrual syndrome, which caused fatigue, pain, and depression. I also had cystic breasts and eye floaters. My hair was getting gray. I chose bad relationships and had an unpleasant job. I decided to join a health support group. [Previously] nothing seemed to improve my life and current group members spoke of improvements and regaining health. Today I have no signs of premenstrual syndrome. I do not feel cysts in my breasts. Although I do get tired, the fatigue has lessened, and feelings of depression were gone within six weeks on the protocol. My eye floaters seem to be diminishing and I notice fewer new gray hairs. I uncluttered all bad relationships, and I allow myself to be close to people and found a new job at a higher wage that I enjoy.

RAINY

I feel more focused and less toxic. I have a healthier, positive attitude toward life in general, and dealing with "problems" has become much easier. I feel much less depressed than usual. I feel more empowered. I do not take life too seriously anymore, and make time for friends and social activities.

JENNIE
Depression has diminished and I have less pain in general. I have more control over my emotions.

CAROL G.
I sleep better and am better able to cope with my nightmares. My depression decreased, and my energy levels have improved. My appetite has improved, and I have lost some weight. My memory and concentration are slowly improving.

JOB
I weighed 210 pounds, smoked three packs of cigarettes a day, drank alcohol, felt depressed, and had knee pains and upper-respiratory infections. One day I looked at the very aged man in the mirror and was shocked. Today I follow Gary Null's protocol. I drink purified water, use supplements, and feel terrific. I haven't had a cold in five years; no more upper-respiratory infections. I follow an organic, vegan diet and do not take vaccines. My neighbors tell me I look forty-five years old. They admire my changes. I appreciate my healthy lifestyle. I am confident and pleased with my life, and I am no longer depressed.

MARIA T.
I was depressed and overweight, uncomfortable with the extra pounds. I held anger in and did not discuss, understand, or share my feelings with anyone. I was afraid to take risks, such as asking for a raise. Being timid and angry was not a good place to be. I knew and trusted Gary Null, so I joined a group to see if I could be happy and make changes. I am on the protocol and love it. My depression lifted as my health increased. I exercise without fear of injury. I lost 20 lbs, and my energy is high. I cope, do not hold anger in, and speak my mind. I spoke up at work and got a raise.

ELAINE
I lose one pound a week. My blood pressure dropped. My hair is shiny. I am not dehydrated nor do I get headaches.

MARIA

Depression and anxiety are very difficult. You get up and do the things you feel you have to do. But you don't feel like you are in the flow of life. My conditions were probably not that apparent to the rest of the world, but I experienced them as very uncomfortable, and they took away from my quality of life. I felt stressed much of the time. I had difficulty concentrating. At times I would forget things. Someone would ask me to do something, and I would forget to do it. I knew there wasn't something wrong with my mind. I felt my lack of focus was due more to my being so hyped up and tense. I felt overwhelmed by ordinary, everyday demands, and I felt exhausted by the end of the day. Many times, after lunch, I would feel really tired, almost like I needed to have a nap. Anxiety and depression seemed to gobble up my energy very quickly. By the end of the day, I was not in the mood for recreational activities. Work wore me out. I would just go home and bug out in front of the boob tube. And I wanted more than that. Once in a while, I would have a drink and notice a difference; I would be able to focus much better. The reason was that the drink helped me relax. But I didn't want to relax that way. I wanted to find an alternative that would really work for me and help me to feel more joy in my everyday experience. I went to several physicians, and they prescribed various medications for me. But I couldn't take medicines. They had all kinds of strange side effects, which were just as bad as the anxiety or the depression. The drugs masked my conditions, but underneath they were still there. All they did was make me feel very sleepy much of the time. I would be sitting at a meeting, dozing off, and I couldn't afford to do that. So I only took medications briefly. I was looking for help when I happened to hear a Gary Null lecture at the Learning Annex. I was very impressed with some of the things I heard about limiting belief systems and how difficult it is to see beyond them. I liked the talk on vegetarianism as well. As a result, I went to see Dolores Perri and was very impressed. Dolores went over my history and concerns. I really enjoyed talking to Dolores because, unlike most physicians I've encountered, she was very relaxed. I didn't get a sense that we were limited by time; we were done when we were done. Basically, I asked my questions and expressed my concerns. It was a very good experience. After we talked, she recommended certain foods, herbs, and supplements. I have been following a nutritional routine for about two and a half months now, and I have definitely noticed a very dramatic shift. In particular, my hypoglycemia has disappeared. That's mostly from getting rid of refined sugars and processed foods. I used to feel very restless and nervous if I didn't eat. That's been stabilized, and I feel much calmer now. My energy level is much, much better with a vegetarian regime, supplements, and herbs. The aloe I've been using is outstanding at picking me up at the beginning of the day. I feel clearer as well. There are subtle differences in my ability to concentrate. And when I go through the day, I feel much calmer. A couple of days ago, I was late for a meeting through no fault of my own. I had to be late for something I thought was very important. Normally, I would be a complete wreck about it. But because of my new regime, I was calm and centered, and I didn't run up the stairs. I just walked in, explained what had happened, sat down, and joined in. In the past, I would have been practically shaking from anxiety. This is a real departure, which I attribute largely to my change in diet as well as to my holistic orientation. I think it's important to know that it's not only a shift in diet that has helped me. I became involved in meditation to clear my mind and help me reach that stillness. I do that in the morning before anything else. In addition, I take a greater interest in the holistic world and participate in seminars. All these different elements help enhance my well-being.

LIZ

Mentally, I am more clear-thinking, making decisions regarding my life and business more quickly, as opposed to laboring over them. I have no depression, but a general feeling of grounding and balance. Affirmations work.

LOUISE

I feel a balance, peacefulness, quietness, and contentment. My depression is gone. This is new for me; I feel joyful. I am now walking two to three miles, four or five times per week. I feel lighter, see the world in a more positive way, and feel content and happier. People are telling me how great I look.

BEATRICE C.

Before

I had lupus for eight years and used prednisone and 13 other pills, which caused me to have an upset stomach. I felt horrible. I had a yeast infection, with liver problems and headaches. I also had low energy. I had five surgeries, and I underwent chemotherapy for my kidney condition. My physicians never suggested diet changes.

Now

Following a specific protocol that uses glutamine, flaxseed oil, and DHEA, and after three hydrogen peroxide injections, I suspended all but one medication. I have higher energy, decreased joint pain, and an improved stomach condition, and my yeast infection has totally cleared up. I do tai chi and yoga, and my depression has gone. My relationships with my friends and family are stronger.

JOAN

Depression is much less. Gary's support group and protocol helped me battle depression. I gained 5 pounds, and I now wake up with more energy. I require less sleep, and there are noticeably fewer muscle-lethargy headaches. I feel wonderful.

DIABETES

MATT

I want to mention my type 1 diabetes. I had an experience throughout the week where my blood sugars have been perfectly normal with minimal amounts of insulin. My reduction in the amount of insulin I take is now at 75 percent or less so I'm only taking 25 percent of what I was taking prior to my arrival here. In one case you did some energy work, on me in particular. I came into the energy work with a 274, no insulin in my body. It was an experiment. And then the consequence of being out three hours later and having dessert: I tested my blood sugar and it was 84. So, I'm a type 1 diabetic? Pretty phenomenal stuff! It's given me amazing reminders of who I am and who I can be.

FRANTZ V.

Before

I had severe diabetes. I was taking insulin and glucophage. I also had high blood pressure and asthma. I then went on the protocol/lifetime diet.

Now

My life has changed tremendously. I have learned to balance my job and my personal life. I have increased my energy levels. I sleep a lot less. My high blood pressure went down. My asthma is gone. I no longer am on any medication for diabetes. And I lost weight: I went from 240 pounds to 205–210 pounds.

DEBORAH

I always had irregular periods and had not menstruated in almost two years. I had been on the pill for years, but went off of it in 2000 due to a 35-pound weight gain. I went off the pill and gradually stopped getting a period. My libido was gone, it was impossible to lose weight around my mid-section, and I got occasional hot flashes. I also experienced depression at the thought of being infertile and the long-term effects of lacking estrogen. All my diabetes was reversed.

ZARA

I am a juvenile diabetic. I used coffee and ate junk food, sodas, etc. I had ongoing diabetic retinopathy; fatty deposits in my eye. I sought healing with a mind-body-spirit approach. It [health support group] opened me to spiritual meditation and finding strength within. I am delighted to report the retinopathy stopped developing, no more fatty deposits. I consulted with my physician three months into the protocol. My exam revealed my eye vessels are stronger and a thicker membrane is growing. I feel vital and energetic since eliminating negative, toxic people in my life.

DAVID P.

My skin color returned to normal. My nails are now growing properly. I have less mucus, and I require less diabetes medication. The sinus problems that caused such discomfort are gone. My hair and eyebrows grew back in their original color. My voice is strong and firm today.

DIGESTIVE PROBLEMS & MEMORY

OMAR

My wife and I joined a support group together. We did not want to lose our stamina as we aged, and we respected Gary Null's knowledge. We intend to raise our family in a healthy environment. I was overweight, which fatigued me. Gastric problems kept me awake at night. My work was stressful, with long hours. I felt annoyed with the friends and family members who interfered in our lives. We embarked on the detox with enthusiasm. Our children enjoyed exploring new foods. I lost 37 lbs, which gave me the energy to enter races. Today, I work fewer days at the hospital and I feel happier. My gastritis is gone. Life is simpler without negative, toxic people in my environment.

RAYMOND

I was tired all of the time, my hair was gray, and I also suffered from irritable bowel syndrome, bloating, and weight gain. After following Gary's protocol, I was able to lose weight, and I no longer have a pot belly. My digestive issues have greatly improved and I no longer feel bloated or have irritable bowel syndrome. I have much more energy, and my hair has stopped growing in gray.

WINSTON

I suffered from a lack of energy, insomnia, and flatulence caused by a spastic colon. My skin looks great, and the liver spots on my neck and chest are barely visible. Hair, nails, and toenails grow quickly and with strength. Constipation, bloating, and indigestion are greatly reduced.

THERESA

I proudly list the following improvements in my health since I began Gary Null's protocol. My poor digestion has improved. I do not feel bloated or suffer from flatulence. I lost 13 lbs. My energy levels have gone way up. I do not require as much sleep as I used to, and I am much happier.

JEAN D

Before

My husband and I began to notice our bodies were not in good condition. He was a meat-and-potatoes man and a very picky eater. Over the years, he was exposed to lead, paint, and cadmium on his job and developed nocturnal seizures, low energy, digestive discomfort, and memory loss. I handled stress badly and was often intolerant. I had a bad accident: my breasts were caught between two doors and throbbed for two years. We followed Gary's protocol in one of his books. We studied urine therapy and acupuncture, and used colonies and sprouts.

Now

Today, my husband has fewer seizures, more energy, and enhanced memory, and he enjoys his new diet. He is enthusiastic and looking forward to his seventy-fifth birthday. We are energetic and without intestinal problems. We handle stress well, because we are no longer toxic. My female organs function as well as they did in my younger years. Our naturopath told me I avoided fracturing a hip during a fall because my bones were well mineralized. We are vegan, eat raw vegetables, juice, and invent nutritious recipes using a dehydrator. I am involved in community affairs. Our outlook is cheerful. We love spreading the word.

SANDY

I came to the program overweight, short of breath, and diabetic. I lost 29 pounds. I walk 2 miles a day without being short of breath, and my diabetes is under control.

DISEASE REVERSAL

LUANNE

As a nurse practicing at least three decades in conventional medicine I've been trained to watch people adapt to whatever illness that they are diagnosed with. And I've witnessed people who actually have lost their whole identity because someone told them that they have a disease. I have had the unique opportunity to watch people deconstruct the illusions in their lives, the identity loss to other people's opinions and descriptions of them. And it is one of the most amazing experiences for me as a health care professional to watch people not adapt anymore to their illness but to transcend it. It's an evolution or devolution, to see them go one step at a time, letting go of one belief that doesn't serve them, then another belief, then another belief. Some of it has to do with their ability to exercise. We have people that have used their age to limit themselves and their ability to go out and do a really good workout. We've had some people use their illness and some people that use their past to justify not going out there and making fundamental changes. So, from where I'm sitting as a nurse I'm seeing people transcend their illnesses. They compensate for the damage that was done and I'm watching people's immune systems getting stronger, their determination to be well getting stronger, their self-esteem is going up, their self-worth going up. And when you're in an environment like this you're surrounded by nature, you're surrounded by a supportive staff and you're surrounded with wisdom. It's not just knowledge, it's wisdom and we all have it but some of us have lost access to it. That's what I've witnessed. And I'm seeing people that are reconnecting with that wisdom and beginning to live their lives consistent with what they're supposed to be doing here, not what someone else told them to do. So it's wonderful as a nurse to watch people take their health back, take their power back and re-access their true identity.

EDEMA—LEGS

MICHAEL, 62 years old

I attended a Gary Null retreat. I learned the benefits of vegetarianism, juicing, supplements, and meditation. In 1994, I became disabled because of carbon monoxide poisoning. I am still in the process of recovery. I no longer work. I cannot see the computer screen. Surgery for two detached retinas affected my eyesight. My blood pressure was extremely high. My heartbeat accelerated to a dangerous level. I took several pharmaceutical drugs to control these conditions. A few years later, I began having seizures and Alzheimer's-like symptoms. Abnormally severe edema in my legs incapacitated me. I was in a coma for 60 days. Nursing home care was considered. My health took an upward turn on the Gary Null protocol. Juicing, stress management, and homework opened me to my potential and purpose in life. I discovered the best of what works, and I realized I was not doing anything worthwhile. Today, I no longer need a compressor for leg edema. My leg size decreased by 30 percent. I sleep less, lost 23 pounds, and exercise with hand weights. I recently received a Bowflex to build my upper body. My blood pressure is lower. My brain speed seems to be faster.

JAY

I have been a holistic dentist and vegetarian for 32 years. I had mood swings and problems concentrating at times, most likely due to sugar and dairy. I was negative on occasion. My hair was graying. My wife and I joined a health support group. We follow the protocol: powders, juices, a lot of liquids, totally organic. My energy increased dramatically, and my mood swings are gone. I maintain a good, positive mental attitude for long periods of time. My concentration stabilized. I notice less gray hair in new growth. We use affirmations, uncluttering, exercise, power walking, and the Nordic Trac. Four of our six children are vegetarians. Gary Null put it all together by formatting a nutritional plan, condensing it, and making it clear. Going to the ranch in Florida caused a major positive change in our lives, and attending the classes, experiencing other energies in a support network, made our successes possible. I recommend the protocol to my patients.

EMOTIONAL CONFIDENCE

MUTABA H.

The biggest change I have experienced since beginning this program has come through focus and eliminating toxic people from my life. I can say no without guilt. My body requires less sleep. My elimination is regular. I have also learned so much more about healing the human body through detoxification. I am truly grateful for this lesson in healing.

MICHAEL

I joined Gary's support group because I wanted to eliminate medications for anxiety and depression. My hair was graying and my complexion was dry and bumpy. I had nervous twitches. I am now vegan and organic, and I juice and exercise without a need for medications. I am aware of mind/body connections. My colitis dissipated as my behavior created changes in body chemistry. The psychological and emotional changes empowered me to study the negative impact of toxic foods and people. I stopped fighting life. Now life supports me. My twitching also stopped from ozone therapy treatments, and my hair is long and healthy. Today I enjoy the new career I have actualized: teaching others self-empowerment

ENERGY

LILLIAN

My energy has really been restored in this bucolic setting. Exercise, power walking, yoga, nutritious food and beverages, lectures from Gary in the evening. So much information to take back with me and to share with others.

LINDA

I take home with me energy, peacefulness, and calmness within myself. I also experienced a talent I didn't know I had in the art class.

WILLIAM

I came here lacking a lot of energy. My energy has really been restored in this bucolic setting.

MARCIA C.

I made changes 47 years ago with Dr. Max Warmbrand, [but more recently] I entered a Gary Null support group overweight, with low libido, and white hair. I rarely exercised. My nails were weak, and my energy was low. I was delighted with the protocol. My energy increased, my nails became stronger, and my once-white hair grew in thicker and in its original brown color. I lost weight in a slow, consistent manner. Today, I am a healthy, energetic woman. I am involved in several new careers: songwriter—one song was recorded—and I am the author of a book based on life-motivating therapy. I am in the process of submitting ideas for an impending radio show for seniors. Life is more fun than it ever was. Part of that is motivating people to jump right in.

MURIEL

I feel fantastic. I have more energy, I think more clearly, and my husband and I both quit smoking.

TOM M.

The reason I decided to join the study is a desire to reach my potential spiritually, physically, and emotionally. To achieve this, I must empower myself. The commitment to the program without compromise is a powerful statement. It says that I am making my own choices in my life, and that these choices are positive and affect every aspect. I am in control. In the past two years, I have been divorced, lost my job, and lost my apartment. The reason that this happened is that I allowed other people to make my decisions for me. Basically, I didn't think enough of myself to express my wants, desires, needs, likes and dislikes, and all the other good stuff that comes along with being a person. I feel that I have come a long way in the past three months, primarily because of the program. Being in control of my decision of what I will and will not put in my body is empowering. I believe the body is sacred and should be treated as such. It is the temple in which we live. Physically I do feel more energetic than I did before. Lack of energy was a problem in the past due to my consumption of large amounts of sweets. Before I was married, I was very spiritual. While I was married, I was less so, due to the demands of being a father, husband, and provider. Now that I am single and possess the solitude necessary for reflection and spiritual growth I am following my path that leads to discovery and wholeness. What I have also discovered is that making positive changes in one aspect of your life leads to positive changes in other areas. Sometimes you don't consciously make positive changes; they just happen, one built upon the other.

LYN W.

My energy levels are up since I started the program. I think more clearly and can better cope with depression. I have a smoother, more regular elimination. Communication with my family is open and positive.

JOEL K.

I have improved in terms of energy, most significantly. I have also found I have much more patience and my relationships have improved. At work, I have become more efficient and I have more energy to do activities on the weekend. All in all, I find that when I keep close to the protocol, I feel and function much better.

ALEXANDRE

One morning I woke up filled with energy. When I started the program, I had a real lack of energy. I was sleeping 10 to 12 hours a night and was always tired by 4 p.m. Now my sleep is down to six to eight hours each night. I still can't believe it. I also lost 10 pounds just from the elimination of sugar, dairy, and wheat. I also maintain a regular exercise program.

FIBROCYSTIC BREASTS

YANICK

I had a history of fibrocystic breasts for 20 years. I was underweight and had hair loss. I took Synthroid and was told I was facing possible thyroid cancer. After six months on the program, my fibrocystic breasts decreased by 50 percent. I gained 2 pounds and exercise five to six days a week. I built muscle. My hair loss lessened, and I no longer use Synthroid.

ELIZABETH

I had candida and a cystofibroid breast. Today I am free of these conditions and feel completely healthy and full of energy. My skin has improved. My hair is thicker. I am happier and have more focus and clarity.

PAULA

I had cystic breast disease for the last 20 years. Four months after becoming a vegetarian and following the detox program, the fibroids are all gone. I lost 5 pounds, my eyes are not dry anymore, and I don't get chest pain after eating certain foods. I have more energy and can get by with fewer hours of sleep per night. I am no longer "righteous."

GENERAL HEALTH IMPROVEMENT

ELLEN

I learned that I am still in there somewhere under all the stuff that has accumulated over the years. I learned it is never too late to get to the things I want to do that I have put off. I remember how good it feels to feel good.

LAURA J. G.

I wanted to write you and thank you for helping me find a new direction in life. I went to your ranch in Naples [Florida] as one person and came home another. I have made permanent changes in my life and I feel terrific. The changes I have gone through are too numerous to list. What I can say is now I feel as if there is nothing I can't do. Thank you so much again. It is truly wonderful, the way you use your gifts.

SIGRID G. E.

Since beginning this anti-aging protocol, the cracking in my knuckles from arthritis is gone. My gums, which looked like raw meat for almost four years, are completely healed. My vision has improved somewhat. There definitely is a threshold. I have an improved relationship with my father, and have gotten rid of some very toxic people—which has made my life much easier. But I have more to go. I have much more energy. Before, I fell asleep at my desk almost every afternoon. At some point, a few months after I started the program, I started to feel like I did many years ago, when I was really young. I am much happier. I used to be hungry all the time, really all the time. Now I can go without eating for a long, long time. I'm hardly hungry, even when I sit down to eat. But I eat. I lost a lot of weight—close to thirty pounds—without effort, and I feel real good about that. I can move about with much more ease. I am very glad all that extra weight is gone. I am more conscious of my spiritual being. I realize that my spiritual needs have to be taken seriously. I have started to read the Bible again. I pay closer attention to what I am doing and try to be in the present, whatever I am doing. I do the activities for the sake of doing and do not look for rewards or approval. I only look for a happier life. I truly believe that to take care of your spiritual needs first is most important, and everything else will fall into place. My spiritual and physical being are now at a better level. I am now closer to where I want to be. Thank you very much for your help!

JACOB

I like loving myself a little. Before I began the program, I had a very low energy level. I needed a sugar boost through the day. My digestion was not great, and the sugar cycle confused my thinking. I have been on the program only three months and have lost 10 pounds. Overall, my energy level is greatly increased. My thinking is much clearer, and I am much more conscious of my interaction with people throughout the day. My body functions have become more regulated. I am much more aware of what and when I choose to eat. Generally, my attitude is much better. I like that I am able to listen better and hear what it is people are saying to me. I am more patient with people and have become more aware of my own needs. I am even able to express them sometimes. Before the program, I was upset with my work, feeling trapped by myself. I felt that my work controlled me and that I had no power. I felt as if I always had to get things done but was never able to feel joy in doing them. Now, after following the program, I am beginning to take more control of my work time. And I have started to take control of my non-work time. I am able now to step back and congratulate myself on small steps taken. I have a more positive view of the future. I like feeling better. I like loving myself a little.

KAREN

I would often have swollen glands and frequent upper-respiratory infections. My energy was low, my hair began to gray, and I was overly tired before my period. My life was complicated with people I today call toxic. I joined a support group and decided to give it all I had. I juiced and became organic, very careful with my food plan. I did the homework and carefully listened to lectures and guest speakers. Today I am in excellent health without colds, premenstrual discomfort, or [being bothered by] the impact of annoying people. My energy is high, and I forgive past errors.

EVA

I just improved my body and that helped me feel better emotionally and spiritually. I have learned to give more care for my body in the future.

MONICA

I lost 3 pounds. I require less sleep. My bronchial condition is corrected. My vision at 71 years of age has remained stable without the need of eyeglasses. Gum health has improved, and nails are stronger and growing more rapidly. My hair roots' color has become speckled brown, black, and gray where it was previously white, and it also grows more rapidly. Skin wrinkles are lessened and skin texture is smoother and softer. Sexually my aging process has been reversed. I am pre-menopausal again. My breasts are fuller and firmer, and my reproductive organs are now self-lubricating.

PAT, 72 years old

I was hospitalized three times for congestive heart disease. I was on oxygen 24 hours a day for emphysema. I weighed 225 pounds. I had arthritis, diabetes, sciatica, and glaucoma, and I used steroids. I came to support group meetings in a wheelchair, with oxygen hookups. Today, I call myself a walking miracle. I follow the protocol, walk daily, no longer use steroids, and even traveled to New York City. It took a while to clean my system out, but vegan organic living was the answer. My neighbors are happy to see me as I leave for my daily stroll. Detoxification works.

GERI L.

My story is long, but I will try to be brief. In February 1996 I went to a holistic medical doctor. My symptoms were: I was tired and "drained" all the time, especially after eating. After days and days of intra-dermal skin tests, it was clear that I was allergic to almost every food and inhalant on the planet. The situation looked bleak. Then I read your book *Who Are You, Really?* in April 1997. It opened my eyes to recognize my true life energy. In your book you give such good examples, and I recognized myself as a dynamic, supportive energy in absolutely the wrong profession. I have been a lawyer for fourteen years. When I joined your study group in July 1997, I was asked to write an answer to the question, "How do I live and experience life?" Looking back on my answer then shows how much I have changed in my thinking. In the summer of 1997, my answer was: "I don't. I'm a workaholic. Life sucks. I'm trapped on a treadmill, worn out, mentally and spiritually dead. "Wow! I cannot believe that was how I answered that question. I was criticizing myself and angry with myself and others. Then, in September 1997, I accepted a full-time teaching position at a graduate school. Then I struggled and questioned, why isn't everything "all better now"? I was carrying two full-time jobs—teaching and lawyering. Today, less than a year later, as I write to you, I am more peaceful and aware. I am in transition and I accept and honor that. Now I see that at first I was trying to make a quick change—to jump from full-time lawyering to full-time teaching. It was impossible to do. I had obligations to finish. I couldn't leave everybody stranded. You taught me to begin to plan for the change. Now my plan is to let go of the old way and make peace with where I was and what I was. I accept and approve of myself. I recognize that I cannot make a radical jump. I was trying to change too fast. Now I'm finding a solution—giving myself time. I'm giving myself time for self-learning, yoga, and meditation. I am saying no to any new law obligations and I'm finishing up with the old obligations. I'm finding a balance here, because now I know that even greater change requires mastery. I'm going some place on a path better than where I was. I am focusing more on being present in the moment. I trust myself and my intuition. Instead of old voices and preconditioning controlling my life, I choose nurturing thoughts. Now, when I meditate each morning, I say to myself I forgive and I am forgiven. All is well. What is it that I need to know about my career? I am peaceful and kind and gentle to myself and I accept that I am in transition, and I don't criticize myself. Thank you, Gary, for this protocol, the nutritional products, self-empowerment videos, and for being so wise that you chose Luanne Pennesi to lead our support group. She is an inspiration to all of us.

FELICIA

I can focus much better. My indigestion is gone. My joint pain is gone. My skin cleared up. I am much slimmer and tight now but not too much.

OLIVE

All of my adult life I have been preparing for tomorrow and the future. I have taken my life so seriously, I did not allow myself time to "play." I have learned to live in the moment, to live for today and to make time for play. It, too, is important.

JOZANA

I was overweight and could not slim down. I had acute heartburn, acid reflux, and angry outbursts. Coping with my teenage son was unbelievably stressful. I wanted to change my life and clear my mind. Since following the protocol, my body is alive and energetic. I unclutter my mind and home daily. I handle coworkers and my son without anger. The incredible homework questions made me think as I never did. I am optimistic, more open and accepting, patient, and less critical. I have traded anger for self-love.

MARY ANN

I gave up wheat, dairy, and sugar. I lost 5 pounds. My relationship to myself and others has transformed. I feel balanced and self-assured. I feel emotionally strong. I am no longer afraid. I feel less controlling of situations and people. I feel less victimized. My bouts with depression are gone. I feel kinder and more compassionate. I don't think before this I was ever aware of how grateful I am. I am able to realize more dreams. They don't seem so out of reach as they used to.

MARCIA D.

I required eight hours of sleep each night and still awoke with low energy. I used to overeat and craved sweets. I often had pains in my body. I did not handle stress well and often worked longer hours, which caused exhaustion. It was difficult saying no to people. The protocol changed these obstacles. My life is far happier and healthier. I require six hours of sleep and feel well rested in the morning. My mind is clear and focused. The exercises defined my leaner body. I am in tune with this healthier eating plan and feel the difference if I go off even slightly. Sugar is not my sweetener. I worked through that addiction using the allowed sweeteners on the protocol. Not overeating and keeping myself clean builds energy. My body pains are gone. My most apparent progress is that I believe in myself, consider my well-being, and say no. I can focus and remain unstressed and calm. I did that with work, and today I enjoy leisure time.

MOLLY

I feel sexy (at 59!), and I'm thinking about companionship. People who haven't seen me blurt out, "My God what have you done to yourself? You look fabulous!" I lost 16 pounds, went down two sizes in clothing, and my abdomen went from 44 to 39 inches. I am much more relaxed, am more able to handle stress, and I need less sleep. My vision is clearer, my hair has gone back to its original color, and I feel 20 years younger. My meditation is now much deeper and richer, and I have less anger and depression. Most days I do twenty-thirty stretching exercises, and I am now willing to challenge my values and beliefs.

RICK, 77 years old

I have been following Gary Null's protocol for the past ten years now. My health has been severely challenged during that time and I have survived each assault. I had surgery many years ago for a hiatal hernia. My diet of vegetables and juices controls this condition. My father and two sisters died from aortal abdominal aneurisms. My brother had one repaired successfully. I was diagnosed with this condition. Surgery was indicated. I prepared myself for six months with a specific protocol. This included a good vitamin regimen, mental and altitudinal insights, and healthy food. During that time I obtained a copy of the surgical procedure from a medical library and realized it was an extensive operation. My internal organs would be removed from my ribs to my pubic bone. My aorta had a balloon type defect, which would be opened and patched. My organs would then be replaced. I meditated on every organ in my body several times before surgery. I was relaxed before and after the procedure. I demanded my body to heal itself. My immune system was at its peak. I survived the surgery well, in excellent condition. I left intensive care in two days and took a bus home a few days later. My physicians were amazed. I explained how I obtained my strong immune system with diet, supplements, and respect for my body. I am now in the process of creating the biggest project of my life: building the world's largest wind farm. Following the Gary Null protocol gave me the strength and energy I must call upon to complete this mission. I encourage seniors to build your energies, both mental and physical, and create new goals, exercise, build your immune system, study, and be a part of your environment.

JOHN

Before I improved by joining a support group, I suffered from rosacea [facial redness], hair loss, dandruff, skin dryness, muscle wasting, overstimulated adrenals, low energy, herpes simplex, elevated cholesterol, kidney weakness, lack of focus, stress, and tinnitus [ringing in the ears].

NATALIE

I lost 50 pounds. I have increased energy. I feel more awake and alert My arthritis has improved and my joints are less painful. Shingles and genital herpes are gone. My allergies have improved and my periods are more regular. I have very little lower back pain and I am not constipated.

BERNIE P.

My week here [at Paradise Gardens] was both the shortest and longest of my life. Short, because I hated to leave. Long because I have rarely, in my sixty-four and a half years, found so much tranquility. Thanks to your teachings I have determined to make a beginning in changing my life. I cannot do it at the pace you suggest, but for my life energy type, it's a start.

WILMA W.

I will be sixty-four years young soon and I was thinking about retirement before I started the program in February. I also lost my job because of downsizing (company moved). Now I feel energized and know that retirement is not what I am looking forward to. In July I will start a twelve-week training program and will join the work world again and life. Physically, I have lost fifteen pounds, converted to a vegetarian diet, and I powerwalk! I feel better now than I have felt for a long time. I did dilation four years ago because of severe angina. I have been free of the angina; I am taking all the recommended supplements and vitamins. I have high blood pressure and cholesterol, am overweight. Spiritually I am more attuned to my surroundings, try to learn more about other people, their customs. Also, I get in touch with my own beliefs and thoughts. Try to help others—if they want my help. When I started the program, I was mostly interested to learn to avoid old-age diseases and to avoid possibly having to go later into an old-age home. Now I know that I do not have to acquire the diseases that most older people succumb to. I want to live an active and healthy life—and now I know that it is possible if I continue the program that we started tonight, and I will continue! It taught me, live a clean and healthy lifestyle: avoid all the bad foods, negative emotions, negative people. I have no problems avoiding the meats, dairy, and my favorite—chocolate. There are some negative people around me, but their negativity has no influence on me, because I do not let it happen. I am now in control of diet, emotions, and my life! I have become more tolerant, see my life in a different light, do not make fast judgments. I am sure that I will overcome my high cholesterol, get off my blood pressure and thyroid medication, reduce to my normal weight. I will be healthy and enjoy my life with my children and friends—old and new—for a long, long time. I want to help other people who are willing to learn from my experience. I want to join others who have the same healthy goals in life. I want to enjoy an active lifestyle, nature walks, power walks. The only way I would not be able to achieve this is by defeating myself with self-doubt and getting off the program and teachings. No doubt there will be set-backs-but I will not let it deter me from achieving my goal!

TED

Fifty pounds of fat is gone. I lost 50 pounds, my body is stronger, my heart is stronger, and my blood pressure is down. I find that my head is clearer. I have not had chronic bronchitis or any colds, and there is a recognizable reduction of mucus in nasal passages. I no longer suffer from heartburn. I feel great! I am energetic and happy. The best part of all of this is that I feel in control of my life. I no longer drink champagne. I've continued the walking program, and I feel my body changing. I've achieved self-esteem, self-reliance, and the notion that I'm the hero in my life. I'm becoming clearer and clearer about how I live my life, and I see how the old ways don't work. I now question why I have certain beliefs. I've reclaimed myself and my life, and I have hopeful and exciting feelings about my future.

LOU I.

For someone with a history of chronic fatigue, committing to a time allotment twice a week to commute to the city was a challenge to me at the start of this program. I also had to adjust to how my family reacted to my lifestyle changes, and I had to get accustomed to the changes in my diet. Physically, the exercise reg-imen took some getting used to. I have learned to have a more positive outlook on life, regardless of any negative events that have happened or that will happen. I have learned to control my temper and not make any decisions if I am in an angry state of mind. I will also admit if I make a mistake, even if I risk embar-rassment. I spend more time with my children and am able to remain patient with them, even if they are whining or nagging. I find that I am more courteous on the road, which is important since I spend ten hours a day driving. I know that my positive attitude will lead to total well-being. Since I began the program, my skin condition [eczema] has improved and my energy seems to be longer-lasting. My senses of taste and smell are improved, so that now I desire less sweet and less salty foods. It seems that I have less gray or white hair than before, and I have fewer body aches, and my vision has improved slightly. Spiritually, I am more willing to help others, even if it inconveniences me. I am also eager to pass on any information that I have learned, if I feel it might benefit the person in need. I know that respecting others' views and opinions without condemning them is an important part of life. Striving to live guilt-free will open up my mind to new learning experiences. At first, dealing with my wife's extremely skeptical view of my participating in this study group was hard to overcome. Being that I had adjusted my diet two years prior to joining the study, it hasn't been too hard to work in the few additional changes. Elimination of wheat and sugar was probably the hardest to overcome, but I have kept them out of my diet. My wife is learning how to cook according to my new diet. She is creating some great-tasting dishes. I feel my health is at about 60 percent now, and I see myself as being closer to 100 percent in a year or less, since I will continue to have a steady desire to do whatever it takes.

RENEE

A big accomplishment for me was giving up my nicotine addiction (two packs daily) and an addiction of 10 to 15 cups of coffee a day. It was difficult in the beginning, but now I feel much better physically and mentally! My energy level has greatly improved, my blood work has improved, and my cholesterol has improved, going from 214 to 187. My triglycerides and PSA levels have also improved. I've incorporated new foods into my diet. I've eliminated dairy entirely, and have less congestion, bloating, and nasal drip. I am currently working on giving up wheat 100 percent. My siblings want to institutionalize my mother. However, I would not allow this to happen and have taken big steps legally and emotionally to avoid this.

MARSHA W. C.

My energy level has improved during this year-and-a-half-long Reversing the Aging Process study. I require less sleep. The ability to maintain a more intense mental alertness, over an extended period of time, has increased. Vision at seventy-one and a half years of age has remained stable, without the need of eyeglasses. Gum health has improved, and my nails are strong and growing more rapidly. Skin wrinkles are lessened and skin texture is smoother and softer. Sexually, my aging process has been reversed. Use of Eternal brought about premenopausal conditions. I experienced sweats, fuller breasts, and vaginal lubrication. Intake of Passion affects my sexual responses. The intensity of those responses are greater. I also experience sexual stimulation from visual sources. These responses are at a level that they had been fifteen years ago. I started taking Greens and Grains recently. Since that time, I lose only a few hairs when I shampoo. My nails are stronger and are growing more rapidly than previously. I'm always searching to determine how I can function more purely in order to manifest my true being. *Who Are You, Really?* made me aware of why I function as a Dynamic Assertive and how to do that more proficiently. You stimulate self-recognition. Especially important is the toxic people I've removed from my environment. Those who are family I have to endure—at times—and have set new rules for dealing with them. May 12, 1998, marked twenty-four years since I became a Nichiren Shoshu Buddhist. The only purpose of chanting "Nan myoho renge kyo" is for personal enlightenment. One can only be to others what they are to themselves. For me, the chanting opens and cleanses energy patterns. Only then can rebuilding of positive energy occur. Thank you, Gary, for being such a devoted host of this fun and joyous voyage.

SHARON

After one year on the program, I have lost 20 pounds and reduced my cholesterol level by over 30 points. Upon hearing Gary was having an orientation for weight management, I finally said to myself, "That's it, no more excuses." The major issue I was faced with was being "slightly overweight" most of my life. But "slightly overweight" turned into "very overweight" after the birth of my three children. I was very lazy, not exercising, and eating everything. Hips and backside became wider, arms were heavier, and my nickname was "thunder thighs." I wondered if I could really follow Gary's healthy protocol. Could I go through the detox and change to a completely different lifestyle? I needed the support of the group. But I also needed the support of my family. Our meals would be taking a whole different turn. I took a deep breath and decided to take it one day at a time. I made a six-month commitment. It is now one year later, and I am thrilled to say that I made it. After one year on the program, I no longer suffer with the excruciating pain from heel spurs. The protocol has helped me immeasurably. After losing 20 pounds, the spurs are almost completely cleared up. I have also reduced my cholesterol level by over 30 points. I started at 190, and at the six-month blood workup it read 157.

MARC C.

I joined a support group to lose weight and change my life for the better. Years ago, I was able to cause positive changes. I seemed to have lost this ability. The homework and group interaction returned this aspect to me. I am an avid skier and ski instructor. Being on the protocol gave me the most rewarding ski season of my life. My students brought an overwhelming amount of positive feedback. I taught the best lessons and received the best tips to date. I received an award for excellence in ski instruction. This year, I was relatively injury-free. During the last four seasons, I experienced injuries that lessened my abilities on the slopes for weeks at a time. I failed a high-level certification exam 14 years ago, but I will retake it this year. The exam will be a learning experience, and my athletic performance is at a high level. My surroundings will be detoxed soon. The group has given me the power to make wonderful changes.

LIZ

I have learned to forgive myself if I make a mistake, and to keep trying.

KEITH

At the age of 51, I am finally starting to live and understand my life. I lost 10 pounds; my mucus drainage has stopped completely; and allergic reactions completely diminished, especially since I changed my diet. I no longer eat meat or dairy. I feel that I am gearing myself to be more positive and see myself as a whole, complete, independent person. I now feel that I am in control of my own needs and destiny.

WANDA

I have learned how to apply discipline, focus, patience, and common sense to all aspects of my life.

HYACINTH F.

Growing up I was taught one way of being healthy: by eating the correct foods. However, on joining the program, I've learned so much about how the body works and is nourished by other nutrients and the process the body goes through. My belief was not quite correct. It was a challenge to change my lifestyle, but mentally I know it was the right change. As the weeks went by, I realized the changes, which were the results of sticking to my diet and knowing it worked for me, the way it was supposed to. I was always ready to help anyone who wanted to make this change in their life, and reaching out to others made me feel good with some satisfaction. I am focused in my thinking and usually set a goal in my mind and really go after it to allow it to happen. The effect of what was told to me in the program made a complete change in my life, and I am able to rationalize problems in the way of health, not any major one, and conquer the problem. Today I am a better person in shape as I feel much healthier than before. Many of the nutrients I took, the juices, and the habit of eating organic vegetables, grains, and fruits gave me phenomenal results. My hair is not as gray as before. Patches have come out with the original black renewed hair, my skin is subtle, firm, and younger-looking. My nails are soft and pink. The arthritis in my fingers diminished, and I don't have those dizzy spells as before. It's my belief that my cholesterol is much lower. I have lost seventeen pounds. I still have to do more in the line of exercises, but this is due to an ailment in the leg. My outlook of appearance is much more appealing to others, as they tell me I look younger. I feel great internally and externally. This physical change is of great importance to me as my health is my happiness. I can do much more at home, as I have more energy, sleep two hours less, and I do not feel fatigued as before. At times, I would feel sloppy on the job, but after attending the classes, I am more alert, think clearly, and am always energetic. I conquer negative emotions by having a passion for what I want, and carrying out my energy to the positive thought. Being here I am more connected with the Higher Being. My prayer life is meaningful to me and others. I share my time with others in their grief and pain, and I can always refer to an encyclopedia, my magnets, and communication with Him. He is always there for me when I need Him. I feel that innermost relationship spiritually. Behavioral patterns have changed, as I do not have any hatred in my heart for people anymore. It does not get me anywhere when I can change the negativity to something positive by assisting and giving myself in a situation. Really, I do find comfort, peace, and satisfaction when I can reflect myself in a manner that would be pleasing to others. They would see and imagine me the way I am. It is my belief that whenever you can do a good deed or say a good word to someone or of them, it is the correct way in mind and body. I am a more focused person in my thinking, and I am able to solve problems I may face on my own. Also, I help others who are in need of it. My body feels more youthful, healthier, and always moving on to a happier life. I am free of sickness and I feel great. I am more spiritually connected and my life is more meaningful of a happier, prayerful life. I have been worried about my high cholesterol due to many years ago and time and again this problem existed. After my body gave me the symptoms last year, as I could not breathe properly, I would take Q1O and smell peppermint oil, but it would persist. This is when I made a decision to solve the problem. After taking the green juices, red stuff, and nutrients, I do not have the breathing problem, so I believe my cholesterol has dropped somewhat. My sister got over her asthma after forty years of her life. She was always in the hospital emergency, and at one time the family thought we would lose her, but she feels great now. I feel much more healthy and I feel I'm living a much more meaningful life. This change was with results and I intend to keep on it all my life. I see there is a way of life taking good foods and with supplements and exercise, one has to be on the way to good health.

PATRICK H.

Since the beginning of my participation in this program, the following has occurred: increased mental clarity; a better sense of overall calm and relaxation; a much-improved outlook on life; an even broader sense of consciousness and self; less crankiness; less fatigue; improved recall and memory; a much-improved ability to cope with stress; faster and more graceful movement; an improved feeling of mental clarity; overall improvements in my level of energy; clearer skin; clearer nasal passages; less excess mucous; improved resting heart rate; decrease in the amount of sleep needed for rejuvenation; improved workout recovery times; a noticeable increase in lean muscle tissue; improved bowel movements, which are also more regular; less sluggishness; more patience; and a decrease in my tonsil size. No longer do I have dark shadows under my eyes. There is significant decrease in pain from peripheral neuropathy in both legs and an extremely remarkable decrease in arthritis pain, both resulting from multiple trauma suffered July 7, 1997. The surgeon who operated on my crushed right calcaneus stated that post-traumatic arthritis was inevitable and that I may have to consider fusion in the future. I haven't gotten sick since I began the program—and that's without a spleen. I can't thank you enough for the knowledge you've bestowed upon me in any other way than to continue to actualize it. Forever I shall be grateful.

NANCY N.

I am no longer constipated, and my overall body pains have subsided.

STACEY T.

How have I changed since I began the program six months ago?

• I now exercise six days a week. When I first started walking, it took me thirty minutes to walk a mile. Now I walk a fifteen- to sixteen-minute mile!

• I've lost more than sixty pounds.

• I have eliminated two toxic people in my life.

• I sleep less and better.

• My skin has cleared up.

• I have better bladder control.

• I don't talk on the phone at night anymore, giving me much more free time. Now I do yoga one night and meditate every night.

• I don't gossip or listen to gossip, and I don't engage in negative conversations.

• I am happier.

• I feel joy.

• I am a better healer, a better doctor, a better human being.

With my mental and physical improvement, my patient numbers have in creased because of my attitude, and because I am physically stronger, I can see more patients. Life is good.

ALBERT

I feel like a new man. I lost 7 pounds. I can walk 10 miles. I sleep less. I help more people on the street and on the job, which feels great. I no longer eat at night.

LAVY

I am more aware of myself. I no longer overreact to others. I feel more confident. No need to smooth things over with people anymore. I simply feel better.

MAVASH

For the first four months of the program, I resisted taking the supplements. All my life, I never took any vitamins and supplements other than what was in the natural foods. I had been eating only natural foods and nothing else. I bought all the required items on the protocol the first night after class. But they stayed on my table untouched for the first four to five months. Finally, I decided that I am in the program already, I might as well go with the flow. I also created more faith and trust in the program. The whole thing was a challenge to my belief system to take factory-made products as foods and as nutritious aids. I was open to change, and new ideas gradually sunk in me over the course of the program. I let it happen. Physically, I am more than ever in touch with my energies within and the energy of other people. Prior to the program the energy field was unknown to me. I took a couple of courses in Pranic healing and in chi gong. Awareness of this issue even helps me in my business. I evaluate the employees who work in my business. During the day, if I observe that they are not present or their energies are low, I send them home to take care of themselves. I didn't do this before. I used to try to get a lot produced during the course of the day. Spiritually, I got in touch with my emotions, which I had piled up under a bunch of factual stuff I had been ignoring how things affect my feelings. I put myself in this program again because I wanted to be in a support group to detoxify and because I have benefitted from the program. I am not finished. I believe that some changes happen as a result of a process and some other changes can occur very fast. The change in eating habits, lifestyle, or spirituality can only happen as a result of a process. They require time and exposure. And the support group provides this for me. I do not have any "obstacles" in my life. I do not look at my life this way. I am looking at where I want to develop to from here and where I want to move on to. I have done everything I've ever wanted to do in my life and I do not have any wish lists to work on, or to be attached to. At this stage of my life, I am inquiring into what I can leave behind and what is my legacy. I want to contribute. I must decide in what way. My passion is in the environment and probably in alternative medicine. I have decided to get out of the business I am in and move on to something that I can directly impact and contribute. That is my challenge. I am in the group because I have benefitted from it. Repeating it will not be the same experience. Probably, more than anything else the group has helped me not to ignore myself emotionally and spiritually. I am also benefitting from detoxifying my body. I have learned a lot of small, detailed, but important information about foods and health.

LINO, 78 years old

My life was going nowhere. I held myself back with bad habits and attitudes. I overused alcohol. I was overweight. Eating fatty flesh foods gave me an almost constant heartburn and fatigue. I felt anxious and angry and not at all content with myself. Gary's protocol was really a radical change. I never drank green juices. In fact, I never ate healthy food. I was not aware of nutrition or meditation. I did not care to look inward or deal with past angers and pain. My life is very different today. I am vegan and organic. I gave alcohol up quickly. The green juices filled an empty space with vitality instead of dulling emotions. I lost thirty pounds. For some reason I feel less or no anger and am relaxed, even content. My eating plan is satisfying and there is after heartburn. I feel and act younger. I look back into my past and wonder why. It was not a lack of self-esteem; it was a lack of body cleansing, natural foods. I found myself.

MELISSA

When I began working with Gary I was extremely toxic. I lived in a toxic environment. I worked in a bar. I had toxic people around me. I was a mess, both mentally and physically. Physically, because I didn't exercise, smoked cigarettes, drank alcohol, and ate all of the bad foods you could possibly put into your body. I didn't sleep well, felt lethargic all of the time, and had low energy. I was 29 years old and burned out. I had one of the worst cases of adult acne you'd ever want to see. It was all over my entire back, face, and neck. It was a condition I had had for 11 years. I attended a Gary Null lecture—actually, I went with my sister to see the lecture. She was the one more interested. After the lecture, Gary approached me and matter-of-factly asked about my skin condition. I told him I had tried everything I knew of, but nothing was working. This was 3 years ago. Today, I am 90 percent free of all of the cystic acne I had for all of those years. My energy level, well, I've never had so much energy. The quality of my friendships and relationships is extraordinary. I have wonderful friendships. I've changed a lot in that I had no self-discipline whatsoever. Now, I'm up early every morning, race-walking and going to the gym. In fact, I am now a state-champion athlete. I'm taking very good care of my body. I am also juicing. I eat all organic produce every day. I don't take many supplements because I find that the juicing takes care of those needs. I am much more open to new ideas. I was a defensive person before. Now, I've learned to step back and put my attitudes and energies into a neutral space. In essence, I've learned how not to personalize when it comes to things that are said and done.

DOUG, 69 years old

I was overweight but considered myself healthy until an abnormal pre-op EKG for gallbladder surgery indicated cardiac problems. I had a quadruple bypass in March 2000. I saw Gary on television and purchased one of his videos and a book. After reading and watching the tape I joined a health support group. I investigated alternative methods to reclaim my health. I had twenty EDTA chelation treatments, became vegan, eliminated sugar, wheat, sodas, and gluten. I shop in a health food store to eliminate sprayed vegetables. I enjoy new information regarding healthier lifestyles. Today I need only six hours of sleep per night, wake up to exercise each morning, and have my large meal midday. I enjoy sharing new insights with others. I am healthy without symptoms of cardiac disease or sinus problems. I am in a new business. I use green and red powders, supplements, protein powders, and magnets. I eliminated carpeting from my home. I plan to study vegetarian cooking and create new recipes.

ANDREW

My hair was thinning. [Since joining a group,] I lost 20 pounds and built great muscle tone. My hair loss stopped, the bursitis in my knee diminished. I no longer need naps in the afternoon. I sleep less and recover from colds quickly. I cured pharyngitis without antibiotics.

RICH V.

My skin tone improved. I lost weight and now run eight miles a day. My sense of smell is improving. My hair grows less gray. I no longer feel a slump of energy at 3 p.m. each day.

DAVID Y.

Physically, this program has given me a pathway onto how to extend my lifespan. How to get away from the American diet, how to cope in this society when you are perceived to be different. This program has given me energy, and an overall feeling that my body is much cleaner. It has helped me see that there is another way to live your life.

ALICE, 61 years old

I had my ovaries removed when I was in my forties. That caused extremely severe menopausal symptoms. I was told it would continue for the rest of my life. I felt extreme abdominal pain, which put me in a depression. Wrinkles and bags developed under my eyes. My energy was low and I had brain fog. The support group and protocol changed all of the above. Because I followed the protocol, used juices, became vegan and organic and looked within, this woman is brand-new. My depression lifted. No more abdominal pain. My skin is less wrinkled and the under-eye bags are gone. I have an enormous amount of energy; the brain fog and cloudy thinking are gone. I realize I am more intelligent than I thought I was. It's as if vitamins and juices washed my brain. I can recommend the protocol with much love and enthusiasm.

BILL

I feel like a new man. I lost 7 pounds. I can walk 10 miles. I sleep less. I help more people on the street and on the job, which feels great. I no longer eat at night.

EDMUND H.

When starting the program, I was pretty well mentally readjusted. Three years ago, my own beliefs were validated as far as not conforming to what the society demands from you, just being a freer thinker with no restrictions. Physically, I work a lot of hours, so I didn't find the time to take care of myself as I should have. On weekends I enjoy outdoor activities. After starting the program, I am more aware of the need for daily exercise for the physical, mental, and spiritual aspect in growing and becoming whole. I've had a hard time in the spiritual area. After having been pushed out of the Catholic Church at an early age, I have had bitter feelings toward the Church and no desire to return. After having children, my wife wanted to bring the children up Catholic, still respecting my feelings. I feel my own spirituality, even though it is not channeled through some bureaucratic system. I am at peace with myself and follow the values I believe are correct. I still feel something lacking in this area, like I need to do more. I am on a new plane of thinking. A higher level, clearer, sharper, more relaxed, able to control anger better. When I wake in the morning, I'm on, not having to wait for a cup of coffee to start to function. It was easy eliminating coffee. Also I feel less limited than before just from my own limitations I put on myself. That's gone—the sky is the limit. I am able to solve problems better just being more focused and less frantic, just clearer thinking. Everything just seems less difficult, enabling me to enjoy life much more. After using protein supplements and weights I am back on track feeling lighter and stronger with more energy and endurance. From time to time I've been having problems with my energy levels. Also, my hair is thicker and faster growing, skin is clearer and healthier looking, nails are thicker. Although not channeling my beliefs through a fixed system, I do feel more at peace with myself. I feel on a higher plane after making these changes in my life. I don't feel I need the rules and regulations from a given religion or the guilt or suffering that's expected of you. Though I feel I would like to find another religion different from what I learned in my past just to expand my mind. The changes I have made were not as difficult for me because I truly want to better myself and make up for the past abuses of my body and the pollution that has accumulated for so long. After making these changes and feeling so much better, it is clear that this is the way I want to live the rest of my life, no doubt. The change was a little different for my wife, who had seen me transform into a new person. She had a hard time adjusting to this, but the change was all positive in my eyes anyway, and now she sees that I am a better, more honest person. I tell it like it is, I don't hold back and accumulate negative emotions. As far as diet goes, I really did not have a hard time eliminating the bad stuff after learning how it affects the body. Though switching to the new diet has been a constant learning process, I still have a way to go. Sometimes I feel weak and tired, most likely from my diet, but it's becoming easier. People look at me drinking my juices and look at me kind of funny, but I don't care because I know I am better off than them just by drinking the juices. My hours at work make it difficult to get the physical part done, but I just make time the best that I can, always being aware of the need to incorporate the physical aspect of the program. It's hard not to make these changes after learning what we have in the program. I find now it's impossible to go back to my old ways. After feeling the positive changes and growing every day and looking forward to a longer, healthier life, it's like I have been reborn. I would also like to run the marathon in 1999, because I don't think I could be ready in 1998. Still I'm going to train now. I love life now. Where everything was pretty much a drag, now I'm on a higher plane looking to go higher and meet harder challenges and learn and better myself as I go and grow through life with my new life's program. Thank you.

BRIAN, 60 years old

I was not certain vegetarianism and nutrients could help me. I was one of those tense corporate people having unpleasant personal relationships. There were pockmarks and eczema on my face. My hair was graying. My eye color changed to a darker shade. I was diagnosed with hypertension. My nails grew slowly. I also had a scar from an old wound that did not lighten. My wife and I joined a support group with amazing results. Hypertension is a thing of the past. My skin had amazing results; no more eczema or facial pockmarks. My gray hair is growing new hair the color of my childhood blond and the receding hairline is reversing. My eyes returned to their blue color. Nails grew in quickly and the scar disappeared. I left the corporate world for a happier life and improved relationships.

JENNIE

I started my change last year when I was undergoing a depressed, crisis state when I recognized that I wasn't able to take care of myself and use the skills that I knew I had. This was because of the anxiety I had and the weakness in my mind and body. I knew that this was a turning point for me. Either I would go back to all of my old ways—medications, doctors, hospitals, for psychiatric conditions that I didn't think I could overcome. It came to that point again and I realized that that wasn't what I wanted. That it was time to find the courage. I had enough self-esteem to ask for help for the support that would really help me. What I did was I decided to go live with friends who had a very structured life, who were very successful. By doing this, I put myself in routines—daily habits that would help me strengthen both my body and my mind. Prior to that, I would have weeks where I wouldn't even get out of bed because I was so depressed. I had clutter in my apartment that would go 8 feet to the ceiling. I just didn't want to get rid of anything. I was on all sorts of different medications. I suffered from chronic pain issues, severe migraines, arthritis symptoms and inflammation in all of my joints, fibromyalgia. They gave me medications to relieve the pain, as well as the other conditions like my thyroid problem. But none of the medications were helping. In addition, I would have panic attacks and I suffered from anxiety that prevented me from answering the phone. This stopped my support system of friends and family who were in a position to help me. I essentially disconnected from them because I felt guilty about my wretched condition. I felt shame and embarrassed. It was not a positive state that I was in. Today, I am a much more disciplined person. I exercise quite a bit now. I eat whole foods, no processed foods. I take supplements every day. I juice daily. I now listen to my body, which frequently tells me which foods to eat. I also pay close attention to hygiene, which a depressed person doesn't always do. I have removed all of the clutter from my life. I am no longer overweight. In fact, I've lost 30 pounds. One of the main reasons that I was able to do this is that Gary told me that I should face my fear of failure. I asked him how I could do this. He said it was simple: I should ride my bicycle from New York to Florida. If I could do that, then I could do anything. Well, I did it alone and in ten days. I am now a championship race walker, who has removed stress from my life. I have removed all of the toxic people from my life.

BOB

I am a recovered alcoholic. It's been about 7 years that I've been off alcohol. At first, I ate a lot of sugar in cakes and things like that. One of the psychological-emotional components of my behavior was that I always had a very difficult time getting started in the morning. The first thing I would think about when I got up was what I was going to eat, which usually included cereal with sugar, a pastry, and sugar-laden coffee. There has been a slow, progressive bettering of my diet, but there has still always been the sugar craving. Sometimes I would be able to get away from it for a week or 2 weeks, but it would always creep back in. Recently, I completed a seven-day fast and a colonic cleansing and I found that after that cleansing process the craving pretty much disappeared. Also, I wake up in the morning feeling rather alert, and I don't have this compulsion to eat sweets. I think that because I am staying away from sugar, I generally am having better days psychologically.

CHRIS M.

My strength and endurance increased. My complexion is clearer.

JOEL

I have more energy and overall get more done from day to day.

BENJAMIN V.

One of the issues I felt difficulty in overcoming was the guilt surrounding my mother's death. I worked with her in her treatment to seek an alternative approach and although she complied initially, in the long run she didn't want to maintain the dietary and lifestyle changes. I felt there were perhaps other ways or approaches I could have pursued in her care in retrospect, but that's all in the past. I felt I could have even contributed to her demise, but I learned I have no control over other people's actions. After four years of living with this guilt I finally let go. Today my father has mild coronary disease, which I feel is partly due to the loss of my mother. I am helping him but understand now that I can explain the options, make suggestions, but ultimately the decision is his own what course he chooses to take. Physical challenges were prematurely aging skin and hair loss, also fifteen or so years of acne. Today my skin is softer, smoother, and more youthful looking. My acne is gone. It is rare to see any hairs on my pillow, because the excessive hair loss has ceased. Finding my purpose in life is an issue I am working on still. But I'm following my instincts and intuition and this is providing insights along the way. Like doing the things I enjoy doing, rather than what I may have been conditioned to do. The forgiveness letters and the emotional work were very helpful in the letting go of the guilt of my mother's death and the past as well. Again, the appearance of my skin, hair, and no longer having any acne is a big improvement. Regular exercise along with dietary changes have made for a better-toned body. Although at one time I trained with weights approximately two to two and a half hours a day, three to four times per week for almost ten years, eventually I slacked off, and today I don't exercise as long so I don't get burned out or bored. I do different things in addition to weight training, biking, mambo dancing, meditating, and have a more balanced approach so I could continue for the long term. The program provided me with options I wouldn't normally consider. Because I've been able to let go of the past I look forward to a brighter future. As a result of the physical and emotional work and changes, I've made more time to focus on the spiritual. Although I'm still not sure what my purpose in life is overall, one aspect has been to serve. As a political activist in my spare time I do work around political prisoners. The people I've come to know, the knowledge I've gained, the personal growth I've experienced have exceeded my contributions, as well as the work I've done for the community advocacy organization. After visiting the stock exchange on Wall Street as a youth, eventually I took a job on Wall Street. I saw myself or created an image for myself that I should be in the business world. Working on Wall Street was an atmosphere that was oppressive and depressing. We worked long hours and then were demoted for our troubles. When I discovered how Wall Street carried its money I realized this was not my ticket out of my perceived poverty. I wanted a life better than my parents, who struggled in factories and odd jobs. I suppose I was overcompensating. I left Wall Street and studied the things I enjoyed—anthropology instead of business. Learned a new language. I am pursuing my interest and intuition, and although I felt a bit apprehensive at first and received many criticisms initially, the changes I've made feel great. I have adopted an organic vegetarian diet, I exercise approximately five days per week. During my fourth month of the program I was feeling somewhat fatigued and began to exercise less, but the extra antioxidants helped. I used to feel stagnant and that I wasn't growing. Today, I am taking on challenges I probably wouldn't have dreamed of in the past—particularly around my activism with regard to political prisoners and other issues. I do temp work for a community advocacy organization and prefer jobs that potentially serve the community. Today I see myself as having a future in which I am open to all sorts of possibilities and not confining myself to preconditioned notions. I find myself willing to explore different things and not just playing it safe as I did in the past. Initially taking risks felt scary and things usually didn't turn out as planned; however I've learned to reflect, learn from the situation, and look for new ways to make improvements. I have learned from the chances I've taken, I feel less apprehensive and look forward more to the challenge. I'm not sure where my pursuits will take me, but at least I'm more open to the unknown and am willing to challenge boundaries, where in the past I probably would have barely even considered, let alone pursued, this. As a result of the changes I've made I feel more connected or engaged to people and things around me. Sort of like being part of a process in the larger scheme of things I'm still learning to comprehend.

LINDA O.

I did not have a disease or major symptoms. I wanted to improve my life and use my physical self in a healthy way. I wanted to grow stronger with age. The protocol made me stronger physically. I feel my health in my energy. I run additional miles without fatigue. My hair and nails are stronger. Keeping a journal made me introspective. I observe life positively. I feel courageous to attempt new projects.

BOB

I was curious about this thing called a detox protocol. I did not feel unhealthy, but I decided to attend a group and see if it impacts me in any way. I wanted to lose some weight but did not like dieting. My blood pressure was a bit high, and I did get headaches. I came to each meeting, and listened and learned. I lost weight without dieting. My waistline is smaller. My blood pressure is normal. I need less sleep, and my headaches are gone. The protocol and science behind it are valid. It was a wonderful experience.

CRIS M.

I have followed Gary's protocol for the last two years. I entered the anti-aging program with fatigue, which impacted my exercise program. Eventually, my strength and endurance increased. My complexion is clearer. My hair loss has reversed. I have a great sense of well-being and personal satisfaction. My outlook has improved in work and in my personal life. Areas of importance have shifted, and I feel focused, alert, and aware.

EUGENE

Three months before joining the study, I was diagnosed with a small melanoma in my right eye. I am legally blind in my left eye. The cancer options were horrendous: removing the eye, treating it with radiation, or leaving it alone, with the chance the cancer would metastasize to my liver. I often had migraine headaches, chronic lower back pain, prostate problems, pain from a rotator cuff injury in my right shoulder and arthritis in a toe. I was overweight. It was time to change strategies and rid myself of these conditions. Gary's words were powerful. I had to become my own authority. Since beginning the protocol, the cancer has not grown in eight months. My migraine headaches virtually disappeared about two months after changing my diet. I lost 35 lbs, and my back has improved. Saw palmetto and other herbs did not relieve my prostate problem in the past, but they are quite effective now. My body is receptive to healing. The other minor conditions have improved. Although my energy level varies, I feel more energetic and younger in a body that knows how to heal itself.

MIKE C.

I have been detoxing for the past year. My life keeps getting better and better. In some ways, I feel like a child again. Gary's uncompromising passion for his beliefs and work and his dedication to the mastery of each day set a powerful role model in my life. I plan to help others grow and improve their lives.

FRANK

I am so glad that I joined Gary's support group. Following his protocol, I lost 9 pounds; my muscle tone, cardiovascular capacity, and digestion have improved. I require less sleep, my allergies are much better and not clogged up. I meditate after work; it clears my head. Exercise has been the easiest part. After doing my cardio exercise, I feel great. I work out at the gym in the mornings and sometimes after work. I walk the golf course instead of riding. Now I trust myself to make decisions, and I go with my gut. My home is less cluttered. I have more of a sense of order. I no longer judge or at least am very aware of doing so if I must. I am now considering moving to a warmer climate. I no longer worry what people think of me. I will not let anyone stop my connection to "my joy." I have disconnected from a lot of negative friends. My faith is even stronger. The positive voice is beginning to overpower the bad.

GINA S.

I am at peace and harmony today. My spirit awakened for the first time since childhood. I have come full circle. Body, mind, and spirit are one. My family has made many life-affirming changes. My father-in-law is beginning to heal. Our children are healthy again. The effects are endless and go much deeper than mere words can express.

BELLA

For 20 years I've had purple spots on my tongue. Now, my tongue has returned to its original color. The vision in my left eye has increased, and I no longer wear a contact lens in the left eye. All of my non-accomplishments in life I blamed on my father, because he mistreated me as a child. I blamed my mother for not going to college after high school. After writing the forgiveness letter, I no longer blame my father. I no longer blame my mother. My personal challenge was the exercise program. In the beginning, it, was the hardest thing for me to do. Now I exercise six days a week. I've also overcome my fear of public speaking. In January, I was the moderator for a fashion show. A year ago I could not have done that. I forever shall be grateful.

NANCY A.

My illness was undiagnosed for a year and a half. It was debilitating. During my stay at Paradise Gardens, I looked at deeper issues. I was able to understand the issues preventing me from achieving health. Gary made me aware of my right to live joyfully and strong. His fierce and unflagging dedication was inspirational, and I am grateful. I look forward to a healthy, strong life.

JOYCE C.

My energy level has gone up. I can get through the day without feeling drowsy. The eczema and constipation improved. My tinnitus symptoms greatly diminished. I lost weight after two months on the program, and my percent of body fat went down almost 10 percent. I did not gain any weight back. My memory has significantly improved. I can now connect the names and faces of my friends. I am calmer and more relaxed.

TOM

I came into a support group to reach my potential and establish goals. I entered the group after a divorce. My job and apartment loss soon followed because I allowed other people to make decisions for me. I gave them power. I entered a study group with an objective of developing the spiritual, physical, and emotional potentials I could not muster alone. An uncompromising commitment to the program would, hopefully, give me the power to make my own choices. I want control, and I have it now by controlling what I will or will not put into my body. I feel my energy without using sugar. Now that I am single and possess the solitude necessary for reflection and spiritual growth, I follow a path toward discovery and wholeness. Positive changes in one aspect of life lead to positive changes in other areas. Good changes can build on each other.

MARK

I joined Gary's support group because I wanted to have more energy. I had gray, thinning hair and osteopenia [low bone density]. I also had abdominal fat, fuzzy vision, and pain in my shoulders. After following his protocol, my hair has begun to grow in darker and thicker, and my bone mass has increased. I also lost weight, and the pain in my shoulders is gone. My vision has also greatly improved.

KEN S.

I work in a prison. This is very stressful work. The impact of this job set me up for tense evenings at home. I felt guilty about my work; it drained my energy. My hair was thinning. I felt this was part of aging. My energy was low. I did not know what to do to rebuild my stamina and change my life. When a support group was formed, I joined it. I follow the protocol and eliminated all allergic foods. I juice, which cleans out my system and gives me energy. I am aware of environmental toxins that can reshape my body and mind. I lost 20 pounds. New hair is growing on my head. My stamina increases daily. The job stress that pulled me down does not impact on my personal life as much as it did. I do not feel guilt about my work. Lately, I think about and question religious doctrine. Things are opening up.

CAROL

I went to Paradise Gardens during the time I had been a support group member for six months. My weight was stable. It was my first step toward fulfillment.

Watching the videotapes and attending Gary's talks led me to the pain I kept in my subconscious. This process made the difference between living an existence and living life to its fullest, at a high energy level. I enjoyed each challenge and learned the joy of walking. At first, I felt I could not do it. Then I stopped thinking and turned the walks into meditations. This unique approach helped me to continue my health journey. I expect I never did anything more important in my life.

PETER

I lost 8 pounds. Thyroid problems are gone. No more depression. I have lots of energy. I need no crutches.

JOSEPHINE

Since starting Gary's protocol, my candida has greatly improved without allergy-like symptoms, my fibroid cysts disappeared, and my adult acne went away.

ANGELA

I lost 5 pounds. Eczema improved and flexibility improved. I have more energy and feel less self-centered.

ANGELO

I am ecstatically happy now. And so is my family! It is my wife who discovered the Gary Null detox program. She is the inspiration for the success we are both experiencing. I was ready for a major change, whatever it was. I'm glad it was this protocol. I had always believed that I was eating properly in the past. However, I was blind to reality. I was getting fatter and fatter, and my health was declining quickly. Since beginning the program five months ago, I have lost approximately 105 pounds. My blood pressure is 120/80, and my cholesterol level has dropped to 158. I feel superb. As I walk, I feel like I am on air, and that I could walk for as long as the day is long. I have much more flexibility. I can perform many of the physical tasks that I could not do before. Before, I could not cross my legs or even tie my shoelaces. Now I can bike, jog, or power walk for long periods of time. I have learned to laugh every chance I get. I still get the job done, but now I am able to enjoy myself at the same time. I will not tolerate any negativity at all. If I am wrong, I have learned to apologize.

MARK M.

The pain I once had in my left testicle has decreased significantly. My energy level has increased. I am energetic all day, into the night. I no longer have to wake up in the middle of the night to urinate. My gray hair is beginning to turn black in areas. I have a great deal of inner peace throughout the day. My memory is sharper. I can remember things that need to be done for myself and others. My focus and concentration are sharper.

SIGRID

I lost 30 pounds.

TRELLINE G.

[Before the program] Stress, weight, hypertension, anemia, and a heavy menstrual period. [With the program] my hair, skin, and nails are strong and healthy. The anemia was life threatening. Today I no longer have this condition, and my periods are normal.

TOM G.

I joined the group to get healthy, regain energy, and develop self-motivation. I have gained far more. My energy returned as I exercised, followed the protocol, and made the appropriate dietary adjustments. My skin is younger looking, and I see the world differently. An old injury that turned into varicose veins is healing. The veins are smaller. I require fewer hours of sleep. Uncluttering really put everything in order. I cleaned my basement for the first time in 15 years and just threw everything out. My wife and I argue less; I bought her a copy of *Who Are You, Really?*, which helped. I intend to stay on the protocol and go to the next level. My family and I thank you. Our lives are happier.

BILL

Before I started the program, I had gallstones and dryness on my fingers. I no longer have any symptoms of gallstones. I lost 3 pounds and my skin is 50 percent less dry, including on my fingers. My immune system is stronger, and I have not had any colds this winter. I see the light at the end of the tunnel. I feel less guilty about saying no. I know what is correct, and I will not be bullied by others. I am also getting less depressed in regards to money.

ROBERT

I developed intestinal problems. My blood pressure was low, there was a tightness in my chest, and I suffered with a chronic, painful skin condition on my hands for 30 years. I am now on the protocol. My first improvement was a rush of energy after eliminating wheat and corn. My hand condition improved; the nails are not pulling away from my skin. My thinning hair is growing. I feel focused and aware of others around, and I aid street people. Writing letters [and thus opening routes of communication] eliminated the pressure in my chest.

MARLENE

I was overweight, which caused a knee joint to swell and become damaged. My blood pressure was high. I always caught colds and flu, and had difficulty recuperating from them. Environmental allergies made me feel sick. I ate dairy and meat. When I had my hair analysis, I was told there was uranium, arsenic, titanium, and commercial dyes in my system. My health diagnosis was so bad I knew I had to do something and that something was announced on Gary Null's radio show. I joined a group. I learned how we damage our body with food and exposure. I was fascinated. Most of the people in the group grew their own illnesses. I followed Gary and Luanne's instructions carefully, one day at a time. Today I am 40 pounds thinner. I can walk freely. I discovered new foods and grains, new breads. I have less sinus discomfort, fewer allergies, no more upper respiratory infections. A sense of well-being is in me. The forgiveness letters and homework gave me insight. I deal with past angers. The classes gave me freedom. I am grateful.

MARIA

At the beginning of the program, I was very tired all of the time. It was difficult for me to get up in the morning. I was tired all day long. My skin had a dark sickly look to it. I had dark circles under my eyes, and my skin would always break out with pimples. My hair was falling out. My body was very thin, and I had no muscle tone. [Now] I have integrated exercise by getting a membership to the YMCA. I also go for walks and ride my bicycle. I have also begun to play the drums in a rock band and have found it to be a fun way to get a great workout. My skin is now much clearer and healthier looking. My body has more muscle tone now that I work out regularly. I also haven't had a cold in the six months of this program. My nose used to be clogged all of the time, but now it is always clear.

I have also had my mercury fillings taken out, which has resulted in a dramatic increase in energy. I have a more positive outlook on life than I used to have. I still fall into negative slumps sometimes, but I am more aware of them so I can I had a job that I absolutely hated. It was a "go nowhere" job in an office in a field that I had no interest in. Luckily for me, I was laid off, which has given me a lot of time to focus on music. My band has been travelling and playing shows with such a great response every place we play. This has given me a sense of satisfaction in being able to do what I love to do. I am a much more happy person spiritually now than ever before. I only surround myself with warm, loving, nurturing people, and I don't tolerate any negative thoughts of my own or from other people. I used to feel that my best days were behind me, but now I feel that they're way ahead of me.

GARY M.

I was 35 pounds overweight. My blood pressure was 180/110, my cholesterol 240. I lost 18 pounds, and now I run the NY marathon.

CYNTHIA

I was a dancer and became an interior designer. I was organic and vegan. I used sugar occasionally and had hypoglycemia. Although I felt disgusted with the waste, toxicity of materials, and disregard in the design field, I was a workaholic and developed septicemia from overwork, travel, and a bad diet. When I left that field, I set out to find myself, and I entered a Gary Null Woman's Issue workshop and studied energy types. Today, I am an acupressure therapist and garden designer. I follow the protocol with more detail, and my hypoglycemia improved. I am energetic, and I have no more bitterness. I am proud and happy in my new professions, and I am in touch with myself. Not honoring oneself allows others to intimidate you.

KENNETH L.

I used to feel no one understood my problem and fear of isolation. I was reticent about meeting with a group of people to improve my life, but I did and felt that the group enhanced my progress. I stayed on the protocol and lost ten pounds. I now feel joy and happiness; I feel really good about myself. I can now easily help other people. Praying and listening to my inner voice brought good results. The protocol cleaned my body and mind.

SUSAN M.

I lost 20 pounds. My skin is smooth, nails strong, and my hair is shiny.

PATRICIA B.

I was diagnosed with myelogenous leukemia during my separation from my abusive husband of 28 years. I was in remission with chemotherapy and attended a Gary Null lecture on "Who you really are." Today I power walk and run three miles five times a week. I do 200 crunches daily. I could not believe I would find the energy to make myself well but I did.

SUSAN M.

Although I was health-conscious, I knew there was room for improvement. I overslept but was low on vitality. I am a busy businesswoman. In the eight months since I began the anti-aging program, I sleep one and a half to two hours less each night and awake with great energy. I lost 20 lbs. My skin is smooth, my nails are strong, and my hair is shiny. I built muscle tone by power walking, yoga, cycling, and Nautilus. I feel more appreciative, with a better perspective. I manage two hectic businesses and four employees calmly, and I enjoy it. I research and pursue new ventures, including a book that may help people. I make time-out and laughter a priority. I am a spur-of-the-moment person, ready for action. Focusing on nontoxic people, I detach with love from the others. Family and friends are curious about my younger look and lifestyle, and I share the protocol with them.

MIRANDA

Since working with Gary, I generally feel better about me. I really have a better attitude. I lost 5 pounds, my energy level is higher, and I feel more alert and rested in the mornings. My cravings for sweets diminished, my ingrown toenails healed, and my scalp dryness eased. I've become more open and confident.

INEZ

She joined the retreat week as a work-study participant. After a consult with Luanne, she had a desire to learn more as she created an organic home. Hypertension and a low thyroid caused her to be cautious about exercise, but she wanted to learn more about physical fitness. She learned how to juice in the kitchen, be totally organic, and prepare vegan meals. Luanne taught her to focus on home hygiene. Andre's exercise class was exceptional, and the eye health lecture improved her eyesight. She found peace and calm that week. With new skills (how to listen to her inner self and create calm), she meditates and creates introspection. Inappropriate issues do not cause her upset when looking beyond and planning a future. Today, she is thinner, healthier, vegan, organic, and working to eliminate occasional "cheating."

JANICE

I had a 10-year-old son but was diagnosed as infertile. I miscarried and could not become pregnant. My periods were heavy. I had Lyme disease, with headaches and joint pain. I was exhausted from all these conditions plus allergies. We ate the typical American nonorganic diet. Good changes came with a Gary Null support group in 2000. I see a 95 percent improvement in all the areas of my health and my life. My periods are normal, my vision is improved, and my allergies are lessened. We eat an organic diet and follow the protocol using Gary's green and red powders. Our family relationships are better, because we are healthy and optimistic.

STUART

I ate flesh foods, but I did not use dairy. I believed this was a sensible diet. I had colitis and cardiac valve prolapse, which required antibiotics before dental work. Although I did get frequent upper-respiratory infections, I considered myself healthy. Something was missing, however, so I decided to join a support group in 1999. I certainly changed my life patterns. Since I became vegan, my energy improved and my perspectives on life issues are healthier. The homework made me aware of my mortality. I get fewer and milder upper-respiratory infections. My colitis is less severe. I work out six days a week, and I use green and red powders. I retired and use my free time to give back to society. I am active in local community affairs.

MONTY

I was an overweight semi-vegetarian. I used dairy and had digestive discomfort. I felt healthy, but I angered easily. I am a trained psychologist and studied Chinese medicine, herbology, and German electro-acupuncture. I lived in Italy for many years. I joined Gary's ·support group to learn the protocol for myself and my patients. I recognized my defensive anger. Today, living vegan, juicing, and enjoying changed eating patterns, I find life to be quite different. I meditate, am self-empowered, set boundaries, and will not expose myself to abuse. My career is beginning to be successful. I make contacts easily. Recalling my former behavior and anger, I realize the support group and detox protocol remolded my life.

BRIAN B.

I could not prioritize my life. I worked 12 hours a day and did not honor my belief system. I used vitamins, exercise, and reaching out to others as my spiritual focus. I will continue to use my supplements and follow the program. I do honor my health and have found comfort in a spiritual power. I will face my problems without fear, because I am more of a complete person. Gary and the group gave me inspiration, insight, and their generosity. I will pass this on to the people in my life. Thank you.

LAURA

My stay at Gary's Florida ranch helped me find a new direction in life. I arrived with my past and present, and came home an enlightened woman. I made permanent changes in my life and feel terrific. My changes are numerous. I feel I can do anything I wish.

JEROME D.

I lost some weight and feel healthier. My skin is softer and more youthful looking. My energy level is way up. My mentality is improving every day. I am now able to cope with events in my life.

ROSE V.

I would like to thank you, Gary, for your constructive criticism of my power walking, as well as for encouraging me to compete eventually in this sport. As for my foot problems, I will follow your advice, because I trust you. I know I will be cured. I would like to let you know, based on my perception, that you are a perfect example of "mens sana in corpore sano." You have given me inspiration to strive for the same, although I wonder how far I will get or when I will feel complete.

SARA

I was interested in avoiding the illnesses my mother suffered in her old age. I had

PMS symptoms for 14 years. My sagging skin aged prematurely with pimples, cysts, and scars. My digestive problems caused bloating. My personal relationships were unpleasant. I read *Get Healthy Now!*, which motivated me to explore sensible methods to relieve my symptoms. I joined the next support group that opened up. I followed the detox protocol, and in time, the results I longed for manifested. I no longer have PMS problems. My skin is tight and less lined. The pimples and discoloration from cysts are fading. I believe the detox cleared these problems, too. My energy increased. The journals and letter writing self-empowered me. I take risks with confidence, not fear. I bicycle, use a rebounder, and belly dance. The new man in my life is far superior to those of the past.

SAMUEL N.

Since I joined the program, I have experienced wonderful changes. I understand the members of my group and I are all from the same source. We receive the same benefits, breathe the same air, receive the same sunshine and rain, and desire the same inner peace. By attending this group, I developed a spiritual awareness I never felt before. I am able to control my emotions, because I am aware that I can return to the spiritual source for guidance. I discovered my mental attitude relaxes my physical body. When interacting with other people, I am less anxious and impatient. I developed an understanding of people. I am most grateful for these improvements in my life within this short amount of time.

MEDINA

I am truly a survivor. I had breast cancer 11 years ago and refused chemotherapy and radiation but used Tamoxifen, which impaired my vision and emotions. I developed polyps, an inflammatory digestive problem, and an ulcer. I was taking too much medication, and it was making me sick. I sought a natural approach to healing-immune enhancement. I gained weight without cause, and my abdomen bloated. It was all wrong, so then I tuned in to *Natural Living* and joined a health support group. After three months on the protocol, my immune system shot up. My digestion improved, without bloating, as I eliminated many foods. The weight is slowly coming off. I feel radiant and wake up 5 a.m. each morning with phenomenal energy to do breathing and meditations with a naturopath. I realize that suppressed emotions of the past and holding on to nonexistent obstacles made me ill. All aspects of my life have fused. I am where I should be.

JOSE

I studied radiography for two years and worked with nuclear isotopes. My radiation badge determined I was exposed. I worried about my health. Information was withheld at work. Prevention training was improper. I ate some vegetables, flesh foods, rice, and beans, but deep within, I knew I had to change my life. I was unable to attend support group meetings, but I followed Gary's information and began the protocol. I used green and red powders, and purchased the weekly specials. I read Gary's books, juice and research supplements and new teas. I became aware of my allergies as I eliminated toxic substances in my diet. My energy is high, my hair is thicker, and my receding hairline is filling in. I teach my family about nutrition and proper diet. Today, I work as a limo driver and tape *Natural Living* to play in my car during the day.

HANK

I was introduced to *Natural Living* in 1980 by my wife. I became vegan at Gary's Texas ranch. I wanted to educate myself and reach my full potential in order to run the 1995 New York City Marathon. I was evolving one step at a time and joined a support group in 1999. I lost 20 lbs. My mental outlook improved, I am decisive, and I focus on realistic goals. I eliminate toxic situations and people. Forgiveness letters cleared the past, and I can enter a free future. Group support was essential. I am now involved in social and political issues, most recently the passage of a school referendum.

JOE G.

I was under major stress and developed twitching muscles. I refused medication. Nocturnal cold sweats and anxiety were difficult. My walking was affected by an Achilles tendon injury. I did not understand true nutrition and needed guidance. There was no better source than Gary Null, and I joined in. The group was a class for me. It was optimism and discovery. As my body cleaned out with the protocol, I improved, as did my behavior. Each meeting taught me the mechanics of our life systems. My muscle twitching stopped. I no longer have cold sweats or feel anxious. The Achilles injury is healing quickly. I enjoy stamina. My family is benefiting from my experience and uses the protocol, too.

KENNETH L.

I was reticent about meeting with a group of people to improve my life, but I did, and my progress was enhanced by these people. The group kept me on the protocol and prevented my usual fear of isolation. I used to feel that no one understands my problem. I lost 10 lbs and feel joy, happiness, really good about myself. I can now easily help other people. Praying and listening to my inner voice brought good results. The protocol cleaned my body and mind.

SHERRY

I wanted to get my life on track. I overextended myself to others, without reciprocation. I ate junk food and had a broken vein in my leg. I joined a health support group to learn about health through nutrition. I learned not only how to eat and what to eat but why we choose this new diet. I began to understand the relationship between the physical and the metaphysical. My family and I are vegan and organic. The vein in my leg healed. I eliminated toxic friends and family from our lives, which allowed me to focus on myself. I use visualization. The relationship with my husband and children is closer, warmer, and more affectionate. We do affirmations and uncluttered our home. With new insights and peace with the past, we are a cohesive family.

MARIE

After my husband died, I tried to adjust to a new lifestyle. I smoked and ate flesh foods, dairy, and sugar. My energy was low, my hair was thinning, and I had scars from earlier acne. I was exposed to asbestos and other chemicals, and developed emphysema, Epstein-Barr disease, and bronchiocytosis. I was a sculptor and inhaled clay dust. Being overweight added to my burden. I felt my energy declining. Listening to *Natural Living* for 10 years opened the world of alternative medicine. I began to take supplements, changed my diet, and had chelation therapy. My response to the food on the protocol was immediate and positive. I am now organic and vegan. Everything tastes so good. I create wonderful desserts: fresh fruit with honey and nuts. I no longer need a leg brace. My hair is thicker, and my skin is lovely. My pulmonary problems have lessened. I lost 8 lbs and will continue to lose weight. I exercise by swimming and walking. Without this protocol, I would have been on an antibiotic one week a month for the rest of my life.

DOW R.

My energy levels have improved. My skin is clearing up. My toenails and skin feel softer. I lost several pounds with no effort.

SUMMER

I always felt tired. I was sick each day, and I had a chronic walking problem because of hip displacement, which fatigued me. I suffered from various allergies. My cholesterol was high. I was depressed. When a health support group started, I felt this was one chance I would not pass up. I had to learn to eat and choose foods according to their compatibility with my body and their nutritional value. I learned how to cleanse my system of toxins and of the abuse of a bad diet. I found peace doing the homework, which forced me to confront painful but important issues that held me back in life. I was motivated and even went on a watermelon fast three times without hunger or fatigue. I use the green powders and juice. Exercising several times a week gives me energy and enthusiasm about life. I can do headstands, and my body is flexible. I go dancing. Also, I am 16 lbs lighter and do not have discomfort walking. My allergies improved. My physician is amazed by my younger, youthful body.

JOE

I follow an organic, vegan diet and do not take vaccines. My neighbors tell me I look 45 years old. They admire my changes. I appreciate my healthy lifestyle. It makes me quite aware of the tremendous amount of obesity today. I am confident and pleased with my life.

ATHENA P.

Cystic Breasts; Depression; Eye Floaters; PMS; Fatigue; Gray Hair
I heard Gary Null's support group members speak on the radio about experiences in the group and on the protocol. I had several conditions to improve and decided to join a group. I suffered with PMS, cystic breasts, depression, eye floaters, fatigue, and graying hair, and I usually was involved in bad relationships. I entered a group with many other people also seeking true health naturally. I detoxified and rebuilt my immune system. The results are no more PMS, cystic breasts, fatigue, and depression, all within six weeks on the program. Uncluttering was crucial. It enabled me to rid my life of negative people and to get closer to those I desired to be with. The eye floaters diminished. I detect no new gray hairs. I changed jobs and have a better salary and work in a happier environment.

DON

The detoxification protocol worked very well for me. My blood pressure dropped to 120/90. I no longer have warts on my hands, and my energy increased tremendously. I walk and climb stairs without getting out of breath. New black hair is growing in without any falling out. My memory has improved and is becoming sharper.

TIM

I no longer have problems sleeping. I have more energy. My eating habits improved. I worry less and have hope for the future. I lost weight without effort and kept it off.

ROBERT

I felt I lost control of myself. I was getting heavier each year, and my muscle decreasing. I did not have the vital energy I once experienced, and I was worried and fearful about my financial situation. I needed guidance to get me back on track. I was not happy with the claims I saw on television or with the many books I read. I did respect Gary Null and entered his support group. The detoxing affected not only my body but also my mind. I shed over 35 lbs and built muscle. I sleep less and have more energy. The lectures and homework opened the true me to myself. I found the strength to forgive, which improved my family relationships. I can do whatever it takes without fear today. This experience is the most effective method of understanding human potential and of gaining respect for our planet. I thank everyone.

AMY

I lost 12 pounds. I no longer have menstrual cramps. My facial skin has never been better. I have a regular exercise routine.

DAVID E.

Before

He listened to *Natural Living* for two years. He had 13 percent body fat. He felt the effects of middle age: he was cynical, had low energy, was dissatisfied with his physical self, felt he looked old, and ate the typical American diet. He was worried about cholesterol but ate meat and restaurant food, and had a poor diet. He was very stressed and had many problems. The shows on *Natural Living* began to influence him to change his life. He abstained from fast food, drank less alcohol, and began to juice organic greens.

Now

He went to Paradise Gardens. He is less self-critical, gave up bad foods and alcohol, and easily accepts himself with a positive attitude. He increased his exercising: he power walks, runs 4-5 miles, is training for a marathon with Gary Null, participates in a running and walking club on Sundays and did 14 miles. He read *Who Are You, Really?* and realizes it was his attitude that once made him feel old. He was asked for proof of age recently to enter a bar to hear a band he enjoys.

OWEN

I was an unhealthy vegetarian. I ate sugar foods and dairy. I assumed my health was good. I never got sick. I listened to *Natural Living* since 1985. One day, I decided to change my health and my life, but I needed parameters. I could not do it alone. I heard testimonials from support group members. They did what I intended to do. They understood the reasoning behind detoxification and rebuilding the body. I wanted to understand it, too. I joined a group. Today, I am not just vegan and organic, but I am an organic cook aware of my reaction to toxic foods. I designed an efficient meal program, and I juice two to three times a day. My body fat is 3 percent, I sleep six hours, and I awake with good energy. I seem to be thinner. We learned to unclutter our lives by uncluttering our environment, and I did that with great benefit. I exercise five times a week and may begin feng shui. Luanne, Gary, and guest speakers gave me an education and stable future. I thank them.

EILEEN F.

Before

Overweight. Hair thin. Nails fragile. Knee would swell due to several accidents. Skin eruptions. Did not sleep soundly.

After

Lost substantial amount of weight. Hair healthy. Nails growing. Knee condition improving. Skin clear. Sleeps well. Is actualizing a new career

ADELE M., 77 years old

Before

Low energy. Allergies. Hair graying. Housewife who wanted to get out.

Now

More energy. Original hair color returning. Allergies not as severe. Has job.

Leads her group, keeps a daily journal, and actualizes change. Developed self-confidence. Enjoys time alone. Engages in self-exploration.

AMY S.

Before

Double heartbeat. Ganglian cyst on wrist, with surgery advised. Nocturnal teeth grinder. Cystic acne. Unhappy with relationships.

Now

Double heartbeat rarely occurs. Ganglian wrist cyst gone. Does not grind teeth at night. Cystic acne gone. Takes stronger role in relationships, no longer following the other person's expectations. Cleaning out life and environment.

CHARLES L., 64 years old

Before

I ate the typical American diet: meat, dairy, sugars. I thought my primary health concern was not being able to gain weight. I began to listen to *Natural Living*. Gary presented valid research. People spoke about their experiences in health support groups. They sounded energetic and happy, as if they created new, free lives. Many of these speakers were my age or older. Their testimonials influenced me to change my life.

Now

I follow a protocol on my own from a book. I use green, red, and protein powders. I no longer put poison in my system from meat. Mine is a natural way of eating. I walk 6 to 8 miles a day and use supplements. Gary Null is my classroom on the air. I gather information daily and put it to use. My health is better today than it was in my younger years.

DEBBIE T.

Cysts diminishing. Weight loss. Gray hair returns to color. My breast cysts are decreasing.

MARIE Q.

I was timid and giving in to other people's opinions and not speaking up for myself. I was happy letting my husband make decisions—at least the small ones. Now I speak for myself and am involved in every aspect. I went to a massage course and will set up my own place in October when I come back from vacation.

I am no longer depressed! I lost fifteen pounds and feel great. The energy is up. No more migraines. The age spots are fading. The edema is much less and I can tolerate the heat better. My arthritis has improved. So has the irregular heartbeat. My skin looks much younger; also my hair looks better. The compliments of other people are proof nobody believes that I am sixty-five. I am exercising aerobics and rebounded and starting weight training. I am reading books about Chinese philosophy and way of life. Nutrition and yoga. I feel connected to the people I care for (older people who need help). This program made me aware that I am great and make good decisions. We consolidated our debt to a low interest rate. I took care of an older sick person against my husband's will and she rewarded me with her life insurance. I feel I can do what I want to achieve. When I began the program I had to stand up to my husband, who does not believe in this program. He fought me tooth and nail and gave me every argument in the world. I convinced him that it was the right thing for me because of my body and my health and that I was going to do it no matter what. He still wants his meat and potatoes, but slowly he tries vegetarian meals. He drinks a juice in the morning and tries tofu. I still have a hard time to get the juicing and exercise in every day. I still have to get more variety in my cooking. I have still a way to go.

BRUCE

Reflecting on my life choices, I have discovered a pattern in the types of women I've had relations with. It spoke volumes about my motivations. I believe my energy level has increased, and I have fewer stomach pains. My dry skin has subsided. I have had only one outbreak of herpes. I find that I am sleeping more regularly. I've decided to take charge of my fate. To do this, I've enrolled in a graduate program at Columbia University where I've met several entrepreneurial students with whom I am in the process of beginning a technology venture.

NEVILLE B.

I have better clarity of my thoughts. My cholesterol dropped, so did my weight, and my muscle tone has improved.

DONNA

I dove right into the protocol. I have lost about 25 pounds. Being overweight only became a problem for me in my adult life. In my thirties I went through a difficult divorce. I was emotionally devastated. I had been smoking and drinking to numb the pain. I decided that I would stop smoking and cut back on the wine. But this became more of a hurdle than I had envisioned. I guess I turned to food to fill the void I felt in my gut. I gained weight steadily and kept it on for over ten years. I was unhappy with the way I looked, but I didn't have the will to do anything about it. I tried a couple of techniques to lose the weight. I tried food combining and met with some success. Shortly after that, I joined the health support group. My general health was not bad, but I was terribly uncomfortable with the extra weight. I dove right into the protocol. I juice every morning. I have eliminated meat, dairy, and wheat. I take all of the supplements and meditate every morning. I also have read books and listened to several tapes recommended by Gary. The one aspect of the protocol that I have been less than consistent with is exercise. Focusing on being positive, setting boundaries, and detaching from toxic relationships has been very liberating. I have been in the program for nine months and I have lost about 25 pounds. I am a new energized person. I have taken control of a situation where I felt dissatisfied and helpless. The protocol has become a way of life.

MILTON J.

When I first joined the support group, I was aware and was struggling to change the way I was conditioned to think. Not just health, but the way I view the world. A lot of the things that were raised in class about guilt and making excuses was taught to me several years ago. Being in this group, in a way, made me see that I have gone a long way. I remember when I had excuses after excuses and never wanted to make any changes. The pain it caused me was great. I wasn't progressing. So when people in the group raise things to me about something I might be doing wrong, I am not so fast to attack them but, always and I mean always, remember that they are coming from the position that they want to make me better. I know that and I know how hard it was for me to get to that stage. It's an everlasting struggle. It is my opinion that the first step is helping yourself and one that I'm willing to take. Over a year ago, I was working out and one day I just stopped. Looking back at it now, I realize I was not motivated. Since joining this group, I realized that my reasons for working out were wrong. I used to work out to look good, and I found myself working out hard. But when I didn't see the results that I wanted, I quit. Working out should not be for looks, but used as a way to stay healthy. It was only when I started to think in those ways that I began to love working out. See, because there was no pressure for time. Every day I went to the gym and benefitted. It made me relaxed, vibrant, and, yes, it made me look good. This group made me see that my mental and physical state is one and the same. I struggle to change my lifelong views and must change my view on staying healthy. P.S. Since joining this group, I feel great, better than I felt in many years.

MICHAEL M.

I started with feelings of guilt. I was apprehensive, spending time in the past. I was influenced by my environment, having trouble actualizing. I felt disorganized, struggling with relationships, commitment, finances, and self-image. Physically, I was gaining weight and feeling achy. My skin was blotchy, hair graying. I was losing my good exercise habits. I was a recovering smoker. I did not think spirit was essential. My spirituality was awakening; I knew it existed, and believed in it. However, it was not an integral part of my life. I have become more aware of my mental process. This has enabled me to see why I was behaving in some negative ways. I lost fifteen pounds; my skin is clearer. My hair seems darker. My digestion is better. I used to have polyps in my lower intestine and they are gone. My life is more affirmed, being able to help others. I feel more worthy. I came to the program to change my diet and attitude in order to detox. I had done some work in these areas previously. However, I seemed to be sliding back to my old ways. The detox program seemed like a good way to get started again. I was a little apprehensive about the completeness of the program. After about two weeks, I changed my diet, leaving behind meat, dairy, and sugar. This was relatively easy in that everybody was supportive. I have to give myself credit for making my family and friends supportive. Listening to Gary, I had been exercising regularly for three years. However, I have stopped exercising. I am still struggling with it even though I am active on the job. I have gained many insights into the meaning of life and actualizing. I see myself integrating more in the future. Right now I feel like I'm letting myself and the group down. I can do a lot better. I see myself joining the running club. Mentally, I think I am getting it. I think I might be able to do more with myself and find more meaning in my life.

OSCAR L.

Mentally, I was chronically depressed. I felt hopeless and lost. When I looked in the mirror I kept thinking and knowing that I was just getting older and uglier and sicker. I was only twenty-one! Each day I would wake up feeling as if I was in an external jail, expecting nothing good to happen, only people who I resented and who didn't love me to meet. I had nowhere to go. I felt that if I didn't have anyone to go somewhere with, it would be pointless to do it by myself. So I stayed home a lot and did nothing. I was so bored with myself, I just slept most of the day. I had to think whether something I would do was productive or not. Trying to only do productive things, like reading about business law all day and having no fun at all made me even more depressed. I wasn't aware at the time that I ended up doing nothing all day because I was so bored. I had nothing to look forward to, nowhere to go, couldn't conceive of what to do, and was always saying to myself that I couldn't do it. I couldn't go to the bookstore in Manhattan because I didn't want to spend the $3 for the train ride. I couldn't get a date because I was too ugly and unlovable. I couldn't be healthy because I didn't have enough money. I couldn't be happy because I was so hopelessly sensitive to criticism and always being made fun of for unknown reasons. I felt sorry for myself a lot. I sang all of my favorite depressing songs over and over to myself. Often I cried before I slept. I hardly ever laughed; I isolated myself from meeting people and didn't smile very much. Another big issue was that I had very low self-esteem. Being a Creative Assertive, I am always somewhat insecure, but I really thought of myself as unworthy of any success. I couldn't even look a person in the eyes when I talked to him. I let people talk to me in condescending ways. I let them tell me how stupid and no good I was, and I believed it. That came from my family. I had no friends. Physically, I was underweight, had acne all over my face, dark circles under my eyes, weak feeling. I had bad indigestion. I couldn't eat grains or starchy foods without having an itchy reaction on my face, with more pimple eruptions afterward. I felt bloated after meals. I ate a lot of fat, which made me feel sluggish, and added to my feelings of depression. I had been weight training at home for about two years, but I could not get any muscle mass. It took all of my strength to squat one hundred pounds ten times. I slept about twelve to fourteen hours a day. I had many outbreaks of herpes cold sores, especially when under emotional stress. Felt tired a lot, wouldn't wake up early in the morning. Spiritually, I was very selfish. Didn't care about anyone but myself. Now I feel good for no reason many times. I look forward to each day, wondering who I will meet. I do my best not to hold grudges. Don't feel sorry for myself, don't tell myself I can't get a date. I say to myself, "Come on, baby, you can do it" instead during difficult times. Don't sing sad songs anymore, only uplifting ones. Can squat 170, deadlift 170 for twenty reps without much trouble. I gained twenty pounds. I am more muscular now, have more endurance. No herpes itch. I think more about helping others. I bought gifts for my sisters for the first time in their entire lives for their birthdays. I don't talk about myself to death to other people, and I have forgiven all the people who hurt me. Not angry and bitter about anything.

ELIZABETH P.

It has been very easy for me to do and follow each step of the program. I have been listening for over eight years and had followed Gary's advice, books, and protocols ever since. This has been an opportunity to do it more in depth. I had been very physically active; this is just a step forward to move my life where I want to be. The program has helped me to focus more on my emotions and feelings and have control over my adventure, instead of focusing on someone else's opinions. It has brought a center to my life as a whole. I am a happier person, I relate to others more easily, and have more flexibility. Mentally, I have a lot more focus and clarity. Everything is a thought away, and I am able to accomplish almost anything that I want to. Physically, I have a lot more energy and feel like I am worth a million! When I started the program on January 16, 1998, I had candida and a cystofibroid breast. Today I am free of it. I feel completely healthy and full of energy. My skin has improved in clarity, it's softer; my hair is fuller and thicker. I feel a sense of wellness, well-being, am happier and more centered. My body looks healthier; I lost some unwanted fat. I am leaner and in great shape. I am pleased to have joined this program. I would recommend it to anyone who would like to improve their health. I am thankful to Gary Null for sharing his time and knowledge with us. Thank you very much and keep up the good work!

BRISEIS G.

Although I had no label-able (or at least labeled) major issues at the start of the program, I noticed, in general, a better mood. Changes got made—I started being firmer about my boundaries, making sure my work got done before taking my daughter out to the playground. Thus, a calmer existence. I had been going away every weekend to avoid my husband (divorce situation). I saw this was draining me and decided to stand my ground. I started giving myself more space from the other "playground moms" who let their kids do things they didn't like and then bemoaned it—and stopped wondering if there was something wrong with me. The fun things—I played a softball game, because I wanted to. I stopped relationships with four people who had lied to me/shown contempt, etc. I seized an opportunity to do something new I wanted to—plastering a house—by offering to help a friend. I had been too busy worrying and thinking I needed to "solve the problem" before doing anything. I noticed that I didn't even consider looking at what was working, positive goal orientation—that in me caution was so strong: "what I want" never even saw daylight above a very pessimistic assumption of "what I can have." I realized this (me) was the biggest influence in making my life bleak. Even though there were some people putting pressure on me that I was blaming—that getting rid of their stuff would only leave me more effectively running from my fear, pain—more comfortably addicted but not joyful. I see people's "stuff" more clearly, helping me let them be more easily, if that seems appropriate, or challenge them if that seems appropriate. Today I told a woman (who I knew *post facto* had abused her child physically and emotionally) who was going to have the child (who I know) evaluated for attention deficit disorder that she needed to face the fact that the child had emotional patterns produced from her experiences and not to be drugging the child to avoid (under the hypothesis "it's genetic") responsibility. I am not unconsciously running around wasting my emotional energy looking for people's approval/attention. I never was a conformist in my behavior, but there was a stress in wanting to be liked.

ANTHONY N.
Spiritually, I felt very alone with no place to turn. I was always looking for something, but failed to touch anything. Very mad for no reason. I am no longer depressed. I don't need to talk about how bad life is because now it is great. I have very little trouble making decisions. I was seeing a person to help me. This I started in October. She said many times that in all her years no one had made the progress I had in such a short period of time. I no longer see her. Physically, my shape has changed dramatically. I went from 195 when we started, with no energy, to 160 now. My weight has been stable for about six weeks. I used to wake up every few hours at night. Now I sleep straight through. I guess this is more mental than physical, or maybe a combination of both. I sleep about five hours a night and have more energy than ever. I take the exercise pretty seriously (actually, it's a lot of fun). Before I had all I could do to get off the couch. I would be winded for nothing. Now I ride a bike about forty minutes every day. I have no more back pain and I can button all of my pants. I was listening to the AM station before Christmas and heard Gary mention new programs forming. This is something I felt I needed but was afraid to do. So what I did was just call before

I had too much time to talk my way out of it. I tell you, from that first meeting on, every day is better than the day before. I have a cabinet shop and my work is no longer painful. I almost look forward to going. I have recently opened a new business also, and it's been a lifelong dream. I no longer see it as impossible. It is a fireworks company and I know now I will have no problem seeing this through. At first my family was afraid I was joining a cult. Now I am asked questions on a daily basis. I receive a lot of support. I had no idea life could be this good. I like to help people around me and look forward to doing as much as I can.

ADELE B.

I was struggling in January—not feeling in sync, needing to move in a direction, not sure about the direction. I knew I was moving in a positive direction but thinking that I needed to make some decisions about my life. I felt more confused, disoriented—why am I doing a lot of things and not happy with the results? Physically, I felt fat and ugly, with a double chin. My complexion was darkening, my back was hurting, my tongue was coated. My clothes didn't lie correctly on my body. I had a smile, but my singing had stopped (sort of—I sing for myself). My digestion was off. I was spiritually connected to higher powers and yet I was still searching. I did not really know how I would spend my next seventy-five years. (I'm forty-eight now). This is my year. I am making more strides in my life than I have perhaps in any other year. I am feeling more clear on a daily basis. I am feeling and thinking and remembering more. I am more in touch with myself. These things have occurred because I want them to and because I am constantly working to have them manifest. I am providing space for mental clarity. I am working on it and it is happening. My body is changing. I am working hard to make it happen. The program, I think, is a major factor. I continue to exercise more and more and I feel good about myself. So far I've probably lost twenty pounds, but muscle takes the place of some of the fat. My complexion is returning to its natural state. My back has fewer blemishes and hurts less often. My breathing is deeper. My memory is improving (somewhat). I can perform more strenuous exercises. I look into the mirror and now I think there is hope. I'm getting pretty again: I'm liking my physical body more. As the fifth child in a family of nine, I have always been the person who tried to bring sanity to insane family situations. Always the one who tried to negotiate, work things out. Striving for balance maybe. The giver. I remember as a teenager I was feeding hungry children (who didn't belong to me) in our community, working with youth. Concerned about making a difference, this spirit led me into counseling, and now for over twenty years I have been counseling and assisting people to change their lives. While very gratifying, I always wanted more. Now I understand as I change myself more, I will be more effective in what I do. As I change me more and I open myself up to what is most gratifying for me, I become more in tune to my needs, and their resolution. I am able to affect more people in a positive manner. I will be communicating to masses of people—motivating, uplifting, and nudging, pushing toward behavior modification.

FIORE D.

In April I was offered a chance to teach piano to a group of adults in an adult education program at a city high school. I accepted and am now teaching a group of thirteen people on Monday nights. A year ago, I probably would have refused to do it, but now that I am doing it, I can see a future—teaching or performing music; getting back into music, doubts and all. I've begun studying with my old music teacher and spending a lot of time at the piano, and deciding how to teach my class. It is something that just happened, but I felt good enough to try it (even though the negative tape was playing in my mind). Another thought occurred to me—if I fail or the job is not renewed, so what? I can keep studying and try to teach elsewhere. This is a big step for me. Physically I have gone from doing little or no exercise to five days a week. I use a NordicTrack, hand weights, and recently began jogging. This is a major step for me because I have always hated exercise, hated gym classes in school, couldn't do most of what was expected, and I had a father who was bigger, stronger, and much more athletic than me. I've always been repelled by gyms and the whole jock mentality. I now am starting to believe that just doing it is important, not how good or how athletic I should be. Spiritually, I am trying to find some connection with life—rather than a just "go with the flow" attitude. I don't accept major religious dogma but am very excited by music, art, theater, etc. Music (composing, performing) is, in one sense, a form of meditation. You need that quiet space. 1 have had to overcome a negative attitude, fostered by a negative or non-supportive family environment—not abusive, but close. I am small, my father was big. I was weak, he was strong. He played sports, I played music. My relatives are generally bigger than me, and this really developed into an inferiority complex. I guess I suffer from what you call the "small man syndrome." All through high school and college I was smallest of my friends. This, combined with a negative attitude, has been very hard to overcome. I am still working on it, a work in progress. I have made some progress and am supported by my wife. I feel this has held me back in life, music relationships, and having a positive outlook. This is definitely a work in progress.

MAGNO O.

At the start of the program, I was almost mentally paralyzed. I thought that my career was over. It was a major challenge to change the outlook of my life. I have many health problems; among the most important were high blood pressure, high cholesterol, enlarged prostate, and hemorrhoids. I was under medical care, and it seemed that treatment was taking me nowhere. I had the belief that for me there was nothing left in life. I was waiting for my Maker to take me away. I reexamined my life. I felt the rush of energy. I restarted my engine. I discovered that there was a life ahead of me. I discovered new interests and I started living again. One of the first things I did with my new burst of energy was start an exercise program. My healthy habits made me lose weight. As I saw my progress, I became more committed to the program. Needless to say, I recuperated my health in every way. I am so amazed that at my age, I am accomplishing things that I thought I never would. I thank God for putting me on the right track of good health. I feel that now I am more in touch with myself. I found new purpose in my life and my energy and optimism is spread to others. Friends and relatives see the changes in me and request my advice. One of the biggest obstacles was inside of me. I have procrastinated for so long that it took a monumental effort to get organized and committed. The second obstacle was clutter in every way. I have examined my life and little by little I started uncluttering my mind of preconceived ideas, or unhealthy habits, and of physical clutter. I became less angry and fearful, and when anger and fear struck me, I've examined my feelings and tried to find out why I was feeling that way. I have forgiven everybody that has hurt me in the past. I understood that the only thing that was hurt was my ego. I have realized that by taming my ego I can free more energy and use it in positive ways. I see myself now and in the future healthy and active, helping other people to reach their goals. I have embarked on new tasks that I never dreamed of. Now I am into biking, camping, and hiking.

SUZANNE Z.

When I called to join the program back at the end of October, I was at the end of my rope. I had been struggling with thoughts of suicide for the past four months and was hoping that being in the program would give me the lifeline I so desperately wanted and needed. I'd been out of work for a year and was feeling hopeless about my situation. I had no unemployment benefits left—my boyfriend was supporting me—and felt useless and worthless. I was seriously considering signing myself into a psychiatric hospital. That is something that I'd never considered in my forty-three years of living, since I know all too well how mental illness is treated and am against using drugs as a first line of treatment (if at all). My first meeting was a bit overwhelming, since I didn't start at the beginning of the group, but I caught up and began the program. It was difficult to afford the supplements, but my boyfriend was supportive and able to help out a bit every week. He was willing to help in any way since it was painful for him to see me in such a state and it made him feel so helpless. The biggest change occurred after a month of being off sugar and dairy. After that point and to this day (eight months later) I have not had the deep depression return. The questions I was asked to answer and reading the life energies book helped me make some major life changes. I applied to, was accepted, and graduated from the Cornell Cooperative Extension Master Gardeners Program. Most people who go through this program are retired because it's held on Wednesdays out on Long Island from 9 a.m. to 4 p.m. Basically, you can't hold a regular nine-to-five job (as I've done for most of my working life) and be in this program. I decided I should just do it now and not wait. I got a job taking care of two children for a friend and was able to have a small income (better than none). I also moved in with my boyfriend of nine years. I also eventually began doing a work/study with the Tri-State Healing Center, working with Diane and Ray, that I enjoyed and appreciated very much. It felt so much better, not having to take more money from my boyfriend. Also, I started a community-supported agriculture organic produce project in my hometown and now have eighty members. I gave lectures, started a CSA newsletter, and helped get an article about CSAs published in *Newsday*. I now need to find a larger location and hope to get another 120 members. These are things I might have dreamed about doing but would never have thought possible. I always thought my place in the universe was to help people with their dreams and that (1) I didn't have any dreams or (2) if I did, there was no way they would come true. This brings me to the present and what I can now say is, I wish I could start the program all over again! The reason is because (like Gary said) I did great with the questions, making life changes, and the spiritual parts, but I didn't deal with the diet and exercise parts of the program as I could/should have. I would like to be a buddy for a new person on the program because I'm a good example of what can happen (great and not so great). I now realize that I want and need to get up to speed with the diet and exercise parts of the program so I am able to keep up with the life changes I've made so far. If I don't, I can see illness around the corner. I won't have the strength to keep up with myself! I realize that I have to get out of my mind (so to speak) and into my body. I had been sexually and physically abused periodically throughout my life, starting as early as age seven (and possibly younger) and stopping approximately twenty years later, and because of that have always had a desire to be bodyless. This program has helped me get my self-esteem to a place where I'm ready to go to the next level of healing. It's all a matter of me getting out of my own way since I am my biggest obstacle. As far as the future goes, I am not sure what it will bring, but I know it's going to be a lot more positive and fun than the first forty-three years. I thank Gary and Luanne, and everyone else connected to this work, many, many, many times.

MIRIAM R., 66 years old

I was an unhappy widow living in a cluttered environment without future goals. I discovered *Natural Living* and began to evolve into the vibrant woman I am today. I sold my large home, which uncluttered my life and opened the door to new experiences. Today I live a happy life. I exercise my body, I am vegan, I ran a five-mile marathon, and I attend track meets with high energy. I am no longer depressed. Life has changed into a positive experience without depression or anger.

WILMA, 69 years old

I had a radical hysterectomy at age 38 and was later diagnosed with chronic fatigue for many years. I refused to take pharmaceutical female hormones and used vitamins for fatigue. My body began to ache with arthritis. I didn't realize I was in a state of acute depression, and I continued to follow the typical American diet. It was difficult to listen to *Natural Living* while I was working, but I had heard the show over the years, and nine years ago I joined a support group. I used biofeedback to prevent blackouts, and medical examinations diagnosed acute angina attacks. Because I was aware of alternative solutions, I decided to have vitamin C drips. The blackouts ceased after chelation. Today I follow the protocol using green and red powders. I attended a Florida retreat. My cardiac, chronic fatigue, and cancer are in total remission. I reject immunizations. I am a life-loving woman who is healthy and in complete control of my life!

PETER A.

When I was young, I suffered from severe chemical and food sensitivities. The orthodox methods (antibiotics for my strep throat) offered no help. Staying off most foods prevented the occurrence of extreme allergic reactions. I still was not feeling good. This was weakening every aspect of my being (cognition, physical strength, moods, state of mind). I had a pale complexion and dark circles under my eyes. When I got involved with Gary Null's allergy program, within two weeks of green juices I was feeling remarkably better. Now it's been nine months and I can eat almost any food. The clarity of my thinking is better. My "light years"—I have no more moodiness, depression, lethargy, or poor complexion. Instead, I feel vital, healthy, and alive. In the future l see myself helping other people through my experience. I will continue to learn about internal energy. Perhaps I will get a PhD in Oriental medicine. I will take my own hardships and the lessons that I learned from them and use them to help others.

STEVEN H.

The obstacle that I had to overcome was that I always followed Null's wellness program, but l was a comfort addict and did things in moderation. Now, I am more disciplined and able to handle the challenge of discomfort. I've been following my health detox program continuously and find it enjoyable and pleasant to do. On the physical level, my dentist told me my gums looked the healthiest he had seen in me when I went for my half-year visit. I told him about your health detox program and the protocols that I took; he wasn't interested. My friends tell me that I look so good, they are inspired to get healthy themselves. I now have a youthful appearance and rejuvenation of glowing skin and hair. I lost about twenty-five pounds and five inches from my waist. I've been cross training almost every day in my rotation routine. I went from walking three miles to jogging five miles. I do about one hour and ten minutes walking and running stairs in a stadium. I bike about sixteen miles on weekends. I'm also weight training and have been taking judo and jujitsu for twenty-five years. I have more energy, strength, vitality, and alertness due to this program. My health is excellent, am never sick or fatigued, and I no longer have sinus problems. Many people and friends have been complimenting me about my well-being and positive attitude. Many come to me seeking health and nutritional advice, but when I tell them what they have to give up (coffee, sugar, smoking, wheat, dairy, alcohol, negative attitude), most change their minds. Some end up making gradual changes, and I help encourage them to do their best. On the emotional level, I use meditation, hypnosis, affirmations, and creative visualization to de-stress. I no longer let toxic people run my life and/or seek their validation. I've been letting go of many things and getting clutter out of my life. I've become more detached from my possessions, am laughing more, and slowing down my lifestyle to the speed of nature, which has increased my awareness. I have become more spiritual, kinder, gentler, humbler since the program began. My intuition and psychic abilities are much sharper from eating, drinking, and juicing organic foods. I'm no longer afraid of challenges and uncertainty in my life: I am better at self-actualizing rather than just talking. I judge people for what they do rather than what they say.

DIDI S.

I started this program at a point where I had become totally obsessed with my weight and body image. This obsession led me to exercise extensively and have such a rigid control over what I ate. There was no joy in any of this for me. My obsession left no room for my family or friends. Everything I did had to fit in around my rigid schedule. This obsession was just replacing a lot of pain I had inside me. If I kept myself busy with exercise and a rigid schedule, I didn't have to deal with any emotions, not sad ones or good ones. I heard Gary Null on the radio for the first time last October, he was talking about detoxification. I know my body wasn't that toxic, but mentally I was struggling. The thing that interested me about what Gary was saying was that his detoxification program was mental as well as physical and spiritual. I joined the next available support group with my husband, because I felt if we could do it together, it would really be helpful. Once starting the group, and following the protocols, my self-esteem started to improve; I started seeing my thought patterns in a new light. If I could replace my negative thoughts with positive ones—what a change might occur! Now I find myself continuously reinforcing positive affirmations to myself and to others, and I believe more and more opportunities are being opened for me. I'm more flexible and relaxed, I'm enjoying myself more, and I'm constantly making changes and looking for ways to improve my life. I have increased my body fat to a much healthier level. My sex drive has increased as well. I have also started to cut back on so much strenuous exercise and add more yoga and learn qi gong, which I needed to help balance me physically. My cholesterol dropped fifty points and my HDL went up to a very healthy ratio. I believe this was due to the elimination of dairy products as I was not eating any other animal products before. I am sleeping about one hour less a day. I used to be a chronic gum chewer and candy eater. I would crave sugar through the day. Now these cravings are gone and I can't imagine ever desiring those things anymore. In the future I see myself becoming more of who I am. I plan to study feng shui, I've started studying qi gong. I plan to continue looking inside myself and questioning things that prevent me from honoring my true self. I'm looking forward to this journey.

KEVIN F.

I first met Gary Null in January 1997. I am amazed at the changes that have occurred since then. I should start by describing the life I led prior to that meeting. I drank ten cups of coffee a day or more. Lunch would be a hero or pizza. Dinner, I could think of nothing better than a burger and french fries washed down with a cold beer—more than one. If not for Chinese takeout, I never would have eaten vegetables. In short, I consumed all the vital chemicals not found in nature. I was a toxic mess, a blob sitting in front of a TV set with one hand on a beer and the other in a bag of chips. I was 380 pounds and killing myself; worse, I was very unhappy. I knew something had to be done, but what? On January 12, 1997, I arrived at Gary's Paradise Gardens, fully committed to do whatever "this nut" wanted for two weeks. That first day, I had no appreciation of the changes I would undergo. For fourteen days, I was happy. I lost sixty pounds. For the first time in my life I was detoxified. In February, I was back in the real world, enjoying a new lifestyle. All my food came from the health food store. I realized a healthy body and a healthy mind went hand in hand. If I put toxic food in my body, I would have a toxic mind.

I now identify myself as a vegetarian. Quite simply, I do not eat meat or dairy. Those few times I cheated, I felt awful. In the past year I have had meat six or seven times, all at social occasions—Christmas or Thanksgiving or when invited to dinner. While I looked forward to these parties and thought I would enjoy the food, I found that I have changed. I no longer like the taste of meat. The next day, it always made me feel sluggish. The next step in my health evolution was to buy a juicer. My days now begin with green tea and vegetable juice. They give me a shot of "energy" I never got from coffee and a Danish. I can and use powdered juice and find them to be very good. I find juicing helps to keep me connected. Gandhi did not have to spin his own cloth. The most important part of my day is exercise. Every day without fail, I work out. I run or walk forty minutes to an hour every morning. In the evening I lift weights or do qi gong. This for me is the most essential part of each day—if I have a hard workout, everything falls into place.

I now set goals for myself; doing this I must be careful—frustration and negative thoughts creep in when I do not achieve these goals in the time limit I set. My life is better than it was and getting better each day. I know that I still have a long way to go, but I will be in good shape soon.

WINSTON W.

When I began the protocol at issue was my general attitude of skepticism regarding whether I would indeed be helped by this program. And whether I was capable of following the protocol laid down was another issue I thought very hard about. How could I manage without eating meat? I was also a worrier, and the general direction of my health was of concern to me. Worrying about my health did not, of course, help the situation—lack of energy and insomnia, also flatulence caused by a spastic colon. There was also stiffness in the legs, which to me indicated a sign of arthritis. Indigestion, dizziness, and leg cramps were virtually a way of life for me, and despite numerous lab tests and doctor's visits, relief at best lasted only for a short time. All of the above contributed to my desire to seek help for my physical condition.

After almost a year in the program, I have become more confident about my health in general and I can see marked improvement in mind, spirit, and body. Having followed the program almost religiously, including the meditation techniques, I find that my mind is more focused and my memory has definitely improved. The most obvious result I have noticed is the increase in my energy level. With only six hours of sleep I can complete a full day without feeling tired or lethargic. My skin is also much smoother than it used to be, and the liver spots that once covered my neck and chest are barely visible. My fingernails, toenails, and hair grow very fast and have to be trimmed more often than before. The constipation, indigestion, and bloating have been greatly reduced.

GILSIA P.

I was glad when I heard of the opportunity to start in a support group with Gary Null. Over the last ten years, I started gaining weight and became a couch potato.

Three years ago, I was diagnosed with hypothyroidism and started using Synthroid pills. I used to get spells of tiredness almost every month that sent me to bed to sleep in order to feel better. I knew that I needed to do something different but did not have enough motivation to do it on my own. That's why getting into the support group was a big difference for me. I can say that the challenges that I was facing when I started the program were dealing with low self-esteem, low motivation to move forward, eating the wrong foods, and being unable to lose weight. I also felt the passion that I used to have when I was younger had diminished. I needed a different perspective in my life. After I started the program and continued the protocol, I felt less tiredness. I am exercising now and I feel great. People tell me that I look thirty-five years old. I am now forty-six, with a grandson. My skin is smooth and I feel young. I don't get headaches and I am in good health. I have some cysts in my breast that I believe will disappear with the change of eating habits. In the past, I used to wear my glasses for reading; now I remove them. My blood test came out much better than the first test. The program has helped me be more relaxed and assertive. When I am facing a problem, I look at it with a different perspective and know that it will be solved, even if it isn't at that particular moment. I get less angry with people and don't feel that I need to compete. My thoughts are more clearly to the point without getting into too much rationalization. Since I started the program, I felt depressed only once and I faced it and it was nothing. My self-esteem has been raised and I am able to look at myself without self-blaming. I feel now more motivated to get involved in different things; to be adventurous and allow the child within me to come up. For example, I heard of a workshop for the preparation of the Latin American Feminist Women Conference, to take place in 1999 in Santo Domingo. Since I am Dominican, I decided to go and find out what it is all about. It was a nice trip and I came away with more knowledge of what is going on concerning women, children, and family issues in Santo Domingo.

MIMI V.

As an artist, 1 felt that my focus was not up to my ability (with the years that I've put into training, more than twenty-five years). Prolific thoughts should have been in prolific works. After listening to Gary Null for three years on the radio, I decided that this could only help me focus and get to the work I needed to do. Since I've been in the program five months, there have been many changes. I have lost ten pounds. My energy, which was low, has increased. I'm not as tired as I was previously. I talk less and finally I find myself listening more to what people are saying (particularly in my family). I did not realize how angry I was until we had to write ten letters to people who caused us some kind of pain. After that exercise I was truly able to let go of the anger and able to speak to my exhaustion without feeling anything, pain or otherwise. While I've always been a mediator, trying to understand why people do the things they do, I no longer care to understand them. I don't need them in my life—now I please myself first. When I began this program I wasn't sure what I wanted to do—become less toxic, enabling me to focus on what I needed to do for me. What's important is that all my life had been the need to create with word or with paint. Two years ago I changed my schedule as a full-time teacher to part-time and replaced my painting full-time. Since then I painted, but not full time. Hence my entrance in the program. I realized I needed to focus my energy and thoughts to create and decided this might be exactly what I needed. It was more than what I envisioned. The questions we had to ask ourselves and answer honestly helped to create an environment for change. I used to be a sweet junkie and now I can walk by cakes, pies, and cookies without feeling deprived. I find I eat many more raw vegetables —something I had not done before. I am rarely tired. I walk now more than I have done in the months before beginning the program. My energy level is higher and I feel great.

BAIJY R.

I did not have any physical constraints that I was aware of. The introduction of the detox program made me aware of my mental restrictions more so than physical. To learn how to focus and not be sidetracked by obstacles was my starting point. I did not know or understand how my energy or relationships would or could affect my perspective of life. This stage of unwillingness allowed me to be happy in my ignorance. I learned how to get toxic people out of my life. I leaned how to strengthen my attitude, be patient, and not respond with negativeness. I look at myself in a new light of happiness and motivation. I have learned how to be happy with myself. Physically, I am stronger from exercising daily. I am a martial artist and I am able to do things other people I work out with are unable to do (handstand pushups, dips, and pushes into having my body parallel with the floor).

MARJORIE A.

At the beginning of the program, I was challenged with learning how to think clearly, to learn to focus and how to plan. Staying away from toxic people and not letting myself get carried away with their problems. It is a slow process, but I'm under control. The challenges that I have at home, in my marriage, I look at with courage, not indifference. The learning process is an everyday affair. My letting go of meat has improved my digestive problems, which I've had since childhood. I found out also that I have an allergy to corn that we consumed daily. Learning to eat organic food has not been easy. My conscience reminds me every time I go against the rules. Letting go of sugar has been great. Detoxifying my system is still an ongoing process—my brain fog is slowly going away.

BARBARA K.

I am an artist. I am very excited. Tomorrow my husband and I are leaving on a two-week Baltic cruise with friends. We were married forty-five years ago. We never did anything fun like this. Our friends do it often. We are both worka-holics, and love what we do. Having fun has been work for us. Also, my diet is limited because of food allergies. I once got amoebic dysentery on a trip. I worried about getting colitis away from home. Gary, I am the woman who told you that twenty years ago the head of gastroenterolgy of a New York City hospital said, "Barbara, get rid of your colon, and get on with your life." I started listening to you. By 1980, I had changed a lot. After my last colonoscopy, I saw a computer printout of the inside of my large intestine. It was "pink and purty." Now, being in the program, my colon is perfect. I question whether there really is such a thing as colitis, or is it just sensitivities to different things? Back to our trip, my husband and I never have been together for two solid weeks without work projects. We will have fun!

MARLENE D.

Following your protocols for the reversing the aging process study has significantly improved my health in many ways. My weight is maintained at 110 pounds effortlessly. It used to fluctuate a lot. It was as high as 130 pounds at one point several years ago. This 110 pounds is the weight I maintained when I was nineteen–twenty-two years old. It's wonderful! I require one hour or more less sleep per night than I did before the study. Now I sleep more soundly and feel more alert and energized during the day. I have gotten no colds or flus since I have been in the program. This is a welcome change! I had been going to a derma-tologist before the study for acne and rosacea. The topical medication he prescribed for rosacea did not help it. Also, he prescribed tetracycline to be taken on an ongoing basis for acne. I refused to take this. I believe that the protocol for the study was a much safer and more effective treatment for acne. Acne is no longer a problem for me and the rosacea has significantly improved. I find that I look and feel younger now than I did before starting the program. People often assume I am ten or more years younger. I'm so grateful for this. My skin is more clear and healthy. My hair is silkier and seems thicker. Also the number of gray hairs growing in is becoming fewer and fewer. This is great. Menstrual pain has lessened very significantly. I used to take Tylenol about every four to six hours for the first forty-eight hours of my menses. I take no medication now whatsoever, and experience at the most only mild discomfort. Also I no longer have the premenstrual puffiness and headaches I used to have. Emotionally, I'm better able to deal with day-to-day stress and traumatic events. In general, I feel more calm and positive than I did before the study. I am fully committed to using what I have learned to maintain my health and perhaps improve it further. I have been sharing what I have learned with others and I'm grateful for the joy of watching them benefit too.

MIGUEL P.

The improvements in my overall health have been amazing. It is difficult to really believe in something until you actually put it into practice and notice the results for yourself. I used to suffer from severe seasonal allergies. During the night, I would not be able to breathe easily since my sinuses would swell and make it difficult to breathe. One nostril would get so clogged that it wouldn't work properly. In a few days I would develop headaches and a bad case of halitosis. This caused me to withdraw from speaking with people at the office, since I did not want them to notice my breath. I had tried going to ENT doctors, but they always told me these were ragweed, pollen, or dust allergies that I had to live with. Then they would give me a prescription for some nasal spray and send me on my way. Needless to say these were only temporary and artificial remedies. Since being on your strict protocol, I have not had these allergic attacks during spring or fall. I have also noticed that my mental sharpness is better now than it was when I was twenty-eight years old (I'm presently forty-one years old). I've noticed this because when I was twenty-eight, I tried going for my master's degree in electrical engineering while working full time. I was not able to focus to the level required for maintaining a B average or better. I've been in graduate school now for three semesters and I have a GPA of 3.25. In this past spring semester, I registered for two courses while working on a project in the office with a very tight schedule and lots of pressure. One of the courses required commuting to the campus thirty minutes away. On both courses I received grades of B. My friends admire my effort, but what they don't know is that I have an edge they don't have; I have more energy, have an optimal diet, and I'm putting all these health benefits to good use. I've also expanded my physical activities to include bicycling and playing tennis. I recently played someone eleven years my junior in a tennis match. I did not get winded and we had to play a tiebreaker. This also I remember not being able to do at age twenty-eight! My emotional well-being was terribly challenged a few months ago, but I think I was able to get through it because of what I've learned from you. I want to thank you very much for all you've done for me and others.

IVON

Being involved with my study group has established a new dimension in my life, which is that I'm a new person. Over the years I do recall you stating that in the order of priority, one's belief system was first and foremost; second, stress management; third, exercise; and diet last. On September 25, 1996, at our first session, you specified that diet represents 15 percent; exercise 10 percent; stress management 25 percent; and behavior 50 percent. This time it was loud and clear—maybe because it was quantified, especially with behavior and stress representing 75 percent of the package. The tools and techniques that were shared in our biweekly meeting were invaluable because it allowed those of us who went through the exercises to get to know more about ourselves and examine our conditioned minds. Also to see where we have been the source of our own suffering and limitations in our lives. I've never been at such peace with myself as I am now, having a "can do" attitude with what matters to me and what is important to me. Reexamining my beliefs, values, and perceptions has provided tremendous benefits with regard to my interactions with others; where they might attempt to manipulate, control, or induce feelings of guilt it has not worked, and not being a victim to these mind games is very empowering. The greatest challenges that I encountered during the entire process was to integrate the suggested dietary intake and consistent exercise with my schedule, so the most number of juices I had gotten to was approximately six. My present occupation requires me to be on the road driving to be in and out on various appointments in various areas, so preparing and taking enough of the juices with me during the day was not as consistent as I would have preferred it to be. In spite of it all, the number of sleep hours that I am able to get by on has reduced to approximately five hours per night. My energy level has never been better and focus with clarity is greater. I am certainly looking forward to going into the advanced stage of the Reversing Aging Process if you decide to continue, because I know there are greater strides I'll be making with the continuous growth and process in my life.

CHARLES M.

I have distanced myself from members of my family who are hostile and negative. I have made many changes on the physical level due to the Reversing Aging Study. I have much less muscle soreness, less lower back pain, which has bothered me for years, and an increase of energy throughout the day. I have better digestion, my skin looks better, and my eyes are clearer. I didn't consider myself overweight, but I went from 192 to 186 pounds, and I am physically stronger. If I get a rare cold, it is of short duration. I have a marked diminishment of allergic reactions. On the emotional and mental level, an improvement in mental alertness. My mind feels stronger, and I have fewer periods of brain fog, and an improved outlook on life because I am proactive. I have more belief in my abilities. I must not only know, I must actualize.

LAURA B.

Since starting this program in January, I have had positive changes both physical and mental. Starting with the physical changes, the constant rash I had on my face from lupus has completely cleared up. I have had the rash for the last two and a half years, and I was told the only way to clear it up was with antibiotics. I also suffered from extreme fatigue. I have cut out 1.5 hours of sleeping. Also migraine headaches that I got often have almost been 100 percent eliminated. My concentration level at work has greatly improved, along with a general feeling of overall calmness. As far as the mental part, this has been my most accomplished detoxing. I have been able to totally eliminate an abusive father and brother from my life. This is the most liberating feeling! I put up with so much from them for years; now that part of my life is gone forever! Having dealt with that situation has also opened my eyes to the kinds of relationships I have been in. All my relationships with men have been abusive. I have never been treated with kindness or respect. I will never let anyone treat me that way again. I have learned that I am good and that I am deserving of kindness and love. This is the greatest feeling. I have also reevaluated my friendships. I have eliminated the ones who were users and takers. I have also uncluttered my household. I have gotten rid of bags and bags of clothing. I have given many knickknack types of junk to an animal group for a garage sale. So many happy and positive things have happened over the last few months, that have changed my life for the better. My life is better now than it has ever been. I am very grateful for this program.

NICK J.

I no longer feel bloated, and my energy level has increased. I lost 20 pounds. I have packed on 5 to 7 pounds of muscle. I run three to four miles a day three to four times a week.

JUNGLIEN C.

I am a hepatitis B carrier and I would like to not be infected with this virus anymore, and have more energy. I feel my energy level is more even. I do not have those high and low yo-yo-like energy levels. I also started having mercury fillings removed, which eliminated this frequent hazy feeling I feel in my brain. I am a person who has problems being consistent and focused. I do get some major goals in my life accomplished but a lot of others I start, then I stop it. I wanted to learn to be fluent in Spanish and I would start studying, but after a few weeks I would stop, and eight years have passed and I still can't speak Spanish. The reason for this behavior I believe is because I am interested in so many things that when I start something, I would be working at it for a while when another activity would appear and distract me. I would stop whatever I was doing and be off on a different path. Then when I look back at my life, I realize that I have accomplished very little. Had I concentrated on one thing at a time I would have accomplished more in the same amount of time. I know my first goal is to heal myself from hepatitis. That means doing what needs to be done listed in the program and obtaining the job that is what I want to do because only then will I feel that I am honoring my life and time. This I feel is an important part of my healing, because the anxiety and guilt that I feel now for not doing what I want affects my healing process. I see myself a year from now filled with energy and health to live every day able to fulfill my goals. I want to feel that every minute of my life is lived with purpose and direction.

IRIS S.

At the start of this program, I was feeling very depressed, because I had been [both holistic and conventional] and felt that they were not really dealing with my whole being—just a few body parts such as my thyroid, liver, etc. I would look around me and just feel so lonely and overwhelmed because it seemed like everyone else was enjoying their lives much more than I was. I really felt stuck and rather hopeless. Physically my body was very depleted. One doctor several years ago told me he didn't know how I made it through the day because I had zero energy in my meridians. I had to force myself to get through each day because I have a husband and two sons. I gave my family all I had and often there was nothing left for me. (I know now that my focus was misdirected.) My hormones were out of balance. My thyroid was not functioning well and my adrenals, lymphatic system, liver, and gastrointestinal systems were all out of balance. I had very bad PMS every month; for almost two weeks out of four I would be achy and bloated. I would go to bed exhausted and wake up just as tired. Spiritually I didn't feel very connected to the world. I guess I felt that life was passing me by and all I had was this struggle called chronic fatigue. I still volunteered and gave my time to causes but always wished I could do more. Mentally I am feeling much more hopeful about my future. I am now convinced that I am a good person and say to myself over and over how proud I am of myself. Even though I feel that I have always been a kind person, I feel that I am even kinder and more giving because I really like, no, love myself. I feel that by saying the affirmations that we were taught I have a much more positive attitude about my abilities. I realize that a big part of my problem has been self-esteem or lack thereof, and now I feel my self-esteem is really blossoming. I feel more confident asking for what I want from other people and am much less shy about talking in public. Another aspect that has improved is that I no longer feel tearful as much as I used to. I know that by feeling stronger mentally I am also helping my immune system to heal. I have been working hard to detoxify my body and have been faithful about doing the program because I knew it would work. Finally I found someone who understood that I am much greater than the sum of my parts. My gastrointestinal system has improved considerably, e.g., I am no longer bleeding rectally and have much fewer episodes of diarrhea. My PMS is down to a day or two as opposed to two weeks of agony. I can get through more days now without the overwhelming need to take a nap in the middle of the day. I have been exercising for about twenty minutes, five to six days a week, and feel a definite improvement in my stamina. My body feels more toned and my muscles feel much stronger. I recently learned that I have the beginnings of osteoporosis and I am also working with a holistic gynecologist to build up my bones. I have taken a deeper interest in my religion and have felt very comforted by being a part of a group. I have been seeking out people to help who are suffering and have given them information about natural forms of healing. Recently I gave four friends information about how to prepare for and recover from the various surgeries they were undergoing using nutritional protocols. They all seemed grateful for my help, and it made me feel very satisfied. I find that I really enjoy helping people. The greatest obstacle that I had to overcome was not believing that I was worth the time to invest in changing my life and healing my problem. At first it was hard to physically get myself to the bimonthly meetings, but once I got there it was always worth the effort. It seemed like an expensive proposition in buying all the supplements, but I changed my priorities and decided that it would be worth all the expense, and I realize it has been. My family, especially my children, did not like all the changes I was making in the food I was buying, but I did it anyway. Now my boys are beginning to respect what I am trying to do because they see that I'm feeling better. I see myself as becoming a happy person totally. I feel very focused as to my goal in improving every part of my life. One of my biggest goals for the future is finding my passion in life, and hopefully finding employment in that field. I feel now that I have the tools necessary to achieve this. Another goal of mine is to totally overcome CFIDS, and actually be healthier than people around me who have no so-called illnesses. I thank the program so much for putting all the necessary components into this study group.

AMY O.

Where do I begin to convey to you how listening to you and being part of the study group has changed my life? It hasn't been easy, and I haven't done it perfectly, but I'm not going to be hard on myself. I've actually done really well, even if I've had my slip-ups. I've lost about twelve pounds and gone down about two or three clothing sizes. I've never felt better. When I really stick to it, I feel the best. The juicing has probably been the best thing that I've incorporated into my daily life. What a difference that has made. I feel more energetic and can get by on less sleep, so I have more of my day to be productive. Just that alone is a major coup! The first thing I noticed, and probably most important to me, was not having any menstrual cramps. My body barely goes through any noticeable changes, and it doesn't disrupt my life the way it used to. I haven't taken any kind of drug—not so much as an aspirin—since beginning the program eight months ago. My facial skin has never been better. I don't even get the one or so monthly breakouts that were just commonplace. I have a pretty regular exercise routine, which is great. I've been able to get rid of a lot of "stuff," including clothes that I had no need for that were just taking up my living space. That's an ongoing process. What I love the most is that people are asking me what changes I've made in my life, and I'm able to share with them what I've been doing. People want to hear this information. Even if they are not ready to make the changes for themselves, they are listening to it and noting what is possible. I'm living proof! I've been talking to people I never thought I would and saying smart things like never before because my confidence level is high. It just makes sense not to eat any animal products, or even use any kind of animal products. It just makes sense to eat a live diet. Processed foods were—and still are—only being produced to make money. There is nothing good about them. Being healthy is so simple, I can't believe the road I had to travel to figure it out. But I'm grateful I've discovered the answers now; it could have been another thirty-seven years. I look forward to sharing information with as many people as I can. That is what is most important—not to hoard this valuable knowledge, but to get it out there among the masses. It can't be said enough. The world will have to change when people start making changes themselves. For this I thank you and look forward to continuing to listen to you and your ideas.

JOEL K.

In the beginning of the program, I felt that I was in a bad state of mind. I felt limited by the hepatitis that I have. Now I don't care about the disease I have in my body. I don't seem to care about my morality as much. I understand that the most important thing is my attitude. If I keep a positive attitude, I know things will be all right. To be aware of myself and the things around me is the only thing that counts. To understand that to have compassion for myself is to have compassion for others and vice versa. Hepatitis was my physical challenge at the beginning of this program. Now the challenge is me and how I can change to be a better person. I guess this is what my challenge has been all along.

MURRAY G.

I have gained awareness that I used to be fearful with other people in interactions with them. In the same context, I had a strong need to be approved of, loved and admired. Now, I no longer fear others and I realize that I do not need love from others. I realize I can, through my own personal positive achievements, manufacture my love for myself, and I have been doing these things and I feel so very, very comfortable in the presence of all others, and I just am. A number of different people say that I look very well. I feel very well generally. I believe my stamina has increased, and I am starting to do some strength exercises for my upper body.

LINDSAY P.-T.

Since beginning this program, for the first time in my life I am able to see myself as a loving, beautiful, complete, whole person, and I see all of these things in myself. I accept myself and I'm making choices because I want to make them. I'm enjoying myself, and exploring all the things I've always wanted to do without fear. I have decided to have closure in all my unfinished business. I've registered to go back to school, and I'm excited about doing that. It's taken me so long. All of a sudden, I have a list of things I want to do, and I'm taking one step at a time. I see myself starting projects—helping children, counseling, and sharing all I know about the changes I have made in my life. I see myself challenging me to run the marathon. I see myself making a transition from living in New York to another space. I have uncluttered my life and I continue to do so. I need less and less accumulation of stuff. Physically, I feel lighter; emotionally, I love myself more and more. I see myself being self-sufficient about the work I want to do—starting an organic cleaning business, learning massage therapy, and doing holistic counseling are the goals I'm focused on for the next five years. I look younger, more energetic. When I started the study, I didn't exercise enough. I was about ten pounds overweight and had no energy by the middle of the day. I had acne on my cheeks and forehead and my skin wasn't healthy at all. By the end of the study, I did the Avon 5K Run and felt wonderful. This propelled me to join the New York Road Runners Club and run in competitions. My skin looks wonderful, and friends and family have commented on how great I look. I never had a problem changing my diet. My issue was the mental/emotional challenge and realizing at this time in my life I'm actualizing my goals and living without stress and negativity, and that co-creating my life is something that is so easy to do. I feel blessed that I'm doing it, negotiating with myself and accomplishing the daily goals I'm setting for myself. I have turned my life around from one of mediocrity to one of purpose and fun.

JULIET H.

I had chronic cysts on my ovaries. Within three months all symptoms of ovarian cyst disease disappeared. My eye bulging is reduced. I no longer have soreness in my throat area and I breathe with comfort.

NORMAN P.

Being on the protocol has helped me physically and mentally. My year-long bouts with allergies have ended. I no longer suffer from seasonal attacks of hay fever brought on by pollen, ragweed, and other allergens. The flu and colds I got with every change of season have also disappeared. Numerous aches and pains experienced when bending down, reaching, or lifting are gone. I sleep better, wake on time, and take these functions for granted, where previously they were unpredictable and problematic. My body has changed considerably, so much so that the list of improvements seems endless to me. But more dramatic has been my change of mind. I no longer suffer from mind fog. My concentration does not lag when listening to someone speak or while reading, and my writing has improved. Since all three are inextricably linked, the change has been hard to believe. I now feel I'm more tolerant and understanding of those I choose to be with. I am able to stand outside myself, seeming to witness changes in behavior and attitude I was not aware of previously. My social skills are such that I no longer see unexplained behavior as threatening or strange. This did not happen overnight, nor did it happen solely because of the diet, the juices, or even the exercises. It happened because both phases of diet and exercise complemented the classes taken and meetings held to clear up questions and problems that occurred during different phases of the program. It was during these meetings that I began to change former concepts of self. Questions were handed out to take home and think about. A lot of thought had to occur before they made sense, and any attempt to answer or even understand them was futile if you—I—did not think hard. These questions dealt with the existence of who you were, or who you thought you were, challenging not only conscious beliefs but ones held without being aware of them. Initially, thought brought on resistance, but the more I grappled with the questions, the more meaningful my responses. They forced in me openness of mind that could no longer cling to the shaky precipice of the easy reply. What has followed has been a profound sense of why and how I dealt with the world around me and where I could obtain some of the answers.

FRANK E.

Eight months after a 20-hour-long brain surgery that left me in intensive care for three days, I joined Gary's health support group and running club. I soon after discontinued steroids, seizure pills, synthroid, laxatives, and antacids. My physician does not understand my physical, emotional, and mental recovery in so short a time.

JOSEPH J. L.

It is a privilege to be part of your research program. Since the first week of applying your protocol, I began to experience a series of changes in my life. My vision has improved; I gained energy, and my memory has improved. Now I have better control of my life. In general, this protocol has helped me to grow physically, emotionally, and spiritually. I hope for more to come!

ANDREW K.

When I came into the study, I was not self-assertive. I would keep my opinions, my emotions, my needs inside to avoid conflict and uncomfortable situations. This was because I always felt "less than" or incapable of doing things. In other words, I had no self-confidence. I failed in college, and my previous image of a gifted, smart student was replaced for many years by a belief that I was no longer special or smart. I decided I couldn't learn anything difficult, so I made this belief come true by not making a 100 percent effort at college. I was afraid to fail; I believed I would fail, and so I failed. This was carried over into all aspects of my life. I adjusted by lowering my expectations—keeping my challenges easily manageable so that I would not fail. Every day I replayed past mistakes, situations when I could have acted better, situations that caused me pain or embarrassment, and I would feel bad all over again. Physically, I had begun to see my metabolism slowing down. Previously, I had no problem maintaining my weight. Now I was gaining weight and looking out of shape. I was beginning to look older than my years. About five years ago, I noticed my hair thinning. While it is not important to have hair, I believed it to be a sign of ill health. I wanted to be so healthy that I could grow a full head of hair. Now that I look back, I had smoked for more than half of my life. I could feel the effects of smoking on my body—reduced endurance, clouded thinking, low self-esteem. I had no ambition or high-energy drive. Since joining the study, I have come to believe that I am both hero and architect of my life. There is no waiting for some magic to happen. I am the magic. With regard to physical conditions, I have lost twenty pounds and have the best muscle tone in my entire life. I have stopped my hair loss. Bursitis in my right knee is greatly diminished. I can exercise more and exert my knee more than before, I don't have the swelling or discomfort I had before. I would have afternoon drowsiness and mental fog between 2 and 4 p.m. I do not have that anymore. I am also able to increase my energy levels through simple breathing techniques—and also because I now believe it is possible for me. I sleep an hour or two less per night. My recovery from infections, colds, or flu is amazing. I was able to rid myself of pharyngitis without any antibiotics in less than a week. Flu would have lasted a week. Now, if I do feel sick I am able to knock it out in two and a half days. All of the symptoms are not as great as before. I am able to exercise longer and with greater ease. Recovery from exercise and exertion is greatly improved, i.e., when I have a heavy workout day, I am not as sore or fatigued the next day. I am able to do several activities in one day and not be exhausted afterward.

ELAINE R.

Thank you for creating this protocol. The changes I was able to make during this protocol were more marked than any changes I have been able to make in several years. When I followed the protocol closely, September through February:

- I lost twelve pounds.
- I lost several inches from my hips and waist.
- My blood pressure dropped to 102/60.
- My self-confidence and energy level rose to a new high.
- My sense of security, that I could cope with new situations, increased.
- I received many comments on my shiny hair.
- People commented on how nice my skin was.
- I had a more focused, steady sense of energy.
- I was less dehydrated.
- I didn't get headaches, whereas before I usually got at least one severe headache a month.
- Overall, I felt more competent, confident, positive, and clear-headed.
- I was able to focus on other goals in my life.

It is clear that my stated goals continue to be missed, despite all of the "preparing" I had done. The act of succeeding in your protocol was the biggest step I have taken in years. I had taken your suggestion to join the weight-loss group, conscious of my desire to lose weight but not really aware of how the extra ten or twelve pounds bothered me. When I succeeded in losing twelve pounds, the psychic burden that was lifted seemed more like a hundred. That, in combination with the pointed exercises that we did in the group, raised my self-esteem, to use that trampled word. I felt better and stronger than ever. I had learned to cope with and compensate for the way I look, except for those few extra pounds, so I would always hide myself. My new mode is, "I feel energetic, attractive, and strong." This was such a palpable improvement for me that I felt like a different person and the people around me really noticed. They saw the physical change immediately, which I thought was funny because as much as the weight bothered me, it was within the norm enough that I didn't think anyone else would notice. But people especially noticed how I seemed stronger and happier. When I lost my job, it was perfect timing, and I was unfazed. As is my tendency, the moment I had more energy, I took on more efforts. In the course of this process, I have come to see myself more clearly. I have always been very energetic and enthusiastic, as well as ultrasensitive. As you can see, that combination can make someone vulnerable. I am a person who lives so much in the moment that I have had trouble with gaining perspective or disciplined long-term thinking, although the level of self-discipline I have shown during long periods of my life for artwork and physical training might seem to belie this. I am a typical creative assertive as described by various traits, but mainly dynamic supportive. The main challenges for me have always seemed to be the practical concerns of taking care of myself, food, clothing, shelter, finances. All of this has led me to a new place in this moment, in reference to the protocol and my life. I am able and strong enough to see "doing my artwork" as the organizing principle, and everything can follow from there.

The protocol requires that I commit to a workout routine, which I can usually do for a limited period of time. The protocol is practical and easy, and I had great satisfaction and success with its routine, i.e., I had a job. Now, I must rise to the challenge of making my own routine and making it long-term—a day at a time. There are other important challenges that face me now that do require courage, as you spoke of the other night, because, as you quoted Henry Emerson Fosdick, "He who chooses the beginning of the road, chooses the place it leads to." There is one other point that I want to address and that is that I went through the weekly questions in the context of other questions that I have been working on and found they are extremely focusing and practical. They really cut to the heart of the matter and are critical to the age-reversing process. When I missed doing them, I really felt the drag in terms of slow grasping of the entire process of the protocol. The questions are pointed, relevant, essential, and practical. For me, the biggest challenge will be to acknowledge the limitation that I cannot do everything and have the courage and consciousness to choose. I really appreciate your giving your time to this process. Thank you.

JOE O.

Since I began to follow this protocol, I have lost twenty pounds—178 pounds, down from 198—without eating any less food. In fact, I eat more healthy food and burn it off more quickly. My sleep is now more restful. I sleep more soundly and wake up more alert than before beginning the program. My hair is growing in a lot faster than before—almost twice as fast, in fact. I am growing new hair in the front of my head, which was bald before, and I had a bald spot on the back of my head but now it is gone. I suffered with lower back pain into my left buttocks, sciatica with pain so bad I could not walk for two days. This is gone now. I think more clearly now, and I think good, positive thoughts. Sexually, I am more alive than ever. My erections last sometimes two hours and I feel more passionate when I make love. It is like I am seventeen all over again. I share more in a physical way with my mate than ever before. Sex is great again, not a chore. I have more physical energy than I ever had before. My muscular strength has almost doubled. I can lift more weight and work out longer with more strength than ever. I can play and work longer without tiring. I was an alcoholic for twenty-two years and every cell in my body was toxic. I have overcome my addiction to sugar and food. I am free of that chain now and eating fresh, organic fruits and vegetables and green juices daily. This has taken away my craving for sugar and has replenished my body. I look forward to each new day with joy and happiness instead of anger, pain, and fear.

DONNY R.

I have learned that I should really watch the things I eat because why would I want to put something harmful into my body? Everything around us has an effect, and it is up to us whether we choose to accept it. I have also learned to take one day at a time and live it to its fullest, and that everyone gives off an energy—some good, some bad, depending on who we are around. We can change this energy, so you don't want to be around people who put themselves down, and you don't want people who feel sorry for themselves around because they can have an affect on us.

JOHN R.

From this program I learned to use my energy more efficiently in a positive way—toward God, my family, and all people—to honor life, spirit, mind, and body. I've also learned that power, money, and greed are things that keep you a prisoner in your life. Nourish your body and mind with foods that provide health, not disease.

VIRGINIA R.

One Sunday morning about a year ago, I woke up, ate breakfast, got dressed, and started to go out. I looked for my car keys but could not find them. I went downstairs to look for my car, and it was missing too. I realized that I had left the keys in the trunk lock and my car had been stolen. Later I was listing to Gary Null and he mentioned the Reversing the Aging Process group. I knew this was what I had to do. I called up, and luckily there was room for me. I had been juicing for almost a year—not organic. I also was taking supplements. I was ready to begin the protocol. Once I began the program, I started to feel better. I didn't get sore throats in the morning after taking 5,000 milligrams of vitamin C at night. I decided that I was going to start living like a human being instead of working all the time like I had been doing. I had taken the month of August off and told my toxic babysitter I couldn't pay him so much. Shortly after I stopped working, I fell in love, and started going out with a man, for the first time since my divorce eight years earlier. I was very happy. I was praying to get my car back and looking for it. One day, I went for a walk and was pulled to go by Our Lady of Mount Carmel Church. I walked a different way than I would have walked ordinarily and miraculously spotted my car. I was so grateful to get it back, and the experience increased my faith in God. Of course the exercise walk was part of the program. Now, I am facing the challenge of building a relationship with my boyfriend and creating harmony between us and my wonderful, exuberant son, Sam. I am working less and spending more time with Sam. I still need to work on my weight and overeating especially when writing for my job. I am sleeping better now, especially if I exercise a lot. Anemia, which had been a problem, has not gotten worse. Also, I still need to work on having more respect for myself and deal even better with toxic people in a calm, confident way and give my knowledge effectively to others. I am a work in progress and I still have a long way to go. At twenty you have the face that God has given you, At forty you have the face that life has given you, and at sixty, you get the face you deserve. Last year, this time

on WBAI Radio, Gary mentioned an orientation and I felt I had to go:
So I showed up with my sidekick and I knew in a flash
He's talking to me—to the Big Apple bimonthly I'd dash.
Just sign on the dotted line so we know you commit,
Show up in your sneakers and shorts and don't try to quit.
If you want to be a fox . . . You're gonna have to detox.
Oy vays uh meer!
No more bagels with a schmear!
As a species we're full of feces.
No dairy, pesticides, caffeine, or wheat,
Your homework will be checked, so don't try to cheat.
I was introduced to aloe Vera, Phil, Sam, Ian and Jill,
All colors, shapes, and sizes—no one's "over the hill."

LISA H.

Since my teen's already a vegetarian so I thought I was cool (huh)
Harboring anger and resentment, parasites, and stubborn as a mule.
Whether in lead be Luanne Pennesi, George, or Gary
Seek in yourself, both the solution and cause
And don't react too quickly, but take time to pause.
When we no longer say and do what we feel and know
We limit our options and counter the natural flow.
Identify and cut loose toxic people in your life
Be it boss, father, mother, neighbor, sister, brother, husband, or wife.
Banish Imbalance and Disharmony and let your love light shine.
Control engaging in meaningless responsibility and "no pearls to swine."
I wanna dance in my magnetic pants.
Where would I be without pycogenol, quercetin and Suprema C?
Having more fun in the buff
Thanks to Red and Green Stuff,
But gotta stay on guard,
Thanks to potent rock hard.
I surrendered my fears,
Shed some tears and took off five years.
It's about dignity of choice
and honoring my inner voice.

Thank you, it's been an honor and privilege to share with this group.
Now it's time to actualize, spread my wings, and fly this coop.
With joy, entitlement, self-esteem, and pride,
Peace, love and Null Trim, it's been one helluva ride!

MURIEL C.

It comes to me as a complete surprise that I am writing this letter to you. It never occurred to me that I would meet you, or even be a client at your healing center, but life is full of surprises. I am grateful for this program because I feel it has put me on the right path and I feel fantastic! I have more energy, think clearer, and, best of all, thanks to hypnosis I have stopped smoking—my husband, too. I have also stopped eating meat and feel very good about this accomplishment. Within this year, I have done a lot of work on myself, of which this program is a very positive part. I continue to work and make many positive changes. Thank you for your insight, courage, and unselfish sharing of your knowledge. God bless you!

DIANA Y.

Where to begin? This program has been a life-changing experience, even though I had begun some of the components of the protocol—detoxing and using nutrition—to control my lifelong asthma symptoms for about a year and a half before joining this group. For most of my life, I had relied on pharmaceutical drugs that appeased my symptoms, made the initial problem worse, and severely damaged my immune system. At the age of twenty-six, I decided to try a more natural approach. My research served me well, and I managed to get off the drugs, but I still had some episodes of breathing difficulty. I was able to control this with herbs and homeopathic remedies, but was disturbed that after all I was doing, this was still happening. Since I started this protocol, I can't even remember the last time I had serious asthma symptoms. I believe the green drinks, not consuming sugar, caffeine (I was truly an addict, convinced that for some people it helped their asthma), or meat, has had a great effect. However, an even bigger difference is in my mental attitude. Having given up wheat, dairy, and processed foods at the beginning of my search for good health, I felt very deprived. When I was upset, stressed, or otherwise not happy with life, I would eat and eat all those things I knew were bad for me and I would feel good, satisfied. Now my attitude has changed completely. I only want to put into my body things that will really nourish me at a cellular level. I listen to what my body is saying when it tells me it wants something sweet and I know now that it needs a little nutrient boost, not a huge slice of chocolate cake. I also take into consideration what is going on emotionally, the power of association, and environment, all of which drive me to eat things that are going to hurt, not heal, my body. Just this past week, I made another breakthrough out of my old thinking pattern. Having had asthma, exercising has already been difficult. My husband had just found a study on exercise-induced asthma and encouraged me to push through the symptoms until the right hormones were released into my body to counteract the wheezing. Well, in our living room, in a very safe way, we tried it, and, lo and behold, it worked! Unbelievable. I have been working out on a lifecycle every day now for a week and I feel great afterward. I just had to pass through that "wall of discomfort". My husband and I are doing this program together. This has given us an opportunity to really look at what is important to us, where we are going, how we plan to get there, while we are still newlyweds. It has brought us closer together as a family, as we make rather unconventional decisions about the food we eat, how we spend our time and our money on health and ourselves, and just how we journey through the rest of our lives together.

ANDREA B.

Participating in Gary Null's anti-aging program has improved my health physically and emotionally. After eliminating dairy foods, sugar, and fried foods from my diet—I was already a vegetarian—my allergies improved and I had fewer colds and better elimination. I also have had more energy and some weight loss. The behavior modification aspect of the program has taught me to be more assertive and confident. I am closer to achieving my goals.

CAROL N.

I had been in a support group for six months. My weight had stabilized and I was getting discouraged. Rather than taking my old path of sabotaging the progress I had made by returning to old ways, I decided to visit Paradise Gardens for a week. I thought my goal was to lose more weight; however, attending the seminars, watching tapes, and attending your talks made me realize that was a limited goal. If I truly committed to the process unfolding before me, I would have the opportunity to start on the road of being a whole person. The pain of the fragmented, unconscious life I had led was overwhelming, and I now know that the process started in this short week will make the difference between a life lived on the side of mere existence and one which will be lived to its fullest at a high-energy level. I liked being challenged. Walking six miles to start and increasing the amount every day was something I didn't think I could do, so I stopped thinking and turned the walks into a meditation. I had not thought of this approach before and it has helped me to go farther. I expect I've never done anything more important in my life.

BEATRICE T.

Before I began this program, I was stuck in a job I disliked. I was unable to produce anything creative. I am now in the process of getting out of this job—I've already handed in my resignation—and I have made plans to reactivate my creative side. Before I began the program, I had arthritis that made it impossible for me to walk from time to time. I have no more arthritic pains. The fungus on my right heel disappeared. My hair, which was thinning, is showing accelerated growth. I have practically no ridges on my fingernails and my energy level is up considerably. Spiritually, I view the future as a good place. My buttons can't be pushed anymore. I can't give you a straightforward account of the obstacles I have overcome, because I do almost everything in an almost somnambulistic, intuitive way. I do have more inspiring dreams than I used to have, and therefore follow a path that is leading me somewhere, but not in that concrete way. When I compare myself now to the way I was a year and a half ago, it is that I moved away from fears and doubt toward hope and optimism, and in some respects, my life has taken on a more constructive form. All your questions gave me an opportunity to deal with issues directly, not my inclination, and therefore just by thinking of an answer, my life has become redirected and rechanneled.

LIZ

I am choosing relationships that are positive. In the six months since beginning the program, I have changed physically, losing 20 pounds and working out four to five days a week. I have incredible energy and am not tired. I sleep less, but the sleep I get is restful. Mentally, I am more clear-thinking, making decisions regarding my life and business quicker, as opposed to laboring over them. I have no depression, but a general feeling of grounding and balance. Affirmations work. I love work! I own my own business, an organic vegan, home-delivery service. Since being a member of the group, I am more organized. No procrastination. Our company has tripled its business. The company has become an extension of my being. I have much more quality play in my life, and I choose very carefully who I'd like to play with. My time is important. Most important, because work is demanding, I truly enjoy my "playtime." As far as relationships go, once again, time is valuable, [and knowing that] made it easy to shed relationships that were toxic and draining. I moved out of a six-and-a-half year relationship to a studio apartment that belongs to me, [and is] serene, peaceful, and beautiful. I am choosing relationships that are positive. Although not every day moves gracefully through my life, each day is growing more enjoyable and fun. This support group has helped change my life to a positive peaceful state of being. A definite catalyst.

GUM INFECTION

ROBERT A.
Before
I had problems with gum swelling and infection (almost always following stress). My dentist told me nothing except that I had a chocolate allergy. I took antibiotics, which caused intestinal problems (candida). Then I had eight fillings removed over the course of 2 years.
Now
I have no more mouth eruptions. My stress levels are still high (I lost my parents), but mouth remains healthy. I just recently found a solution to my intestinal problems at the Metropolitan Wellness Center.

HAIR LOSS STOPPED

JOE M.
I sought healing for my allergies and loss of hair. I did not turn to medications. I felt there had to be another way to stop these conditions. I came into a support group for these problems but learned much more. My experiences in a health support group opened me to my potential and unexplored strengths and joy. I follow the protocol and use juices. I can feel my body react to the detox. My allergies are greatly relieved. I feel energetic, and I require less sleep. My hair loss stopped. Today, I eat more than ever, and I experience real taste and health. I read my body.

HEADACHES

BARBARA

I was labeled disabled for four years. Migraine headaches caused me to be bedridden, and I used pain medication for a spinal disc injury. I was swollen after eating my usual meat, wheat, sugar, coffee, and dairy. My cholesterol was high. Candida plagued my body. I threw up after meals and was stressed by anxiety attacks. One day, after reading one of Gary's books, I saw him on PBS. I joined a support group in 1994. I attended classes open to change, and after two weeks on the protocol being vegan, organic, and never returning to toxic foods, the change began. I exercise in a rehab center for my back problem. Probiotics and sensible eating eliminated throwing up. I am a vegetarian cook and intend to study vegetarian meal preparation. My back pain is sporadic and not as acute. I am still in recovery but use no medication. I never looked at life as I do now.

JAYNE

I am migraine-free. My circulation has improved in my fingers and toes, and I have lots of energy. My sleep has improved, and I wake up energized.

NATALIE K.

I no longer have tension headaches and the severity of cold sores has diminished.

ELAINE

The changes I made since the onset of the protocol exceed any I made in several years. For a month or two, I had a difficult time sticking to the program. In that short time, I gained a few pounds and experienced exhaustion. My headaches returned. Now that I am fully committed to the protocol, I lose 1 lb a week and inches from my hips and waist. My blood pressure dropped to 102/60. My self-confidence, energy, and sense of security increased. My hair is shiny. I am not dehydrated, nor do I get headaches. I feel competent, confident, positive, and clear-headed, with an ability to focus on life goals.

HEMORRHOIDS

ART G., 67 years old

Blood pressure normalized. No more hemorrhoids. My cholesterol went from 260 to 180. My hemorrhoids have gone. My vision has improved. I have no more constipation. I have lost 18 lbs and run three marathons.

HEPATITIS VIRAL LOAD REDUCED

EDWIN M.

My hepatitis C viral load reduced from 7 million to 4 million since following Gary Null's protocol. I think clearer; my brain fog and mental and physical fatigue are reduced. The aches and pains in my knees and ankles are gone. My weight reduced by 40 lbs. I find my mental and physical clarity enhanced, and I have more energy and strength. I seem to need at least two hours less sleep.

HYPOGLYCEMIA

DORA

I considered my eating plan to be healthy. I thought meat and dairy gave me good protein and calcium. I enjoyed wheat breads. As time went on, I developed cysts in my breasts and was diagnosed as hypoglycemic. I did not feel well, and I wondered if my diet impacted my physical system. Motivated by a fear of future illnesses, I joined a support group. The teachings and protocol gave me the answers I needed. I quickly lost 8 lbs. The lumps in my breast are gone, and I have no more pain. I am vegan and organic. My dog and I enjoy green and red juices and powders. I do not test as hypoglycemic. I can skip meals. With daily yoga and exercise, I have wonderful energy. My skin is moist; people compliment my glow and happier attitude. My hair and nails are healthy. I sleep well, and I am aware of potential toxic people and situations. My goals are financial independence and business success. My family is beginning to follow the protocol.

IMPROVED MEMORY

JOYCE C.

My memory has significantly improved. I can now connect the names and faces of my friends. I am calmer and more relaxed. My energy level has gone up. I can get through the day without feeling drowsy.

RITA

I had heard about Gary Null from a friend who had been listening to his daily radio program in New York. I decided to go to his office, where he had mentioned there would be a support group. I was showing signs of Alzheimer's that were getting worse and worse. I was overweight, and I had blotches of skin discoloration all over my body. I thought Gary's protocol was too harsh to try, so I decided not to go on it. After a few months, however, when my condition got worse, I went back to his office and immediately began the program. I had not exercised for quite some time. Now, every day, I would set aside time to walk. My bowel habits became more regular, and suddenly I was remembering things that I used to forget. I could easily recall the names of friends I would run into on the street, whereas before I would have difficulty doing so. I feel that Gary's protocol has given me my life back, for it doesn't matter how good of shape your body is in if your mind is forgetful.

PAT

I feel better now than I did in my 20s. I am 42 now. I lost 20 pounds. My skin is clearer, my energy increased. I feel greater mental stability. Dry skin on my feet cleared up, thinning hair improved, allergies are gone. I have not had a cold or flu since I started the protocol. I need less sleep yet wake up refreshed.

SCOTT D.

I am a construction worker. I felt I was losing stamina and did not know if I could handle my work. I felt my body age. I ate the typical American diet, without labeled illnesses. One day, I listened to *Natural Living* and discussed the show with a friend. I decided to join a group. Today, I can keep up with younger coworkers, my physical endurance has increased. Injuries and pulled muscles heal quickly. I juice, and I keep to the protocol more and more as time goes by. I exercise and find myself seeking new directions. My forgiveness letters allowed me true introspection, and I focus on myself, avoiding all toxic situations.

INFERTILITY

MOIRA

I had an eating disorder. My body fat level was low. I was an athlete: a runner and a hockey player. I could not ovulate and was diagnosed as infertile. I tried the orthodox treatment and found it ineffective, with unpleasant side effects. My husband and I joined a health support group in 2000. After four months on the protocol, I ovulated and conceived. I feel my hormonal system is now stronger. I had a natural birth, but I experienced postpartum depression. My doctor labeled me clinically depressed. I was advised to discontinue nursing and to use medication. I rejected this and continued nursing. My health returned six months postpartum with exercise and meditation. My family and I are vegan. We juice and use only organic food. We stick to the protocol. I research postpartum depression and reach out to women suffering with this condition.

JOINT PAIN & ANXIETY

IRIS

Before joining Gary's support group, I was overweight, which caused pain in my knees and joints. I felt anxious all of the time, angry and overworked. I would also grind my teeth at night and wake up with jaw pain. After being in Gary's support group, I lost weight. My knees and joints no longer ache. I no longer grind my teeth, and I have a more positive outlook on life without the anxiety and anger that were plaguing me.

PATTY

I had no energy. My skin was dry and thinning, and I was gaining weight and losing muscle. My body felt stiff, and I had floaters blocking my vision. Gary's protocol helped me build muscle and lose weight. My joints no longer feel stiff, and my vision has improved greatly now that the floaters have disappeared: I have much more energy now and I feel great.

LYME DISEASE—IMPROVEMENT

PHILIP G.

My health began to improve six years ago when I was introduced to Gary Null's nutritional protocol. I had symptoms of Lyme disease. Being physically ill and exhausted, I had a rotten attitude. I did want to improve my life. I gradually experimented with Gary's concepts and became healthier. I took responsibility for myself and did not depend on others for care. I will not hand myself over to professionals anymore—auto mechanics or medical. I research and listen to their advice before taking action. I feel better since beginning this journey, and I continue to improve.

NATALIE K.

I suffered with bothersome tension-type headaches, which sometimes became debilitating migraines. I also had recurrent cold sores; one episode involved one of my eyes, resulting in a cornea-scraping procedure. Since joining the group, I have been eating a primarily vegetarian diet, including fish. I eliminated caffeine and sugar. I can state that I no longer have tension headaches, and the severity of my cold sores has diminished. I will continue working on eliminating them. I feel very fortunate. I am an optimistic person, and I feel loved and respected in all of my relationships. I am an intelligent, supportive woman with a natural desire to learn new things. I have learned many new concepts in the group and by reading *Who Are You, Really?* I see changes in my physical health and awareness of my surroundings. Understanding my life energies further empowered me, with insight and understanding.

MARIJUANA DETOX

ANDRE B.

He was in a support group years ago but did not follow the protocol. He decided to go to the retreat because he was mentally fatigued and could not give up marijuana. He learned to exercise in a workshop and began drinking juices to rebuild his body. He needed this push to establish self-confidence and gain the willpower to stop using marijuana. The people, environment, and lectures made a positive impact. He has not smoked marijuana since he left the retreat. He is following the protocol, and he is juicing. In order to stick to the program, he eliminated toxic and negative people from his life. His positive attitude and determination to renew his life intelligently, without emotions, reveals the building of self respect.

MENTAL CLARITY

CATHY T.

I was bedridden for two weeks with Epstein-Barr disease and could not walk more than three minutes at a time. I lost some of my memory. I returned to work but only put in five hours a day, and went to bed as soon as I returned home.

Stair climbing was difficult. My physician could do no more and suggested I do independent research. A homeopathic examination revealed food sensitivities. The day I watched Gary on PBS changed my life. I donated to the station and soon joined a support group. Today I carefully follow the protocol. I gave up chocolate without difficulty. At first the new food choices were difficult to accept, but today I am vegan and feel 100 percent better. I work seven hours a day and exercise after work. I walk one and a half hours and am training to race walk in the New York Marathon. I still need eight hours of sleep, possibly because of Epstein-Barr, but my waking hours are productive. With a clear mind, good memory, energy, and concentration, I plan future occupations in art and volunteer work.

FAYE MARIE L.

I had a "fuzzy" toxic head. I also had a lack of focus. The intensive focus on body, mind, spirit became clear in manifestation. I feel I have more focus and motivation and a new sense of who I am. My awareness is heightened. I believe I am moving toward divine health.

PATRICK H.

My recall and memory is sharp. My skin is clear. I have less nasal mucous, an improved resting heart rate. My tonsil size decreased. No longer do I have dark circles under my eyes and pain from peripheral neuropathy in both legs has diminished as has arthritic pain. I have not been ill since I started the program.

KAREN

I learned that my mental limitations take my life away. I convinced myself that I have physical limitations. I learned I have the brain power to bust through these barriers and live to my fullest potential.

MENOPAUSE

MARIA R.

I was prescribed Prozac for post-menopause syndrome by my gynecologist. I gained weight and lost energy. My hair and nails were weak. I had difficulty sleeping, and I felt depressed. I thought I followed a sensible eating plan. I did not connect food and aging. I began the detox protocol carefully and followed it diligently. I wanted to reverse my aging and clean my system out. I lost weight and am keeping it off. I have good energy. My hair and nails are growing to pre-menopausal thickness and strength. I discontinued the Prozac when I began the protocol and am not depressed. I sleep well, look well, and get healthier each day

MERCURY REDUCTION

JULIE C.

She attended one retreat in the past. She was ready for a new beginning. Her dog was 10 years in remission from cancer, thanks to an alternative veterinarian. There was much to learn about health and nutrition. Gary's lectures expanded her mind. She learned that life does not have to be routine and boring. The issues were exactly what she needed to explore: energy dynamics and alternative dimensions. She wanted to apply these issues practically and went on a media fast for one week, listening to music but not television. She had choices and was not alone. During this time, she was diagnosed with hepatitis C. Today, she works as a buyer and is an environmental activist. She and her husband decluttered their home, rescued five cats, and adopted two dogs. She admits to following the protocol 98 percent, tempted by the free-range chicken she prepares for her animals. The family, human and nonhuman, uses green and red powders, juices, and many supplements. She sees an alternative physician for her hepatitis, and the mercury level in her blood is half the level of two years ago. Her last eye examination revealed 20/20 vision for the first time.

MOODINESS, NEGATIVITY, ANGER

FRED M.

I used drugs and was melancholy, with tendencies to cling to and control people. I reacted to others with anger and felt unpleasant toward them. My decisions were based on that which was best for others. I could not understand why I behaved this way. I wanted a happy life. I discovered my body was reacting to the drugs and toxic foods I consumed. The protocol provided me with a method of starting all over again, cleaning my body and my mind out. Little by little, I lost my need to control people and to strike out in anger. Uncluttering my environment made me aware of the rational possibilities ahead, beginning with a clean slate. I now think before reacting to people. I feel positive. My relationships improved.

PATRICIA

I have a psychiatric history that spans more than 30 years. I have a goiter and an inflamed thyroid from lithium and mild tardive dyskinesia [involuntary movements] from Stelazine. Today I am off all psychiatric drugs. I am off lithium and Wellbutrin and Stelazine. I feel balanced, happy, and excited by life. I am less confused and clearer in my thinking, with improved recall.

O.L.

I was underweight, and I had behavior problems. I had a lot of unresolved past issues that caused anger and brooding. I often engaged in negative thinking. It was time to change. Since following the protocol, my emotional and physical health improved. My skin is smooth, and I have more energy. I gained 10 lbs and lift weights. Recovery from heavy exercise is faster today. I wake up mornings with clarity. The homework questions helped me eliminate unpleasant memories and resentments. I let go of people who do not accept me, and I find myself seeking and obtaining new relationships, having fun, laughing. The guidance of Gary, Luanne and my fellow group members is appreciated. I am very thankful.

MULTIPLE SCLEROSIS

TEXAS DOCTOR

There is a woman here with end stage MS. She was written off by the medical community—my colleagues. She comes from a family, many of whom are physicians in traditional medicine. She was given no options other than to make the best out of the rest of her life. When she first got here, she couldn't walk. She was in a wheelchair. She couldn't move her legs. Each day she started progressing and by the end of the retreat not only was she not in a wheelchair, she was walking with a walker and then at the very end of the retreat she was able to walk without a walker. It's nothing short of a miracle. And I would love if the rest of the medical community could at least witness some of this and start to use it in their practice. I'm so happy to see these patients get better.

KENNETH

I've been diagnosed with probable MS, and joined the health support group for people with neurological disorders. It has been a life-changing experience. For me to be a part of this health support group, I needed to first ask myself one question, "Do I want to get well?" I would retreat to this question whenever anything I had to do to get me well took me out of my comfort zone. Being able to answer "YES" made it easier to make changes. Because I've answered yes to everything, I am much better today. The heavy metals that plagued my body are almost completely eradicated compared to six months ago. My cognitive functions have also improved greatly. I no longer have any symptoms. This is not about symptom suppression for me anymore. I will follow through with the protocol to the point of elimination. Reverse the lesions in the brain, and remove the worry about the protein in the spine that triggers MS symptoms. My original neurologist will wonder what happened, and what I did. The protocol is a series of therapies and lifestyle changes working in chorus to get you better than well.

PARKINSON'S DISEASE

THOMAS G., 70 years old
Parkinson's symptoms improved
Before
I suffered from Parkinson's disease, hypertension, skin problems, herpes simplex outbreaks, and arthritis. I became aware of the importance of nutrition and studied various theories, but my physical problems continued. My Parkinson's symptoms caused me shame in public. I could not write. I typed with two fingers. My hands trembled when I put food in my mouth. I was advised to take medications. My past experiences with drugs were unpleasant. I refused them. I went on Gary's protocol and learned the specifics of diet and organics, the biochemical necessity of green juices and grasses, and the importance of attitude and beliefs.
Now
It was when I combined supplements with my diet that things began to look up. I honor myself, unclutter my life of people and objects, and share this important knowledge with others. I am alert, without past negative influences. Green and red powders keep me going. These are my happiest and proudest times. I intend to live another 70 years.

JOSEPH
My doctors had given up on me. They didn't tell me that, but I could see it in their eyes and hear it in their voices. They told me that I had Parkinson's and that there was no cure for it. They told me that Janet Reno and Muhammad Ali had

forms of it, and they were leading productive lives. This may sound strange, but the thing I feared the most about my condition was being unable to stop my shaking. This may sound selfish, but it is true. I visited Gary in his office on Seventy-second Street and Broadway, where he had me go get my blood work done. Then he designed a program for me that changed my life. At first, I did not think I could go through with it. Now, I know I can. Although my shaking has not completely gone away, it has lessened a great deal. My wife is amazed at my progress, and I look forward to living the rest of my life knowing that one day, I will not be shaking at all.

BARBARA

I came here because my husband developed mild Parkinson's. It is absolutely spectacular here. I was thrilled when I saw everything. We have absolutely fantastic food. The preparation of and the staff that make the food, are so loving so kind. Everybody here showed us so much love and kindness. That's exactly what we needed when we were here. My husband is getting stronger and stronger all the time. He is now on the road to recovery. He starting to walk a little and take steps a bit bigger. He's also starting to hold himself a little better. We're going to keep up the good eating and we're going to keep up our calmness. So now I'm completely relaxed and it's the first time in many, many years that I can say I'm relaxed.

PERIMENOPAUSAL

JANET F.

Was perimenopausal but now gets hot flashes and her period
Before
A college teacher, I was a longtime listener of *Natural Living*. I was never totally committed to change. I had low energy, I saw aging in my future, and I wanted group support. Though I was a vegetarian, I ate dairy, sugar, and wheat. I had insomnia and indigestion, and I was constipated.
Now
I joined a health support group in August 1999 and gave up dairy, sugar, and wheat. At first, I felt weird. I lost 15 lbs slowly. My hair is 3 inches longer, shinier and thicker. I was peri-menopausal but began to get hot flashes and my period. My period continues to come and go. I lost my sugar craving. I have charges of

energy. I eat my big meal at midday. I use green powders. My skin texture has improved, and I get no more age spots. My eye floaters are gone. I feel the writing and homework are as important as the dietary aspect and are responsible for my life changes. I create an area for introspection, and I love being in a group of positive people.

RETREAT APPRECIATION:
REJUVENATION & LIFE-CHANGING EXPERIENCE

BRIAN

I feel for the first time that I was able to realign my energy with my authentic self. And I feel confident leaving here that I'm going home with clarity, inspiration, and amazing energy.

LLOYD

This is the third experience that I've had with Gary with regards to retreats and I must say that they just get better and better. I strongly advise anyone who wants to make a major change in life to seek the retreats out. I'm grateful to Gary especially for his spiritual input. It has made a significant difference in my life. Very positive.

JIM

I wish I could stay another week. I have learned a lot about nature, its balance and keeping things in harmony. I have a lot of tools that I will take home with me as far as gardening, cooking, and exercise.

CAITLIN

I've learned about the powers of positive energy, learned a lot about myself through reflection being by myself and take the time to think about the important things in my life, setting goals for myself. The food was great. I had the pleasure of being in the kitchen a lot, learned many different techniques and lots of recipes.

GERALD

I've been searching for answers for the last three years as to where I want to end up in my older days. I came to the retreat and I finally got the answer. It's been a very beautiful experience, the scenery has been immaculate, it is something I always dreamed of and I thank Gary for giving me that insight. Now I am ready to move on to the next level. I could not have asked for a better experience than this.

KB

I cannot put into words the amazing and wonderful experience here at Gary Null's retreat. I came here physically debilitated. Today I feel 90 percent better. I'm able to do what I couldn't do before. I have participated in a race that I have never imagined I would ever be able to take part in. I would have never had the courage had I not come. I've learned so much and now I want to be a viable part of my community as a result of the information that I've had here. This is better than any vacation I could ever have taken in the world. And I've traveled the world. Now I know that life is about living and I've learned how to do so here at this retreat.

BARBARA

The beauty of the place is hard to describe beyond: exquisite. But it's not just the beauty of the place, it's the energy of the place. The food is organic and it's cooked with so much love and you feel it, it's delicious. The environment. As far as the people working here everyone is supportive and following in the same direction that you're going and helping to carry through what your beliefs are. I just wish for anyone who is on this journey that they would take the opportunity to do this.

LUANNE

This has to be one of the most bucolic, one of the most healing environments that I've ever been in and here is the place where I am probably for the first time in my life connecting with nature like I never have before. And there's a sense of relaxation and a sense of bliss that I didn't know that I could even experience. And I'm watching other people go through this in their own way and while all this is going on, I'm enjoying whole live organic foods. There's no meat, no dairy, no sugar, no processed foods but instead we're getting whole live foods prepared in a way that I never had before. We are getting some of the most delicious gourmet vegan meals that have been prepared by the specialty chefs. And mouthwatering delicious meals that are satisfying. We're outdoors and exercising every morning, all of us walking in one big group. Power walking outside as the sun is coming up and then we're doing yoga right on the most beautiful lake with swans. It's just quite frankly nothing like I have ever experienced before. It is just one of the most amazing experiences of my life and I'm so grateful and so thankful to have been here.

TOM

I've just completed a week at Gary's retreat. Right now I feel extremely peaceful. It's been a week of many experiences. I've enjoyed it extremely and I would advise anyone who wants to have a rewarding experience and have a soulful search to go here.

JOHN

The week that I've just spent here, had so much fun in the pool, just walking around and seeing this beautiful villa that Gary has created, with hummingbirds, butterflies everywhere with guinea hens running around making noise but they are just so joyful to watch. The energy here is really high and the food is off the chart. Meals each day are prepared by these gourmet chefs, it's vegan. If you are not a vegan and not eating this way I feel sorry for you. It's really delicious food. And the lectures at night, they force you to open your mind and think. I can't think of a better place where I would rather be than here, just taking in all this beauty. I hope you get a chance to do this; you ought to do this at least once.

ROB

It's nice to speak with people who are open-minded, relaxed, comfortable, and positive. Excellent food and the atmosphere throughout the whole landscape.

JON Q.

I came down to Gary's villa to train some people as far as physical training and water training as well but like all the other retreats of Gary's you just get overwhelmed with the surroundings, the lake, the trees, the animals. I've been here for two weeks now and I think Gary's going to have to get security to kick me out of here! This is always a great experience, the weather's been great, the people have been incredible. The energy is very, very, very high. I'm looking forward to my next visit down here to Gary's villa.

ADAM

It's hard to put into words the experience because everything has been so overwhelmingly phenomenal. Everything about this place is magical. The food is absolutely amazing. I love to cook and cook a lot of dishes. This week I've been inspired to study vegan cooking and take my cooking to another level. I've been energized more than I've ever been. The running has been great. I'm not used to running four miles, and today it felt like it was almost effortless. I've lost some weight and I feel much lighter and much happier. Gary's lectures are phenomenal. His insights and wisdom are nourishing. It's very, very powerful, the things he has to say. I'm just enjoying my experience here very much and I think is going to be life-changing for anybody that decides to come.

SUSAN

This has been the most authentic thing that I've ever done in my life. I'm a chef by trade, but the whole world of veganism, which I've dabbled in before, has been pretty bland to me and this has opened up my eyes. I have not been hungry. I have not lacked anything or had cravings for any of the regular foods that I would normally eat. The amount of reflective time as well as interactive time with other people and the programs has been just outstanding. I want to say that the animals have been awesome here as well as looking up and seeing vast amounts of sky in varying shapes and colors.

DANIEL

The food was tremendous, all vegan. I am a vegan but had a pretty poor diet. I feel like I am going to leave here and not make the foolish compromises that I do in my diet and my regimen of life, with exercise and meditation and some dreams or goals that I have, things that are visions of empowerment or contribution that I have not addressed as strongly as I should have done. I feel now empowered to begin with a resolution and efficiency hereafter.

FRED

I had a fantastic time in a beautiful environment. The food was fantastic. The vegetarian food was prepared excellently and there were a lot of ideas that I could take with me to make simple vegetarian meals. I picked up a lot of ideas and practices on living a vital, full vibrant life. I look forward to incorporating a lot of the approaches and ideas in my life.

JEMMA

I have been a natural practitioner for over thirty years. I came here because this is a time in my life for a new beginning for me. This was the very best decision that I could ever make. Everyone on the staff was supportive and loving and very constructive. The environment is loving and nurturing. Through Gary's guidance I learned to go in and allow nature to heal me. I'm just very grateful for this opportunity. Everything is so lovely and pristine and balanced. I'm taking much with me. I know that I'm capable of a new beginning in my life.

MELINDA

I've just spent a week at Gary's retreat and it was a unique and extraordinary experience in a beautiful environment. I'm going to be taking home a lot of new information on how to incorporate vibrant eating habits and exercise that is fulfilling in so many ways. It was a full experience and I will be coming away with a lot of new information.

RAYNEY

This was a very rich learning experience with daily lectures and power walks and exercise which made us feel good. The energy and the love we all received from this beautiful environment were incredible.

ANDREA

I would like to thank Gary for allowing us to see that the sky is the limit. We can go beyond our potentials in so many areas. I'll take all that I've learned back to grow for myself and my family. And, as I heard Gary mention, "as you grow you help someone with you" so along with my family I will make sure that I have other people who can grow along the way and help someone along the way, and make sure to pass it along to someone who is worth the while.

RON

I'm coming away with a bigger smile, a larger heart, a lot of information to chew on, aim to go out into the world with a better attitude and try to make myself and hopefully humanity a little bit better.

PEDRO

I've wanted to come to the retreats for some years now. I went through a lot of things in my personal life. I lost some people and had a bad breakup. This experience has been so unique. I've never been one to run, I've never been one to get up at five in the morning. Not only am I getting up at five and running, I was actually falling behind all week and this morning I actually was the leader of the pack. In fact, I was probably about two blocks in front of everybody. I didn't break a sweat so that really impressed me. Also, Gary did some energy work on me. It makes sense now but all these emotions came rushing out. A lot of mixed emotions but after the fact I just felt cleansed. It was a cleaning of the mind, body, and soul. I must have lost about maybe 8 lbs by now between the yoga, the pool, exercising. It just brings you back to life. You're brand-new again, you're reborn. If I had to do it again—it's not even a matter of having to—I would love to do this again! I recommend this to everyone. The food, I'm lost for words. The food is absolutely amazing. I don't think I've ever gone two days without meat. It's been seven days and I don't miss it. There's nothing about chicken, beef, ribs—just don't miss it. I've basically wiped the slate clean in my life. This is a brand-new beginning. And I thank everybody for co-creating this experience with me.

FERNETTA

I am on a journey. And it was a pleasure to come to Gary's retreat. One of the outstanding segments was to be authentic and stand in your truth. That was awesome. The food was outstanding. I was hesitant and afraid to eat vegan because I did not know it could taste so good. It is AWESOME. I've had a dessert that's the best I've ever had in my life because not only was it wonderful to taste, but it was healthy for my body. The information here I am going to use going forward and this was a positive step in my life.

SUSAN

I am so pleased with myself that I made this decision to invest my time in coming to the Gary Null retreat. It's very easy for me to take care of others and meet the needs of others. So this was a very big change for me and a very life-affirming and0-life changing experience for me.

DAVE

The setting here is really amazing. The staff is friendly and open. There were a lot of people that were healed. It was interesting seeing the changes in people. The food was phenomenal; it really again made me more determined to fully commit to being vegan.

RICH

The energy here is really fantastic. If you need to heal this is the place to come. It's very serene and yet it's a lot of fun. I laughed a lot this week and cried a little bit and it was very healing for me. It's what you put into it you get out of it and I really enjoyed it.

JOE

I made a New Year's resolution to make healthier choices. The retreat was a tipping point for me not to make unhealthy choices.

PAULINE

The spiritual aspects were tremendously moving and yet so personal and the lectures that Gary gave every night were eye-opening. I'm coming away challenged to do more and start a new chapter in my life, with my family and with work. It's really lifted my spirits a lot.

CHRIS

I'm a veteran and I was tinkering on the edge of suicide. I was putting my fears in order while putting a smile on my face for everybody. But I thank Gary for giving me this time to breeze and to breathe, and really let loose and just—breathe—and it has really changed my life. He's given me the tools to go back and once again try to live a full life.

REGULATION OF MENSTRUAL CYCLE

KATE

Period regulated

Before

I was a vegetarian for years but ate dairy, sugar, and wheat. I was an insomniac, had indigestion, was constipated, and had floaters in my eyes. I had age spots on my skin, and my hair and skin were unhealthy. I was a college teacher and a long-time listener of Gary's show, but I never totally committed. I needed a group support. With low energy and aging in my future, my career as a professional singer was out the door.

Now

I have lost 15 lbs and no longer have a sugar craving. My hair is longer and thicker, and my age spots are gone. My skin improved, I am more energetic, and my eye floaters have disappeared. I joined a support group and love being with positive people. I follow the protocol and have eliminated toxic foods. At first I felt weird. I eat a large meal at midday. The green powder gives me a large charge of energy. Although I have been perimenopausal for many years, my hot flashes have resumed and my period has returned. I feel my hormones are active. I ended a toxic marriage and healed my relationship with my son. I uncluttered, cleaned, up my finances, and feel responsible for my life.

REPRODUCTIVE HEALTH

KARIN

I was nearsighted and experienced severe premenopausal symptoms the week before my period, including night sweats, insomnia, and mood swings. Gary's support group helped relieve these symptoms and improve my vision.

DIANE P.

Cervical dysplasia improving

I was diagnosed with cervical dysplasia (CIN 2—moderate). After following Gary's protocol, the cervical dysplasia went to CIN 1, which is classified as mild. On the last colposcopy, the gynecologist saw nothing to biopsy. I am confident that the cervical dysplasia will be reversed. I now have radiant skin and hair, more energy, a general sense of well-being, and no more colds and flu.

MARGARET W.

I was plagued with a long-term yeast infection. My personal relationship did not satisfy me, but I held onto it. Life was not empowering. I felt I was not going anywhere. I joined a support group and was amazed to see other people like me searching for a happier and healthier life. None of us understood where we went wrong. I juiced and detoxed with optimism. My yeast infection and the accompanying lethargy is over. I feel happy and energetic. I ended my toxic relationship without guilt. I am mentally and spiritually awakened. I fell in love with running and power walking, and I am training other people to use them. This is a wonderful time.

ROCHELLE K.

My PMS symptoms drastically declined. I no longer feel sad, and I have little fatigue and almost no bloating, cravings, or feelings of nausea. Overall, I feel good energy and sleep fewer hours at night. I lost about 10 lbs after cutting out junk food and improving my diet.

TARA

I no longer need medication for my menstrual cramps.

RESPIRATORY PROBLEMS

RUBEN

I did not like the way I felt or looked. My skin broke out with infectious cysts. I needed long nighttime rests. My weight gain coincided with frequent outbreaks of colds and flu, and my hair developed a dry unpleasant texture. In a short amount of time, I lost 12 pounds and the skin cysts cleared up. My hair is soft and healthier. I do not have respiratory infections anymore. I sleep less and enjoy waking hours more. The protocol really worked for me.

ANN L.

My concern for several medical conditions brought me into a detoxification group. We met weekly. The group dynamic was powerful. I wanted to participate in rebuilding and regaining health. I had mitral valve prolapse, and I had several upper respiratory infections and gum problems each year. Cleaning my body and rebuilding my immune system turned my health around. I follow the protocol carefully. It is all in my hands. I do not have mitral valve prolapse or colds and flu. I have no more gum problems. My energy returned. I participate in new activities, such as studying botany and leading bird-watching groups. I can control old, negative habits, and carefully choose people who will enhance my life.

ALICE, 73 years old

When I came into a Gary Null health support group, I had an acute allergy from cortisone injections into my scalp for alopecia. I had many upper-respiratory infections during the year. I needed to sleep long hours to feel rested. My eyes were dry, a condition which was annoying and uncomfortable. It took a while to adjust to my new eating plan. I never realized true taste before. My body felt cleaner after a month. Best of all, I no longer have alopecia. Symptoms of the cortisone allergy are subsiding. My eyes are healthier. I wake up refreshed, full of energy, with less sleep. I am uncluttering my home environment, drinking green drinks, and re-reading the group class assignments. When I think of where I was before, I am ecstatic about where I am now.

TERRY

I tried to be vegetarian. I did not eat flesh foods, but I did eat fried foods, breads, pizza, and muffins. I had asthma and refused to use an inhaler. My hair was thinning. My intake of water was low, and my job stressed me. I joined a support group in 2000. I lost 7 lbs detoxing, and I became organic. My energy increased. I am calmer and sleep less. My hair grows in thicker, and I seem to be less stressed between jobs. I discovered my spiritual side, and I use quality time well. By uncluttering, I set boundaries. Now, I handle people well, without getting involved in toxic situations. I make thought-out meals for family dinners and do not react to adverse remarks. I find I am attracted to people on a cellular level. Exercising and sports are on my agenda. My asthma attacks come faster and leave easier. I identify their cause. Respiratory infections heal quickly. I returned to school, and I made a list of future accomplishments.

TED J.

I made many positive changes as a result of attending Gary Null's support group. I always used nutritional supplements. Today, I understand the relationship between the emotional, spiritual, and physical. I used to have upper-respiratory infections and needed naps during the day. I endured stress in my professional life, and I wasted time on petty things. I increased my knowledge of the interdependence of food, biochemistry, and emotional and environmental factors in the support group. Upper-respiratory infections ceased when I gave up dairy. My energy is maintained all day without naps or long sleeps. I changed my professional life. I own my own business—professional training. It is very satisfying. I often demonstrate techniques in the new support groups. I no longer waste time.

RICHARD

I noticed that I got a lot of upper-respiratory infections when I gained weight. Also, my energy dropped, and I needed more sleep. My skin was dry and often was problematic. I was not happy, and I had a negative outlook. I heard about Gary

Null and listened to his show. The results of the people who completed the support groups were too good to be true, but I gave it a shot and joined.

I learned many things, but most of all, I learned it is not difficult to become healthy. It is simple and enjoyable. Physical and emotional health developed for the first time in my life. I lost 20 lbs, and I have good energy because of it. I do not need to sleep as long as I used to. I no longer cough up phlegm. My skin is smooth and moist. I threw out unnecessary objects and people. These are positive actions that I handled successfully without stress. I am proud of that.

ALICE D.

My immune system was weak. I caught many upper-respiratory infections. I required long hours of sleep each night. Many years ago a physician injected cortisone into my scalp. We soon discovered I was allergic to the drug and I developed alopecia [bald spots]. My eyes were dry, and I was generally uncomfortable with myself. I began support group sessions and stuck to the protocol and affirmations. I soon noticed I no longer had colds and flus. I slept less and awoke refreshed. My eye condition is improving and I am aware of the relationship between uncluttering and getting my life in order. I am happy to report my life is indeed satisfying. The protocol and teachings brought success.

VERONICA

I ate junk food and was a heavy coffee drinker. I was hypoglycemic and fainted frequently. My skin had ugly eruptions. I cried easily and had low energy. I had several allergies. I heard Gary speak about Paradise Gardens and the experiences people had there, improving their insights and health. It sounded beautiful. I signed up for the trip. That was the beginning of a new, wonderful life. I learned how to power walk and exercise, how to juice and prepare healthy foods and fruits, and how to plan meals. I lost 15 lbs. Eventually, all my upper-respiratory infections and skin problems disappeared. I still follow the diet, juice during the day, eat fruits in the evening and make one well-planned meal a day. I am now a marathon runner. My energy is without limit. I am healthy.

CHERYL

I developed severe allergies and upper-respiratory infections. I was consumed with family issues, which made me angry and anxious. Negative people annoyed me. My past caused anger. I could not express my feelings or deal with them.

The support group and protocol allowed me to see myself and my life on many levels. I developed a healthier life, without colds and other respiratory illnesses. I am now vegetarian, juice, meditate, and see my loved ones with compassion. I understand my anger and anxieties. They are gone. The past no longer plays over and over again in my mind. I actualized a new, successful career as a freelance editor, which means no toxic office environment. I am active in political causes, especially violence against women, using hotlines and shelters.

RESISTENCE TO COLDS

RICARDO

I was constantly sick with colds and the flu, my hair was thinning, I lost my energy, and I was getting fat. I overreacted to people who were critical of me and never dealt with situations correctly. I changed my eating habits and followed Gary's protocol. I no longer get the cold and flus anymore, my hair is thicker, and I have the energy of my youth. I did not diet, I just followed the protocol and lost weight. I feel clarity and handle people effectively. That's maybe because I found my self-esteem. It was a major improvement for me.

RETINOPATHY

ZARA B.
Retinopathy in remission
Before
I was a vegetarian and had juvenile diabetes. I consumed coffee, junk food, sodas and such. I had diabetic retinopathy and fatty deposits in my eye. I consulted a "health coach" for alternatives and to control my diabetes, but saw this as a bandage rather than healing. I wanted a mind-body-spirit approach. I began Gary's protocol, and this opened me up to spiritual meditation and personal strength.
Now
My retinopathy is in remission. I no longer have fatty deposits after three months on supplements. I use acupuncture and drink green juices that are organic. Medical examinations revealed that my eye vessels are stronger and that a thicker membrane is growing.

SINUS PROBLEMS, HYPERTENSION & ASTHMA

DIANE G.
Sinusitis, hypertension, and asthma gone
I was a New York City paramedic diagnosed with occupational asthma. I inhaled a mixture of bleach and ammonia during a medical pickup and developed a condition called osteopenia from prednisone. My vision diminished, my hair began to turn gray, and my skin peeled as if it were ash. I was stressed, had insomnia and sinusitis, and slept three hours a night. I retired from the fire department because of the accident, and I joined a support group. Today, I am a vegetarian, I am organic, and I juice. I am no longer suffering with sinusitis, hypertension, or asthma. My black hair is returning, my skin is lovely, and my vision has improved. I sleep six hours a night, and I am calm and happy. My family joined a food co-op. My vitality and energy have zoomed up. I work out in an adult ballet class, study flamenco, and will perform in a recital. I also rollerblade, do spin cycles, and am studying toward a rabbinical career.

NEVEA V.
I no longer have sinus infections or colds, my skin looks great, and my menstrual periods are normal.

JOEL
I lost 8 pounds. I lost 2 inches off my waist line. Two percent body fat is gone. My hair and skin look better, and my eyes are clearer, and less fatigued. My hair is shinier. The redness on my face has faded.

LEDA
I used to get serious sinus infections three times a year, and now I rarely do. My skin was very dry and has become very smooth. I was diagnosed with rheumatoid arthritis and I hardly have any symptoms anymore. My sense of hearing has increased dramatically.

NEVA
I eliminated food allergies when I eliminated wheat, dairy, and processed foods. I learned about, and now feel the benefits of, eating a healthy diet. I no longer have sinus infections or colds, my skin looks great, and my menstrual periods are

normal. One major change is listening to my body. If I feel a major change, it is because I consumed something I am allergic to. The program and protocol put me on the right track.

SKIN CONDITIONS

LINDA L.

I was able to eliminate several problems with Gary Null's protocol in a healthy, normal way. My acne and cysts cleared up. I used to produce a lot of phlegm, and I do not now. My hands and feet are not cold. The spider veins in my legs are less apparent. The dark circles and broken blood vessels around my eyes are reduced. The intestinal bloating of the past is gone. How's that for success?

PEGGY

I was slightly overweight. My symptoms were uncomfortable: skin outbreaks, cysts and eruptions on my arms, and premenstrual syndrome. These conditions did not fit into my projection of a happy future. That is why I joined a support group and learned a totally new way of life. Today, my facial skin is clear, the eruptions on my arms are gone, and the annoying sinusitis is over. It is a pleasure to be healthy. I intend to remain so.

JENNIFER

I have so much more energy. The cysts I used to get on my back and chest are gone. I feel like I am standing taller. I feel slender. I feel great. I lost 10 pounds!

JOANNE

I was quite negative. This drained my energy. My skin was not clear, I had backaches, and I could not confront heavy emotional issues. I did not help myself or others. I was not certain if detoxification could help these problems, but I joined a support group. I really enjoyed and benefited from the group meetings. I became organic and vegan, and I love the lifestyle. I feel healthy, and my skin looks wonderful. The lectures and writing assignments were educational and psychologically healing. Exercise improved my back problems and energized me. I now look at life with a positive eye and can undertake world issues that will help others. I let my negativity go.

JOAN

When I had the opportunity to get into Dr. Null's program, I made the decision to do it. By the fourth month, I lost 12 pounds. I drink five glasses of organic vegetable juices a day. My family and I eat organically now. I feel things are starting to go in the right direction. My big lesson is learning to take time for myself. Now I'm learning to get out in the sun and exercise. I am learning to have patience with myself. I do attribute the weight loss to the diet, the love I have for myself, and the pride I have in what I'm doing.

MOISHE

Shyness, guilt, and low self-esteem were replaced with self-respect and personal control. An acne condition and weak nails have cleared. The arthritis that hampered me is 70 percent improved. I no longer need drops for dry eyes. I used to take injections two or three times a week without improvement for several allergies. I had difficulty walking in the toxic city air. These problems either diminished or are completely gone. I look 10 years younger. My facial skin is clear and healthy.

JOHN C.

My body changed with each birthday. My skin tone was sallow, almost yellow. I had a general, daylong fatigue and would get hay fever, which drained my energy. My body could not defend itself, and I was ready to commit to change. I signed up for a support group. The protocol and meetings expanded my reasoning, thinking, and sensitivities. I am energetic; I have no more fatigue. My skin is healthy. My hay fever bouts lessened and are manageable. Uncluttering changed me emotionally. I dream less, feel well-grounded, and have released past angers with forgiveness letters, meditation, and prayer.

DELIA

When I started with Gary's support group, I was constantly tired, my hands and feet were itchy, and my skin was extremely dry. I was a smoker and experienced frequent bronchitis, a chronic cough, and I could not breathe deeply. I also had high blood pressure and sciatica in my right leg, experienced constipation, and lost my night vision. After following Gary's protocol, I feel so much better. I have lost weight and learned to eat well and exercise, and now have much more energy. My skin has become much suppler and no longer itches. My blood pressure has decreased, and my sciatica has improved. A lot of my issues related to my smoking have eased. I am able to breathe better; I no longer get bronchitis; and my cough is gone. My eyesight and digestive issues have also improved greatly.

FRAN, 65 years old

My skin condition embarrassed me. The sagging moles and dark age spots on my body saddened me. The energy I used to enjoy decreased with age. Tests indicated high LDL and HDL levels. I watched my hair change color and noticed my mental functions decrease. The reasons for these unpleasant changes were explained to us in meetings of the support group. The foods we eat, water we drink, and thoughts we think all contribute to body malfunctions. I learned reasons for detoxification: why we need it and what we will experience as we begin. I realized I suffered from years of bad eating. Today I follow the protocol and always will. The result is a new healthy and optimistic me. Facial moles are gone, my skin is tighter and age spots faded. My attitude and body are more youthful. New hair grows in dark brown. Also my blood tests went from high risk to normal. I am full of energy and open to change without fear. The support group gave my life back to me.

JANICE

I had major skin eruptions and cysts on my arms. I would get unpleasant PMS symptoms each month. Sinusitis was persistent. I wanted to lose weight and sought a sensible approach to end these symptoms without medications. I felt optimistic about Gary Null's approach. He certainly expanded my knowledge through his radio show. I jumped at the chance to enroll in a support group. I found the detoxification aspect pleasant to follow. The spiritual lessons changed my attitude. My skin is clear and eruption-free, and the arm cysts are gone. I have no more sinusitis and my PMS symptoms are less severe. I lost 10 lbs, and I am focused and more positive. I meditate with tai chi.

PATRICIA

My skin cleared up. It is smooth and soft now. I have more energy. My varicose veins are lightening up. I lost 10 pounds. I am down a size and a half. I feel so good exercising.

STRESS RELIEF

ANDREA

I've truly been blessed being here. It has truly been an experience for me. It's not just about living the healthy lifestyle; it is understanding that the energy you portray good or bad affects not only us but the people around us. It is so clean. You can tell the difference in the way you breathe versus when I'm in New York City. You learn to connect more with who you are. You have quiet time; something you don't always experience when you're in the city. But this is what you experience when you come on a retreat such as this. I would encourage anyone who is looking for a different type of vacation. This is one you will truly and enjoy and come away learning more that you can even imagine.

THYROID

WARNETTA A.

Thyroid normalized. Carpal tunnel syndrome and cataracts gone.

Before

I listened to Gary's show for many years before I actualized the information. My cholesterol and blood pressure were elevated, but my primary concern was obesity: my weight was 209. I wore a size 22, and I was diagnosed with an underactive thyroid, low energy, osteoporosis, osteoarthritis, cataracts, and carpal tunnel syndrome. Gary explained that detoxification must precede dieting in order for the dieting to be effective. That made a lot of sense to me, so I went with the protocol.

Now

I weigh 150 lbs and maintain it. Recent physical examinations ruled out an abnormal thyroid, carpal tunnel syndrome, and cataracts. I take lutein and blueberry capsules, and I threaded a fine needle today without difficulty. My cholesterol and blood pressure are slightly elevated but not abnormal. I have no symptoms of osteoarthritis or osteoporosis. I exercise three times a week with a senior class in a Buddhist temple. I buy organic food, and I stopped eating meat and eat fish instead. Ingredient labels shocked me. I am more aware of the unnecessary amount of salt in products. I share my new knowledge with people interested in regaining their health. I was determined to enjoy life in good health, and I do now, with great, positive energy.

TUMOR REGRESSION

WILLIAM

I came down to Gary's retreat feeling stressed and trying to get back on track. All I can say is what a wonderful atmosphere to de-stress. I feel like I have been helped immensely. It's made a good impact on me, validated some things I wasn't sure about. Coincidentally, I have a mass or tumor on my back and I didn't really come down here for that. I had some energy work done and I can't believe it, it seems like it has gone down at least one half. I know that sounds unbelievable but it's unbelievable to me also. All very positive, very informative. I feel invigorated. I'm just so glad I came. I had no idea it was going to be like this and I was going to feel like this.

MARTHA

I went down there expecting to learn about vegan food and just to lie around like what you would expect at a resort but I gained much, much more. I had the most wonderful time. It was a life-changing experience. I was around good people, good energy, beautiful surroundings, clean water, and good food. What I gained was a lifestyle change. We had exercise, yoga, meditation in the most beautiful surroundings. I gained so much insight into how to correct things in my life. The environment was also very spiritual. We had spaces for meditation, we had yoga and art and all of those things and wonderful staff. I learned about exercise. We had a personal trainer to teach us how to do power walking. The most important thing I gained was, I went down to the retreat with a breast tumor about the size of half an orange. I didn't tell anyone I was coming with that. And there was wonderful energy there. I noticed overnight that the tumor was at least half. I didn't tell anyone that I had cancer when I went down there and no one there was diagnosed or treated for any disease but this is what happened when the energy work was done, I mean; just the concept of energy working like that was just phenomenal. I know a lot of people will not believe it but I'm glad I was able to witness it for myself. In addition to myself there were at least three other people who came on the retreat with similar experiences as mine and they also had the experiences of having the tumors reduced by at least half or more, overnight. That is unprecedented. I am so grateful for the opportunity to have gone to the retreat because I was given new lifestyle changes that I will incorporate into some of the things I was already doing and it's just a wonderful thing, it's a blessing. I would encourage anyone, even if you are healthy, to have the experience. It was wonderful.

DAISY

Gary was not aware of my illness or my sickness. When I went there—the energy, the walking, communicating with other people. It just helped so much. The exercise, the yoga classes, everything was just perfect for me and for other people. It was amazing for me how people were so enthralled with what was happening. As for me, my last day there I had a hard lump under my arm, about the size of a quarter. I never expressed it to anyone, not a physician, no one. It had been there for maybe a couple of months and I'm taking a shower and I'm feeling under my arm and I'm not feeling anything. I say maybe this is not right. So I went and put more soap and I'm washing again—and when I finished I just lay down across the bed and started thanking God for what had happened. Only God knows what happened. No one else knows. I never expressed it to anyone, my condition. Not even my husband. No one. It has stayed gone. But I was so grateful to have had the opportunity to go there and see what was happening. So much energy, birds, the air, the water. It was just amazing.

DIANE P.

Prior to seeing Gary on PBS, I never heard of him. A dark spot on my mammogram was suspicious. The specialist wanted to biopsy my breast. I objected and bought one of Gary's books. This began a tremendous education in all areas of my life. My diet, life, and relationship with animals changed. I followed the detox in one of Gary's books. My breast specialist was quite distressed. I soon entered a support group and followed the protocol carefully. After one year, I returned for another mammogram. The spot was gone. My blood pressure medication was lowered, and I will soon discontinue it altogether. I meditate, use yoga, power walk, exercise, and attend cardio exercise. Spirituality and self-empowerment are very effective motivators for change and self improvement. My family had an attitude shift, and we reclaimed power by home schooling our child and not returning her to the atmosphere created by 9/11. My mother went through cardiac surgery and is on the protocol. Her cardiologist is amazed with the improvement in her walking stress test, cholesterol level, and blood pressure. My husband's hair no longer falls out and appears thicker than it was originally.

ERNESTINA P.

Fatty tumors gone

Before

I had fatty tumors under my arm and on my thighs. I was overweight, with low energy and joint pain. I took pain relievers, and I was tense. I held onto past angers.

Now

I am pain-free, and the fatty tumors are gone. I have lost 30 lbs.

ALIM A.

Three of the tumors I once had are no more; another one has decreased in size. My skin is softer and smoother. My stomach is smaller. I feel more energetic. I exercise regularly.

ULCERATIVE COLITIS

CHRISTOPHER B.

Ulcerative colitis healed

Following your protocol, I had my ulcerative colitis healed. Prior to going to your retreat, I was unaware that there were people out there who could actually heal other people. My life has changed immeasurably.

URINARY TRACT INFECTION

NORA

I was plagued with a urinary tract infection that would not clear up. I had infections in my mouth and was tired most of the day. My skin began to look older, and my hair, weaker. I held a fast-paced job, which exhausted me, and I held on to anger from the past. I became part of an active health support group. The group energy and lectures were of great benefit. I keep to the protocol and drink juices, take supplements, and eat organic and vegan. All my infections cleared up. I am less tired, my skin improved, and my hair grows in healthier and thicker. Doing less, slowing my pace, simplifies my day. I have a positive outlook and put the past where it belongs—in the past, not in my mind.

WEIGHT LOSS / OBESITY

DOROTHY

During the program, I lost 50 lbs and many inches. My bra and shoe sizes are reduced, and I am five dress sizes smaller. My skin tone and elasticity improved, and my energy level increased. I had several haircuts in the past month. I handle stress and negativity; this increased my self-esteem. Meditation time is important, as is reading and reflection, not only at the end of the day but whenever I require it. I set future goals, focusing on solutions and personal needs. I use affirmations in the present tense during the day, accepting myself without denial. I am confident of positive solutions, without negative factors. My strengths are far greater than I once thought. I am a work in progress, and forgive, learn my lessons, and leave the garbage.

LIZ M.

I lost 20 pounds. I have incredible energy and no exhaustion. I sleep fewer hours, but have restful sleep. I am not depressed.

LIZA S.

I am a teacher and would get angry at my students. On the program I lost 25 pounds and have more strength and less pain. My skin is good. I can tolerate my students without anger. My new viewpoint and positive energy seems to be rubbing off on them.

OLIVER

I weighed 238 pounds. My cholesterol and blood pressure were elevated. I had pain in my chest, pain in my knees and ankles, and frequent heartburn. I was embarrassed by brown age spots on my skin and my eyesight was off. My weight went from 238 pounds to 188 pounds within 5 months. Blood pressure and cholesterol values were lower. I exercise one to two hours daily, meditate, and use juices and supplements with great enthusiasm. No longer do I have chest pains or heartburn. I feel energetic, less astigmatic, and my hair and nails are healthier. The support group ended but my life just began.

CHARLOTTE

I have definitely enjoyed the [anti-aging] protocol. I have lost almost thirty-five pounds. I am not hungry and I feel really strong. I am much happier and more content with myself and my life in general. I have a positive attitude toward things in general. I have also been gaining more respect from my peers.

JANE
My life was sluggish. I was overweight and always tired, which caused me to sleep too long. My eyesight was impaired with floaters and there were spots on my facial skin. I became an exhausted, negative woman. I joined Gary Null's support group and through the detoxing cleaned up my life. I lost weight and am two dress sizes smaller. I enjoy renewed energy and require less sleep. After being post-menopausal for five years, I began menstruating again. This makes me feel normal and happy. Facial spots are fading, hair is growing in healthy, eye floaters have diminished, and I have a positive attitude.

STEVEN
I lost 25 pounds. My hair and skin have rejuvenated. I use meditation, hypnosis, affirmations, and creative visualization to de-stress.

MIMI
I lost 10 pounds.

KRISTI A.
My attitude and body transformed. I lost 83 pounds.

ALEXANDRIA
I lost 16 pounds and gained much more energy. My feelings of deep anger that would eventually depress me have subsided. My friends and family have all commented on the change. I am more muscular. I never thought I would love exercise but now I do!

KEVIN
I lost 60 pounds in 14 days. Exercise is primary on my agenda.

KENNETH
I carried around too much weight on my body. I was uncomfortable, with pain in my shoulder from an injury. My asthma often held me back. These problems

made me angry and pessimistic. I often had temper tantrums sometimes with violence. My confidence and esteem were low. The juicing, homework, vegetarian diet, lectures, and confidence in me the people in the group showed got me through the first few weeks. I am vegan and enjoy my lifestyle now. I learned a lot about myself by answering the questions. I thought about my relationships. I lost over 35 lbs. My nose no longer runs all day, my asthma seems to be controlled, and I do not try to keep up with others. My life is uncluttered, and so is my head.

LIZA S.

I have lost 25 pounds and have less pain from fibromyalgia and arthritis. I am mentally clearer and much more focused. I have more energy yet I sleep a lot less.

KEITH

I was quite unhappy with my life. I had to lose weight and thought that was the problem. I did not feel I could accomplish much. Where was I going, not doing anything constructive? I was not sure lectures and a change of diet would help. Things were that bad, so what did I have to lose? I joined a support group. Many group participants entered that door wondering if this would work. We knew the information and teaching would be correct, but could we do it? I did it, and so did everyone else. What a change from day one to graduation. I lost 10 lbs and maintain it. I don't feel alone, and I look forward to planning a better future. I actually feel happy and have learned to listen to my inner voice. The experience has reshaped me. I know I have self-determination, and I am wild about the protocol.

FLORENCE H.

I lost weight and feel more energetic. I follow the protocol with enjoyment.

LARRY

Carrying around a heavy body caused me exhaustion and fatigue. I never exercised, and I ate the typical American diet. I often had heartburn, probably from the sugar in sodas and the bad food. It took me some time to get used to drinking juices, but the explanations and respect shown to the people in the group made me enthusiastic. I began to feel the energy growing. I went with it totally: I am organic, vegan, and exercise. I run and power walk. My hair is growing in darker.

I lost 20 lbs, and my digestion improved. I still follow the protocol, using the powders and supplements, and I love my new body and lifestyle. Thank you, Luanne and Gary, for helping us understand that our lives are in our hands.

SANDY

I came to the program overweight, short of breath, and diabetic. I lost 29 pounds. I walk 2 miles a day without being short of breath, and my diabetes is under control.

ANDREA V.

Lost 75lbs

Before

She weighed 300 lbs. and wore size 24–26. Although she had no diagnosed illnesses, she was exhausted, had painful varicose veins and back problems, was nauseated after meals, had bad digestion, and was lactose intolerant. She ate flesh foods and dairy. She listened to *Natural Living* and joined a support group.

Now

She lost weight, going down to 225 pounds and size 18. She developed a sense of values in the group and can say no. She feels centered and empowered within her truth. She juices, uses powders, and takes supplements. She discovered a new world of health food stores. She chooses products carefully, reads labels, and does not use canned products. As a creative cook, she enjoys translating old recipes into vegan meals, using grains. She discusses the availability of this lifestyle with others. Her family acknowledges her progress. Her mother now uses supplements.

MICHAEL

I lost 15 pounds, my skin and hair color improved.

RALPH

I felt well-balanced and healthy even though I functioned in a hyperactive mode. I slept eight hours a night but awoke feeling tired. I was slightly overweight and needed good dietary and behavioral changes. What better way toward health than a Gary Null support group? I jumped right in. Detoxing brought miracles to my life. I lost weight and am now 6.2-percent body fat. I feel clean, healthy, and energetic when I awake and throughout the day. I sold my company and entered a PhD program. I created a method of teaching the trumpet. I believe these changes were manifested by uncluttering my home and life.

ADELE

I was unhappy about my weight and double chin and darkening complexion. After following the protocol, my memory improved. The most wonderful difference this program gave me is seeing my body change. I lost 25 pounds and gained muscle.

ANGELO Q.

Lost 100 lbs

Before

He was 300 lbs and had high cholesterol and blood pressure. He had high hemoconiosis (abnormal hemoconia count in blood), hepatitis B, and discoloration around his eyes. He used an inhaler and had eczema, bleeding knuckles and elbows, and hemorrhoids. He felt sluggish and fatigued, and had pain with simple movements. He listened to *Natural Living* and joined a support group with his wife in 1999.

Now

All the above-mentioned ailments are gone. He lost 100 lbs. He has constant energy and runs, race walks, power walks, skates, does aerobics, and trains in a gym. He lost one shoe width size. His skin and hair improved, and he needs more frequent haircuts. He has had no additional graying of his hair. He follows the protocol, juicing and using green and red powders. He creates organic vegetarian menus with his wife. He finds he easily completes tasks, and he is on a wild uncluttering spree. He does image consulting today. His children are slowly adapting to his lifestyle.

ALEXANDRA M.

Before

I was dissatisfied with my body. My energy was low, and I was very overweight. My acquaintances and friends were depressing me to the point of irritability. I had a fear of public speaking and did not know where to turn for guidance. I joined a health support group. Gary Null was informative on the radio, but I could not apply this information in a constructive way.

Now

I lost 16 lbs without dieting. My increased energy made me feel young again. I need less sleep, and I find I am not distracted by other people's petty, unimportant issues. My house was uncluttered; having fewer objects gave me space and a feeling of freedom. My toxic relationships were dismissed; my self-esteem replaced them. I learned to be the real me, healthy and vital.

MAREY C.

Before

I was overweight and had weak hair. My skin was wrinkling, and I had herniated disks in my neck that caused severe pain. My muscle tone was low, and I suffered from upper respiratory infections. I was always fatigued and pessimistic.

Now

Following Gary's protocol, I have lost 20 lbs, my hair is healthier, and I have fewer wrinkles. I have less pain from the herniated disks in my neck. My muscle tone has improved, and I no longer have head colds or sinus infections. I feel I am stronger, calmer and more positive.

EVA

I lost 35 pounds. I am no longer depressed and bloated. Pain has subsided. My back never hurts anymore.

SUSAN

I lost 20 pounds, my skin is smoother, my hair is shinier, and my nails are stronger. I am much stronger with much more muscle tone.

NICK

I no longer feel bloated, and my energy level has increased. I lost 20 pounds. I have packed on 5 to 7 pounds of muscle. I run three to four miles a day three to four times a week.

LIZA

I have lost 25 pounds and have less pain from fibromyalgia and arthritis. I am mentally clearer and much more focused. I have more energy yet I sleep a lot less.

GARY

I have clearer thinking. I lost 11 pounds. I have more energy. My skin tone glows. My breathing is much better. My attitude towards life has improved greatly.

MARY E.

I decided to get my life together, lose weight and enjoy life. I just did not know how to do it. One day, Gary announced the opening of a health support group. Several people spoke about their positive changes in the group and their ongoing accomplishments. I registered, and my life is not the same. I had fibroids, painful periods and bloating. I wore a size 20 dress and could not stick to a "diet." I was not happy spending long hours on a job I did not like. Detoxification and eliminating dairy and other allergens seemed more difficult than it actually was. I found many choices to replace the old foods. My new diet is varied and delicious. No longer do I get painful periods and bloating. I do not have fibroids, and I wear a size 10 dress. I still lose weight just eating naturally. I will not interact with negative people, and I have a job I enjoy.

ANDREA M.

Before

I was dissatisfied with my body. My energy was low, and I was very overweight. My acquaintances and friends were depressing me to the point of irritability. I had a fear of public speaking and did not know where to turn for guidance. I joined a health support group. Gary Null was informative on the radio, but I could not apply this information in a constructive way.

Now

I lost 16 lbs without dieting. My increased energy made me feel young again. I need less sleep, and I find I am not distracted by other people's petty, unimportant issues. My house was uncluttered; having fewer objects gave me space and a feeling of freedom. My toxic relationships were dismissed; my self-esteem replaced them. I learned to be the real me, healthy and vital.

DIMITRIOS

I was too heavy and wanted to lose weight in a healthy way. I worried about things more than they required, and I would get involved in bad relationships, without the proper tools to handle them. I joined a support group and immediately began the protocol. I lost 15lbs, and I retained this loss when the group ended. I work out three times a week and have built new muscle. I developed confidence and self esteem. Doctors do not intimidate me anymore. I no longer listen to commercial radio. I hardly watch television, but fill my time with soccer, dance lessons and I lost 15 pounds and retained this loss. I work out three times a week. 1 hardly watch television. I love running and walking.

VIOLA

I was afraid and confused. I was overweight and stuck in an home situation. The hours stuck in self-doubt left me with a fear being crazy. There was no one to talk to and nowhere to turn. At first [when I joined a Null self-help group and heard about the dietary changes that were being advocated] I felt "How can I give up all the food I ate my whole life?" Then I remembered how stuck I was, so I vowed to go on Gary Null's program totally. I lost weight and became a vegetarian. My children and I thrive on the program. I will not ever again tolerate verbal abuse. I set firm boundaries. My children and I recently moved to another state and now we have a peaceful home. Uncluttering the past brought new friends into our lives.

STACEY T.

I lost more than 60 pounds. I sleep less. My skin cleared up, and I have bladder control. I practice yoga and meditation.

Index